Stackey

The Language of Medicine

A Write-In Text Explaining Medical Terms

Davi-Ellen Chabner, B.A., M.A.T.

Third Edition

1985
W. B. Saunders Company
Philadelphia • London • Toronto • Mexico City • Rio de Janeiro • Sydney • Tokyo

W. B. Saunders Company: West Washington Square
Philadelphia, PA 19105

1 St. Anne's Road
Eastbourne, East Sussex BN21 3UN, England

1 Goldthorne Avenue
Toronto, Ontario M8Z 5T9, Canada

Apartado 26370—Cedro 512
Mexico 4, D.F., Mexico

Rua Coronel Cabrita, 8
Sao Cristovao Caixa Postal 21176
Rio de Janeiro, Brazil

9 Waltham Street
Artarmon, N.S.W. 2064, Australia

Ichibancho, Central Bldg., 22-1 Ichibancho
Chiyoda-Ku, Tokyo 102, Japan

Available from the publisher is a set of audio tapes that reproduce the words found in the Pronunciation of Terms sections at the ends of the chapters. Short definitions accompany the dictated words.

The Language of Medicine ISBN 0-7216-1184-2

Last digit is the print number: 9 8 7 6 5 4 3 2

To Bruce and Betty,
for their guidance and unwavering confidence

and

To Mary Ann,
for her courage and friendship

PREFACE

Welcome to the third edition to *The Language of Medicine*! This new edition is the product of constant revision and evaluation, not only by myself and my medical terminology students, but by the many instructors who, along with their students, have used the two previous editions and have contributed valuable suggestions and comments. The success of the two previous editions has been due, in large measure, to the honest and careful appraisal given by medical terminology instructors and their students during the past eight years.

I have written this book with the needs of different types of students in mind. These people include allied health professionals such as medical assistants, medical technologists, physical therapists, dental assistants, medical-technical writers, radiological technicians, medical transcriptionists, medical librarians, hospital personnel, insurance examiners, nursing and premedical students, and all laypeople interested in understanding the terms used by their doctors. No previous knowledge of biology, anatomy, or physiology is presumed or needed, and any student, at the high school level or beyond, should be able to read and understand the text. Not only is a knowledge of medical terminology helpful to people in their jobs, but it is also valuable to all health consumers. Being able to decipher a doctor's report and ask relevant questions adds to the confidence of patient and family.

You have chosen to study the medical language in a unique way. This text combines a workbook format with comprehensive factual information. Because I believe that writing is a valuable key to learning, in each chapter you will have ample opportunity to complete written exercises (answers are also provided), label diagrams, complete meanings of terms, and fill in review sheets to test your understanding. This workbook format is combined with simple, nontechnical explanations of medical terms and descriptions of anatomy, physiology, and pathology. Thus, medical words are not presented for rote memorization in a dictionary-like fashion, but are explained in their proper context, which is the structure and function of the human body in health and disease. When you complete this text you will have finished a *workbook* of medical terminology and will still have a comprehensive *reference* for daily use on the job.

Those who are familiar with the text will find its basic format unaltered. The initial chapters (1 to 4) are concerned with the fundamentals of word analysis, orientation to the body as a whole, and common suffixes and prefixes. Chapters 5 to 17 explore the systems of the body. Each of these chapters has a similar format: anatomical and physiological terminology, combining forms, pathological terminology, clinical procedures, laboratory tests and abbreviations, exercises and answers, pronunciation of terms, and review sheets. Chapters 18 to 21 deal with specialized medical areas—cancer medicine (oncology), radiology, nuclear medicine, and radiotherapy, pharmacology, and psychiatry.

In the two previous editions, a medical paper was presented in an early chapter as an example of the use of medical words in context. In this edition, that same medical paper is presented at the end of the book (Chapter 22) as a culmination of a series of new Practical Applications sections in chapters 6 through 21. These sections are short examples of the use of medical language in case reports, operative and diagnostic lists, autopsy records, drug descriptions, laboratory and x-ray reports, and other medical contexts.

Timely new terms, such as NMR (MRI), oncogenes, AIDS, and PET scanning have been added in this edition, while terms that are rarely used have been omitted. Emphasis has been placed on explaining a term completely when the literal meaning of the term won't suffice. Thus, "anemia," whose literal meaning (lacking in blood) differs from its actual meaning, is explained as a blood condition of a deficiency of the number of red blood cells or the hemoglobin content of the red cells.

The glossary includes an "English to Medical Terms" section in this edition. This list gives the medical term counterpart to English terms.

The teacher's guide contains a series of multiple-choice questions for each chapter.

Audio cassettes to accompany the text are available.

Undeniably, the study of medical terminology requires diligence and commitment of time and effort. The rewards are many, though, and this text aims at bringing the language alive by making the study interesting, logical, and easy to follow. Please do not hesitate to communicate your comments and criticisms. I will take them into consideration in future editions.

Thank you for choosing this text; work hard, but have fun with *The Language of Medicine.*

DAVI-ELLEN CHABNER

ACKNOWLEDGMENTS

My editor, Elizabeth J. Taylor, has skillfully guided this book through its first and now third editions. She initially recognized its potential and clearly understood how it would best serve the needs of students and teachers. I have always relied on her good judgment, editorial skills, and loyalty. Over the years, she has become a valued editor, mentor, and friend.

Kathleen Moore, who expertly typed the teacher's guide and helped assemble the index and glossary, has once again been a perceptive sounding board for all aspects of my work. Meadie Osborne, of the Training and Development Branch of the National Institutes of Health, organized my classes for the past years and I am grateful for her fine managerial skills. She has consistently supported medical terminology courses and is responsible for the successful training of NIH employees in this area.

My husband, Bruce A. Chabner, M.D., once again read many chapters and offered valuable advice about content and style. My brother, James L. Rosenzweig, M.D., and my uncle, Norman M. Simon, M.D., meticulously reviewed the endocrine and urinary system chapters, respectively, and I am grateful for their helpful comments and suggestions.

Through the years, many teachers of medical terminology have communicated their ideas about the book and I am indebted to them, beyond words, for their practical advice. My thanks to: Mary Basile, RRA, Claudia Tessier, CMT, Judy Beall, R.N., Jean Hough, Carol Warden, CMA-A, Marcia Lewis, R.N., Shirley Carr, OTR, Nancy Snodgrass, Lesha Yerka, R.N., and Arlene Cafferty.

Lastly, but perhaps primarily, I am grateful for the responses and enthusiasm of my students. To all of you, past and present, who spend hours with me and with *The Language of Medicine*, I am thankful for the opportunity to work with you, and to share in the excitement of learning.

DAVI-ELLEN CHABNER

CONTENTS

CHAPTER 1

BASIC WORD STRUCTURE

In this chapter you will:

- Become familiar with basic objectives to keep in mind as you study the medical language;
- Divide medical words into their component parts;
- Find the meaning of basic combining forms, prefixes, and suffixes of the medical language; and
- Use these combining forms, prefixes, and suffixes to build medical words.

This chapter is divided into the following sections:

I. Objectives in Studying the Medical Language
II. Basic Word Structure
III. Combining Forms, Suffixes, and Prefixes
IV. Exercises
V. Pronunciation of Terms

I. OBJECTIVES IN STUDYING THE MEDICAL LANGUAGE

There are three major objectives to keep in mind as you study medical terminology.

1. To Analyze Words Structurally. Your goal is to learn the **tools** of word analysis which will make the understanding of complex terminology easier. For example, we will learn to divide words into basic elements such as **roots**, **suffixes**, **prefixes**, **combining vowels**, and **combining forms**. With this knowledge of word construction and the meanings of the specific word elements, even the longest and most complicated terms can be handled and understood.

You may or may not already know the meanings of the following terms, but this is how we will learn to analyze them structurally:

GASTROENTEROLOGY GASTR/O/ENTER/O/LOGY

GASTR — root; O — combining vowel; ENTER — root; O — combining vowel; LOGY — suffix

The root **gastr** means **stomach**
The root **enter** means **intestines**
The suffix **-logy** means **process of study**
The combining vowel **o** links root to root and root to suffix

The entire word (always reading the meaning of terms starting from the suffix **back** to the first part of the word) means: **the process of study of the stomach and intestines.**

ELECTROCARDIOGRAM   ELECTR/O/CARDI/O/GRAM

root (ELECTR), combining vowel (O), root (CARDI), combining vowel (O), suffix (GRAM)

The root **electr** means **electricity**
The root **cardi** means **heart**
The suffix **-gram** means **record**

The entire word means: **the record of the electricity of the heart.**

Try another:

ONCOGENIC   ONC/O/GEN/IC

root (ONC), combining vowel (O), root (GEN), suffix (IC)

The **root onc** means **tumor**
The root **gen** means **producing**
The suffix **-ic** means **pertaining to**

The entire word means: **pertaining to tumor producing.**

Note that the combining vowel (o), usually placed between the root and suffix, is **dropped** in this word because the suffix (ic) begins with a vowel. However, combining vowels are usually **retained** between two **roots** in a word even if the second root begins with a vowel. For example:

gastroenteric   not   gastrenteric

root (gastr), combining vowel (o), root (enteric)

To summarize: Three important rules to remember as you study the medical language are:

(a) Read the meaning of medical terms from the suffix back to the first part of the word.
(b) Drop the combining vowel (usually o) before a suffix beginning with a vowel: gastric **not** gastroic.
(c) Retain the combining vowel between two roots in a word.

2. To Correlate an Understanding of Word Elements with the Basic Anatomy, Physiology, and Disease Processes of the Human Body. This text will continually emphasize not only the division of terms into structural elements but also the relationship of the medical words to the functioning of the body, in both health and disease.

For example, the term **hemat/o/logy** means the study of the blood. This term, however, will mean more to you as you learn the many different components of blood, how they function in the body, and the various disease conditions associated with blood. This text is structured so that the terms presented have relevance to the anatomy, physiology, and disease processes of the body. Memorization of terms, while essential to retention of the language, should not become the primary objective of your study.

3. To Be Continually Aware of Spelling and Pronunciation Problems. Spelling is especially critical in the medical language because many words are pronounced alike but spelled differently and have entirely different meanings. For example:

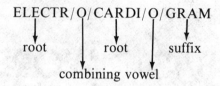

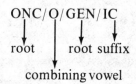

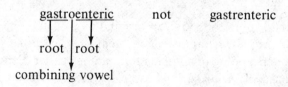

ileum is a part of the small intestine

and

ilium is a part of the pelvic, or hip, bone

It should be obvious as well that a misspelled word may give the wrong meaning to a diagnosis. For example:

hepat/oma: tumor of the liver; an abnormal growth of cells

hemat/oma: blood tumor; a mass, or collection, of blood under the skin

Words spelled correctly but incorrectly **pronounced** may be easily misunderstood. For example:

urethra (ū-RĒ-thră)	is the urinary tract tube leading from the urinary bladder to the external surface
ureter (ū-RĒ-tĕr) or Ū-rē-tĕr)	is one of two tubes leading from the kidney to the urinary bladder

Figure 1-1 illustrates the difference between the urethra and ureters.

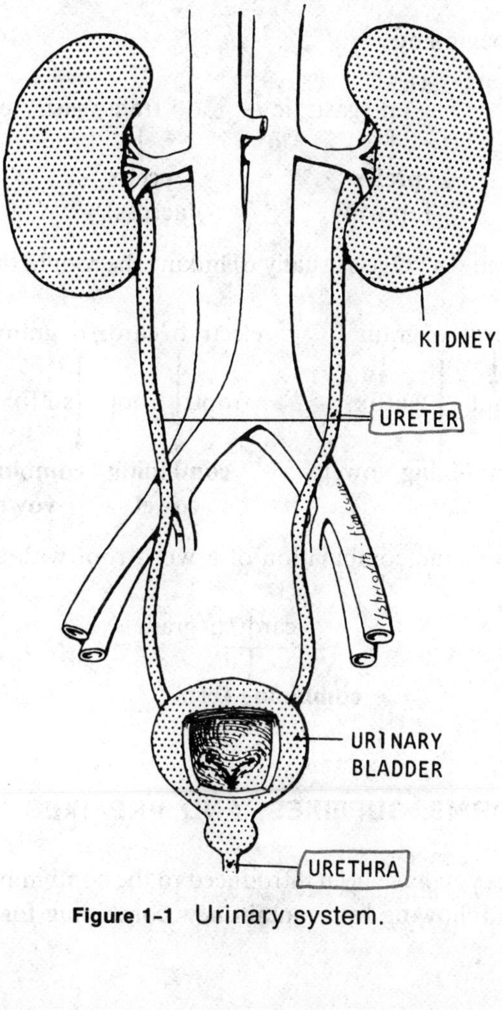

Figure 1-1 Urinary system.

II. BASIC WORD STRUCTURE

Studying medical words is very similar to learning a new language. The words at first sound strange and complicated although they may stand for commonly known English terms. The words **gastralgia**, meaning "stomach ache," and **ophthalmologist**, meaning "eye doctor," are examples.

The medical language is fascinatingly logical in that each term, complex or simple, can be broken down into its basic component parts and then understood.

These basic component parts of medical words are:

1. **Word root:** foundation of the word

gastr/ic
root
(stomach)

2. **Suffix:** word ending

gastr/itis — **suffix** (inflammation)
gastr/ic — **suffix** (pertaining to)

3. **Prefix:** word beginning

epi/gastr/ic — **prefix** (above)
trans/gastr/ic — **prefix** (across)

4. **Combining vowel:** a vowel (usually o) linking the root to the suffix or to another root

cardi/o/gram — root, **combining vowel**, suffix
electr/o/cardi/o/gram — root, **combining vowel**, root, **combining vowel**, suffix

5. **Combining form:** the combination of a word root with the combining vowel

cardi/o/gram
combining form

III. COMBINING FORMS, SUFFIXES, AND PREFIXES

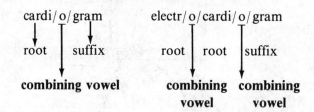

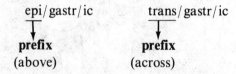

In previous examples you have been introduced to the combining forms gastr/o (stomach) and cardi/o (heart). The following lists contain new combining forms, suffixes, and prefixes with examples of medical words using those word parts. Your job is to write the **meaning** of the new medical word in the space provided. As you do this, you may want to put slashes through the words to divide them clearly into their individual parts.

Don't forget to consult the pronunciation sheet at the end of the chapter which contains an alphabetical list of most new terms. To test your understanding of word parts and terminology, complete the exercises on pages 10 to 16 and check your answers on pages 16 to 17.

Combining Forms

Combining Form	*Meaning*	*Terminology*	*Meaning*
aden/o	gland	adenoma	tumor of a gland
		-oma means tumor.	
		adenitis	inflammation of a gland
		-itis means inflammation.	
arthr/o	joint	arthritis	inflammation of a joint
bi/o	life	biology	study of life
		-logy means process of study.	
carcin/o	cancerous	carcinoma	cancerous tumor
		A carcinoma is a major type of cancerous tumor; carcinomas grow from epithelial (skin) cells that cover the outside of the body and line organs, cavities, and tubes within the body.	
cardi/o	heart	cardiology	study of the heart
cephal/o	head	cephalic	pertaining to the head
		-ic means pertaining to.	
cerebr/o	brain, cerebrum	cerebral	pertaining to the cerebrum
		-al means pertaining to. The cerebrum is the largest part of the brain. A cerebrovascular accident (CVA) occurs when damage to blood vessels in the cerebrum leads to injury to cerebral nerve cells. This condition is also called a stroke.	
cis/o	to cut	incision	process of cutting into
		in- means into; -ion means process.	
		excision	process of cutting out
		ex- means out.	

Combining form	Meaning	Terminology
crin/o	secrete (to form and give off)	endocrine glands secrete hormones w/in body *Endo- means within; endocrine glands secrete chemicals (hormones) directly into the bloodstream while other glands (exocrine glands) secrete chemicals (such as saliva, sweat, and tears) into tubes that lead to the outside of the body.*
cyst/o	urinary bladder	cystoscopy examination of the urinary bladder *-scopy means process of visual examination.*
cyt/o	cell	cytology study of cells
derm/o dermat/o	skin	hypodermic below the skin *hypo- means under, below.* dermatosis condition of skin *-osis means abnormal condition.*
electr/o	electricity	electrocardiogram record of electricity in heart *-gram means record.*
encephal/o	brain	electroencephalogram record of electricity in the brain
enter/o	intestines (usually small intestine)	enteritis inflammation of the sm. intestines
erythr/o	red	erythrocyte red blood cell
gastr/o	stomach	gastrectomy removal of stomach *-ectomy means removal.* gastrotomy cutting into the stomach *-tomy means process of cutting.*
gen/o	producing, produced by	carcinogenic producing cancer
gnos/o	knowledge	diagnosis state of complete knowledge *dia- means complete; -sis means state of. A diagnosis is made after sufficient information has been obtained about the patient's condition.* prognosis state of before knowledge *pro- means before. The prognosis is a prediction about the outcome of the illness; it is determined after the diagnosis has been made.*

gynec/o	woman, female	gynecology study of women
hem/o hemat/o	blood	hematoma collection of blood *A hematoma is a collection (mass) of blood outside blood vessels. In this term, -oma does not mean "tumor" in the sense of a growth of cells. A hematoma occurs when blood is lost from blood vessels and collects as a mass in a cavity or organ or under the skin.*
hepat/o	liver	hepatitis inflammation liver
iatr/o	treatment	iatrogenic produced by treatment
leuk/o	white	leukocytic white blood cell
nephr/o	kidney	nephrotomy incise kidney
neur/o	nerve	neurosis condition of nerves - abnormal
onc/o	tumor	oncology study of tumors
ophthalm/o	eye	ophthalmoscopy examine eye w/ scope
oste/o	bone	osteoarthritis inflammation of bones + joints
path/o	disease	pathologist disease specialist *-ist means a specialist.*
ped/o	child	pediatric pertains to child treatment
physi/o	nature	physiology study of the nature of things *study of the nature of things (organs); how they work*
psych/o	mind	psychosis abnormal condition of mind *A more serious abnormal mental condition than neurosis.*
radi/o	rays, x-rays	radiology study of x-rays
ren/o	kidney	renal pertaining to kidney *Ren/o (Latin) and nephr/o (Greek) both mean kidney; ren/o is used with -al to describe the kidney, while nephr/o is used with other suffixes and prefixes to name abnormal conditions and operative procedures of the kidney.*
rhin/o	nose	rhinitis inflammation of the nose

sarc/o	flesh	sarcoma tumor of connective tissue
		Sarcoma is a type of cancerous tumor; sarcomas grow from cells of "fleshy" connective tissue such as muscle, fat, and bone.
secti/o	to cut	section to cut ~~in~~ into
		An incision.
thromb/o	clot	thrombocyte clotting cell
		Thrombocytes, also called platelets, are blood cells that help in the formation of a clot.
tom/o	to cut	gastrotomy incision of stomach
ur/o	urine, urinary tract	urology study of urinary tract

Suffixes

Suffix	*Meaning*	*Terminology* *Meaning*
-ac	pertaining to	cardiac pertaining to the heart
-al	pertaining to	neural pertaining to nerves
-algia	pain	arthralgia pain in a joint
-cyte	cell	leukocyte white blood cell
-ectomy	excision	adenectomy excision of a gland
-emia	blood condition	leukemia ______
		Increase in number of cancerous white blood cells.
-gram	record	electroencephalogram ______
-ia	condition	erythremia ______
-ic	pertaining to	gastric ______
-ist	one who specializes in	nephrologist ______
-itis	inflammation	cystitis ______
-logy	process of study	endocrinology ______

-oma	tumor, mass	hepatoma ________
-opsy	process of viewing	biopsy ________ *The removal and microscopic examination of a small amount of living tissue.*
-osis	abnormal condition	leukocytosis ________ *-osis means slight increase when used with blood cell terms.*
-scope	instrument to visually examine	gastroscope ________
-scopy	process of visually examining	gastroscopy ________
-sis	state of, condition	diagnosis ________
-tome	instrument to cut	osteotome ________
-tomy	process of cutting	rhinotomy ________
-y	process	gastroenterology ________

Prefixes

Prefix	*Meaning*	*Terminology*	*Meaning*
a-, an-	no, not	anemia	decrease in erythrocytes *Literally, a condition of being without blood. Obviously an anemic person has blood, so the literal definition is not accurate. Anemia means a decreased number of erythrocytes or amount of hemoglobin in the erythrocytes.*
auto-	self	autopsy	examine a dead body *The examination of a dead body (with one's own eyes) to determine the cause of death and nature of disease.*
ana-	up, apart	anatomy	cutting apart *Cutting up or apart to understand the structure of things.*
dia-	through, complete	diagnostic	knowing completely *-tic means pertaining to.*

endo-	within	endocrinologist endocrine specialist
epi-	above	epidermic above the skin
ex-	out	excision cut out; remove
exo-	out	exocrine glands glands which secrete out of body
hyper-	excessive, above	hyperemia lg. blood flow to body pt *An unusually large amount of blood flow to a part of the body.*
hypo-	below, deficient	hypogastric pertaining to below the stomach
peri-	surrounding	pericardium structure surrounding the heart *-um means a structure*
pro-	before	prognosis prediction about a condition's outcome
re-	back	resection removal *an excision*
retro-	behind	retrogastric pertaining to behind the stomach
trans-	across	transgastric pertaining to across from the stomach

IV. EXERCISES

A. Complete the following:

1. Word beginnings are called prefixes.
2. Word endings are called suffixes.
3. The foundation of a word is called the word root.
4. A letter linking a suffix and a root or two roots in a word is called the ~~combining form~~ vowel
5. The combination of a root and a combining vowel is known as the combining form.

B. Using slashes (/), divide the following terms into component parts; write the word root; and give the meaning of the entire medical term:

	Root	*Meaning*
1. adenoma	adeno	gland
2. cerebral	cerebro	cerebrum
3. pathogenic	patho	disease
4. hypogastric	gastro	stomach
5. leukocytic	leuko	white
6. rhinitis	rhino	nose
7. arthrotomy	arthro	joint
8. hepatitis	hepato	liver

C. Using slashes, divide the following terms into component parts; identify the combining forms; and give the meaning of the entire term:

	Combining Form	*Meaning*
1. carcin/o/genic	carcino	cancer producing
2. electro/encephal/o/gram	electroencephalo	record of brain electricity
3. oste/o/tome	osteo	instrument to cut bone
4. erythr/o/cyt/osis	erythrocyt	condition of abnormal red cells
5. nephr/o/logist	nephro	one who studies kidneys
6. encephal/o/pathy	encephalo	disease of brain
7. bi/ology	bio	study of life
8. physi/o/logy	physi	study of the nature of things

D. Find the suffixes in the following words and give the meaning of the entire term:

	Suffix	*Meaning*
1. leuk/emia	emia	blood condition (excess white cells)
2. gastr/ectomy	ectomy	removal of stomach (part or whole)

3. hema/toma — oma — mass of blood
4. neph/ritis — itis — inflammation of kidneys
5. gastro/scope — scope — study the stomach w/ scope
6. derma/tosis — osis — skin condition
7. psycho/genic — genic (ic) — pertaining to being caused by the mind
8. neur/algia — algia — pain of nerves

E. Identify the prefixes in the following terms and give the meaning of the entire term:

	Prefix	*Meaning*
1. ana/tomy	ana	cut up (study of structure)
2. peri/carditis	peri	inflam. around heart
3. retro/gast/ric	retro	behind stomach
4. hypo/dermic	hypo	under the skin
5. hyper/emia	hyper	excessive blood
6. endo/crine	endo	secrete within
7. dia/gnosis	dia	complete knowledge
8. pro/gnosis	pro	before knowledge

F. The following are some of the fields of medicine with which you should be familiar. First use vertical slashes to divide up the words into root, combining vowel, and suffix; and then give the meaning of the term:

1. Ur/o/logy — study of urinary system
2. Gynec/o/logy — study of women
3. Hemat/o/logy — study of the liver
4. Onc/o/logy — study of tumors
5. Nephr/o/logy — study of kidneys
6. Cardi/o/logy — study of the heart

7. Neurology study of nerves / nervous system
8. Dermatology study of skin
9. Radiology study of x-rays
10. Ophthalmology study of eyes
11. Gastroenterology study of the stomach & intestines
12. Endocrinology study of endocrine system
13. Psychiatry study of the mind
14. Pediatrics study of children

G. Give the meaning of the following combining forms:

1. aden/o gland
2. leuk/o white
3. cephal/o ~~brain~~ head
4. arthr/o joint
5. cerebr/o cerebrum
6. cyt/o cell
7. oste/o bone
8. dermat/o skin
9. erythr/o red
10. encephal/o brain
11. bi/o life
12. physi/o mind
13. path/o disease
14. rhin/o nose
15. nephr/o kidney
16. carcin/o cancer
17. gnos/o knowledge
18. onc/o tumor
19. tom/o to cut
20. gynec/o woman
21. hepat/o liver
22. cyst/o bladder

H. Fill in the suffixes for the following English terms:

1. Inflammation ITIS
2. Resection, or surgical removal ECTOMY
3. Section OTOMY

4. Condition (usually abnormal) OSIS

5. Process of study OLOGY

6. Instrument to examine visually SCOPE

7. Instrument to cut TOME

8. One who specializes in OLOGIST (IST)

9. Pertaining to IC AL AC

10. Blood condition EMIA

11. Tumor OMA

12. Pain ALGIA

13. Record GRAM

14. Cell CYTE

15. Process of viewing OPSY

I. Give the prefixes for the following English terms:

1. Surrounding PERI
2. Across TRANS
3. Complete, through DIA
4. Above HYPER, EPI
5. Before PRO
6. Within ENDO
7. Excessive HYPER
8. Deficient HYPO
9. Self AUTO
10. Up ANA
11. Behind RETRO
12. Outside, outer EXO
13. Back RE
14. Out EX
15. No, not, without A, AN

J. Build medical terms: (These may seem hard, but don't give up!)

1. Blood mass (tumor) hematoma

2. Inflammation of a gland adenitis

3. Record of the electricity of the heart electrocardiogram

4. Abnormal condition of clotting cells (slight increase in numbers)
thrombocytoses

5. Pertaining to across the stomach transgastric

6. Study of the skin (and its diseases) dermatology

7. Head pain cephalalgia

8. Instrument to cut bone osteotome

9. Removal of the stomach gastrectomy

10. Instrument to visually examine the eye opthalamascope

11. To view life (removal of living tissue for microscopic examination) biopsy

12. Inflammation of bones and joints osteoarthritis

13. One who specializes in the study of tumors oncologist

14. Pertaining to producing disease pathogenic

15. Incision of the stomach gastriotomy

16. Process of viewing the urinary bladder cystoscopy

K. *Give the meaning for the following terms:*

1. Autopsy to examine a dead body

2. Nephrotomy to incise a kidney

3. Erythremia high no number of red blood cells

4. Oncogenic pertaining the production of tumors

5. Cephalic pertaining to the brain

6. Gastric section pertaining to an incision of the stomach

7. Gastric resection pertaining to an excision of the stomach

8. Cystitis inflammation of the urinary bladder

9. Hepatoma tumor of the liver

10. Anemia (no blood) lack of blood cells

11. Leukemia (white blood) increase in w. blood count

12. Carcinoma cancerous tumor

13. Thrombosis condition of clot formation

14. Sarcoma tumor in tissue

ANSWERS

A.

1. Prefixes
2. Suffixes
3. Word root
4. Combining vowel
5. Combining form

B.

1. aden/oma—tumor of a **gland**.
2. cerebr/al—pertaining to the **brain**, or **cerebrum**.
3. path/o/gen/ic—pertaining to **disease producing**.
4. hypo/gastr/ic—pertaining to under the **stomach**.
5. leuk/o/cyt/ic—pertaining to **white** (blood) **cells**.
6. rhin/itis—inflammation of the **nose**.
7. arthr/o/tomy—incision of a **joint**.
8. hepat/itis—inflammation of the **liver**.

C.

1. carcin/o/gen/ic—pertaining to producing **cancer**.
2. electr/o/encephal/o/gram—record of the **electricity** in the **brain**.
3. oste/o/tome—instrument to cut **bone**.
4. erythr/o/cyt/osis—abnormal condition (slight elevation in number) of **red** (blood) **cells**.
5. nephr/o/logist—one who specializes in the study of the **kidney**.
6. encephal/o/pathy—disease condition of the **brain**.
7. bi/o/logy—process of studying **life**.
8. physi/o/logy—process of studying the **nature** of things (how they work). A physiologist studies the normal functioning of organs.

D.

1. leuk/emia—**blood condition** of excessive numbers of cancerous white blood cells. *There will be instances of terms which defy simple definitions by structural analysis. In those cases, as with the term "leukemia," you will have to understand not only how the word is constructed but also a more complete meaning of the term. Your dictionary should help with those terms.*
2. gastr/ectomy—**removal** of the stomach.
3. hemat/oma—mass of blood; collection or swelling of blood.
4. nephr/itis—**inflammation** of the kidney.
5. gastr/o/scope—**instrument to examine** the stomach.
6. dermat/osis—**abnormal condition** of the skin.
7. psych/o/gen/ic—**pertaining to** being produced by the mind.
8. neur/algia—**pain** of nerves.

E.

1. ana/tomy—process of cutting up. Anatomy is the study of the **structure** of living things.
2. peri/cardi/tis—inflammation of the pericardium (the sac **surrounding** the heart). *Note that one i is dropped when -itis is preceded by a root ending in a vowel.*
3. retro/gastr/ic—pertaining to **behind** the stomach.
4. hypo/derm/ic—pertaining to **under** the skin.
5. hyper/emia—blood condition—**increased** flow to a region.
6. endo/crine—secretion **within**. *Glands are classified as to their method of secretion. Some glands are endocrine, meaning they produce hormones which enter the bloodstream directly and thus influence organs and other glands all over the body; examples are the pituitary, adrenal, and thyroid glands. Other glands are exocrine, meaning they produce chemicals which leave the gland via ducts and travel to cavities which lead to the outside of the body; examples of exocrine glands are tear, digestive, and sweat glands.*
7. dia/gnosis—state of **complete** knowledge. *The root gnos is linked to the suffix -sis (meaning state of or condition). A diagnosis is made on the basis of extensive knowledge about the patient—family history, laboratory tests, x-rays, urinalysis, physical examination.*
8. pro/gnosis—state of **before** knowledge. *A prognosis is made by a doctor after a diagnosis about the nature of the patient's illness. It is a prediction (knowledge) before) about the outcome of the disease.*

dermatosis	dĕr-mă-TŌ-sĭs
diagnosis	dī-ăg-NŌ-sĭs
electrocardiogram	ē-lĕk-trō-KĂR-dē-ō-grăm
electroencephalogram	ē-lĕk-trō-ĕn-SĔF-ă-lō-grăm
encephalopathy	ĕn-sĕf-ă-LŎP-ă-thē
endocrine	ĔN-dō-krĭn
endocrinology	ĕn-dō-krĭ-NŎL-ō-jē
epidermic	ĕp-ĭ-DĔR-mĭk
erythremia	ĕr-ĭ-THRĒ-mē-ă
erythrocytosis	ĕ-rĭth-rō-sĭ-TŌ-sĭs
exocrine	ĔK-sō-krĭn
gastrectomy	găs-TRĔK-tō-mē
gastric resection	GĂS-trĭk rē-SĔK-shŭn
gastric section	GĂS-trĭk SĔK-shŭn
gastroenterology	găs-trō-ĕn-tĕr-ŎL-ō-jē
gastroscope	GĂS-trō-skōp
gastroscopy	găs-TRŎS-kō-pē
gynecology	gī-nĕ-KŎL-ō-jē or jĭn-ĕ-KŎL-ō-jē
hematology	hē-mă-TŎL-ō-jē
hematoma	hē-mă-TŌ-mă
hepatitis	hĕp-ă-TĪ-tĭs
hepatoma	hĕp-ă-TŌ-mă
hyperemia	hī-pĕr-Ē-mē-ă
hypodermic	hī-pō-DĔR-mĭk
hypogastric	hī-pō-GĂS-trĭk
iatrogenic	ī-ăt-rō-JĔN-ĭk
leukemia	lo͞o-KĒ-mē-ă
leukocytic	lo͞okō-SĬT-ĭk
nephritis	nĕ-FRĪ-tĭs
nephrologist	nĕ-FRŎL-ō-gĭst
nephrology	nĕ-FRŎL-ō-jē
nephrotomy	nĕ-FRŎT-ō-mē

neuralgia	nū-RĂL-jă
neurology	nū-RŎL-ō-jē
neurosis	nū-RŌ-sĭs
oncology	ŏn-KŎL-ō-jē
ophthalmology	ŏf-thăl-MŎL-ō-jē
ophthalmoscope	ŏf-THĂL-mō-skōp
osteoarthritis	ŏs-tē-ō-ăr-THRĪ-tĭs
osteotome	ŎS-tē-ō-tōm
pathogenic	păth-ō-JĔN-ĭk
pathologist	pă-THŎL-ō-jĭst
pediatric	pē-dē-ĂT-rĭk
pericarditis	pĕr-ĭ-kăr-DĪ-tĭs
pericardium	pĕr-ĭ-KĂR-dē-ŭm
physiology	fĭz-ē-ŎL-ō-jē
prognosis	prŏg-NŌ-sĭs
psychiatry	sī-KĪ-ă-trē
psychosis	sī-KŌ-sĭs
radiology	rā-dē-ŎL-ō-jē
renal	RĒ-năl
retrogastric	rĕ-trō-GĂS-trĭk
rhinitis	rī-NĪ-tĭs
rhinotomy	rī-NŎT-ō-mē
sarcoma	săr-KŌ-mă
thrombocytosis	thrŏm-bō-sī-TŌ-sĭs
transgastric	trănz-GĂS-trĭk
urology	ū-RŎL-ō-jē

REVIEW SHEET I

This review sheet and the others following each chapter are complete lists of the word elements and important terms contained in that chapter. The review sheets are designed to pull together the terminology and to reinforce your learning by giving you the opportunity to write out the meanings of the words and test yourself. Check the answers you are unsure of with the information in the chapter or in the glossary at the end of the book.

Combining Forms

aden/o	______________	gen/o	______________
arthr/o	______________	gnos/o	______________
bi/o	______________	gynec/o	______________
carcin/o	______________	hem/o	______________
cardi/o	______________	hemat/o	______________
cephal/o	______________	hepat/o	______________
cerebr/o	______________	iatr/o	______________
cis/o	______________	leuk/o	______________
crin/o	______________	nephr/o	______________
cyst/o	______________	neur/o	______________
cyt/o	______________	onc/o	______________
derm/o	______________	ophthalm/o	______________
dermat/o	______________	oste/o	______________
electr/o	______________	path/o	______________
encephal/o	______________	ped/o	______________
enter/o	______________	physi/o	______________
erythr/o	______________	psych/o	______________
gastr/o	______________	radi/o	______________

ren/o	________	secti/o	________
rhin/o	________	thromb/o	________
sarc/o	________	tom/o	________
ur/o	________		

Suffixes

-ac	________	-itis	________
-al	________	-logy	________
-algia	________	-oma	________
-cyte	________	-opsy	________
-ectomy	________	-osis	________
-emia	________	-scope	________
-gram	________	-scopy	________
-ia	________	-sis	________
-ic	________	-tome	________
-ist	________	-tomy	________
-y	________		

Prefixes

a-, an-	________	hyper-	________
ana-	________	hypo-	________
dia-	________	peri-	________
endo-	________	pro-	________
epi-	________	re-	________
ex-	________	retro-	________
exo-	________	trans-	________

CHAPTER 2

TERMS PERTAINING TO THE BODY AS A WHOLE

In this chapter you will:

- Define terms which apply to the structural organization of the body;
- Identify the body cavities and recognize the organs contained within those cavities;
- Locate and identify the anatomical and clinical divisions of the abdomen;
- Locate and name the anatomical divisions of the back;
- Become acquainted with terms which describe positions, directions, and planes of the body; and
- Find the meanings for new word elements and use them to understand new medical terms.

This chapter is divided into the following sections:

Since this is a long chapter, special study sections have been included in each section of the text to help you learn the meanings of terms.

I. STRUCTURAL ORGANIZATION OF THE BODY

The Cell

The cell is the fundamental unit of every living thing (animal or plant). Cells are everywhere in the human body—every tissue, every organ, is made up of these individual units.

Similarity in Cells. All cells are similar in that they contain a gelatinous substance composed of water, protein, sugar, acids, fats, and various minerals. This substance is called **protoplasm**. Several parts of a cell are described below and pictured schematically in Figure 2-1 as they might look when photographed with an electron microscope. Label the structures on Figure 2-1 as you learn how they function as part of the activity in the cell:

(1) *Cell membrane.* This structure surrounds and protects the internal environment of the cell, determining what passes in and out of the cell.

(2) *Nucleus.* The nucleus is the controlling structure of the cell. It controls the way a cell reproduces and contains genetic material that determines the functioning and structure of the cell. All the material within the nucleus is called **nucleoplasm** or **karyoplasm** (kary/o = nucleus).

(3) *Chromosomes.* These are 23 pairs of thin strands of genetic material (DNA) located within the nucleus of a cell. These 23 pairs of chromosomes contain regions known as **genes** which determine our hereditary makeup. The DNA within chromosomes regulates the activities

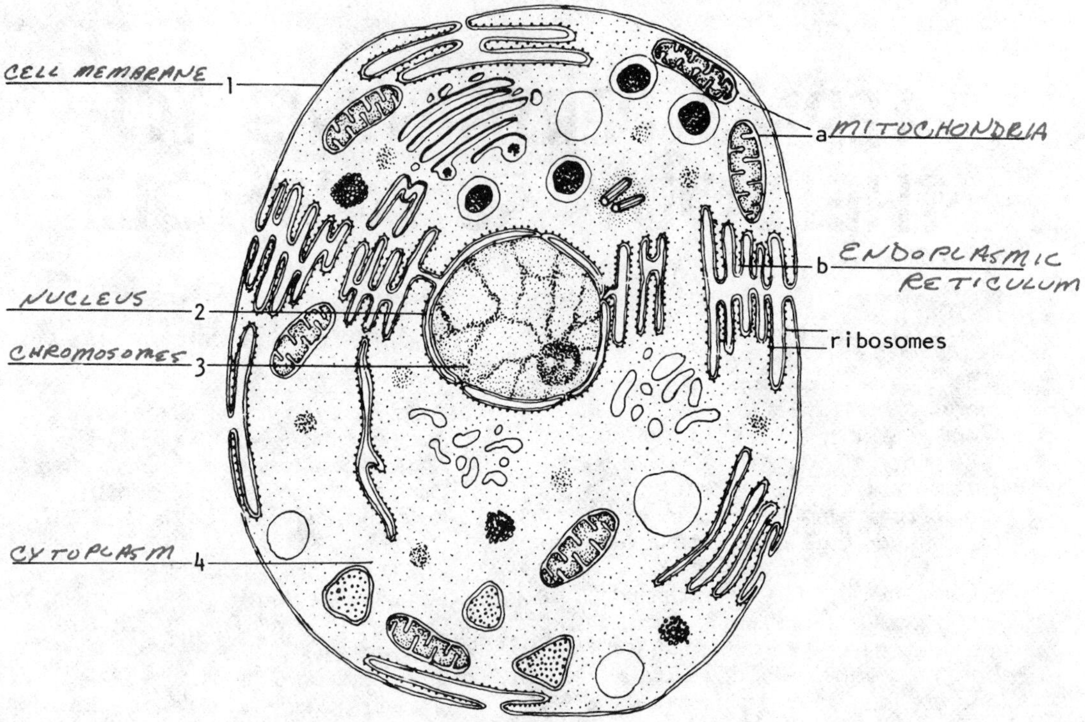

Figure 2-1 Major parts of a cell.

of each cell by guiding the formation of another substance, called RNA, which can leave the cell nucleus, enter the cytoplasm, and direct the activities of the cell.

Chromosomes can be studied and classified as to size, arrangement, and number. This classification is called a **karyotype**. Karyotyping of chromosomes is useful in determining whether chromosomes are normal in number and structure. Figure 2-2 shows a karyotype or chromosome "map."

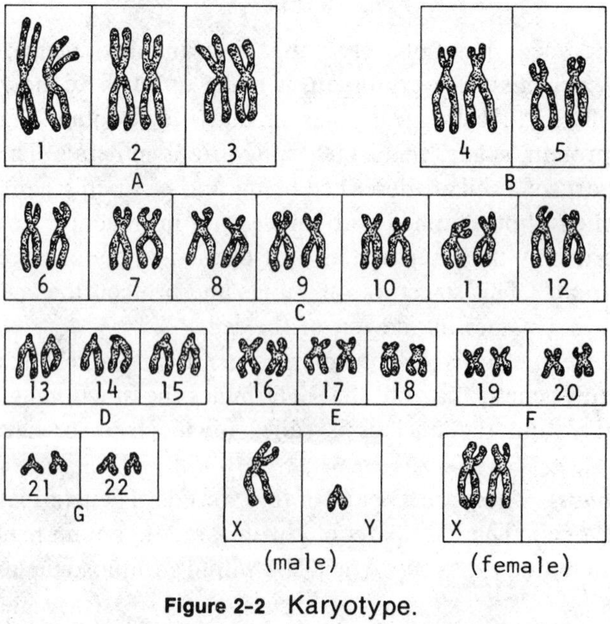

Figure 2-2 Karyotype.

(4) *Cytoplasm.* Cytoplasm is all the protoplasmic material outside the nucleus. It carries on the work of the cell (in a muscle cell, it does the contracting; in a nerve cell, it transmits impulses). The cytoplasm contains:

(a) *Mitochondria*—small bodies which carry on the production of energy in the cell by burning food in the presence of oxygen. This process is called **catabolism** (cata = down; bol = to cast or throw). During catabolism complex food materials are broken down into simpler substances and energy is released.

(b) *Endoplasmic reticulum*—a series of canals within the cell. Some canals contain small bodies called **ribosomes** which help make substances (proteins) for the cell. This synthesizing (building-up) process is called **anabolism** (ana = up; bol = to cast). Together the processes of catabolism and anabolism constitute the total **metabolism** of the cell. Metabolism means the sum of the building-up processes (anabolism) and breaking-down processes (catabolism) in a cell.

STUDY SECTION 1

These are the important terms introduced in this first section of text. Make sure that you can spell each term and know what each term means. It may help you to practice writing the terms correctly.

protoplasm	The material of the cell, including the cytoplasm, nucleoplasm, and membranes.
nucleoplasm	The protoplasm within the nucleus.
karyoplasm	Nucleoplasm.
cytoplasm	Protoplasm that is outside the nucleus and within the cell membrane.
cell membrane	The structure surrounding and protecting the cell; it determines what enters and leaves the cell. SEMI-PERMEABLE
nucleus	The structure that contains genetic material (chromosomes) and controls the activities of the cell.
chromosomes	Twenty-three pairs of rod-shaped structures in the nucleus; each contains DNA.
genes	Regions of DNA found within each chromosome. There are thousands of genes on each chromosome.
DNA	Deoxyribonucleic acid, the hereditary chemical found within each chromosome.
karyotype	A picture of the chromosomes in a cell nucleus; chromosomes are arranged in numerical order.
mitochondria	Small structures found in the cytoplasm; they carry on the process of catabolism (burning food to release energy in the cell).

catabolism	The process in which nutrients are chemically burned (broken down) to release energy.
endoplasmic reticulum	Canals within the cytoplasm; ribosomes are found on them.
ribosomes	Small, round structures on the endoplasmic reticulum; site of anabolism.
anabolism	The process by which proteins are built up or synthesized (protein synthesis).
metabolism	The sum of the chemical processes in a cell; includes anabolism and catabolism.

Difference in Cells. Cells are different, or specialized, throughout the body to carry out their individual functions. For instance, a muscle cell is long and slender and contains fibers which aid it in contracting and relaxing; an epithelial, or skin, cell may be square and flat to provide protection; a nerve cell may be quite long and have various fibrous extensions which aid it in its job of carrying impulses; a fat cell contains large, empty spaces for fat storage. These are only a few of the many types of cells in the body. Study the different types of cells pictured in Figure 2-3 and label the **nerve** cell, **epithelial** cell, **fat** cell, and **muscle** cell.

Tissues

A tissue is a group of similar cells working together to do a specific job. A **histologist** is one who specializes in the study of tissues. Some types of tissues are:

Epithelial Tissue. Epithelial tissue is located all over the body as lining for internal organs, in exocrine and endocrine glands, and as the outer surface of skin covering the body.

Muscle Tissue. Voluntary muscle is found in arms and legs and parts of the body where movement is voluntary, while involuntary muscle is found in the heart and digestive system, as well as other places where movement is not under conscious control.

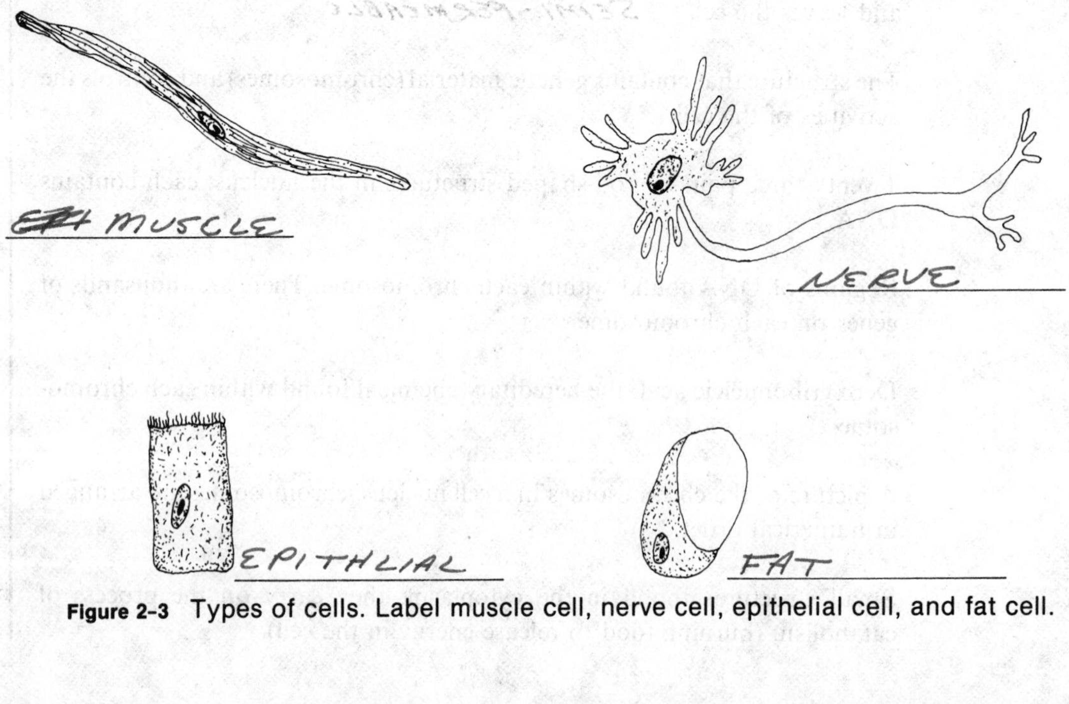

Figure 2-3 Types of cells. Label muscle cell, nerve cell, epithelial cell, and fat cell.

Connective Tissue. This can be fat (also called **adipose** tissue), **cartilage** (elastic, fibrous tissues attached to bones), bone, or blood.

Nerve Tissue. Nerve tissue conducts impulses all over the body.

Organs

These are structures composed of several kinds of tissue. For example, an organ like the stomach is composed of muscle tissue, nerve tissue, and glandular epithelial tissue. The medical term for internal organs is **viscera** (singular: **viscus**). Examples of abdominal viscera (organs located in the abdomen) are the liver, stomach, intestines, pancreas, spleen, and gallbladder.

Systems

These are groups of organs working together to perform complex functions. For example, the mouth, esophagus, stomach, and small and large intestines are organs that compose the digestive system.

Examine the list of ten body systems below and become familiar with some of the organs within each system:

System	*Organs*
Digestive	Mouth, pharynx (throat), esophagus, stomach, intestines (small and large), liver, gallbladder, pancreas.
Urinary, or excretory	Kidneys, ureters, urinary bladder, urethra.
Respiratory	Nose, pharynx, larynx (voice box), trachea (windpipe), bronchial tubes, lungs.
Reproductive	Female: Ovaries, fallopian tubes, uterus, vagina, mammary glands. Male: Testes and associated tubes, urethra, penis, prostate gland.
Endocrine	Thyroid gland, pituitary gland, sex glands (ovaries and testes), adrenal glands, pancreas (islets of Langerhans), parathyroid glands, pineal gland, thymus gland.
Nervous	Brain, spinal cord, nerves, and collections of nerves.
Cardiovascular	Heart, blood vessels (arteries, veins, and capillaries), lymphatic vessels and nodes, spleen, thymus gland.
Muscular	Muscles.
Skeletal	Bones and joints.
Integumentary	Skin, hair, nails, and associated glands (sweat and sebaceous or oil glands).

II. BODY CAVITIES

A body cavity is a space within the body which contains internal organs (viscera). Label Figure 2-4 as you learn the names of the body cavities. Some of the important viscera contained within those cavities are listed as well.

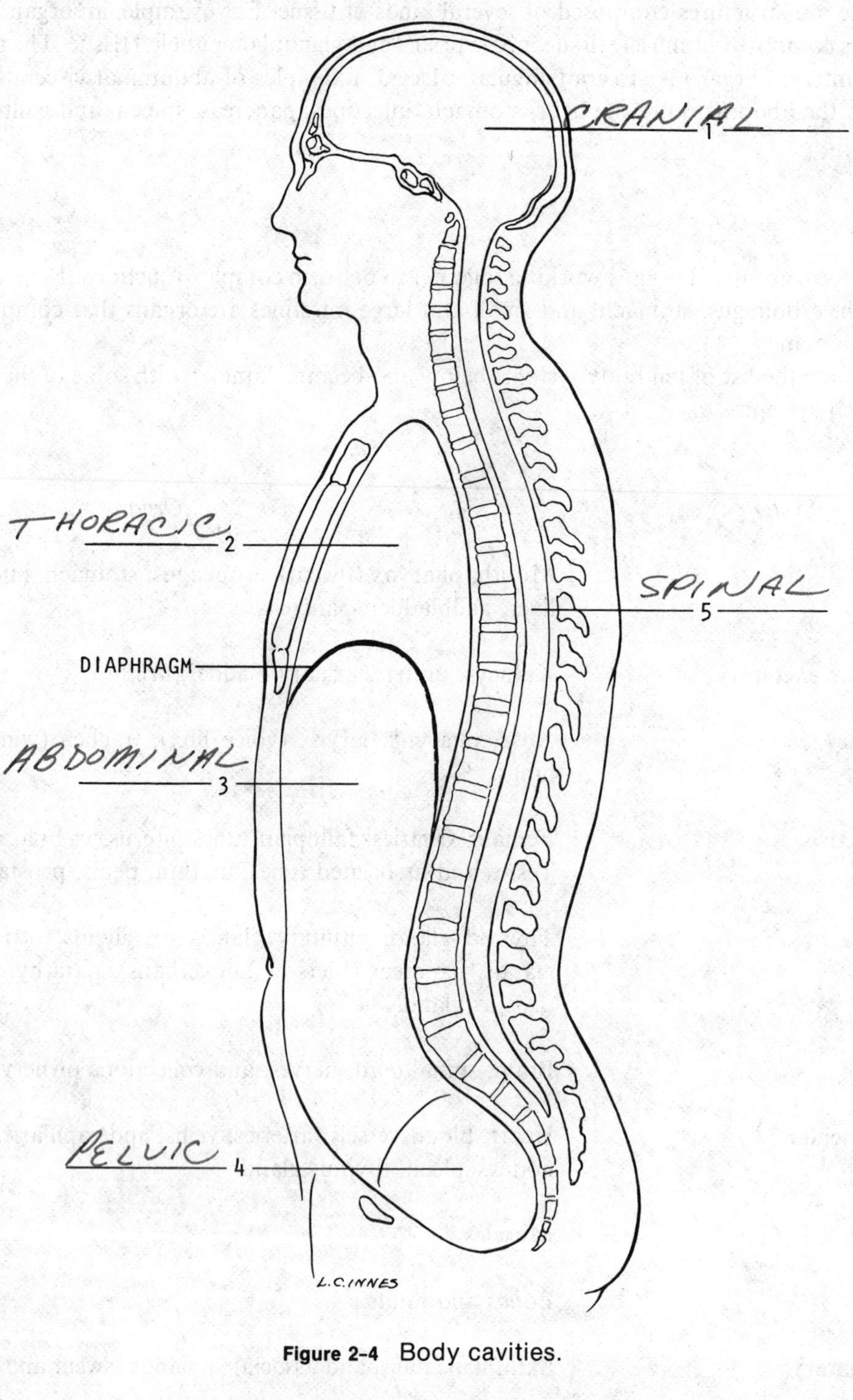

Figure 2-4 Body cavities.

Cavity	*Organs*
(1) **Cranial**	Brain
(2) **Thoracic**	Lungs, heart, esophagus, trachea, thymus gland, aorta (large artery).

The thoracic cavity can be divided into two smaller cavities:

(a) The **pleural cavities**—the areas surounding the lungs. Each pleural cavity is lined with a double-folded membrane called **pleura**; visceral pleura is closest to the lungs, and parietal pleura is closest to the outer wall of the cavity.

(b) The **mediastinum**—the area between the lungs. It contains the heart, aorta, trachea, esophagus, and thymus gland.

Study Figure 2-5, which reviews the divisions of the thoracic cavity.

(3) **Abdominal**	Stomach, small and large intestines, spleen, liver, gallbladder, pancreas.

The **peritoneum** is the double-folded membrane surrounding the abdominal cavity (see Figure 22-3). The kidneys are two bean-shaped organs situated at the back (retroperitoneal area) of the abdominal cavity on either side of the backbone.

(4) **Pelvic**	Urinary bladder, urethra, ureters; uterus and vagina in the female.
(5) **Spinal**	Nerves of the spinal cord.

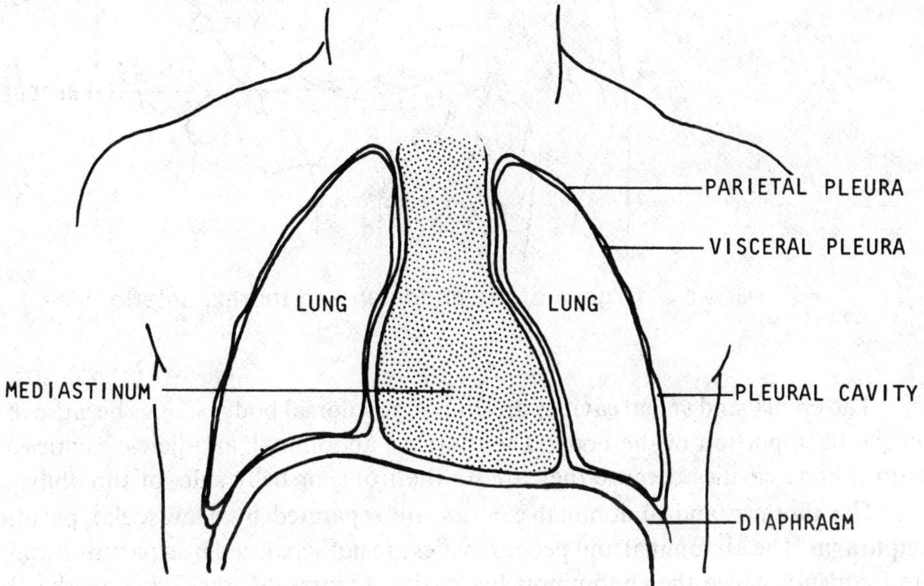

Figure 2-5 Divisions of the thoracic cavity.

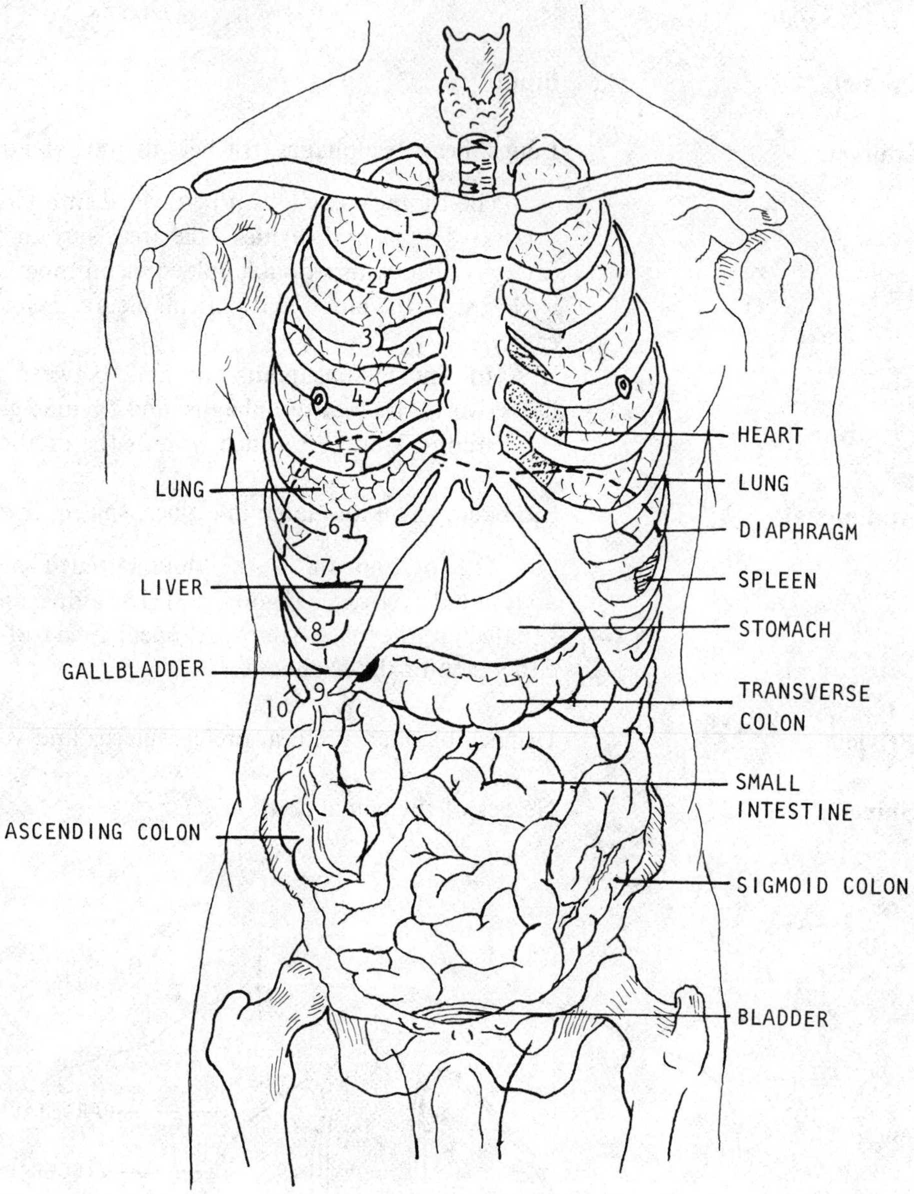

Figure 2-6 Organs of the abdomen and thorax, anterior view.

The cranial and spinal cavities are considered **dorsal** body cavities because of their location on the back portion of the body. The thoracic, abdominal, and pelvic cavities are considered **ventral** body cavities because they are on the front, or belly side, of the body.

The thoracic and abdominal cavities are separated by a muscular partition called the **diaphragm**. The abdominal and pelvic cavities are not separated by a partition and together they are frequently called the abdominopelvic cavity. Figures 2-6 and 2-7 show the abdominal and thoracic viscera from anterior (ventral) and posterior (dorsal) views.

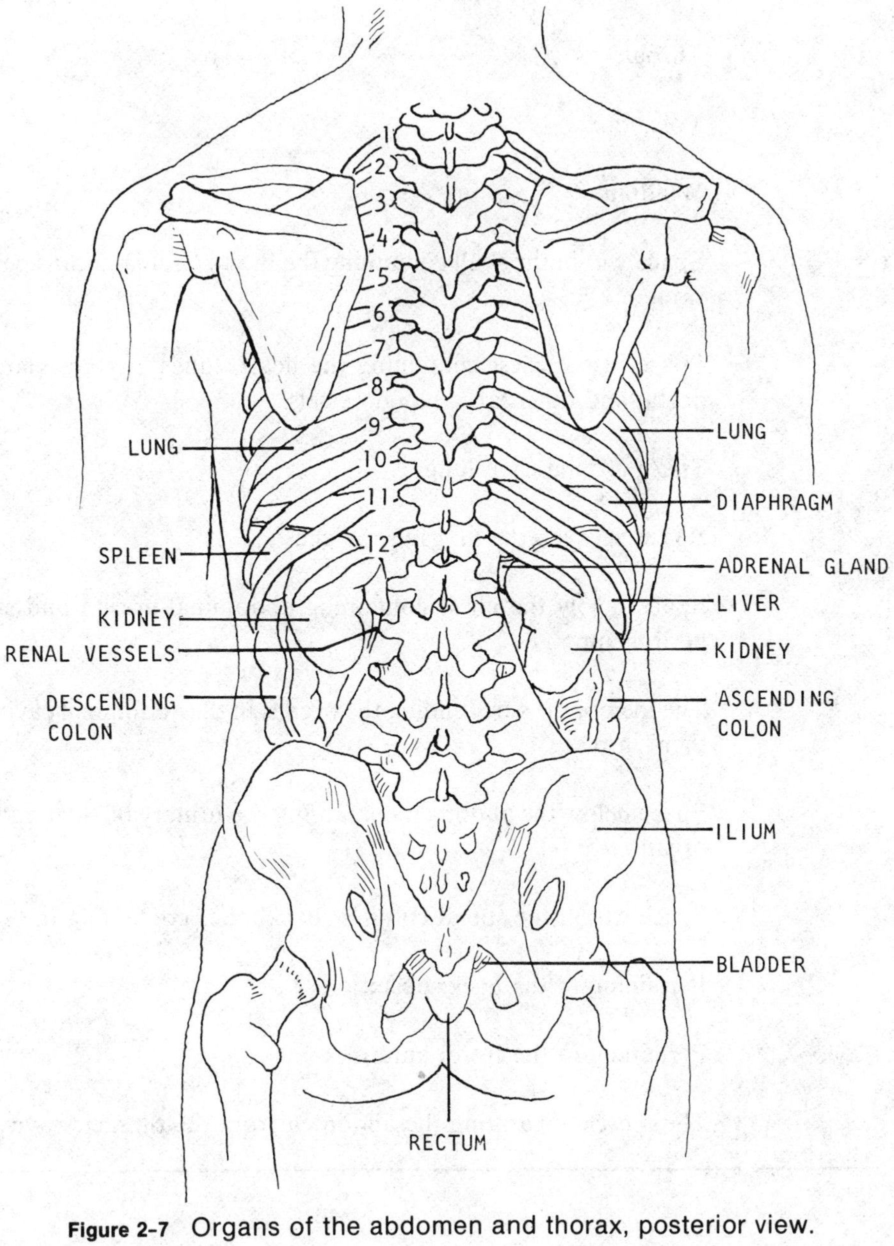

Figure 2-7 Organs of the abdomen and thorax, posterior view.

STUDY SECTION 2

epithelial	Pertaining to skin cells; cells that form the outer layer of skin and the lining of body cavities, glands, secretory tubes, and internal organs.
histologist	One who studies tissues.
adipose	Pertaining to fat.
cartilage	Flexible connective tissue found in joints, around the trachea, in the nose, and in the external ear.

viscera	Internal organs.
pharynx	Throat.
larynx	Voice box.
trachea	Windpipe.
cranial cavity	Space within the skull containing the brain. Cranial means pertaining to the skull.
thoracic cavity	Space in the chest containing the heart, lungs, thymus gland, esophagus, aorta, and other large blood vessels.
pleural cavity	Space around each lung.
mediastinum	Space between the lungs in the chest.
abdominal cavity	Space below the chest containing abdominal viscera and surrounded by peritoneum.
peritoneum	The membrane surrounding the organs in the abdominal cavity and holding them in place.
pelvic cavity	Space below the abdomen containing the urinary bladder and reproductive organs.
spinal cavity	Space within the spinal column (backbone) containing the spinal cord.
dorsal	Pertaining to the back; posterior.
ventral	Pertaining to the front; anterior.
diaphragm	The muscle separating the abdomen from the thoracic cavity.

III. ANATOMICAL DIVISIONS OF THE ABDOMEN

Label Figure 2-8 as you learn the anatomical divisions of the abdomen. These divisions are used in anatomy texts to describe the regions in which organs and structures are found.

(1) Hypochondriac regions (upper lateral regions beneath the ribs).
(2) Epigastric region (region of the stomach).
(3) Lumbar regions (two middle lateral regions).
(4) Umbilical region (region of the navel or umbilicus).
(5) Inguinal (iliac) regions (lower lateral regions).
(6) Hypogastric region (lower middle region, below the umbilicus).

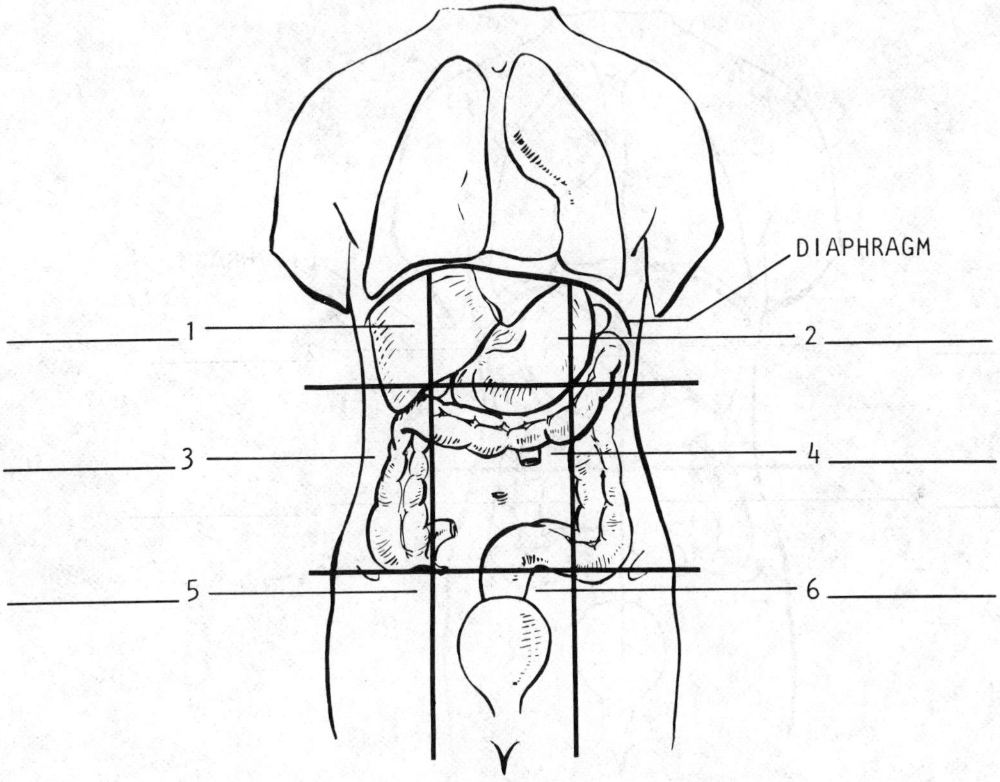

Figure 2-8 Anatomical divisions of the abdomen.

IV. CLINICAL DIVISIONS OF THE ABDOMEN

Label Figure 2-9 as you identify the clinical divisions of the abdomen. These terms are used to describe the divisions of the abdomen when a patient is examined in clinic (at bedside).

(1) **Right upper quadrant, RUQ.** Contains the right lobe of the liver, gallbladder, and parts of the large and small intestine.

(2) **Left upper quadrant, LUQ.** Contains the left lobe of the liver, stomach, pancreas, spleen, and parts of the large and small intestine.

(3) **Right lower quadrant, RLQ.** Contains parts of the large and small intestine, appendix, right ureter, right ovary and uterine (fallopian) tube.

(4) **Left lower quadrant, LLQ.** Contains parts of the small and large intestine, left ureter, left ovary and uterine (fallopian) tube.

V. ANATOMICAL DIVISIONS OF THE BACK (SPINAL COLUMN)

The back is separated into divisions corresponding to regions of the spinal column. The spinal column is composed of a series of bones extending from the neck downward to the tailbone. Each bone is called a **vertebra** (plural: vertebr<u>ae</u>).

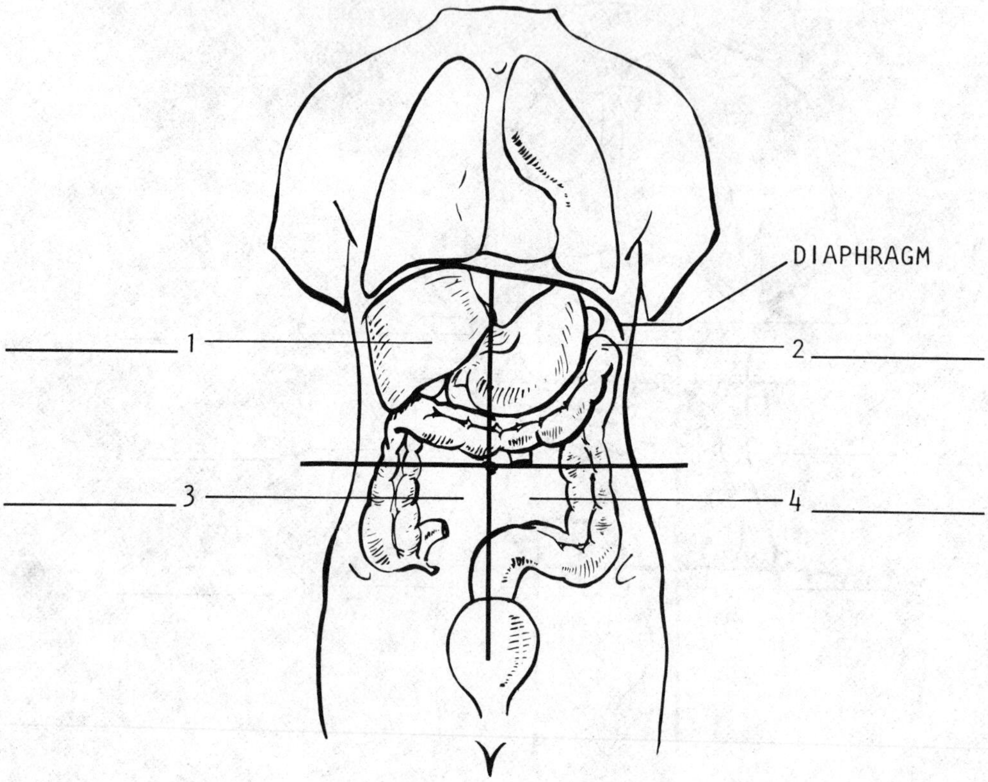

Figure 2-9 Clinical divisions of the abdomen.

Label the divisions of the back on Figure 2-10 as you study the following:

Division of the Back	*Abbreviation*	*Location*
(1) **Cervical**	C	Neck region. There are 7 cervical vertebrae (C1–C7).
(2) **Thoracic**	T or D (D = dorsal)	Chest region. There are 12 thoracic vertebrae (T1–T12). Each bone is joined to a rib.
(3) **Lumbar**	L	Loin or flank region (between the ribs and the hip bone). There are 5 lumbar vertebrae (L1–L5).
(4) **Sacral**	S	Five bones (S1-S5) are fused to form one bone, the sacrum.
(5) **Coccygeal**		The **coccyx** (tailbone) is a small bone composed of 4 fused pieces.

An important distinction should be made between the **spinal column** (the vertebrae) and the **spinal cord** (nerves running through the column). The former is bone tissue, while the latter is composed of nerve tissue.

The spaces between the vertebrae (intervertebral spaces) are identified according to the two vertebrae between which they lie; e.g., L5-S1 lies between the 5th lumbar and the 1st sacral vertebrae. An intervertebral cartilaginous (made of cartilage) **disk** (disc) lies between each vertebra and acts as a pad to absorb shocks and make movement easier.

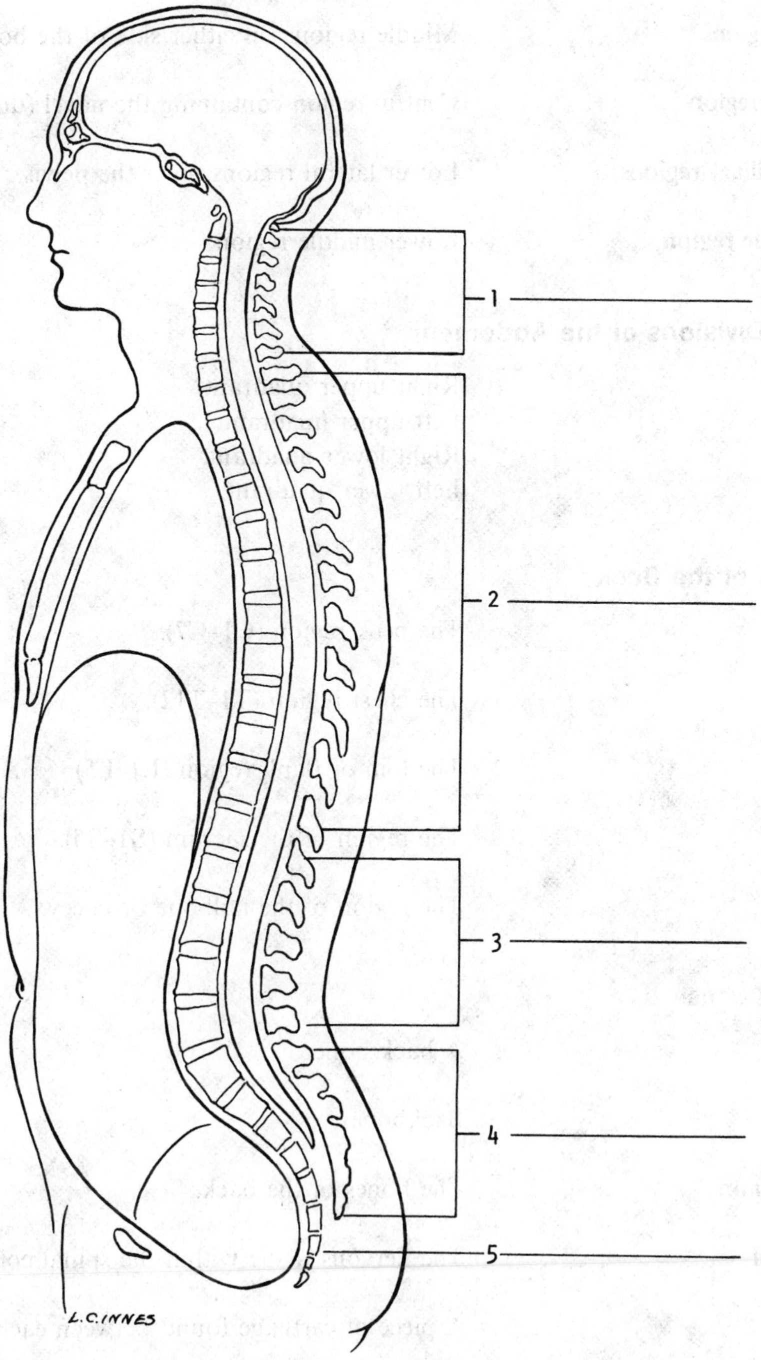

Figure 2-10 Anatomical divisions of the back (spinal column).

STUDY SECTION 3

Anatomical Divisions of the Abdomen

hypochondriac regions	Upper lateral regions beneath the ribs.
epigastric region	Upper middle region containing the stomach.
lumbar regions	Middle regions on either side of the body.
umbilical region	Central region containing the navel (umbilicus).
inguinal (iliac) regions	Lower lateral regions, near the pelvis.
hypogastric region	Lower middle region.

Clinical Divisions of the Abdomen

RUQ	Right upper quadrant.
LUQ	Left upper quadrant.
RLQ	Right lower quadrant.
LLQ	Left lower quadrant.

Divisions of the Back

cervical	The neck region (C1–C7).
thoracic	The chest region (T1–T12).
lumbar	The loin or flank region (L1–L5).
sacral	The region of the sacrum (S1–S5).
coccygeal	The region of the tailbone or coccyx.

Related Terms

vertebra	A back bone.
vertebrae	Backbones.
spinal column	The bones of the back.
spinal cord	The nervous tissue within the spinal column.
disk	A piece of cartilage found between each vertebra.

VI. POSITIONAL AND DIRECTIONAL TERMS

Afferent — Conducting **toward** a structure. *Example: Veins are called afferent vessels since they take blood toward the heart.*

Efferent — Conducting **away from** a structure. *Example: Arteries are efferent blood vessels since they take blood away from the heart.*

Anterior (ventral) — **Front** of the body. *Example: The abdomen is located anterior to the spinal cord.* Ventral and anterior mean the same position in the human.

Posterior (dorsal) — **Back** of the body. *Example: The posterior lobes of the brain are in the back of the head and are called the occipital lobes.* Dorsal means the same position as posterior.

Central — Pertaining to the **center**. *Example: The heart is located in the central portion of the thoracic cavity; it lies between the lungs in the mediastinum.*

Deep — Away from the surface. *Example: The lesion penetrated deep into the abdomen, away from the surface of the body.*

Superficial — Near the surface. *Example: The wound was a superficial one, just penetrating the skin.*

Distal — Away from the beginning of a structure; away from the center. *Example: At its distal end, the thigh bone (femur) joins with the knee cap (patella).*

Proximal — Pertaining to the beginning of a structure. *Example: The proximal end of the femur joins with the pelvic (hip) bone.*

Inferior (caudal) — Away from the head; situated below another structure. *Example: The feet are the caudal parts of the human body.*

Superior (cephalic) — Pertaining to the head; situated above another structure. *Example: In a cephalic presentation of the fetus, the head comes through the birth canal first.*

Lateral — Pertaining to the side. *Example: The little toes are lateral to the big toes.*

Medial — Pertaining to the middle or nearer the median plane of the body. *Example: In the anatomical position (see Figure 2-11) the palms of the hand are faced outward and the fifth finger lies medial to the other fingers.*

Supine — Lying on the back.

Prone — Lying on the belly.

VII. PLANES OF THE BODY

A plane is an imaginary flat surface. Label Figure 2-11 as you study the terms for the planes of the body:

(1) **Frontal** Vertical plane which divides the body or structure into anterior and posterior portions.

(2) **Sagittal** Lengthwise vertical plane which divides the body or structure into right and left portions. The midsagittal plane divides the body into right and left halves.

(3) **Transverse** Plane running across the body parallel to the ground (horizontal). It divides the body or structure into upper and lower portions.

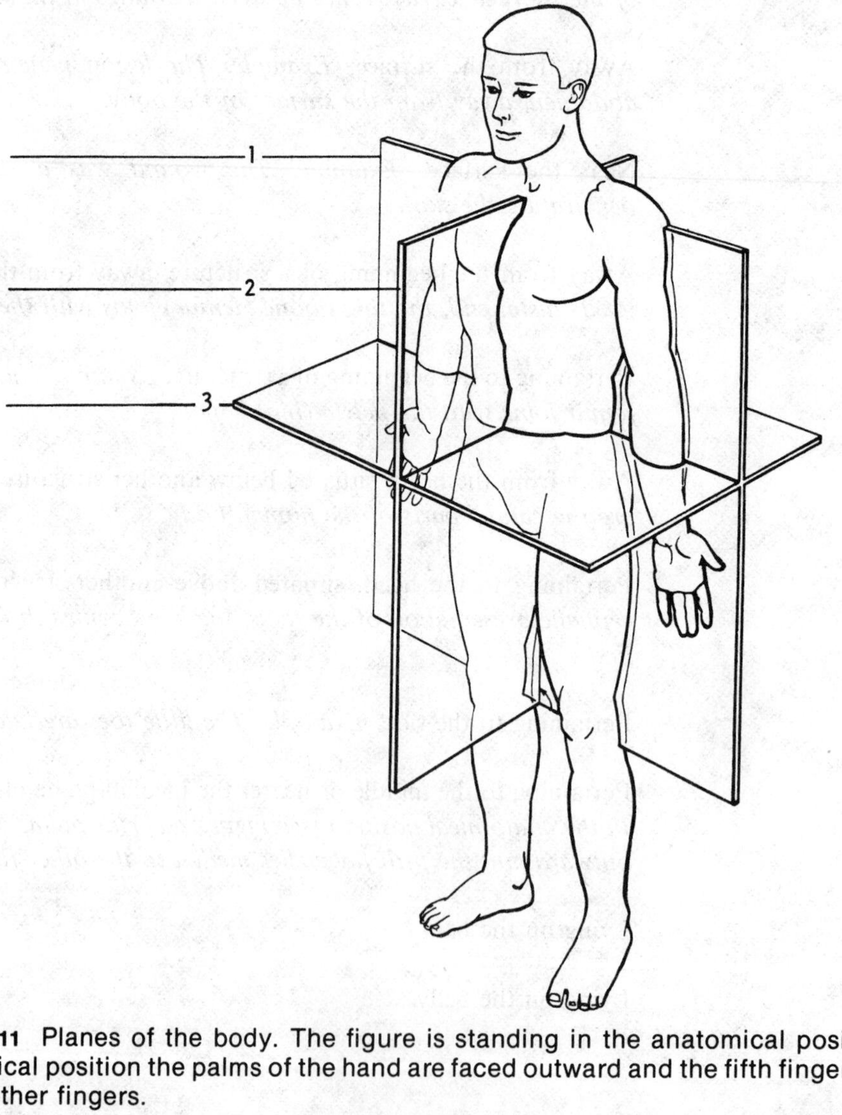

Figure 2-11 Planes of the body. The figure is standing in the anatomical position. In the anatomical position the palms of the hand are faced outward and the fifth finger lies medial to the other fingers.

STUDY SECTION 4

afferent	Conducting toward a structure.
efferent	Conducting away from a structure.
anterior	Front of the body (ventral).
posterior	Back of the body (dorsal).
central	Pertaining to the center.
deep	Away from the surface.
superficial	Near the surface.
distal	Away from the beginning of a structure; away from the center.
proximal	Pertaining to the beginning of a structure.
inferior	Away from the head; below another structure (caudal).
superior	Toward the head; above another structure (cephalic).
lateral	Pertaining to the side.
medial	Pertaining to the middle.
supine	Lying on the back.
prone	Lying on the belly.
frontal plane	Vertical plane dividing the body or structure into an anterior and posterior portions.
sagittal plane	Vertical plane dividing the body or structure into right and left portions.
transverse plane	Horizontal plane dividing the body or structure into upper and lower portions.

VIII. COMBINING FORMS, PREFIXES, AND SUFFIXES

Write the meaning of the medical term in the space provided.

Combining Form	*Meaning*	*Terminology*	*Meaning*
abdomin/o	abdomen	abdominal	pertaining to abdomen
adip/o	fat	adipose *-ose means pertaining to.*	pertaining to fat
anter/o	front	anterior *-ior means pertaining to.*	pertaining to the front
bol/o	cast, throw	anabolism *-ism means process.*	~~process of throwing up~~ process of protein syn.
caud/o	tail, lower part of the body	caudal	pertaining to the lower body
cervic/o	neck *(of the body or of the uterus)*	cervical	pertaining to the neck
chondr/o	cartilage *(type of connective tissue)*	chondroma *This is a benign tumor.*	cartilaginous tumor
		chondrosarcoma *This is a malignant tumor. The term sarc indicates that the malignant tumor is a type of flesh or connective tissue.*	cartilageous malignant tumor
chrom/o	color	chromosomes *These cell structures absorb the color of dyes used to stain the cell; som/o means body.*	colored bodies
coccyg/o	coccyx (tailbone)	coccygeal	pertaining to the tailbone
crani/o	skull	craniotomy	incision of skull
dist/o	far	distal	pertaining to being distant
dors/o	back portion of the body	dorsal	pertaining to the back

hist/o	tissue	histology study of tissue
ili/o	ilium *(part of the pelvic bone)*	iliac pertaining to the ilium *See page 31 for a picture of the ilium.*
inguin/o	groin	inguinal pertaining to the groin
kary/o	nucleus	karyoplasm formation of the nucleus *-plasm means formation.*
later/o	side	lateral pertaining to the side
lumb/o	lower back, loin *(side and back between the ribs and the pelvis)*	lumbosacral lower back tumor
medi/o	middle	medial pertaining to the middle
my/o	muscle	myoma muscle tumor
nucle/o	nucleus	nucleic pertaining to nucleus
pelv/o	hip, pelvic cavity	pelvic pertaining to the hip
poster/o	back, behind	posterior behind
prot/o	first	protoplasm formed first
proxim/o	near	proximal nearness
sacr/o	sacrum	sacral pertaining to the sacrum
sarc/o	flesh	myosarcoma muscle tumor (malignant)
spin/o	spine, backbone	spinal pertaining to the back
spondyl/o	vertebrae	spondylitis inflammation of the vertebrae *Use spondyl/o when building medical words about condition or diseases of the vertebrae.*
thel/o	nipple	epithelium ______ *This tissue, originally identified as covering nipples, is found as outer and inner skin covering throughout the body.*
thorac/o	chest	thoracic pertaining to the chest

ventr/o	belly side of the body	ventral pertaining to the belly
vertebr/o	vertebrae, backbones	vertebral pertaining to vertebrae
viscer/o	internal organs	visceral pertaining to internal organs
ana-	up	anabolic pertaining to protein syn.
cata-	down	catabolism break down of nutrients
epi-	above	epigastric upper stomach region
hypo-	below	hypochondriac upper lateral region *The Greeks blamed organs (liver and spleen) in the hypochondriac region of the abdomen as the origin of imaginary, psychosomatic illnesses. Hence, the term hypochondriac, a person with unusual anxiety about his or her health and with symptoms not attributable to any disease process.*
inter-	between	intervertebral between vertebrae
meta-	change, beyond	metabolism process of changing
sub-	under, below	subcutaneous ________

Some new suffixes introduced in this chapter are:

-iac	pertaining to	-ium	structure
-ior	pertaining to	-ose	pertaining to
-ism	process	-plasm	formation

IX. EXERCISES

A. Build medical words:

1. Process of study of tissues histology
2. Pertaining to the skull cranial
3. Incision into the chest thoracotomy
4. Pertaining to the loin lumbar

5. Pertaining to under the stomach hypogastric

6. Pertaining to the neck cervical

7. Pertaining to below the cartilage subchondriac

8. Abnormal condition of vertebrae spondylosis

9. Pertaining to internal organs visceral

10. Pertaining to the side lateral

11. Pertaining to the middle medial

12. Process of food breakdown to produce energy ("casting down")

~~catabl~~ catabolism

13. Tumor of muscle myoma

14. Inflammation of skin dermatitis

B. *Give the answers called for:*

1. Where is the mediastinum? space bet. lungs in thoracic cavity

What organs are contained within the mediastinum? heart,

~~esop~~ esophagus, & trachea

2. What does sacroiliac mean? pertaining to lower back & ilium

3. Where are the inguinal regions of the abdomen? low region - near pelvis

4. Give the meanings of: cephal/o head

encephal/o brain

crani/o skull

cerebr/o cerebrum / brain

cervic/o neck

5. What is adipose tissue? fat tissue

6. What is epithelial tissue? skin tissue

7. What is the endoplasmic reticulum? site of ribosomes

What are ribosomes? site of protein synthesis (anabolism)

8. Describe the location and function of chromosomes. in nucleus heredity

C. Give the ***opposites*** *of the following terms:*

1. deep superficial
2. afferent efferent
3. proximal distal
4. ventral dorsal
5. posterior anterior
6. caudal cephalic
7. supine prone

D. Identify the following planes:

1. Which plane divides the body into anterior and posterior portions?

FRONTAL

2. Which plane divides the body into upper and lower portions?

TRANSVERSAL

3. Which plane divides the body into left and right halves?

SAGITTAL

E. Fill in the blanks:

1. The bones of the spinal column are called vertebrae
2. One of these bones is called a vertebra
3. Two combining forms for this structure are spondylo / vertebro
4. What does L5–S1 mean? ______

F. Complete the following sentences using medical terms expressing position or direction:

1. The left lung lies ______ to the heart.
2. The upper arm bone (humerus) joins at its ______ end with the elbow.

endoplasmic reticulum	ĕn-dō-PLĂZ-mĭk rĕ-TĬK-ū-lŭm
epigastric	ĕp-ĭ-GĂS-trĭk
epithelial	ĕp-ĭ-THĒ-lē-ăl
epithelium	ĕp-ĭ-THĒ-lē-ŭm
frontal	FRŬN-tăl
histology	hĭs-TŎL-ō-jē
hypochondriac	hī-pō-KŎN-drē-ăk
hypogastric	hĭ-pō-GĂS-trĭk
iliac	ĬL-ē-ăk
inguinal	ĬNG-gwĭ-nal
intervertebral	ĭn-tĕr-VĔR-tĕ-brăl or ĭn-tĕr-vĕr-TĒ-brăl
karyotype	KĂR-ē-ō-tīp
larynx	LĂR-ĭnks
lumbar	LŬM-băr
lumbosacral	lŭm-bō-SĀ-krăl
mediastinum	mē-dē-ăs-TĪ-nŭm
metabolism	mĕ-TĂB-ō-lĭzm
mitochondria	mī-tō-KŎN-drē-ă
myalgia	mī-ĂL-jă
myoma	mī-Ō-mă
nucleic	nū-KLĒ-ĭk
nucleoplasm	NŪ-klē-ō-plăzm
nucleus	ŇU-klē-ŭs
pelvic	PĔL-vĭk
pharynx	FĂR-ĭnks
pleural	PLŌŌR-ăl
posterior	pōs-TĒR-ē-ŏr
prone	prōn
protoplasm	PRŌ-tō-plăzm
proximal	PRŎK-sĭ-măl
ribosome	RĪ-bō-sōm
sacral	SĀ-krăl

sacrum	SĀ-krŭm
sagittal	SĂJ-ĭ-tăl
spondylitis	spŏn-dĭ-LĪ-tĭs
subcutaneous	sŭb-kū-TĀ-nē-ŭs
supine	sū-PĪN or SŪ-pīn
thoracic	thō-RĂS-ĭk
thoracotomy	thō-ră-KŎT-ō-mē
trachea	TRĀ-kē-ă
transverse	trănz-VĔRS
umbilical	ŭm-BĬL-ĭ-kăl
ventral	VĔN-trăl
vertebra	VĔR-tĕ-bră
vertebrae	VĔR-tĕ-brā
vertebral	VĔR-tĕ-brăl or vĕr-TĒ-brăl
viscera	VĬS-ĕr-ă
visceral	VĬS-ĕr-ăl

REVIEW SHEET 2

Combining Forms

Give the meaning:		*Give the combining form:*	
abdomin/o	abdomen		groin
adip/o	fat		nucleus
anter/o	front (Top)		side
bol/o	throw		lower back, loin
caud/o	tail		muscle
cervic/o	neck		hip bone
coccyg/o	tail		first
crani/o	skull		sacrum
dist/o	distance		flesh
dors/o	back		vertebra (2)
hist/o	tissue		
ili/o	ilium		chest
ventr/o	front		internal organs

Suffixes

-tomy		-plasm	
-ectomy		-oma	
-osis		-itis	
-ose		-ism	

Prefixes

ana- ____________ hypo- ____________

cata- ____________ meta- ____________

inter- ____________ epi- ____________

Label the anatomical divisions of the abdomen:

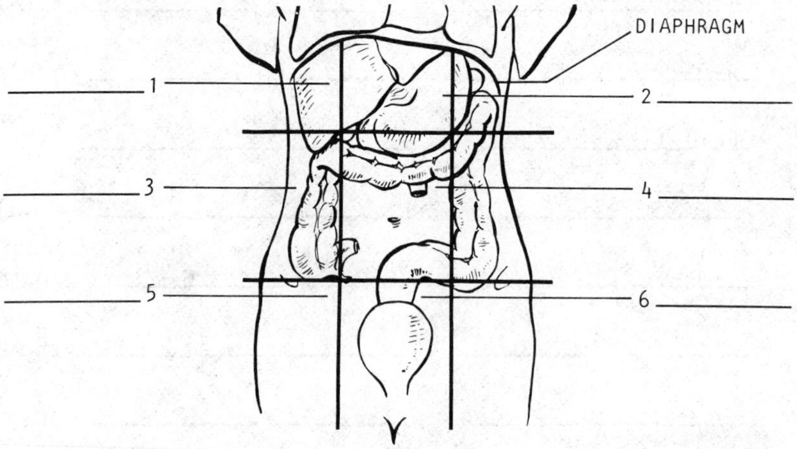

Name the anatomical divisions of the spinal (vertebral) column:

Neck region ____________ Region of the sacrum ____________

Chest region ____________ Tailbone region ____________

Lower back (loin) region ____________

Name the planes of the body:

Vertical plane which divides the body into anterior and posterior portions

____

Horizontal plane dividing the body into upper and lower portions

____

Vertical plane dividing the body into right and left portions

____

Name the positional and directional terms:

Pertaining to the head (above another structure) ________________

Away from the beginning of a structure ________________

Conducting toward ________________

Conducting away from ________________

In front of the body ________________

Away from the head (below another structure) ________________

Pertaining to the beginning of a structure ________________

Away from the surface ________________

Back of the body ________________

Pertaining to the side ________________

Near the surface ________________

Pertaining to the center ________________

Pertaining to the middle or midline ________________

Lying on the back ________________

Lying on the belly ________________

From the following list of terms, pick the one which fits the definition best:

ribosomes	pleural cavity	anabolism
mediastinum	endoplasmic reticulum	metabolism
mitochondria	chromosomes	
diaphragm	catabolism	

________________ Structures in the cytoplasm of the cell which produce energy by chemically burning food in the presence of oxygen.

________________ Contains the hereditary material (DNA) of the cell.

________________ Building-up, or synthesizing, process in the cell.

________________ Contains the heart and other structures between the lungs in the thoracic cavity.

______________________ Process in the cell whereby food is burned to release energy.

______________________ Structures in cytoplasm of cell which are the site of protein synthesis.

______________________ Surrounds the lungs in the thoracic cavity.

______________________ Network of canals in the cytoplasm of a cell.

______________________ Total of building-up and breaking-down processes in cell.

______________________ Muscular wall dividing the abdominal and thoracic cavities.

CHAPTER 3

SUFFIXES

In this chapter you will:

- Define new suffixes and review those presented in previous chapters;
- Gain practice in word analysis by using these suffixes with combining forms to build and understand terms; and
- Name and know the functions of the different types of blood cells in the body.

The chapter is divided into the following sections:

I. Introduction
II. Combining Forms
III. Suffixes and Terminology
IV. Appendices
V. Exercises
VI. Pronunciation of Terms

I. INTRODUCTION

This chapter has three purposes. The first is to teach many of the most common suffixes in the medical language. As you work through the entire book, the suffixes mastered in this chapter will appear often. An additional group of basic suffixes is presented in Chapter 6.

The second purpose is to teach new combining forms and use them to make words with suffixes. Your analysis of the terminology in Section III of this chapter will increase your medical language vocabulary.

The third purpose is to expand your understanding of terminology beyond basic word analysis. The appendices in Section IV give explanations of many terms listed. In particular, emphasis is placed on learning the names and functions of different types of blood cells. These terms are basic to the vocabulary of a person working in the paramedical field.

II. COMBINING FORMS

Read this list and underline those combining forms which are unfamiliar.

abdomin/o	abdomen
acr/o	extremities, top, extreme point
acu/o	sharp, severe, sudden
amni/o	amnion (sac surrounding the embryo in the uterus)
angi/o	vessel
arteri/o	artery
arthr/o	joint

axill/o	armpit
bronch/o	bronchial tubes (two tubes, one right and one left, which branch from the trachea to enter the lungs)
carcin/o	cancer
chem/o	drug, chemical
chir/o	hand
chondr/o	cartilage
chron/o	time
col/o	colon, large intestine
cutane/o	skin
cyst/o	urinary bladder
dactyl/o	fingers or toes
encephal/o	brain
eosin/o	rosy, dawn-colored
gon/o	seed
granul/o	granules
hepat/o	liver
hydr/o	water
isch/o	to hold back
lapar/o	abdomen, abdominal wall
laryng/o	larynx (voice box)
lymph/o	lymph *(lymph is clear fluid that bathes tissue spaces and is contained in special lymph vessels and nodes throughout the body)*
lith/o	stone, calculus
maxill/o	upper jaw
morph/o	shape, form
muc/o	mucus
myel/o	bone marrow, spinal cord *(context of usage indicates which meaning is intended)*
necr/o	death (of cells or whole body)
ophthalm/o	eye
oste/o	bone

ot/o	ear
peritone/o	peritoneum
phag/o	to eat, swallow
phil/o	like, love, attraction to
phob/o	fear
plasm/o	development, formation
pneum/o	lungs
rect/o	rectum
ren/o	kidney
splen/o	spleen
staphyl/o	clusters, grapes
strept/o	twisted chains
thorac/o	chest
thromb/o	clot
tonsill/o	tonsils
trache/o	trachea (windpipe)
ven/o	vein

III. SUFFIXES AND TERMINOLOGY

Noun Suffixes. The following is a list of the most common noun suffixes. A medical term is given to illustrate the use of the suffix. The basic rule for building a medical word is that the combining vowel, such as **o**, is used to connect the root to the suffix, with the exception that the combining vowel is **not** used before suffixes that begin with a vowel. For example: gastr/itis, **not** gastr/o/itis.

Suffix	*Meaning*	*Terminology*	*Meaning*
-algia	pain	arthralgia	____________
		otalgia	____________
		neuralgia	____________
-cele	hernia[1]	rectocele	____________
		cystocele	____________

[1]See Appendix A

-centesis	surgical puncture to remove a fluid	thoracocentesis (thoracentesis) ______
		amniocentesis ______
		abdominocentesis ______ *Also called paracentesis.*
-coccus (plural: -cocci[3])	berry-shaped bacteria	streptococcus[2] ______
		staphylococcus[2] ______
-cyte	cell	erythrocyte[4] ______
		leukocyte ______
		thrombocyte ______
-dynia	pain	gastrodynia ______
-ectomy	removal, excision	laryngectomy[5] ______
-emia	blood condition	anemia[6] ______
		ischemia[7] ______
-genesis	condition of producing, forming	carcinogenesis ______
		oncogenesis ______
-gram	record	electroencephalogram ______
		myelogram ______ *Myel/o means spinal cord in this term.*
-graph	instrument for recording	electroencephalograph ______
-graphy	process of recording	electroencephalography ______

[2]See Appendix B
[3]See Appendix C
[4]See Appendix D
[5]See Appendix E
[6]See Appendix F
[7]See Appendix G

-itis	inflammation	bronchitis ______
		tonsillitis ______
-logy	study of	ophthalmology ______
-lysis	breakdown, destruction, separation	hemolysis ______
-malacia	softening	osteomalacia ______
		chondromalacia ______
-megaly	enlargement	acromegaly[8] ______
		splenomegaly[9] ______
-oma	tumor	hepatoma ______
		myeloma ______
		Myel/o means bone marrow in this term.
-opsy	to view	biopsy ______
-osis	condition, usually abnormal	necrosis ______
		hydronephrosis ______
		erythrocytosis[10] ______
-pathy	disease	cardiomyopathy ______
-penia	deficiency	erythropenia ______
-pexy	fixation, putting in place	nephropexy ______
-phobia	fear	hydrophobia ______
		A symptom and common name for rabies.
		acrophobia ______

---

[8] See Appendix H
[9] See Appendix I
[10] See Appendix J

-plasia	development, formation	chondroplasia ____________
-plasty	surgical repair	thoracoplasty ____________
-poiesis	formation	hematopoiesis ____________
		myelopoiesis ____________
		Myel/o means bone marrow here.
-ptosis[11]	drooping, sagging, prolapse	visceroptosis ____________
-sclerosis	hardening	arteriosclerosis ____________
-scope	instrument for examination	endoscope ____________
-stasis	stopping, controlling	metastasis ____________
		Meta- means beyond. A metastasis is the spreading of a malignant tumor beyond its original site to a secondary organ or location.
		hemostasis ____________
-stomy	new opening	colostomy ____________
-therapy	treatment	hydrotherapy ____________
		chemotherapy ____________
-tome	instrument to cut	osteotome ____________
-tomy	incision, section	laparotomy ____________
-trophy	nourishment, development	hypertrophy ____________
		Cells increase in size, not number.
		atrophy ____________
		Cells decrease in size.

The following are shorter noun suffixes which are usually attached to roots in words:

-ia	condition	leukemia ____________

[11]See Appendix K

-y	condition, process	nephropathy	
-ole	little, small	arteriole[12]	
-ule	little, small	venule	
-or	one who	chiropractor[13]	
-er	one who	radiographer	
-ist	one who specializes in	nephrologist	
-um, -ium	structure, tissue	pericardium	

Adjective Suffixes. The following are adjective suffixes:

Suffix	*Meaning*	*Terminology*	*Meaning*
-ic	pertaining to	dactylic	
		osteogenic	
		chronic	
	What does acute mean?		
-tic	pertaining to	necrotic	
-al	pertaining to	peritoneal	
-ac, -iac	pertaining to	cardiac	
		hypochondriac	
-ar	pertaining to	glandular	
-ary	pertaining to	submaxillary[14]	
		axillary	
-eal	pertaining to	laryngeal	
-ose	pertaining to	adipose	

[12]See Appendix L
[13]See Appendix M
[14]See Appendix N

-ous	pertaining to	mucous ____________________
	What is mucus?[15] ____________________	
-oid	resembling	lithoid[16] ____________________
		epidermoid ____________________
		An epidermoid carcinoma is composed of cells that resemble epidermis.

IV. APPENDICES

Appendix A

A hernia may be a bulging forth, or protrusion, of an organ or the muscular wall of an organ through the cavity which normally contains it. Some examples of hernias are a hiatus hernia (stomach protrudes upward into the mediastinum through the esophageal opening in the diaphragm; see Fig. 5-15) and an inguinal hernia (part of the intestine protrudes downward into the groin region and commonly into the scrotal sac in the male; see Fig. 5-15). A rectocele is a hernial protrusion of part of the rectum toward the vagina, and a cystocele is a hernial protrusion of the urinary bladder toward the vagina (Fig. 3-1).

Appendix B

Streptococci are berry-shaped bacteria which grow in twisted chains. One group of streptococci are responsible for such conditions as "strep" throat, tonsillitis, rheumatic fever, and certain kidney ailments while another group cause infections in teeth, in the sinuses (cavities) of nose and face, and sometimes in the valves of the heart.

Staphylococci are bacteria which grow in small clusters, like grapes. Staphylococcal lesions

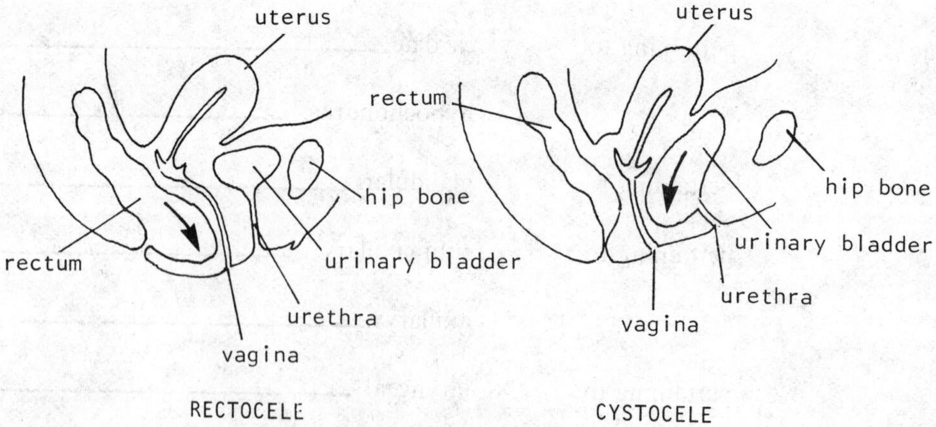

Figure 3-1 Left, Cystocele. Arrow points to downward displacement of the urinary bladder. Right, Rectocele. Arrow points to downward displacement of the rectum.

---

[15]See Appendix O
[16]See Appendix P

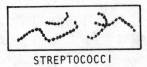

STREPTOCOCCI STAPHYLOCOCCI

Figure 3-2 Types of coccal bacteria.

may be external (skin abscesses, boils, styes) or internal (abscesses in bone and kidney). (An abscess is a collection of pus, white blood cells, and protein, which are present at the site of infection.) Figure 3-2 illustrates the pattern of growth of streptococci and staphylococci.

Other bacteria that are coccal in shape include **pneumococci** (pneum/o = lungs), which are the most common cause of bacterial pneumonia in adults, and **gonococci** (gon/o = seed), which infest the reproductive organs and cause gonorrhea.

Appendix C

Words ending in -us commonly form their plural by dropping the -us and adding -i. Thus, nucleus becomes nuclei and coccus becomes cocci (kok-sī). A guide to formation of plurals is found in the glossary at the end of the book.

Appendix D

Study Figure 3-3 as you read the following to note the differences among the three different types of cells in the blood.

1. **Erythrocytes** (red blood cells). These cells are made in the bone marrow (soft tissue in the center of some bones in the body) and are important in that they transport oxygen (O_2) from the lungs through the bloodstream to the cells all over the body. The oxygen is then used up by body cells in the process of converting food to energy (catabolism). **Hemoglobin**, containing iron (globin = protein), is an important protein in erythrocytes which helps to carry the oxygen as it travels through the bloodstream. Erythrocytes also carry away carbon dioxide (CO_2), a waste product of catabolism of food in cells, from the body cells to the lungs where it is expelled in the process of breathing.
2. **Leukocytes** (white blood cells). There are several types of leukocytes:
   (a) **Granulocytes** (cells with granules in their cytoplasm) are formed in bone marrow. There are three types of granulocytes:
      (1) **Eosinophils** (granules stain red with acid stain) are thought to be active and elevated in allergic conditions such as asthma.
      (2) **Basophils** (granules stain blue with basic stain). The function of basophils in the body is unclear.
      (3) **Neutrophils** (granules stain blue and red [purple] with neutral stain) are called **polymorphonuclear leukocytes** (poly = many; morph/o = shape or form) because the nucleus has many forms or shapes. The function of polymorphonuclears is defense of the body against bacteria by means of phagocytosis. These cells are called **polys** as an abbreviation.
   (b) **Agranulocytes** (cells without granules in cytoplasm) are produced by lymph nodes and spleen. There are two types of agranulocytes:
      (1) **Lymphocytes** (lymph cells) fight disease by producing antibodies and thus destroying foreign material. They may also attach directly to foreign material and destroy it.

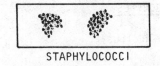

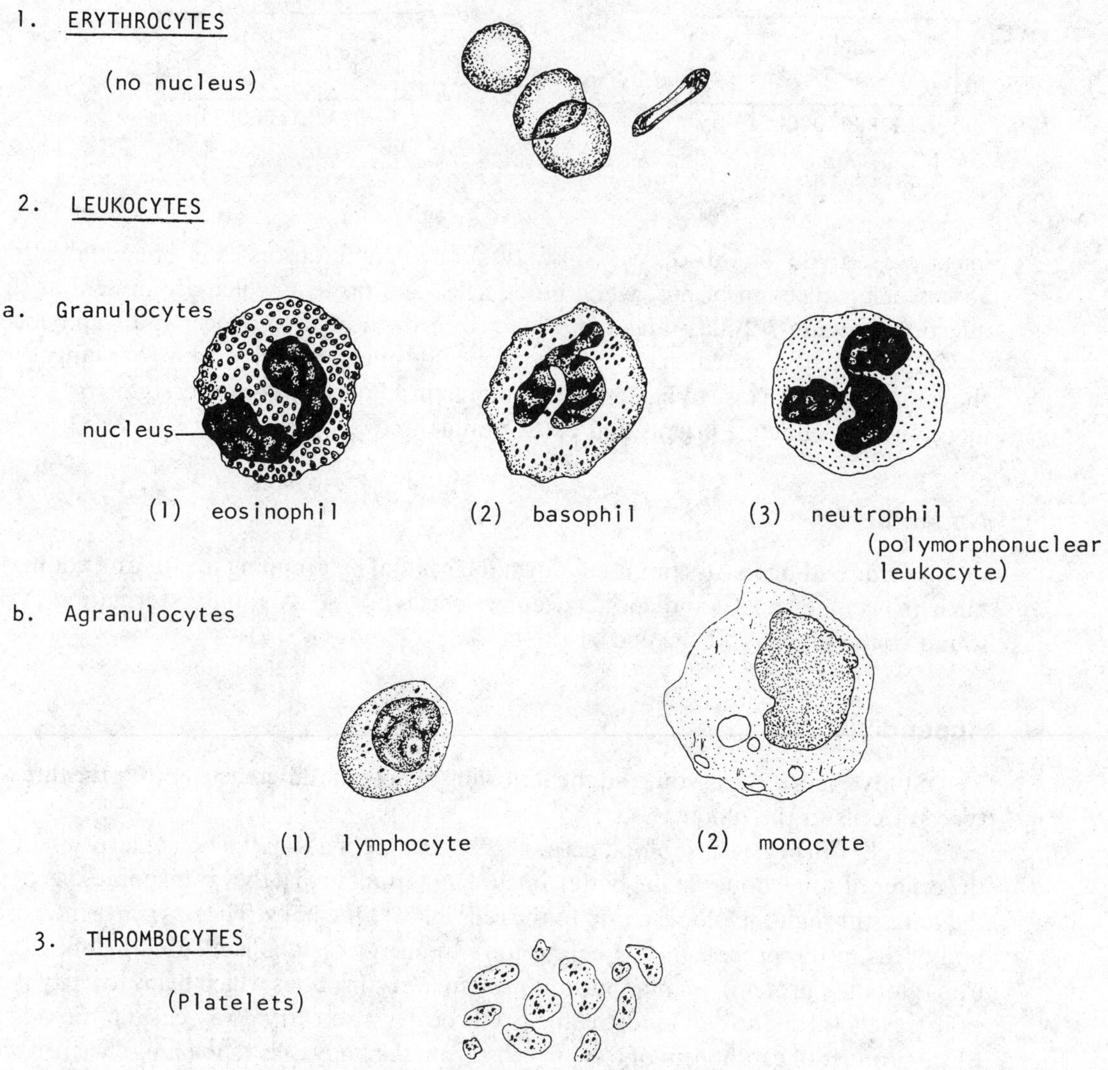

Figure 3-3 Types of blood cells.

(2) **Monocytes** (cells with a very large nucleus) ingest (phagocytose) and destroy foreign material.

3. **Platelets** or **thrombocytes**. These tiny cells, formed in the bone marrow, are necessary for blood clotting.

Appendix E

Pronunciation clue: The letters **g** and **c** are soft (as in ginger and cent) when followed by an **i** or **e**, and are hard (as in good and can) when followed by an **o** or **a**.

For example: laryngitis (lăr-ĭn-JĪ-tĭs)

laryngocele (lă-RĬNG-gō-sēl)

Appendix F

Anemia literally means "no blood." In medical language and usage, anemia refers to a medical condition in which there is a **reduction** in the number of erythrocytes or amount of hemoglobin in the circulating blood. There are many different kinds of anemias, classified on the basis of the many different problems which can arise with red blood cells, their circulation, and content. **Aplastic** (a = no; plas = formation) **anemia** is a severe type in which the bone marrow fails to produce not only erythrocytes, but leukocytes and thrombocytes as well.

Appendix G

Tissue that becomes **ischemic** loses its normal flow of blood and thus becomes devoid of oxygen. The ischemia can be caused by mechanical injury to a blood vessel, by blood clots lodging in a blood vessel, or by the gradual closing off (occlusion) of a vessel due to arteriosclerosis (hardening of the arteries).

Appendix H

Acromegaly is an example of an endocrine disorder. The **pituitary gland** attached to the base of the brain produces an excessive amount of growth hormone after the completion of puberty. Hence, a person with acromegaly is of normal height, because the long bones have stopped growth after puberty, but has an abnormally large growth of bones and tissue in the hands, feet, and face. An excessive amount of growth hormone before completion of puberty produces excessive growth of long bones (gigantism) as well as acromegaly.

Appendix I

The spleen is an organ in the left upper quadrant of the abdomen (below the diaphragm and to the side of the stomach). It is composed of lymph tissue and blood vessels. Its job is to manufacture blood cells the substances to fight disease, and to dispose of dying red blood cells. If the spleen must be removed, other organs carry out these functions.

Appendix J

When **-osis** is used as a suffix with blood cells, it means an abnormal condition in which there is a slight increase in number of circulating blood cells. When **-emia** is used as a suffix with blood cells (-cyte is usually dropped, as in leukemia), the condition is an abnormally high or excessive increase in number of blood cells. For example, erythrocyt<u>osis</u> means an elevation of red blood cells, but erythr<u>emia</u> is an excessively high increase of red blood cells.

Appendix K

The suffix **-ptosis** is pronounced TŌ-sĭs. The rule is that when two consonants begin a word, the first is silent. If the two consonants are found in the middle of a word, both are pronounced. For example visceroptosis (vĭs-ĕr-ōp-TŌ-sĭs). The term ptosis is often used alone to mean a sagging or **prolapse** (pro = before, forward; lapse = to slide) of an organ or part.

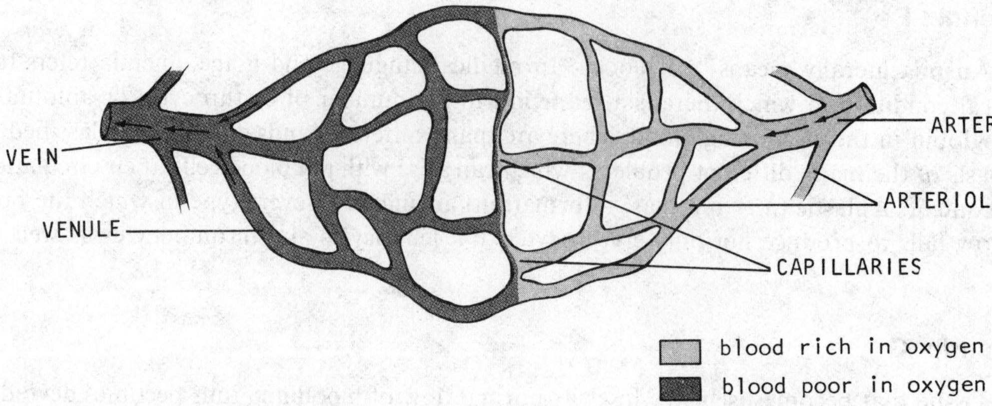

Figure 3-4 Relationship of blood vessels.

Appendix L

The relationship between an artery, arterioles, capillaries (tiniest of blood vessels), venules, and a vein is illustrated in Figure 3-4.

Appendix M

A **chiropractor** is a specially trained person who manipulates the bones of the vertebral column to relieve pressure on nerves.

Appendix N

Submaxillary means under the upper jaw (maxilla) and actually refers to the lower jaw bone.

Appendix O

Mucus is a sticky secretion produced by mucous membranes and glands. It contains a protein called mucin, water, salts, and other substances. Mucosa is another term for a mucous membrane.

Appendix P

The combining from **lith/o** refers to a **stone**, or **calculus**, within the body. Stones are usually composed of mineral salts.

V. EXERCISES

A. Construct medical words:

1. Instrument to visually examine the larynx ______________________
2. Pain in the fingers ______________________

3. Enlargement of the liver ______
4. Surgical repair of nerves ______
5. Incision of the chest ______
6. Deficiency of white blood cells ______
7. Softening of the brain ______
8. One who specializes in the study of the eye ______
9. New opening of the kidney ______
10. Fear of extremities (heights) ______
11. Formation of red blood cells ______
12. Formation of bone ______
13. Condition of hardening of arteries ______
14. Prolapse of the kidney ______
15. Fixation of the internal organs ______
16. Removal of tonsils ______
17. Resembling a stone ______
18. Small vein ______
19. Small artery ______
20. Tumor of the liver ______

B. *Give the meaning of the following medical terms:*

1. mucus ______
2. otitis ______
3. staphylococci ______
4. arthropathy ______
5. ischemic ______

6. laryngectomy ______________________________

7. peritoneal ______________________________

8. hypertrophy ______________________________

9. otalgia ______________________________

10. cardiomegaly ______________________________

11. eosinophil ______________________________

12. hydrocele ______________________________

13. bronchoscopy ______________________________

14. thrombocytopenia ______________________________

15. electroencephalography ______________________________

16. mucosa ______________________________

17. tracheostomy ______________________________

18. angiogenesis ______________________________

19. myelogram ______________________________

20. myeloma ______________________________

C. *Test your knowledge by giving the meaning of the following* ***noun*** *suffixes:*

1. -gram ______________
2. -plasty ______________
3. -osis ______________
4. -itis ______________
5. -genic ______________
6. -graphy ______________
7. -oma ______________
8. -graph ______________
9. -tome ______________
10. -emia ______________
11. -coccus ______________
12. -trophy ______________
13. -tomy ______________
14. -ectomy ______________
15. -stomy ______________
16. -megaly ______________

carcinogenesis	kăr-sĭ-nō-JEN-ĕ-sĭs
cardiomyopathy	kăr-dē-ō-mī-ŎP-ă-thē
chemotherapy	kē-mō-THĔR-ă-pē
chiropractor	KĪ-rō-prăk-tŏr
chondromalacia	kŏn-drō-mă-LĀ-shă
chondroplasia	kŏn-drō-PLĀ-zē-ă
chronic	KRŎN-ĭk
colostomy	kō-LŎS-tō-mē
cystocele	SĬS-tō-sēl
dactylic	dăk-TĬL-ĭk
electroencephalogram	ē-lĕk-trō-ĕn-SĔF-ă-lō-grăm
electroencephalograph	ē-lĕk-trō-ĕn-SĔF-ă-lō-grăf
electroencephalography	ē-lĕk-trō-ĕn-sĕf-ă-LŎG-ră-fē
eosinophil	ē-ō-SĬN-ō-fĭl
epidermoid	ĕp-ĭ-DĔR-moyd
erythrocytosis	ĕ-rĭth-rō-sī-TŌ-sĭs
erythropenia	ĕ-rĭth-rō-PĒ-nē-ă
gastrodynia	găs-trō-DĬN-ē-ă
hematopoiesis	hē-mă-tō-poy-Ē-sĭs
hemolysis	hē-MŎL-ĭ-sĭs
hemostasis	hē-mō-STĀ-sĭs
hydronephrosis	hī-drō-nĕ-FRŌ-sĭs
hydrophobia	hī-drō-FŌ-bē-ă
hydrotherapy	hī-drō-THĔR-ă-pē
hypertrophy	hī-PĔR-trō-fē
ischemia	ĭs-KĒ-mē-ă
laparotomy	lăp-ă-RŎT-ō-mē
laryngeal	lă-RĬN-jē-ăl or lăr-ĭn-JĒ-ăl
laryngectomy	lăr-ĭn-JĔK-tō-mē
laryngotomy	lăr-ĭng-GŎT-ō-mē
leukopenia	lo͞o-kō-PE-nē-ă
lithoid	LĬTH-oyd

lymphocyte	LĬM-fō-sīt
monocyte	MŎN-ō-sīt
mucus	MŬ-kŭs
myelogram	MĪ-ĕ-lō-grăm
myeloma	mī-ĕ-LŌ-mă
myelopoiesis	mī-ĕ-lō-poy-Ē-sĭs
necrosis	nĕ-KRŌ-sĭs
nephrologist	nĕ-FRŎL-ō-jĭst
nephropathy	nĕ-FRŎP-ă-thē
nephropexy	NĔF-rō-pĕk-sē
neutrophil	NŪ-trō-fĭl
oncogenesis	ŏn-kō-JĔN-ĕ-sĭs
ophthalmology	ŏf-thăl-MŎL-ō-jē
osteogenic	ŏs-tē-ō-JĔN-ĭk
osteomalacia	ŏs-tē-ō-mă-LĀ-shă
osteotome	ŎS-tē-ō-tōm
otalgia	ō-TĂL-jă
paracentesis	păr-ă-sĕn-TĒ-sĭs
peritoneal	pĕr-ĭ-tō-NĒ-ăl
platelet	PLĀT-lĕt
pneumococcal	nū-mō-KŎK-ăl
polymorphonuclear	pŏl-ē-mŏr-fō-NŪ-klē-ăr
splenomegaly	splē-nō-MĚG-ă-lē
staphylococci	stăf-ĭ-lō-KŎK-sī
streptococcus	strĕp-tō-KŎK-ŭs
submaxillary	sŭb-MĂK-sĭ-lăr-ē
thoracentesis	thō-ră-sĕn-TĒ-sĭs
thoracoplasty	thō-ră-kō-PLĂS-tē
thrombocytopenia	thrŏm-bō-sī-tō-PĒ-nē-ă
tonsillitis	tŏn-sĭ-LĪ-tĭs
venule	VĔN-ūl
visceroptosis	vĭs-ĕr-ŏp-TŌ-sĭs

REVIEW SHEET 3

Noun Suffixes

-algia	______	-opsy	______
-cele	______	-or	______
-centesis	______	-osis	______
-coccus	______	-pathy	______
-cyte	______	-penia	______
-dynia	______	-pexy	______
-ectomy	______	-phobia	______
-emia	______	-plasia	______
-er	______	-plasty	______
-genesis	______	-poiesis	______
-gram	______	-ptosis	______
-graph	______	-sclerosis	______
-graphy	______	-scope	______
-ia	______	-stasis	______
-ist	______	-stomy	______
-itis	______	-therapy	______
-logy	______	-tome	______
-lysis	______	-tomy	______
-malacia	______	-trophy	______
-megaly	______	-ule	______
-ole	______	-um	______
-oma	______	-y	______

Adjective Suffixes

-ac ______
-al ______
-ar ______
-ary ______
-eal ______
-ic ______
-oid ______
-ose ______
-ous ______
-tic ______

Combining Forms

Give the combining form:

joint ______
cancer ______
head ______
brain ______
kidney ______
nerve ______
tumor ______
eye ______
ear ______
nose ______
peritoneum ______
armpit ______
red ______
liver ______
muscle ______
spinal cord or bone marrow ______
windpipe ______
chest ______
neck ______
clot ______
tonsil ______
death ______
spleen ______

Give the meaning:

chondr/o ______
oste/o ______
acr/o ______
acu/o ______
col/o ______
cutane/o ______
bi/o ______
lith/o ______

chir/o	______	lapar/o	______
muc/o	______	dactyl/o	______
laryng/o	______	eosin/o	______
arteri/o	______	hydr/o	______
chron/o	______	gon/o	______
maxill/o	______	isch/o	______
phil/o	______	granul/o	______
phob/o	______	strept/o	______
rect/o	______	staphyl/o	______
radi/o	______	abdomin/o	______
pneum/o	______	viscer/o	______
leuk/o	______	morph/o	______
ren/o	______	ven/o	______

Prefixes

a-, an-	______	hyper-	______
auto-	______	meta-	______
hypo-	______	sub-	______

CHAPTER 4

PREFIXES

In this chapter you will:

- Define basic prefixes used in the medical language;
- Analyze medical terms which combine prefixes and other word elements; and
- Learn about the Rh condition as an example of an antigen-antibody reaction.

The chapter is divided into the following sections:

I. Introduction
II. Combining Forms and Suffixes
III. Prefixes and Terminology
IV. Appendices
V. Exercises
VI. Pronunciation of Terms

I. INTRODUCTION

This chapter on prefixes, like the preceding chapter on suffixes, is designed to give you practice in word analysis and provide a foundation for the study of the terminology of body systems that follows.

The list of combining forms, suffixes, and their meanings in Section II will help you analyze the terminology in the rest of the chapter. The appendices are included to give more complete understanding of the terms and to explain the words with reference to the anatomy, physiology, and diseases of the body.

II. COMBINING FORMS AND SUFFIXES

amni/o	amnion, sac in which the embryo develops
cib/o	meals
cis/o	to cut
cost/o	rib
duct/o	to lead, carry
furc/o	forking, branching
gloss/o	tongue
glyc/o	sugar
morph/o	shape, form

mort/o	death
nat/i	birth
nect/o	to bind, tie, connect
norm/o	rule, order
ox/o	oxygen
secti/o	to cut
seps/o	infection
somn/o	sleep
son/o	sound
the/o	to put, place
thel/o	nipple
thyr/o	shield; the thyroid gland must have resembled (-oid) a shield to those who named it.
top/o	place, position, location
tox/o	poison
ven/o	vein
-blast	embryonic, immature
-crine	to separate, secrete
-cyesis	pregnancy
-drome	to run
-fusion	to pour
-grade	to go
-lysis	to break, separate
-meter	to measure
-partum	birth, labor

-plasia	formation, development
-phoria	to bear, carry
-physis	to grow
-pnea	breathing
-rrhea	flow, discharge
-stasis	to stop, control
-trophy	nourishment, development

III. PREFIXES AND TERMINOLOGY

Prefix	*Meaning*	*Terminology*	*Meaning*
a-, an-	not, without	apnea	________________
		anoxia	________________
ab-	away from	abnormal	________________
		abductor[1]	________________
ad-	toward	adductor	________________
		adrenal glands[2]	________________
ana-	up, apart	anabolism	________________
		analysis	________________
ante-	before, forward	ante cibum (ac)	________________
		ante partum	________________
anti-	against	antisepsis[3]	________________
		antibiotic[4]	________________

[1]See Appendix A
[2]See Appendix B
[3]See Appendix C
[4]See Appendix D

		antigen[5] ________________
		In this word, anti stands for antibody.
		antibody ________________
		antitoxin ________________
auto-	self	autogenous ________________
bi-	two	bifurcation ________________
		bilateral ________________
brady-	slow	bradycardia ________________
cata-	down	catabolism ________________
con-	with, together	congenital anomaly[6] ________________
		connective ________________
contra-	against, opposite	contraindication ________________
		Contra- means against in this term.
		contralateral[7] ________________
		Contra- means opposite in this term.
de-	down, lack of	dehydration ________________
dia-	through, complete	diameter ________________
		diarrhea ________________
		dialysis[8] ________________
dys-	bad, painful, difficult	dyspnea ________________
ec-, ecto-	out, outside	ectoderm[9] ________________
		ectopic pregnancy[10] ________________

[5]See Appendix E
[6]See Appendix F
[7]See Appendix G
[8]See Appendix H
[9]See Appendix I
[10]See Appendix J

en-, endo-	in, within	endoderm ______
		endoscope ______
		endocrine ______
epi-	upon, on, above	epithelium ______
eu-	good, well	eupnea ______
		euphoria ______
ex-	out, away from	exophthalmia[11] ______
hemi-	half	hemiglossectomy ______
hyper-	excessive, above, beyond	hyperplasia[12] ______
		hypertrophy ______
		hyperglycemia ______
hypo-	deficient, under	hypodermic ______
		hypoglycemia ______
in-	not	insomniac ______
in-	in	incision ______
infra-	below, inferior	infracardiac ______
inter-	between	intercostal ______
intra-	within	intravenous ______
macro-	large	macrocephalic ______
mal-	bad	malignant ______
		malaise ______
meso-	middle	mesoderm ______
meta-	change, beyond	metamorphosis ______
		Meta- means change in this term.

[11]See Appendix K
[12]See Appendix L

		metastasis ______________
		Meta- means beyond in this term.
micro-	small	microscope ______________
pan-	all	pancytopenia ______________
para-	near, beside, abnormal	parathyroid[13] ______________
		paralysis ______________
per-	through	percutaneous ______________
peri-	surrounding	pericardium ______________
		periosteum ______________
polio-	gray matter of the brain or spinal cord	polioencephalitis ______________
		poliomyelitis ______________
poly-	many	polymorphonuclear ______________
		polyneuritis ______________
post-	after, behind	post mortem ______________
		postnatal ______________
pre-	before, in front of	precancerous ______________
pro-	before	prodrome[14] ______________
pseudo-	false	pseudocyesis ______________
re-	back	relapse ______________
		-lapse means to slide, fall. A disease or its symptoms return after an apparent recovery.
		remission ______________
		-mission means to send. Symptoms lessen and abate.
retro-	behind, back	retroperitoneal ______________

[13]See Appendix M
[14]See Appendix N

		retrograde[15] ______
semi-	half	semiconscious ______
sub-	under	subcostal ______
supra-	above	suprathoracic ______
		suprarenal glands ______
syn-, sym-	together, with	syndactylism ______
		synthesis ______
		syndrome[16] ______
		Before the letters b, p, and m, syn becomes sym.
		symbiosis[17] ______
		symmetry ______
		symphysis[18] ______
tachy-	fast	tachypnea ______
trans-	across	transfusion ______
ultra-	beyond, excess	ultrasonography[19] ______

IV. APPENDICES

Appendix A

Abductors are muscles which draw the limbs **away** from the center of the body, while adductors are muscles which draw the limbs **toward** the center of the body.

Appendix B

The adrenal glands are endocrine glands located above each kidney. They are sometimes called suprarenal glands (supra = above). They secrete chemicals called hormones which affect the functioning of the body.

Appendix C

Noun suffixes like **-sepsis** which end in **sis** can be made adjectives by dropping the **sis** and adding **tic**. Hence, **antisepsis** becomes **antiseptic**. The prefix anti- is pronounced an-tuh; the prefix ante- is pronounced an-tee.

[15] See Appendix O
[16] See Appendix P
[17] See Appendix Q
[18] See Appendix R
[19] See Appendix S

Appendix D

An antibiotic is an agent which destroys or inhibits the growth of microorganisms (small living things). Penicillin is an example of an antibiotic.

Appendix E

An antigen is a substance, usually foreign to the body (such as a poison, virus, or bacterium), that stimulates the production of antibodies. Antibodies are protein substances developed by the body in response to the presence of foreign antigens. For example, the flu virus (antigen) enters the body, causing the production of antibodies in the bloodstream. These antibodies will then attach to and destroy the antigens (viruses) which produced them. The reaction between an antigen and antibody is called an **immune** reaction (immun/o means protection). Sometimes antibodies can be developed against proteins that are not foreign, but are already a part of the body. These antibodies cause autoimmune disorders marked by inflammation and injury to body cells.

Another example of a familiar antigen-antibody reaction is the Rh condition. A person who is Rh^+ has a protein coating (antigen) on his or her red blood cells (RBC). This antigen factor is something that the person is born with and is normal for him or her. A person who is Rh^- has normal red blood cells as well, but they do not carry the Rh factor antigen.

If an Rh^- woman and an Rh^+ man conceive an embryo, the fetus may be Rh^- or Rh^+. A dangerous condition arises only when the embryo is Rh^+. During delivery of the first Rh^+ baby, some of the baby's blood cells containing antigens may escape into the mother's bloodstream. This sensitizes the mother and causes her to produce antibodies against the new Rh^+ antigens in her blood. Because this occurs at delivery, the first baby is not generally affected and is normal at birth.

Difficulties arise with the second Rh^+ pregnancy. If the embryo is Rh^+ again, during pregnancy the mother's acquired antibodies will enter the infant's bloodstream and attack the infant's red blood cells (Rh^+). The infant's RBC's are destroyed and the infant attempts to compensate for this loss of cells by making many new immature red blood cells (erythroblasts). The infant is born with a condition known as **erythroblastosis fetalis**, also known as hemolytic disease of the newborn (HDN). One of the clinical symptoms of erythroblastosis fetalis is jaundice, or yellow skin pigmentation. The jaundice results from the excessive destruction of red blood cells, which causes a substance called bilirubin (chemical pigmentation produced when hemoglobin of red blood cells is broken down) to accumulate in the blood.

To prevent erythroblastosis fetalis, Rh immune globulin is given to the mother within 72 hours after each Rh^+ delivery or after every abortion and miscarriage if the father is Rh^+. The globulin destroys Rh^+ cells that have escaped into the mother's circulation, and thus prevents sensitization of the mother and formation of Rh^+ antibodies, so that future babies will not develop erythroblastosis fetalis. Figure 4–1 reviews the antigen-antibody reaction in the Rh condition in diagrammatic fashion.

Appendix F

An anomaly is a structure or organ which is irregular in formation (malformation). Examples of congenital anomalies are missing fingers or toes and heart defects.

Appendix G

The effect of a stroke (cerebral ischemia or necrosis) on the limbs of the body is **contralateral**. This means that if the brain damage is located on the right side of the brain, the patient

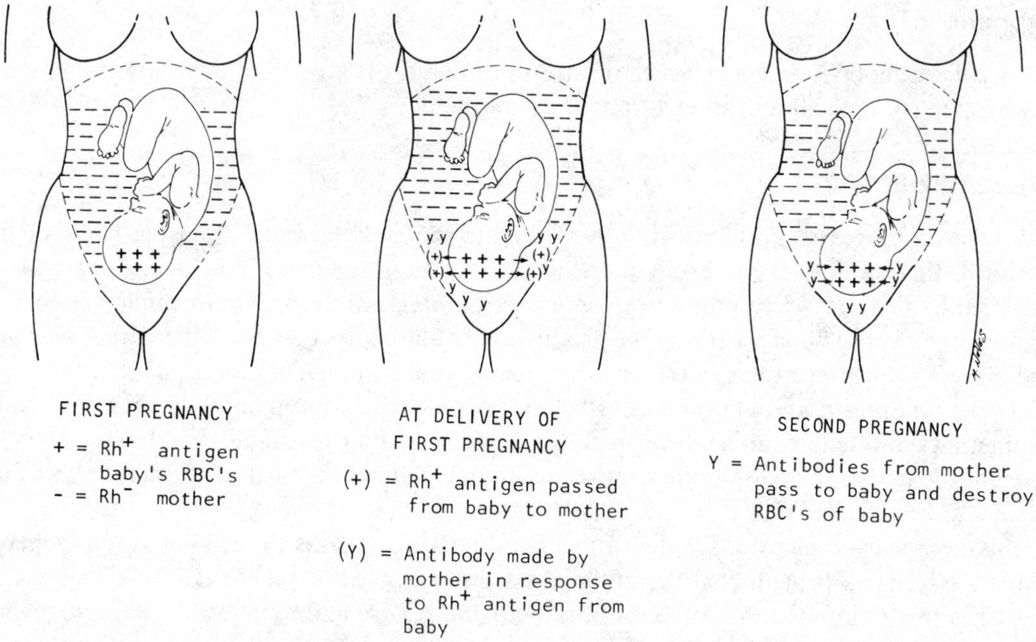
FIRST PREGNANCY
+ = Rh+ antigen baby's RBC's
- = Rh- mother
AT DELIVERY OF FIRST PREGNANCY
(+) = Rh+ antigen passed from baby to mother
(Y) = Antibody made by mother in response to Rh+ antigen from baby
SECOND PREGNANCY
Y = Antibodies from mother pass to baby and destroy RBC's of baby

Figure 4-1 Rh condition as an example of an antigen-antibody reaction.

will have paralysis on the left side of the body. The muscles on one side of the body are controlled by nerves from the opposite side of the brain.

Appendix H

Dialysis literally means "complete separation." A dialysis machine (artificial kidney) can completely separate out from the blood the harmful waste products of the body which are normally removed by the urine.

Appendix I

The **ectoderm**, **endoderm**, and **mesoderm** are the three layers of cells which form in the early stages of growth of the embryo. At this early stage of development, the embryo consists of an outer layer of cells called **ectoderm** (these cells specialize to become nerve cells in the brain and spinal cord and cells in the ears, eyes, nose, and skin); a middle layer of cells called **mesoderm** (these cells give rise to connective tissue such as bone, fat, cartilage, muscle, and blood); and an inner layer of cells called **endoderm** (these cells specialize to become the cells which line the digestive organs, liver, pancreas, lungs, bladder, and glandular tissue of the body).

Appendix J

In a normal pregnancy, the embryo develops within the uterus. In an **ectopic pregnancy**, the embryo is implanted outside the uterus—most commonly it is found in the uterine (fallopian) tubes, and sometimes in the ovary or abdominal cavity.

Appendix K

Exophthalmia is an abnormal protrusion of the eyeball. It is commonly associated with enlargement of the thyroid gland.

Appendix L

Hyperplasia refers to increase in size of an organ by virtue of increase in cell numbers. **Hypertrophy** also means increase in size of an organ or tissue, but in the context of an increase in individual cell size and development.

Appendix M

There are four parathyroid glands located on the dorsal side of the thyroid gland. The parathyroids are endocrine glands which produce a hormone and function entirely separately from the thyroid gland.

Appendix N

Prodrome means symptoms of disease (such as rash or fever) which appear before and signal the onset of an approaching more severe illness.

Appendix O

In a **retrograde** pyelogram, a contrast medium, or dye, is injected into the tubes of the urinary system (ureters) so that it flows back up into the renal pelvis region of the kidney. X-ray pictures are then taken.

Appendix P

A **syndrome** is a group of signs or symptoms which commonly occur together and indicate a particular disease or abnormal condition. An example of a syndrome is Horner's syndrome, characterized by ptosis of the eyelid, enophthalmos, and a cool, dry face on the affected side due to nerve damage.

Appendix Q

Symbiosis refers to the living together in close association of two organisms, either for mutual benefit or not. The bacteria which normally live in the digestive tract of humans are an example of symbiosis. **Parasitism** is an example of symbiosis in which one organism benefits, while the other does not.

Appendix R

A **symphysis** is a type of joint in which the bony surfaces are firmly united by a plate of cartilage. An example is the junction where the pubic bones of the pelvis have grown together.

Appendix S

Ultrasonography is a diagnostic technique using ultrasound waves (inaudible sound waves) to produce an image or photograph of an organ or tissue. The ultrasonic echoes are recorded as they pass through different types of tissue.

V. EXERCISES

A. Test yourself by filling in the meaning of the following prefixes:

1. anti- ______
2. pro- ______
3. meta- ______
4. sub- ______
5. con- ______
6. meso- ______
7. ab- ______
8. peri- ______
9. dys- ______
10. para- ______
11. retro- ______
12. dia- ______
13. pan- ______
14. ante- ______
15. contra- ______
16. infra- ______
17. inter- ______
18. intra- ______
19. hyper- ______
20. in- ______
21. ana- ______
22. cata- ______
23. poly- ______
24. pseudo- ______
25. mal- ______
26. ultra- ______
27. tachy- ______
28. brady- ______
29. eu- ______
30. auto- ______

B. What prefix means the same as:

1. per- ______
2. hemi- ______
3. contra- ______
4. pre- ______
5. con- ______
6. infra- ______
7. a-, an- ______
8. intra- ______
9. ex- ______
10. supra- ______
11. cata- ______
12. retro- ______

C. *Give the meaning of the following terms:*

1. dysplasia ____________________
2. transcostal ____________________
3. anomaly ____________________
4. exocrine ____________________
5. chondrodystrophy ____________________
6. antiseptic ____________________
7. intravenous ____________________
8. epicardium ____________________
9. bifurcation ____________________
10. diarrhea ____________________
11. amniocentesis ____________________
12. pseudocyesis ____________________
13. diagnosis ____________________
14. prognosis ____________________
15. prodrome ____________________

D. *Give the meanings of the following suffixes and combining forms:*

1. -stasis ____________________
2. -meter ____________________
3. -scopy ____________________
4. -tome ____________________
5. -rrhea ____________________
6. -blast ____________________
7. -oid ____________________
8. -emia ____________________
9. -dynia ____________________
10. -ectomy ____________________
11. -pnea ____________________
12. amni/o ____________________
13. peritone/o ____________________
14. gloss/o ____________________

15. glyc/o ____________________ 18. cost/o ____________________

16. lapar/o ____________________ 19. seps/o ____________________

17. tox/o ____________________ 20. nephr/o ____________________

E. *Give the meaning of the following terms. These may be difficult, but you can figure them out by using your knowledge of prefixes. Be sure to check your answers.*

1. euthanasia (hint: thanas = death) ____________________
2. agenesis ____________________
3. contraception ____________________
4. dysfunction ____________________
5. asymmetrical ____________________
6. perfusion ____________________
7. anti-inflammatory ____________________
8. deoxygenation ____________________
9. prolapse ____________________
10. semicomatose ____________________
11. antenatal ____________________
12. anaerobic (hint: aer = air) ____________________

ANSWERS

A.

1. against
2. before
3. beyond, change, between
4. under
5. with, together
6. middle
7. away from
8. surrounding
9. bad, painful, difficult
10. near, beside, abnormal
11. behind
12. through, complete
13. all
14. before
15. against, opposite
16. below
17. between
18. within
19. excessive
20. not, in
21. up
22. down
23. many
24. false
25. bad
26. beyond, excess
27. fast
28. slow
29. good
30. self

B.

1. dia-
2. semi-
3. anti-
4. ante-, pro-
5. syn-
6. sub-, hypo-
7. in- (when it means not)
8. endo-
9. ec-
10. hyper-, epi-
11. de-
12. post-, re-

C.

1. Bad formation—abnormal tissue development.
2. Across the ribs.
3. Without rule; structure which is unusual or irregular.
4. To separate out—glands which secrete substances **out** into ducts, e.g., tear, sweat, mammary.
5. Poor, bad development of cartilage.
6. Against infection (**sis** becomes **tic** in the adjective form).
7. Pertaining to within a vein.
8. Above the heart.
9. Forking, branching into two.
10. Flow through—water flows through the large bowel instead of being reabsorbed into the body.
11. Surgical puncture of the amnion (the sac in which the embryo develops). This procedure is done to examine the cells of the embryo.
12. False pregnancy.
13. Complete knowledge about a patient's illness.
14. Probable course or outcome of a patient's disease.
15. Symptoms which appear before and signal the onset of a more severe disease.

D.

1. Stopping, controlling.
2. To measure.
3. Process of visual examination.
4. Instrument to cut.
5. Flow, discharge.
6. Embryonic, immature.
7. Resembling.
8. Blood condition.
9. Pain.
10. Removal, excision.
11. Breathing.
12. Amnion—sac in which the embryo develops.
13. Peritoneum—membrane around abdominal cavity.
14. Tongue.
15. Sugar.
16. Abdominal wall, abdomen.
17. Poison.
18. Rib.
19. Infection.
20. Kidney.

E.

1. Dying easily, quietly, and painlessly. The term is also used to refer to the willful ending of life in persons with incurable disease (mercy killing).
2. Failure of an organ or part to develop.
3. Against conception (the union of the egg and sperm and implantation of the embryo in the uterus).
4. Bad function—any abnormal or impaired function of an organ or part.
5. Pertaining to lack of symmetry of organs or parts on opposite sides of the body.
6. To pour through—for example, injecting blood or fluid into an artery to supply an organ or tissue with nutrients and oxygen.
7. Against inflammation.
8. Lack of oxygen.
9. To slide forward; to sag.
10. Half-conscious—a state of unconsciousness from which a patient may be aroused.
11. Before birth.
12. Without air (oxygen)—having the ability to grow in an oxygen-free environment.

VI. PRONUNCIATION OF TERMS

abductor	ăb-DŬK-tŏr
adductor	ă-DŬK-tŏr
adrenal	ă-DRĒ-năl
analysis	ă-NĂL-ĭ-sĭs
anoxia	ă-NŎK-sē-ă
ante cibum	ĂN-tē SĒ-bŭm
ante partum	ĂN-tē PĂR-tŭm
antibiotic	ăn-tĭ-bī-ŎT-ĭk
antibody	ĂN-tĭ-bŏd-ē

antigen	ĂN-tĭ-jĕn
antisepsis	ăn-tĭ-SĔP-sĭs
antitoxin	ăn-tĭ-TŎK-sĭn
apnea	ĂP-nē-ă or ăp-NĒ-ă
autogenous	ăw-TŎJ-ĕ-nŭs
bifurcation	bī-fŭr-KĀ-shŭn
bradycardia	brăd-ē-KĂR-dē-ă
congenital anomaly	kŏn-JĔN-ĭ-tăl ă-NŎM-ă-lē
contralateral	kŏn-tră-LĂT-ĕr-ăl
dehydration	dē-hī-DRĀ-shŭn
dialysis	dī-ĂL-ĭ-sĭs
diameter	dī-ĂM-ĕ-tĕr
diarrhea	dī-ă-RĒ-ă
dyspnea	DĬSP-nē-ă or dĭsp-NĒ-ă
ectoderm	ĔK-tō-dĕrm
ectopic pregnancy	ĕk-TŎP-ĭk PRĔG-năn-sē
epithelium	ĕp-ĭ-THĒ-lē-ŭm
euphoria	ū-FŎR-ē-ă
eupnea	ŪP-nē-ă or ūp-NĒ-ă
exophthalmia	ĕk-sŏf-THĂL-mē-ă
hemiglossectomy	hĕm-ē-glŏs-SĔK-tō-mē
hyperglycemia	hī-pĕr-glī-SĒ-mē-ă
hyperplasia	hī-pĕr-PLĀ-zē-ă
hypertrophy	hī-PĔR-trō-fē
hypodermic	hī-pō-DĔR-mĭk
hypoglycemia	hī-pō-glī-SĒ-mē-ă
infracardiac	ĭn-fră-KĂR-dē-ăk
insomniac	ĭn-SŎM-nē-ăk
intercostal	ĭn-tĕr-KŎS-tăl
intravenous	ĭn-tră-VĒ-nŭs
macrocephalic	măk-rŏ-sĕ-FĂL-ĭk

malaise	mă-LĂZ
mesoderm	MĔZ-ō-dĕrm
metamorphosis	mĕt-ă-MŎR-fŏ-sĭs
metastasis	mĕ-TĂS-tă-sĭs
pancytopenia	păn-sī-to-PĒ-nē-ă
paralysis	pă-RĂL-ĭ-sĭs
parathyroid	păr-ă-THĪ-royd
percutaneous	pĕr-kū-TĀ-nē-ŭs
periosteum	pĕr-ē-ŎS-tē-ŭm
polioencephalitis	pō-lē-ō-ĕn-sĕf-ă-LĪ-tĭs
poliomyelitis	pō-lē-ō-mī-ĕ-LĪ-tĭs
polymorphonuclear	pŏl-ē-mŏr-fō-NŪ-klē-ăr
polyneuritis	pŏl-ē-nū-RĪ-tĭs
post mortem	pōst MŎR-tĕm
postnatal	pōst-NĀ-tăl
prodrome	PRŌ-drōm
pseudocyesis	soo-dō-sī-Ē-sĭs
retrograde	RĔT-rō-grād
retroperitoneal	rĕt-rō-pĕr-ĭ-tō-NĒ-ăl
subcostal	sŭb-KŎS-tăl
suprarenal	sōō-pra-RĒ-nal
suprathoracic	sōō-pră-thō-RĂ-sĭk
symbiosis	sĭm-bē-Ō-sĭs
symphysis	SĬM-fĭ-sĭs
syndactylism	sĭn-DĂK-tĭ-lĭzm
syndrome	SĬN-drōm
synthesis	SĬN-thĕ-sĭs
tachypnea	tă-KĬP-nē-ă or tăk-ĭp-NĒ-ă
transfusion	trăns-FŪ-zhŭn
ultrasonography	ŭl-tră-sŏn-ŎG-ră-fē

REVIEW SHEET 4

Prefixes

a-, an-	________	in-	________
ab-	________	infra-	________
ad-	________	inter-	________
ana-	________	intra-	________
ante-	________	macro-	________
anti-	________	mal-	________
auto-	________	meso-	________
bi-	________	meta-	________
brady-	________	micro-	________
cata-	________	pan-	________
con-	________	para-	________
contra-	________	per-	________
de-	________	peri-	________
dia-	________	polio-	________
dys-	________	poly-	________
ec-, ecto-	________	post-	________
epi-	________	pre-	________
eu-	________	pro-	________
ex-	________	pseudo-	________
hemi-	________	re-	________
hyper-	________	retro-	________
hypo-	________	semi-	________

sub-	______	tachy-	______
supra-	______	trans-	______
syn-, sym-	______	ultra-	______

Combining Forms

amni/o	______	norm/o	______
cib/o	______	ophthalm/o	______
cis/o	______	ox/o	______
cost/o	______	ren/o	______
duct/o	______	secti/o	______
furc/o	______	seps/o	______
gloss/o	______	somn/o	______
glyc/o	______	son/o	______
hepat/o	______	the/o	______
later/o	______	thyr/o	______
morph/o	______	tom/o	______
mort/o	______	top/o	______
nat/i	______	tox/o	______
necr/o	______	ven/o	______
nect/o	______		

Suffixes

-blast	______	-fusion	______
-crine	______	-grade	______
-cyesis	______	-lysis	______
-drome	______	-meter	______

-partum	__________	-pnea	__________
-plasia	__________	-rrhea	__________
-phoria	__________	-stasis	__________
-physis	__________	-trophy	__________

CHAPTER 5

DIGESTIVE SYSTEM

In this chapter you will:

- Name the organs of the digestive system and describe their locations and functions;
- Describe some disease processes which affect these organs; and
- Define combining forms for organs and the meaning of related terminology using these word parts.

The chapter is divided into the following sections:

I. INTRODUCTION

The digestive system, also called the **alimentary** or **gastrointestinal tract**, begins with the mouth, where food enters the body, and ends with the anus, where solid waste material leaves the body. The primary functions of the organs of the digestive system are threefold.

First, complex food material which is taken into the mouth must be **digested**, or broken down, mechanically and chemically, as it travels through the gastrointestinal tract (passageway). Digestive **enzymes** are substances that speed up chemical reactions and help in the breakdown (digestion) of complex nutrients. Complex proteins are digested to simpler **amino acids**; complicated sugars are reduced to simple sugars, such as **glucose;** and large fat molecules are broken down to **fatty acids** and **triglycerides.**

Second, the digested food must be **absorbed** into the bloodstream by passing through the walls of the small intestine. In this way, valuable nutrients, such as sugar and amino acids, can travel to all the cells of the body. Within the cells, nutrients are catabolized (burned) in the presence of oxygen to release energy stored within the food. Amino acid nutrients are used to anabolize (build) large protein molecules which are needed for growth and development of cells. Fatty acids and triglycerides are also absorbed through the walls of the small intestine but enter lymphatic vessels rather than blood vessels. These digested fats eventually enter the bloodstream as lymph vessels join with blood vessels in the upper chest region.

The third function of the digestive system is to **eliminate** the solid waste materials that cannot be absorbed into the bloodstream. These solid wastes, called **feces**, are concentrated in the large intestine and finally pass out of the body through the anus.

II. ANATOMY OF THE DIGESTIVE SYSTEM

Oral Cavity

The alimentary tract begins with the oral cavity, or mouth. Label Figure 5-1 as you learn the major parts of the oral cavity.

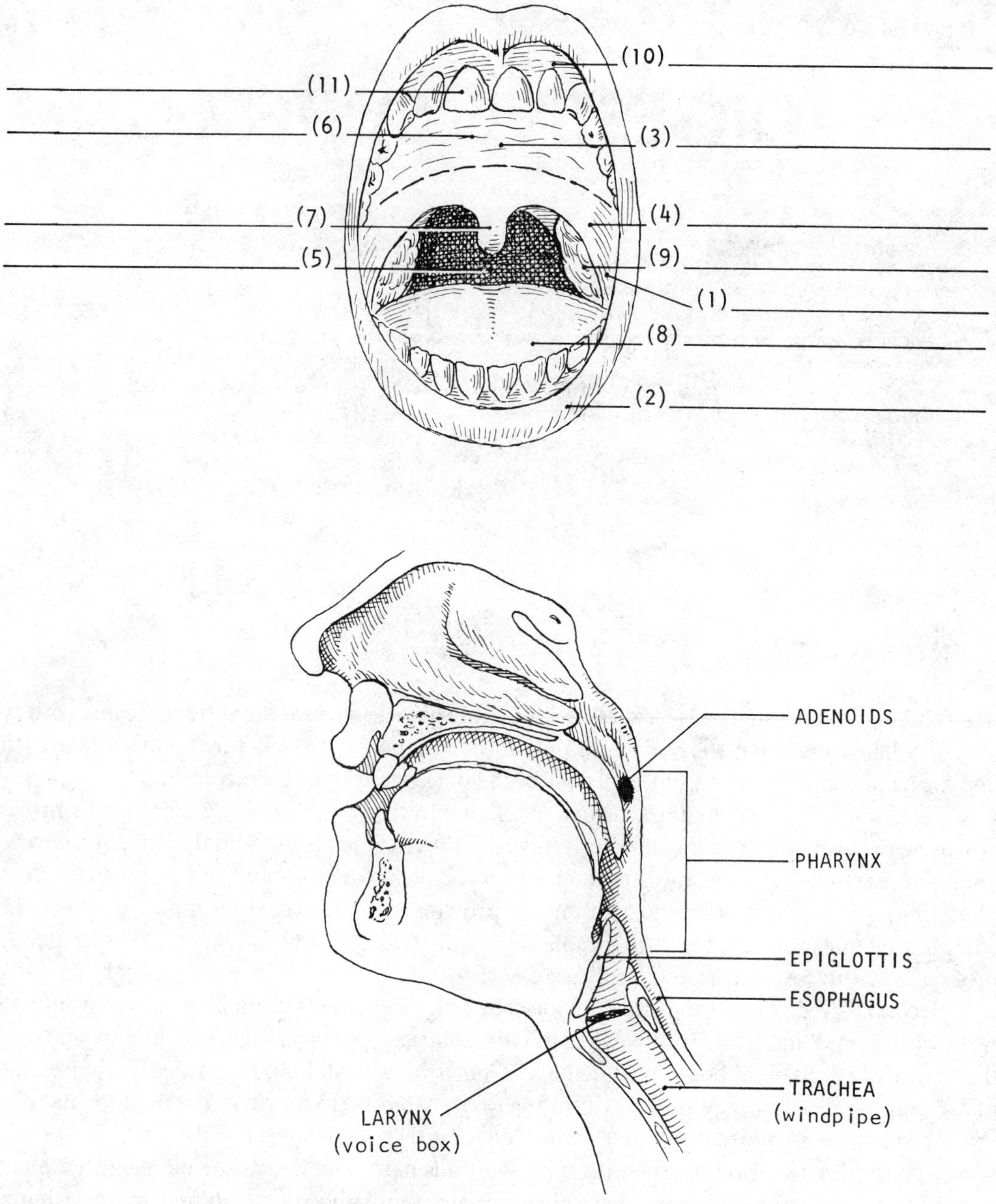

Figure 5-1 Oral cavity and throat.

The **cheeks** (1) form the walls of the oval-shaped oral cavity, and the **lips** (2) form the opening to the cavity.

The **hard palate** (3) forms the anterior portion of the roof of the mouth, while the muscular **soft palate** (4) lies posterior to it and separates the mouth from the **pharynx** (throat) (5). **Rugae** (6) are the irregular ridges in the mucous membrane covering the anterior portion of the hard palate. Hanging from the soft palate is a small, soft tissue called the **uvula** (7). The word uvula means "little grape." The structure functions to aid in producing sounds and speech.

The **tongue** (8) extends across the floor of the oral cavity and is attached by muscles to the

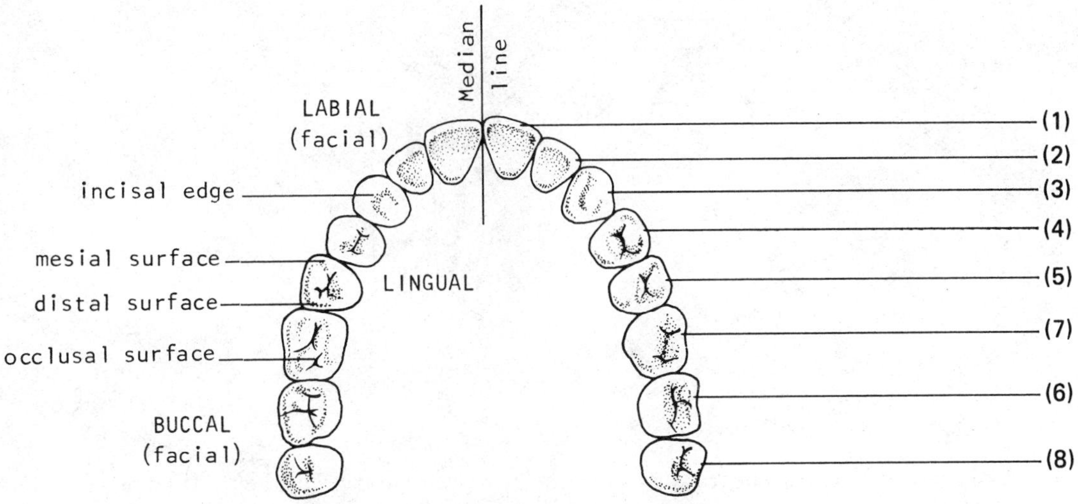

Figure 5-2 Permanent teeth within the dental arch.

lower jaw bone. It moves food around during **mastication** (chewing) and **deglutition** (swallowing). The tongue is covered with a series of small projections called **papillae** which contain cells, called taste buds, that are sensitive to the chemical nature of foods.

The **tonsils** (9) are masses of lymphatic tissue located in depressions of the mucous membranes in the walls of the pharynx. They act as filters to protect the body from the invasion of microorganisms and produce lymphocytes, which are white blood cells able to fight disease.

The **gums** (10) are made of fleshy tissue and surround the sockets in which the **teeth** (11) are found. Figure 5-2 shows a dental arch with 16 permanent teeth (there are 32 permanent teeth in the entire oral cavity). Label the figure with the following names of teeth:

(1) central incisor
(2) lateral incisor
(3) cuspid or canine
(4) first bicuspid
(5) second bicuspid
(6) first molar
(7) second molar
(8) third molar, or wisdom tooth

Dentists use special terms to describe the surfaces of teeth. These are indicated on the left side of Figure 5-2. The surface lying nearest the lips, for incisors and canines, is called the **labial** surface (labi/o means lip). The corresponding surface on bicuspids and molars is called the **buccal** surface (bucc/o means cheek). Some dentists refer to both the labial and buccal surfaces as the **facial** surface (faci/o means face). Opposite to the facial surface, all teeth have a **lingual** surface (lingu/o means tongue). The **mesial** surface of a tooth lies nearest to the median line and the **distal** surface is farthest from the median line. Bicuspids and molars have an additional **occlusal** surface (occlusion means to close) which comes in contact with a corresponding tooth in the opposing arch. A sharp **incisal** edge is found on incisors and cuspids.

Figure 5-3 shows the inner anatomy of a tooth. Label it as you read the following description:

A tooth consists of a **crown** (1), which is above the gum, and a **root** (2), which is embedded in the bony tooth socket. The outermost protective layer of the crown is called the **enamel** (3). Enamel is a dense, hard, white substance—the hardest substance in the body. Underneath the enamel is a layer which extends throughout the crown and is the main bulk of the tooth. It is called the **dentin** (4). Dentin is a yellowish color and is composed of bony tissue which is softer than enamel. The dentin in the root is covered by a protective and supportive layer called **cementum** (5).

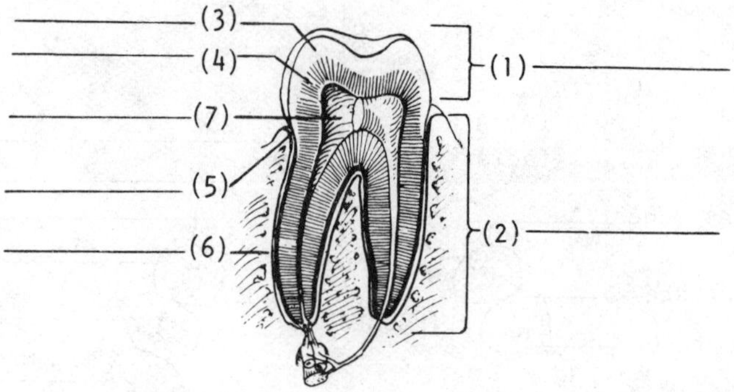

Figure 5-3 Anatomy of a tooth.

A **periodontal membrane** (6) surrounds the cementum and holds the tooth in place in the tooth socket.

Underneath the dentin is a soft, delicate layer in the center of the tooth; this is called the **pulp** (7). Within the pulp canal (also called the **root canal**) are blood vessels, nerve endings, connective tissue, and lymph vessels. When there is disease or abscess (pus collection) in the pulp, root canal therapy may be advised. The tooth is opened from above and the root canals are cleaned of nerves, blood vessels, and debris. The pulp is then disinfected and filled with a material to prevent entrance of microorganisms and decay.

Around the oral cavity are three pairs of **salivary glands** (see Figure 5-4). These exocrine glands produce a fluid called **saliva** which contains important digestive **enzymes**. Saliva is released

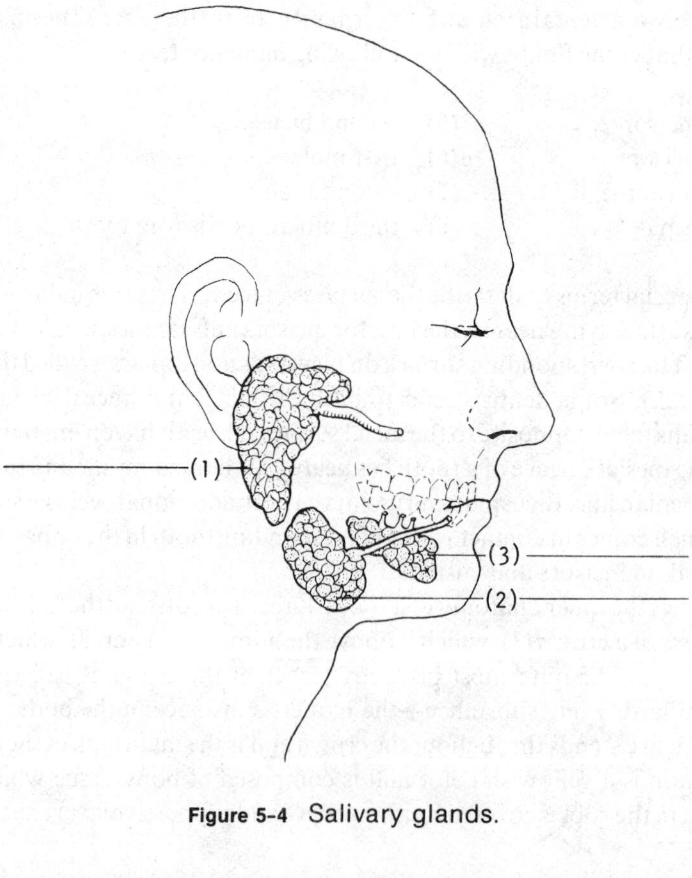

Figure 5-4 Salivary glands.

from the **parotid** gland (1), **submaxillary** (also called submandibular) gland (2), and **sublingual** gland (3) on each side of the mouth. Narrow ducts carry the saliva into the oral cavity.

Figure 5-5 traces the passage of food through the alimentary tract after it leaves the mouth. Label the figure as you read the following descriptions of organs.

Pharynx

Food passes from the mouth to the **pharynx** (throat) (1). The pharynx is a muscular tube lined with a mucous membrane. It serves as a common passageway for air from the nasal cavity to the larynx (voice box), as well as for food going from the mouth to the **esophagus** (2). A flap of tissue called the epiglottis covers the opening to the larynx and prevents food from entering the windpipe (trachea) when deglutition (swallowing) occurs (see the lower portion of Figure 5-1).

Esophagus

The esophagus is a 9- to 10-inch muscular tube extending from the pharynx to the stomach. It aids in swallowing and moves the food along. **Peristalsis** is the name of the involuntary,

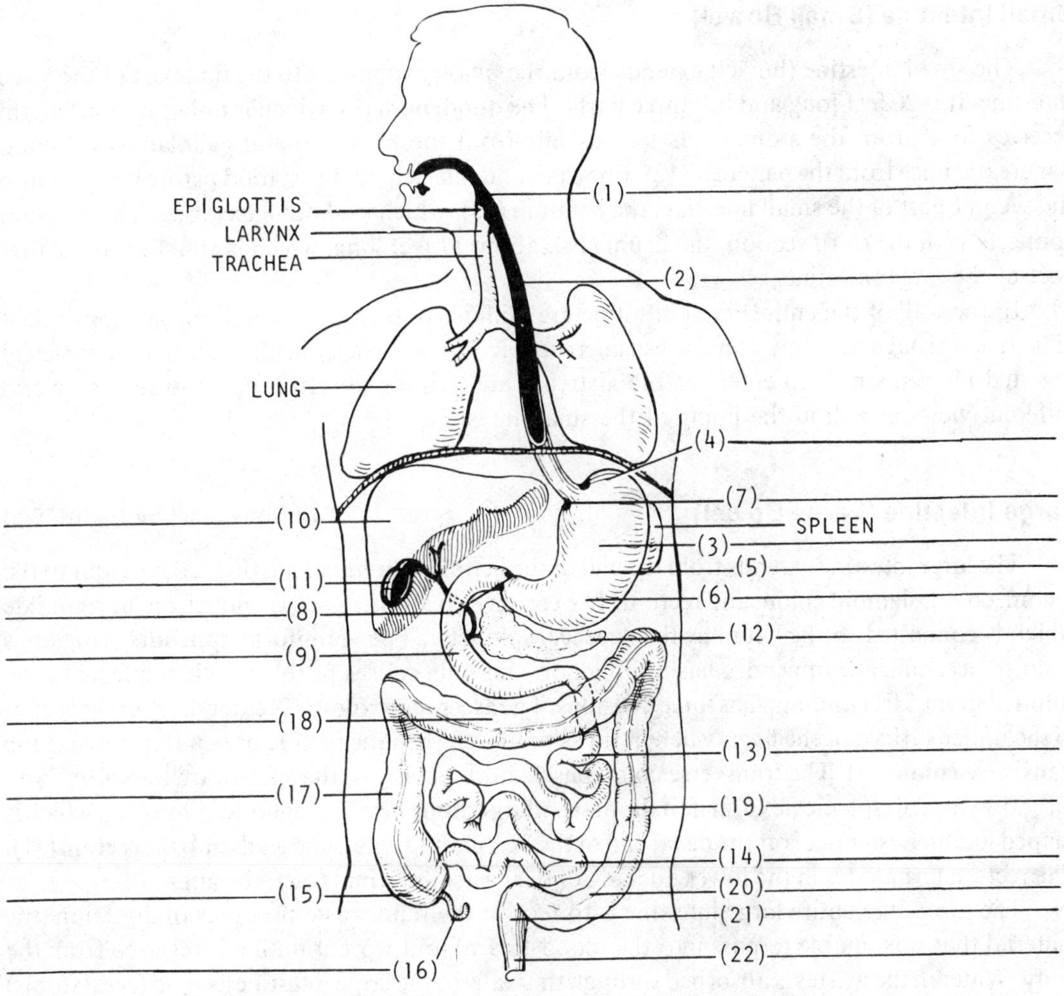

Figure 5-5 The digestive system.

progressive, wavelike contraction of the esophagus (and other gastrointestinal tubes) that propels the food through the system.

Stomach

Food passes from the esophagus to the **stomach** (3). The stomach is composed of a **fundus** (4), **body** (5), and **antrum** (6). The openings into and from the stomach are controlled by rings of muscles called **sphincters**. The **cardiac sphincter** (7) relaxes and contracts to move food from the esophagus into the stomach, while the **pyloric sphincter** (8) allows food to leave the stomach when it has been sufficiently digested. **Rugae** are the folds in the mucous membrane (**mucosa**) lining the stomach. Digestive glands, producing enzymes and hydrochloric acid, are located within these folds.

The role of the stomach is to prepare the food chemically and mechanically so that it can be received in the small intestine for further digestion and absorption into the bloodstream. Food does not enter the bloodstream through the walls of the stomach. The stomach controls the passing of foods into the first part of the small intestine so that it proceeds only when it is chemically ready and in small amounts.

Small Intestine (Small Bowel)

The small intestine (bowel) extends from the pyloric sphincter to the first part of the large intestine. It is 20 feet long and has three parts. The **duodenum** (9), which is only 1 foot in length, receives food from the stomach as well as **bile** from the **liver** (10) and **gallbladder** (11) and pancreatic juice from the **pancreas** (12). Enzymes and bile help to digest food before it passes into the second part of the small intestine, the **jejunum** (13), which is about 8 feet long. The jejunum connects with the third section, the **ileum** (14), about 11 feet long, which is attached to the first part of the large intestine.

In the wall of the entire small intestine are millions of tiny, microscopic projections called **villi**. It is through the tiny capillaries (microscopic blood vessels) in the villi that completely digested nutrients pass to enter the bloodstream and lymph vessels. Figure 5-6 shows several different views of villi in the lining of the small intestine.

Large Intestine (Large Bowel)

(Continue labeling Figure 5-5)

The large intestine extends from the end of the ileum to the anus. It is divided into four parts: cecum, colon, sigmoid colon, and rectum. The **cecum** (15), or first part, is a pouch on the right side which is connected to the ileum by the ileocecal sphincter. The **vermiform appendix** (16) hangs from the cecum. The appendix has no function and only causes problems when infected. The **colon** is about 5 feet long and has three divisions. The **ascending colon** (17) extends from the cecum to the under surface of the liver, where it turns to the left (hepatic flexure or bend) to become the **transverse colon** (18). The transverse colon passes horizontally to the left toward the spleen, and turns downward (splenic flexure) into the **descending colon** (19). The **sigmoid colon** (20), which is shaped like an S (sigma), is at the distal end of the descending colon and leads into the **rectum** (21). The rectum terminates in the lower opening of the gastrointestinal tract, the **anus** (22).

The job of the entire large intestine is to receive the fluid waste products of digestion (the material that was unable to pass into the bloodstream) and store it until it is released from the body. Water in the wastes is absorbed through the walls of the large intestine as solid **feces** (stools) are formed.

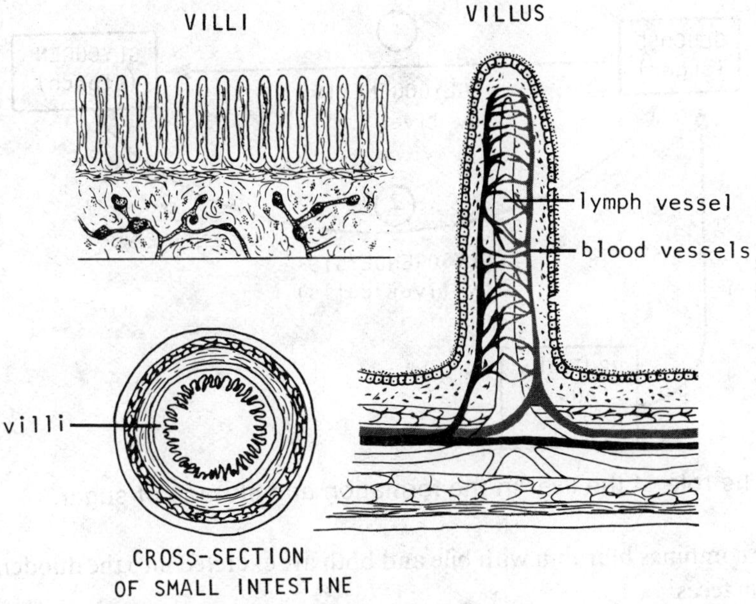

Figure 5-6 Villi in the lining of the small intestine.

Liver, Gallbladder, and Pancreas

Three important additional organs of the digestive system are the liver, gallbladder, and pancreas. Although food does not pass through these organs, each plays a crucial role in the proper digestion and absorption of nutrients. Label Figure 5-7 as you study the following:

The **liver** (1), located in the right upper quadrant (RUQ) of the abdomen, manufactures a thick, yellowish brown, sometimes greenish, fluid called **bile**. Bile contains cholesterol (a fatty substance), bile acids, and several bile pigments. One of these pigments is called **bilirubin**. Bilirubin is a waste product of hemoglobin destruction (which occurs in the liver as red blood cells

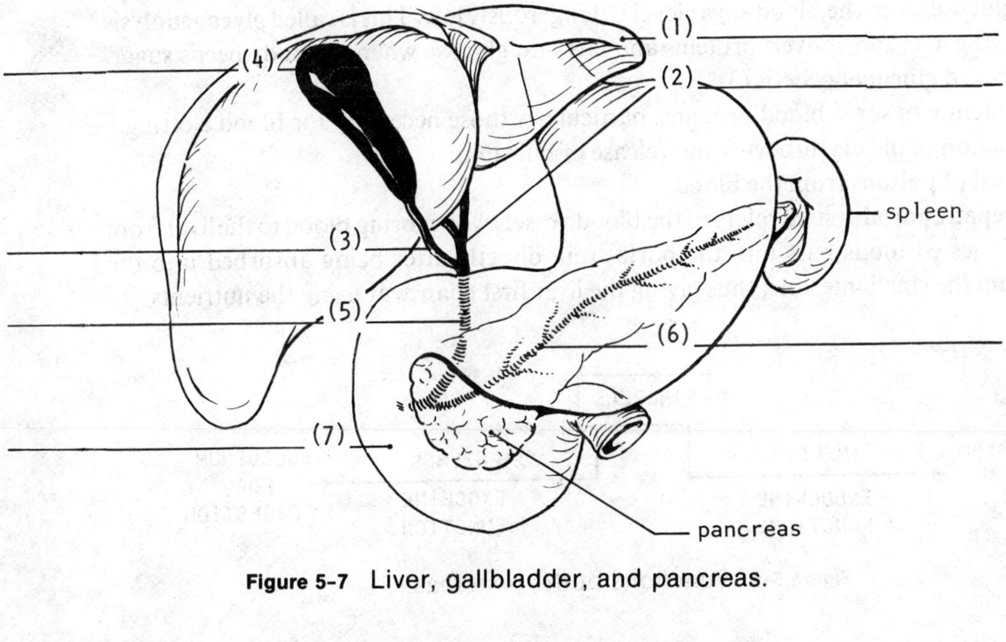

Figure 5-7 Liver, gallbladder, and pancreas.

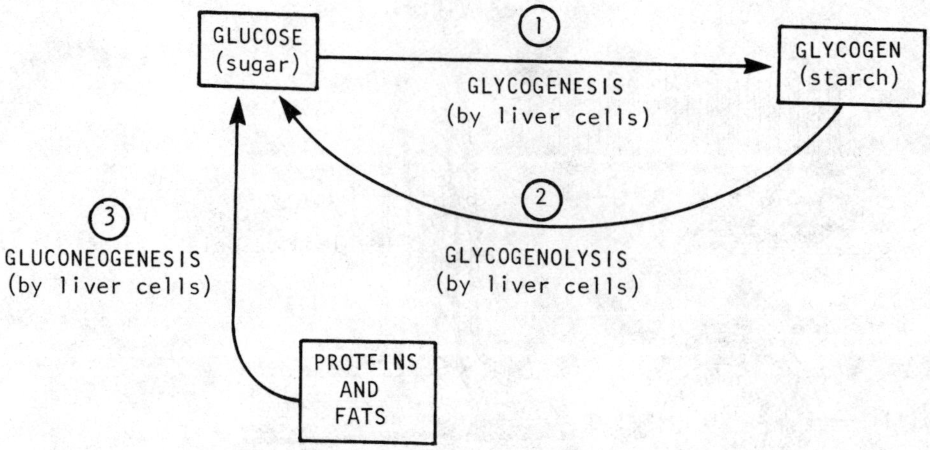

Figure 5-8 The role of the liver in the formation and storage of sugar.

are destroyed). The liver combines bilirubin with bile and both are excreted into the duodenum, finally leaving the body in feces.

Bile is continuously released from the liver and travels down the **hepatic duct** (2) to the **cystic duct** (3). The cystic duct leads to the **gallbladder** (4), a pear-shaped sac under the liver, which stores and concentrates the bile for later use. After meals, in response to the presence of foods in the stomach and duodenum, the gallbladder contracts, forcing the bile out the cystic duct into the **common bile duct** (5), which joins with the **pancreatic duct** (6) just before the entrance to the **duodenum** (7). The duodenum thus receives a mixture of bile and pancreatic juices.

Bile has a detergent-like effect on fats in the duodenum. It breaks apart large fat globules so that enzymes from the pancreas can digest the fats. This action is called **emulsification**. Without bile, most of the fat taken into the body would remain undigested.

The liver, besides producing bile, has several other vital and important functions. Some of these are:

1. Keeping the amount of **glucose** (sugar) in the blood at a normal level (see Figure 5–8). The liver removes excess glucose from the bloodstream and stores it as **glycogen** (starch) in liver cells. This is called **glycogenesis** (1). The liver can also reverse the process and convert the glycogen in storage into glucose when the blood sugar level is dangerously low. This is called **glycogenolysis** (2). In addition, the liver can convert proteins and fats into glucose when the body needs sugar. This process is called **gluconeogenesis** (3).
2. Manufacture of some blood proteins, particularly those necessary for blood clotting.
3. Destruction of old erythrocytes and release of bilirubin.
4. Removal of poisons from the blood.

The term **hepatic portal system** refers to the blood vessels which bring blood to the liver from the intestines. Digested foods pass into the portal vein directly after being absorbed into the bloodstream from the small intestine, thus giving the liver first chance at using the nutrients.

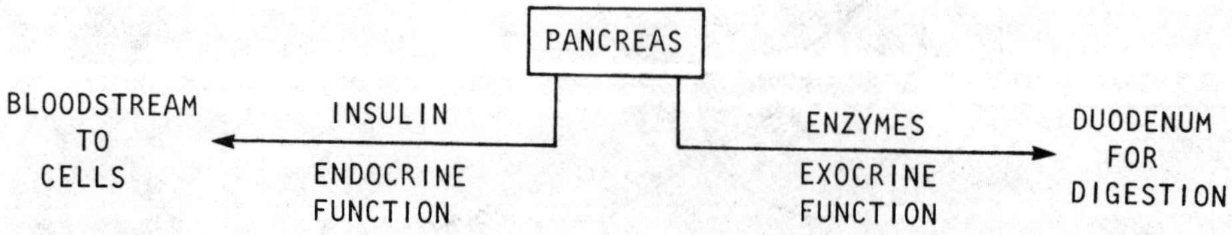

Figure 5-9 Functions of the pancreas.

The **pancreas** is both an exocrine and endocrine organ. As an exocrine gland (secreting into a tube leading outward), it produces pancreatic juices filled with enzymes (**amylase** and **lipase**) to digest food. These pass into the duodenum through the pancreatic duct.

As an endocrine gland (secreting into the bloodstream), the pancreas secretes **insulin**. This hormone is needed to help release sugar from the blood to be used by the cells of the body. Figure 5–9 reviews these functions of the pancreas.

Figure 5–10 is a flow chart following the pathway of food throughout the gastrointestinal tract.

III. VOCABULARY

This list will help you review many of the new terms introduced in the text. Short definitions will reinforce your understanding of the terms. See the list at the end of the chapter for help in pronouncing the more difficult terms.

absorption Passage of materials into the bloodstream.

alimentary tract The digestive system; aliment means food.

amino acids Small substances which make up proteins and are produced when proteins are digested.

amylase Enzyme (-ase = enzyme) from the pancreas to digest starch (amyl = starch).

antrum Lower part of the stomach.

anus Lower opening of the digestive tract.

bicuspid teeth Two premolar teeth distal to the cuspid (canine) on each side of a dental arch; bi = two, cusp = point.

bile Digestive juice made in the liver and stored in the gallbladder.

bilirubin Pigment released by the liver in bile; produced from the destruction of hemoglobin.

bowel Intestine.

canine Cuspid; canine means doglike.

cecum First part of the large intestine.

cementum Bonelike supportive tissue that surrounds the dentin in the root of a tooth.

colon Large intestine; ascending, transverse, and descending parts.

common bile duct Carries bile from the liver and gallbladder to the duodenum.

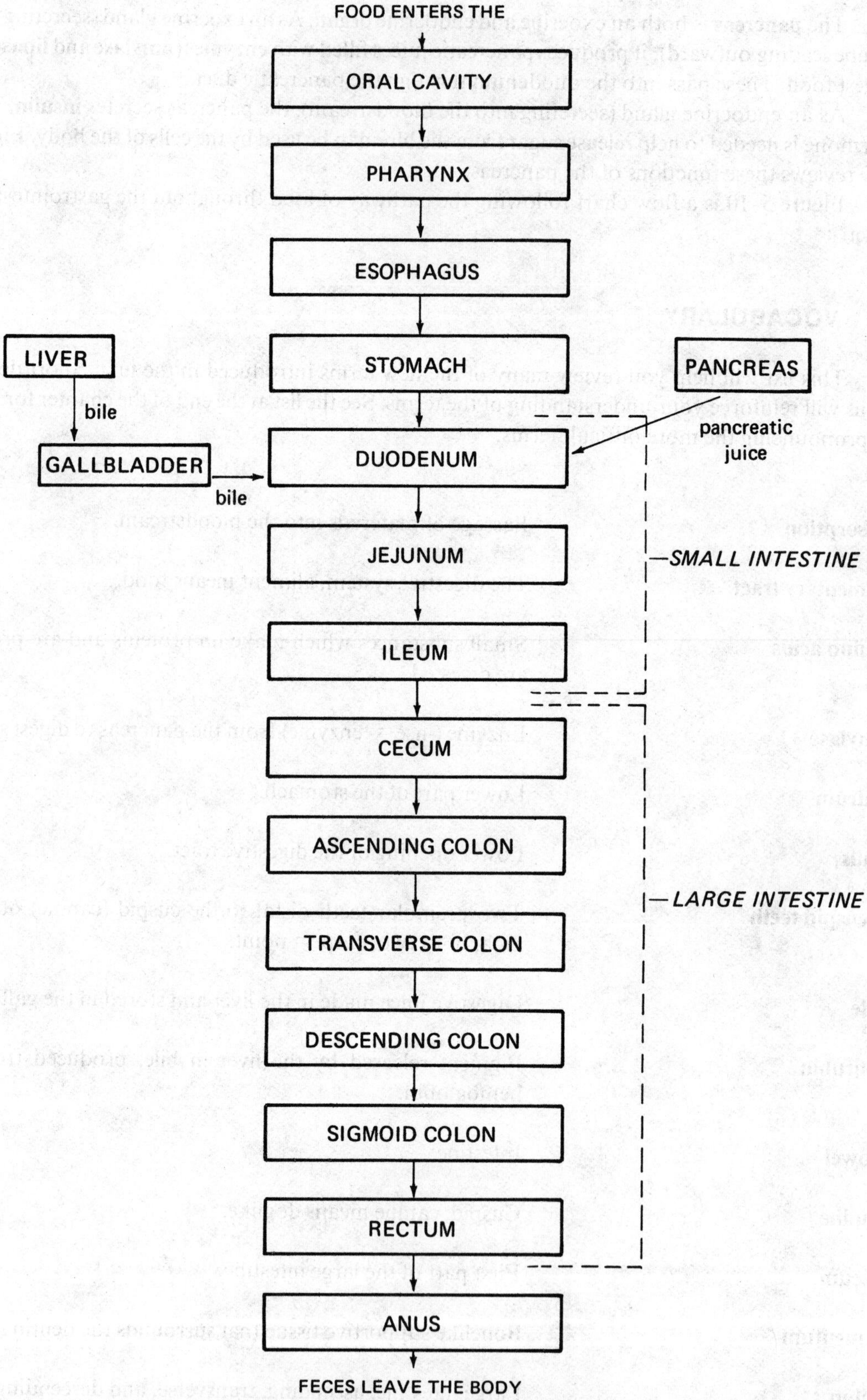

Figure 5-10 Pathway of food through the digestive tract.

cuspid	Canine tooth; the cuspids of the upper jaw are called eyeteeth.
deglutition	Swallowing.
dentin	Major tissue composing teeth, covered by enamel in the crown and by cementum in the root.
digestion	Breakdown of complex foods to simpler forms.
duodenum	First part of the small intestine. Duo = 2, den = 10; the duodenum measures 12 inches in length.
emulsification	Breaking up of large fat molecules.
enamel	Hard, outermost layer of a tooth.
enzyme	A chemical that speeds up a reaction between substances. Digestive enzymes help in the breakdown of complex foods to simpler foods.
esophagus	Tube connecting the mouth to the stomach.
etiology	Study of the cause of disease.
fatty acids	Substances produced when fats are digested.
feces	Solid wastes; stools.
fundus	Upper, rounded part of the stomach.
gallbladder	Small sac under the liver; stores bile.
glucose	Simple sugar.
glycogen	Animal starch; glucose is stored as glycogen.
hepatic portal system	The capillary networks of the intestines and liver which are connected via the portal vein. The portal vein brings nutrient-rich blood to the liver from the intestines.
hydrochloric acid	Substance produced by the stomach; necessary for digestion of food.
ileum	Third part of the small intestine.
incisor	One of four front teeth in the dental arch.
insulin	Hormone produced by the pancreas.
jejunum	Second part of the small intestine. The Latin *jejunus* means empty; this part of the intestine was always empty when a body was examined after death.

lipase	Pancreatic enzyme necessary to digest fats.
mastication	Chewing.
palate	Roof of the mouth.
pancreas	Organ under the stomach; produces insulin (for transport of sugar into cells) and enzymes (for digestion of foods).
papillae	Small elevations on the tongue.
parotid gland	Salivary gland near the ear.
peristalsis	Wavelike contractions of the tubes of the alimentary tract.
pharynx	Throat.
pulp	Soft tissue within a tooth.
pylorus	Area of the pyloric sphincter; distal region of the stomach.
rectum	End of the colon.
rugae	Ridges on the hard palate and wall of the stomach.
saliva	Digestive juice produced by salivary glands.
salivary glands	Parotid, sublingual, and submaxillary (submandibular) glands.
sigmoid colon	Lower part of the colon; shaped like an S.
sphincter	Ring of muscles.
triglycerides	Products of fat digestion.
uvula	Soft tissue hanging from the soft palate.
vermiform appendix	Blind pouch hanging from the cecum.
villus; villi	Tiny microscopic projections in the walls of the small intestine to absorb nutrients into the bloodstream.

IV. COMBINING FORMS AND RELATED TERMINOLOGY

Help with pronunciation of this terminology can be found in the pronunciation list at the end of the chapter.

Combining Form	*Structure or Substance*	*Terminology*	*Meaning*
or/o stomat/o	mouth	oral	
		stomatitis	
bucc/o	cheek	buccal mucosa	
labi/o cheil/o	lip	labial	
		cheilosis	
dent/i odont/o	tooth	dentibuccal	
		periodontist	
		endodontist *Does root canal therapy.*	
		orthodontist *Orth/o means straight.*	
gingiv/o	gum	gingivitis	
lingu/o gloss/o	tongue	lingual	
		glossotomy	
palat/o	palate	palatoplasty	
uvul/o	uvula	uvulectomy	
tonsill/o	tonsil	tonsillectomy	
sial/o	saliva	sialolithiasis *-iasis means abnormal condition and is commonly used with lith/o.*	
sialaden/o	salivary gland	sialadenitis	

submaxill/o	lower jaw	submaxillary ______
		maxill/o = upper jaw
pharyng/o	throat	pharyngeal ______
		Note that the final g is softened by adding an e between the suffix -al and the root.
esophag/o	esophagus	esophagogastric ______
		______
		esophageal ______
gastr/o	stomach	gastralgia ______
celi/o	belly, abdomen	celiac ______
enter/o	small intestine	parenteral ______
		Par- (from para) means opposite or other than in this term. Parenteral injection of material can be intravenous, subcutaneous, or intramuscular.
		mesentery ______
		The mesentery is a membrane which, like a fan, holds together and connects the small intestine to the dorsal body wall. See Figure 5–11. The mesentery is a part of the peritoneum. The peritoneum (peri = surrounding, tone/o = stretch) stretches around the abdominal viscera and lines the abdominal cavity.
		enterostomy ______
		enteric anastomosis ______
		______
		An anastomosis is a new surgical connection between segments of an organ. An enteroenterostomy is the same procedure as an enteric anastomosis. See Figure 5–11.
duoden/o	duodenum	duodenal ______
jejun/o	jejunum	jejunostomy ______
		______
ile/o	ileum	ileitis ______

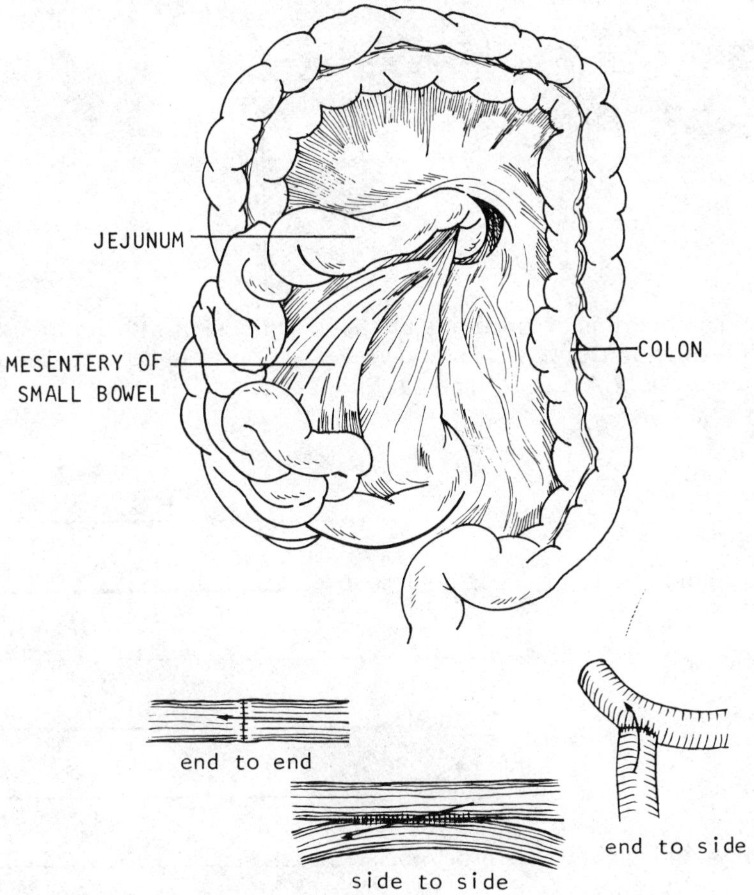

Figure 5-11 Mesentery and three types of anastomoses.

cec/o	cecum	ileocecal sphincter ______________________ ______________________
append/o appendic/o	appendix	appendicitis ______________________ appendectomy ______________________
col/o colon/o	colon	colostomy ______________________ *-stomy, when used with only one combining form, means an opening to the outside of the body. (See Figure 5–12.* colocolostomy ______________________ ______________________ *An anastomosis of one part of the colon to another section of the colon.*

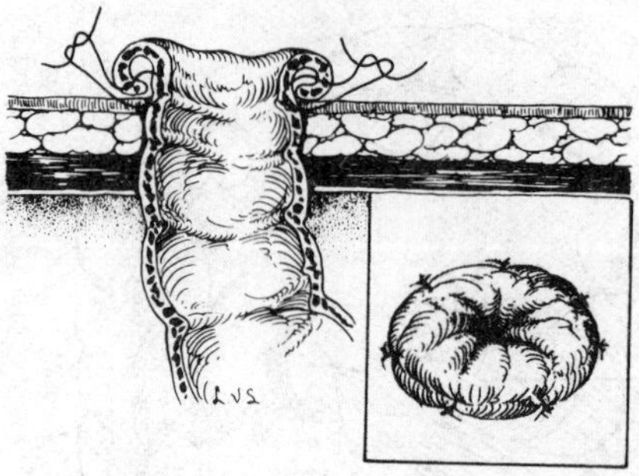

Figure 5-12 Colostomy. The margins of the stoma are fixed to the skin with sutures. (From Schrock, T.R.: Large intestine. In Dunphy, J.E., and Way, L.W.: Current Surgical Diagnosis & Treatment. 5th ed. Los Altos, CA, Lange Medical Publications, 1981.)

		colonic
sigmoid/o	sigmoid colon	sigmoidoscopy
rect/o	rectum	rectocele
an/o	anus	anorectal
proct/o	anus and rectum	proctologist
hepat/o	liver	hepatocholangioduodenostomy
chol/e bil/i	gall, bile	cholelithiasis
		biliary
		The biliary tract includes the organs (liver and gallbladder) and ducts (hepatic, cystic, and common bile) that secrete, store, and empty bile into the duodenum.
cholecyst/o	gallbladder	cholecystectomy
choledoch/o	common bile duct	choledochotomy
bilirubin/o	bilirubin	hyperbilirubinemia

pancreat/o	pancreas	pancreatitis ________________
peritone/o	peritoneum	peritoneoscopy ________________
		________________
pylor/o	pylorus, pyloric sphincter	pyloroplasty ________________
		________________
splen/o	spleen	splenomegaly ________________
amyl/o	starch	amylase ________________
gluc/o glyc/o	sugar, glucose	gluconeogenesis ________________ *Sugar is formed by liver cells from fats and proteins.*
		hyperglycemia ________________
		________________
glycogen/o	glycogen, animal starch	glycogenesis ________________
		glycogenolysis ________________
		________________
lip/o steat/o	fat, lipids	lipolysis ________________
		steatorrhea ________________ *Fats are improperly digested and appear in the feces.*
-ase	enzyme	lipase ________________
-iasis	abnormal condition	choledocholithiasis ________________
		________________
-prandial	meal	postprandial ________________

V. PATHOLOGY OF THE DIGESTIVE SYSTEM

Pronunciation of these terms can be found in the pronunciation list at the end of the chapter.

anorexia Lack of appetite.

oral leukoplakia — White plaques or patches (-plakia means plaques) on the mucosa of the mouth. This is a precancerous lesion which may lead to a malignant lesion.

dental caries — Cavities in teeth; caries means decay.

aphthous stomatitis — Inflammation of the mouth associated with small ulcers. This condition, the cause of which is unclear, is also called **canker sores**.

herpetic gingivostomatitis — Inflammation of the mouth and gums by infection with the herpes virus. This condition is also called **cold sores** or **fever blisters**.

periodontal disease — Inflammation and degeneration of gums, teeth, and surrounding bone; also known as **pyorrhea** (py/o means pus). Gingivectomy may be necessary to remove pockets of pus in gums and allow new tissue to form.

cleft palate — Congenital split in the roof of the mouth; lip may be affected as well.

regurgitation — Return of solids and fluids to the mouth from the stomach.

Heartburn is a burning sensation caused by reflux (flowing back) of acid from the stomach into the esophagus.

achlorhydria — Lack of hydrochloric acid in the stomach. This condition may be produced by chronic gastritis or carcinoma of the stomach.

cirrhosis — Chronic disease of the liver with degeneration of liver cells.

Alcoholism combined with nutritional deficiency is a common **etiological** (eti/o means cause) factor, but infection and poisons are factors as well. Hepatomegaly occurs first, but eventually the liver becomes smaller as hepatocytes die and scar tissue forms. The root cirrh means orange-yellow and refers to the jaundiced discoloration of the patient's skin as the liver malfunctions and bilirubin is not eliminated from the body.

hepatitis — Inflammation of the liver caused by virus or damage to the liver from toxic substances.

There are 3 types of viral hepatitis: **Hepatitis A** (caused by type A virus and formerly called infectious hepatitis) is spread through water and food, and the virus is excreted in feces. **Hepatitis B** (caused by type B virus and formerly called serum hepatitis) is acquired from transfusions and via body fluids such as tears, saliva, and semen. There is now a vaccine that provides immunity to type B hepatitis and is recommended for hospital personnel, dentists, laboratory technicians, and persons requiring frequent transfusions. **Non-A, non-B hepatitis** is not caused by the A or the B type virus. This disease is like type B hepatitis and can be transmitted by blood transfusion. In both non-A, non-B and chronic hepatitis B, liver enzymes may be elevated in the blood indicating damage to liver tissue. Symptoms include malaise (tiredness and bodily discomfort), joint pain, and in severe cases, nausea, anorexia, and jaundice.

jaundice

Yellow-orange coloration of the skin and other tissues.

Jaundice, also called **icterus**, results from excessive accumulation of bilirubin in the bloodstream and can occur in three major ways: (1) Obstruction of bile passageways prevents bilirubin from leaving the body in bile (i.e., cholelithiasis). (2) Malfunction of liver cells, as in cirrhosis, hepatitis, or hepatic carcinoma, impairs the liver's ability to combine bilirubin with bile. Bilirubin thus remains in the bloodstream. (3) Excessive destruction of erythrocytes, as in erythroblastosis fetalis and other anemias, creates abnormally high levels of bilirubin in blood.

esophageal varices

Swollen, twisted veins around the distal end of the esophagus.

Increased blood pressure in the hepatic portal system (from cirrhosis, for example, which causes damage to vessels in the liver) can lead to enlarged, twisted esophageal veins with danger of hemorrhage (bleeding).

ulcer

Sore or lesion (wound) of mucous membranes or skin.

Gastric and duodenal ulcers are examples. They occur when acid and juices from the stomach digest damaged mucous membranes. Treatment includes drugs to weaken the effect of hydrochloric acid, vagotomy (cutting the vagus nerve, which stimulates acid secretion in the stomach), and pyloroplasty to increase the size of the duodenal orifice (opening).

ulcerative colitis

Chronic inflammation of the colon with presence of ulcers.

Nervous tension and anxiety may be etiological factors. Ileostomy may be needed in severe cases to drain the intestinal contents to the outside of the body.

Crohn's disease

Inflammation of the intestinal tract, commonly of the terminal (end) portion of the ileum.

Crohn's disease (named for gastroenterologist Burrill Crohn) is a chronic relapsing inflammation with diarrhea, abdominal cramping, and fever. It is similar to ulcerative colitis and both are considered types of **inflammatory bowel diseases** (IBD). Crohn's disease, believed to be caused by a virus or autoimmunity (antibodies attack the body's own cells), is treated with drugs (anti-inflammatory steroids) to promote healing of lesions. Surgical removal of the diseased portion, with anastomosis of the remaining intestinal parts, may be needed.

dysentery

Painful, inflamed intestines.

The condition commonly occurs in the large intestine. Ingested food containing bacteria (shigellae) or amebae (one-celled organisms) can lead to colitis, diarrhea, and pain.

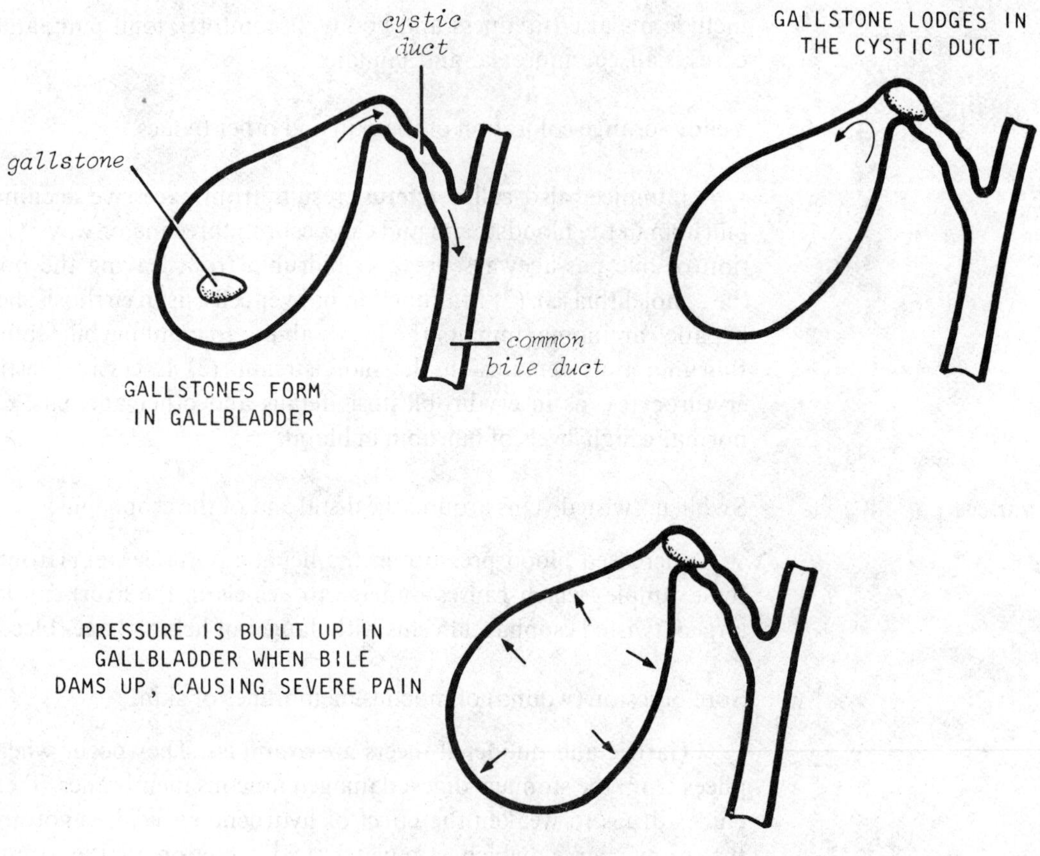

Figure 5–13 Gallstones.

gallstones

Hard collections of bile that form in the gallbladder and bile ducts.

Calculi can become lodged in the neck of the gallbladder or in the ducts leading to the duodenum. Pressure builds up in the gallbladder, pain is experienced, and infection may follow. Treatment is cholecystectomy or choledocholithotomy. Recent procedures use endoscopes to snare stones and remove them. In addition, a drug (chenodeoxycholic acid) is now administered orally to decrease cholesterol synthesis in the liver and also cause dissolution of existing gallstones. Figure 5–13 shows how gallstones can block the cystic duct and cause pain.

diverticula

Abnormal side pockets in a hollow structure such as the intestine.

Common sites are the sigmoid colon and duodenum. If inflammation (diverticulitis) occurs, diverticulectomy may be necessary as treatment. Figure 5–14 illustrates diverticula.

hernia

Protrusion of an organ or part through the wall of the cavity which contains it.

An **inguinal hernia** occurs when a small loop of bowel protrudes through a weak place in the lower abdominal wall or groin. A **hiatal hernia** is a protrusion of part of the stomach through the esophageal opening in the diaphragm. Figure 5–15 shows inguinal and hiatal hernias.

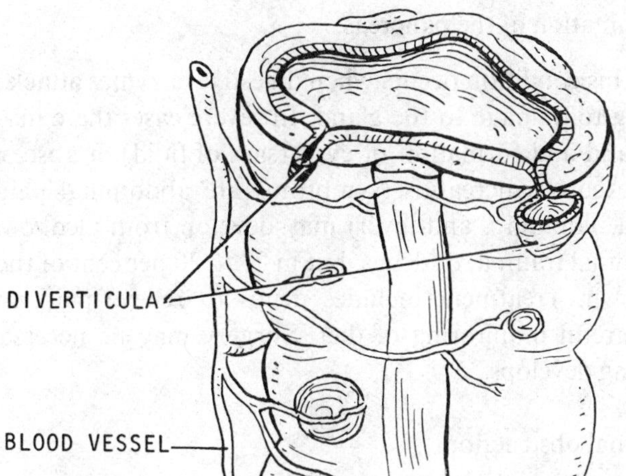

Figure 5-14 Diverticula of the large intestine. The mucous lining bulges through the muscular wall to form a diverticulum.

ascites Abnormal accumulation of fluid in the peritoneal cavity.

This condition, also called **dropsy**, occurs when fluid seeps out of the bloodstream and into the peritoneal cavity. Etiological factors are cirrhosis, tumor, infection, and heart failure.

melena Black stools; feces containing blood.

steatorrhea Excessive amounts of fat in the feces.

This symptom is often seen in pancreatic disease when fat absorption is impaired.

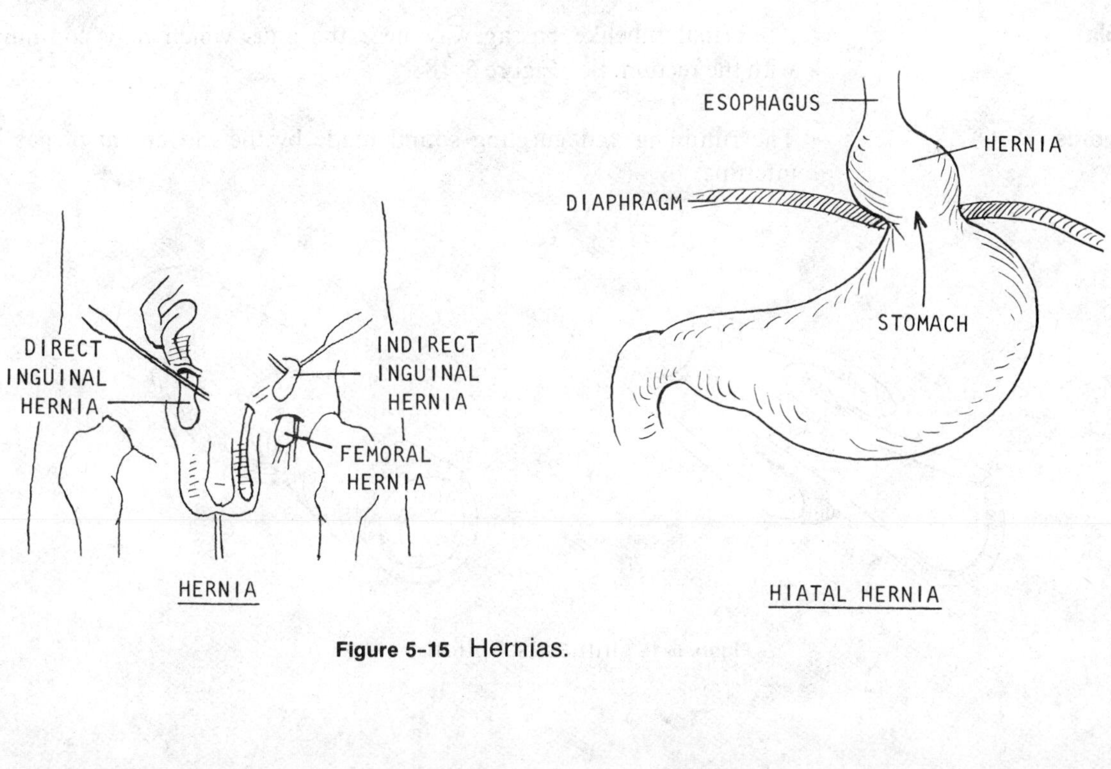

Figure 5-15 Hernias.

pancreatitis

Inflammation of the pancreas.

This condition occurs when digestive enzymes attack pancreatic tissues, leading to damage to the gland. In severe cases there may be bleeding into the gland and formation of cysts (sacs of fluid) or abscesses (collections of pus). Acute pancreatitis (symptoms are abdominal pain and tenderness, nausea, vomiting, and fever) may develop from alcohol abuse, gallstones, abdominal trauma, or drugs, but in 20 to 30 per cent of the cases the cause is unknown. Treatment includes drugs to relieve pain, intravenous fluids, and careful monitoring of diet. Surgery may be necessary when cysts or bleeding develops.

ileus

Intestinal obstruction.

Causes of ileus include hernia, tumor, failure of peristalsis, and abnormal twisting of the intestine.

intussusception

Telescoping of the intestines.

The condition occurs most commonly in children and usually in the ileocecal region. Surgical resection of the intussusception and creation of an end-to-end anastomosis are the treatment. Figure 5–16 illustrates intussusception (intus = within, susception = to receive).

volvulus

Twisting of the intestine upon itself.

An operation can be performed to untwist the loop of the bowel. Figure 5–17 illustrates volvulus.

colonic polyposis

Polyps (small growths) protrude from the mucous membrane of the colon. Figure 5–18 shows two kinds of polyps.

anal fistula

Abnormal tubelike passageway near the anus which may communicate with the rectum. See Figure 5–18.

borborygmus

The rumbling and gurgling sound made by the movement of gas in the intestine.

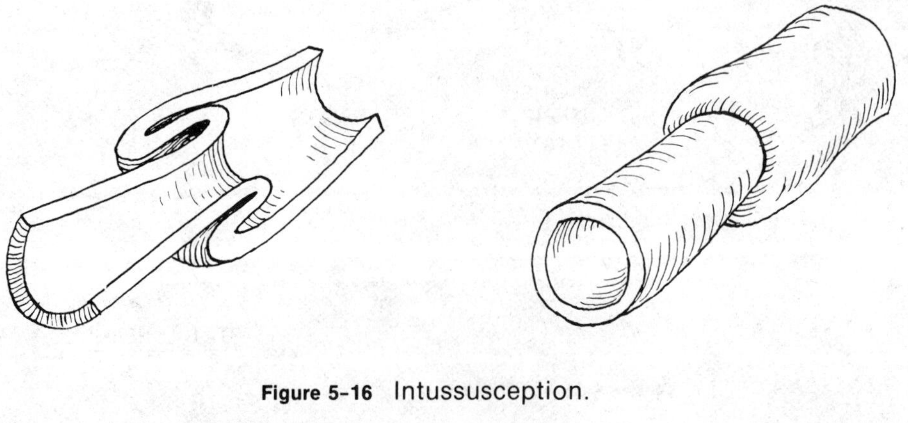

Figure 5–16 Intussusception.

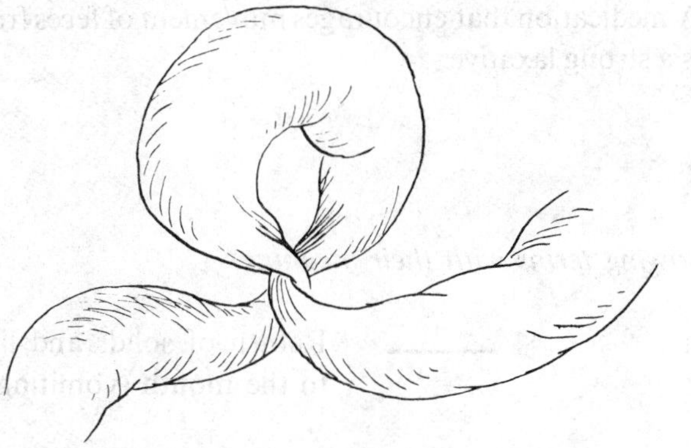

Figure 5-17 Volvulus.

constipation	Difficult, delayed defecation caused by slow peristaltic movement of the bowels, or dry and hard stools.
eructation	The act of belching or raising gas from the stomach.
flatus	Gas expelled through the anus.
hemorrhoids	Swollen or twisted veins in the rectal region.
irritable bowel syndrome	A group of symptoms (diarrhea alternating with constipation, lower abdominal pain, and bloating) associated with stress and tension. Also called spastic colon or mucous colon.

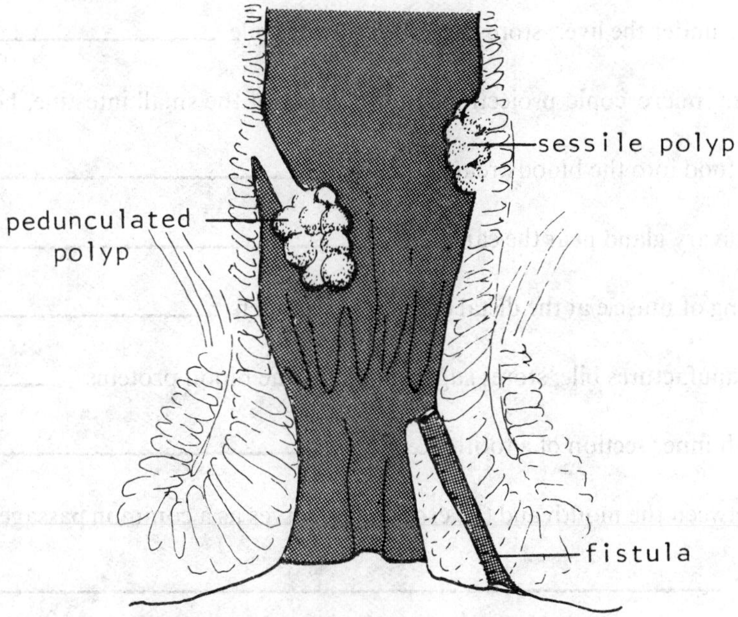

Figure 5-18 Polyps and anal fistula.

laxative A medication that encourages movement of feces from the colon. A *cathartic* is a strong laxative.

VI. EXERCISES

A. Match the following terms with their meanings:

1. deglutition ______ Return of solids and liquids from the stomach to the mouth (vomiting).
2. absorption ______ Breakdown of complex substances.
3. mastication ______ New connection between segments of an organ or tube.
4. digestion ______ Wavelike movements of digestive tubes.
5. peristalsis ______ Breaking up large fat molecules.
6. emulsification ______ Passage of nutrients into the bloodstream and lymphatic vessels.
7. anastomosis ______ Swallowing.
8. regurgitation ______ Chewing.

B. Identify the digestive system structure from the following description:

1. Sac under the liver; stores and concentrates bile ______________________
2. Tiny microscopic projections in the lining of the small intestine; help in absorption of food into the bloodstream ______________________
3. Salivary gland near the ear ______________________
4. Ring of muscle at the distal end of the stomach ______________________
5. Manufactures bile; stores sugar; makes some blood proteins ______________________
6. Soft inner section of a tooth ______________________
7. Between the mouth and the esophagus; serves as a common passageway for food and air ______________________
8. First part of the small intestine ______________________

9. Third part of the small intestine ____________________

10. Behind the stomach in the LUQ; produces enzymes to digest food and also a hormone called insulin ____________________

11. Second part of the small intestine ____________________

12. Hard, outermost layer of a tooth ____________________

C. *Give the meanings of the following terms:*

1. endodontist ____________________
2. oral surgeon ____________________
3. periodontist ____________________
4. orthodontist ____________________
5. lingual ____________________
6. buccal ____________________
7. facial ____________________
8. enzyme ____________________
9. occlusal ____________________
10. mesial ____________________

D. *Name the teeth in the dental arch, beginning at the medial line:*

1. ____________________ 5. ____________________
2. ____________________ 6. ____________________
3. ____________________ 7. ____________________
4. ____________________ 8. ____________________

E. *Build medical terms:*

1. Pertaining to under the tongue ____________________
2. Inflammation of a salivary gland ____________________

3. Blood condition of excessive bilirubin ____________

4. Pertaining to the throat ____________

5. Removal of a tonsil ____________

6. Enlargement of the liver and spleen ____________

7. Hernia of the rectum ____________

8. New opening between the ileum and the cecum ____________

9. Incision into the common bile duct ____________

10. Prolapse of the gallbladder ____________

11. Visual examination of the anal and rectal region ____________

12. Condition of disease of the small intestine ____________

13. New opening into the colon ____________

14. Surgical repair of the lips ____________

15. Pertaining to the cheek ____________

16. Pain in a tooth ____________

17. Inflammation of the gums ____________

18. Study of the causes of disease ____________

19. After meals ____________

20. Removal of the pancreas ____________

F. *Give the meaning of the following medical terms:*

1. gastroscopy ____________

2. stomatitis ____________

3. celiomyalgia ____________

4. colorectostomy ____________

5. esophagotomy ____________

6. sigmoidopexy ______________________________

7. duodenal ______________________________

8. sialolithiasis ______________________________

9. cholecystectomy ______________________________

10. pancreatitis ______________________________

11. pharyngoplasty ______________________________

12. alimentary tract ______________________________

13. hepatic portal system ______________________________

14. amylase ______________________________

15. lipase ______________________________

16. glycogen ______________________________

17. glycogenesis ______________________________

18. glycogenolysis ______________________________

19. gluconeogenesis ______________________________

20. palate ______________________________

G. *Describe the following gastrointestinal disorders:*

1. diverticulosis ______________________________

2. esophageal varices ______________________________

3. intussusception ______________________________

4. cirrhosis ______________________________

5. ulcer ______________________________

6. dysentery ______________________________

7. peritonitis ______________________________

8. hiatal hernia ______________________________

9. volvulus ______________________________

10. pancreatic carcinoma ______________________________

11. ulcerative colitis ______________________________

12. hepatitis ______________________________

13. colonic polyposis ______________________________

14. anal fistula ______________________________

15. pancreatitis ______________________________

16. Crohn's disease ______________________________

H. *Name the following medical symptoms related to the digestive system:*

1. black stools ______________________________

2. white plaques on mucous membranes ______________________________

3. lack of appetite ______________________________

4. fatty stools ______________________________

5. condition of low blood sugar ______________________________

6. lack of hydrochloric acid ______________________________

7. abnormal collection of fluid in the peritoneal cavity ______________________________

8. orange-yellow condition of the skin ______________________________

9. intestinal obstruction ______________________________

10. reflux of material from the stomach to the mouth ______________________________

11. discharge of pus (associated with periodontal disease) ______________________________

12. difficult, delayed defecation ______________________________

13. gurgling sound made by movement of gas in intestines ______________________________

14. belching; raising gas from the stomach ______________________________

15. gas expelled through the anus ______________________________

alimentary	ăl-ĕ-MĔN-tăr-ē
amino acids	ă-MĒ-nō ĂS-ĭdz
amylase	ĂM-ĭ-lās
anorectal	ā-nō-RĔK-tăl
anorexia	ăn-ō-RĔK-sē-ă
antrum	ĂN-trŭm
anus	Ā-nŭs
aphthous stomatitis	ĂF-thŭs stō-mă-TĪ-tĭs
appendectomy	ăp-ĕn-DĔK-tō-mē
appendicitis	ă-pĕn-dĭ-SĪ-tĭs
ascites	ă-SĪ-tēz
biliary	BĬL-ē-ār-ē
bilirubin	bĭl-ĭ-RŌŌ-bĭn
borborygmus	bŏr-bō-RĬG-mŭs
buccal mucosa	BŬK-ăl mū-KŌ-să
cecum	SĒ-kŭm
celiac	SĒ-lē-ăk
cementum	sē-MĔN-tŭm
cheilosis	kī-LŌ-sĭs
cholecystectomy	kō-lē-sĭs-TĔK-tō-mē
choledocholithiasis	kō-lĕd-ō-kō-lĭ-THĪ-ă-sĭs
choledochotomy	kō-lĕd-ō-KOT-ō-mē
cholelithiasis	kō-lē-lĭ-THĪ-ă-sĭs
cirrhosis	sĭr-RŌ-sĭs
colostomy	kō-LŎS-tō-mē
constipation	kŏn-stĭ-PĀ-shŭn
Crohn's disease	krōnz dy-ZĒZ
deglutition	dē-glōō-TĬSH-ŭn
dental caries	DEN-tăl KĀR-ēz
dentibuccal	dĕn-tĭ-BŬK-ăl
diverticula	dĭ-vĕr-TIK-ū-lă
duodenum	dū-ō-DĒ-nŭm or dū-ŎD-dĕ-nŭm

dysentery	DĬS-ĕn-tĕr-ē
emulsification	ē-mŭl-sĭ-fĭ-KĀ-shŭn
endodontist	ĕn-dō-DŎN-tĭst
enteric anastomosis	ĕn-TĔR-ĭk ă-năs-tō-MŌ-sĭs
enterostomy	ĕn-tĕr-ŎS-tō-mē
eructation	ĕ-rŭk-TĀ-shŭn
esophageal	ĕ-sŏf-ă-JĒ-ăl
esophagogastric	ĕ-sŏf-ă-gō-GĂS-trĭk
esophagus	ĕ-SŎF-ă-gŭs
etiology	ē-tē-ŎL-ō-jē
fistula	FĬS-tū-lă
flatus	FLĀ-tŭs
gingivitis	jĭn-jĭ-VĪ-tĭs
glossotomy	glŏ-SŎT-ō-mē
gluconeogenesis	gloo-kō-nē-ō-JĔN-ĕ-sĭs
glycogen	GLĪ-kō-jĕn
glycogenesis	glī-kō-JĔN-ĕ-sĭs
glycogenolysis	glī-kō-jĕ-NŎL-ĭ-sĭs
hemorrhoids	HĔM-ō-roydz
hepatitis	hĕp-ă-TĪ-tŭs
hepatocholangioduodenostomy	hĕp-ă-tō-kō-lăn-jē-ō-dū-ō-dĕ-NŎS-tō-mē
herpetic	hĕr-PĔT-ĭk
hiatal hernia	Hī-Ā-tăl HĔR-nē-ă
hydrochloric	hī-drō-KLŌR-ĭk
hyperbilirubinemia	hī-pĕr-bĭl-ĭ-roo-bĭ-NĒ-mē-ă
icterus	ĬK-tĕr-ŭs
ileitis	ĭl-ē-Ī-tĭs
ileocecal	ĭl-ē-ō-SĒ-kăl
ileum	ĬL-ē-ŭm
ileus	ĬL-ē-ŭs
intussusception	ĭn-tŭs-sŭs-SĔP-shŭn
jaundice	JĂWN-dĭs

jejunostomy	jĕ-jo͞o-NŎS-tō-mē
jejunum	jĕ-JO͞O-nŭm
labial	LĀ-bē-ăl
laxative	LĂK-să-tĭv
leukoplakia	lo͞o-kō-PLĀ-kē-ă
lingual	LĬNG-gwăl
lipase	LĪ-pās or LĬP-ās
lipolysis	lĭ-PŎL-ĭ-sĭs
mastication	măs-tĭ-KĀ-shŭn
melena	mĕ-LĒ-nă or MĔL-ĕ-nă
mesentery	MĔS-ĕn-tĕr-ē
palate	PĂL-ăt
palatoplasty	PĂL-ă-tō-plăs-tē
pancreas	PĂN-krē-ăs
pancreatitis	păn-krē-ă-TĪ-tĭs
papillae	pă-PĬL-ē
parotid	pă-RŎT-ĭd
periodontal disease	pĕr-ē-ō-DŎN-tăl
peristalsis	pĕr-ĭ-STĂL-sĭs
peritoneoscopy	pĕr-ĭ-tō-nē-ŎS-kō-pē
pharyngeal	fă-RĬN-jē-ăl or făr-ăn-JĒ-ăl
pharynx	FĂR-ĭnks
polyposis	pŏl-ē-PŌ-sĭs
postprandial	pōst-PRĂN-dē-ăl
proctologist	prŏk-TŎL-ō-jĭst
pyloroplasty	pī-LŌR-ō-plăs-tē
pylorus	pī-LŌR-ŭs
pyorrhea	pī-ō-RĒ-ă
regurgitation	rē-gŭr-jĭ-TĀ-shŭn
ruga	RO͞O-gă
saliva	să-LĪ-vă
sialadenitis	sī-ăl-ăd-ĕ-NĪ-tĭs

sialolithiasis	sī-ă-lō-lĭ-THĪ-ă-sĭs
sigmoid colon	SĬG-moyd KŌ-lŏn
sigmoidoscopy	sĭg-moy-DŎS-kō-pē
sphincter	SFĬNGK-tĕr
splenomegaly	splē-nō-MĔG-ă-lē
steatorrhea	stē-ă-tō-RĒ-ă
stomatitis	stō-mă-TĪ-tĭs
tonsillectomy	tŏn-sĭ-LĔK-tō-mē
ulcer	ŬL-sĕr
uvula	Ū-vū-lă
uvulectomy	ū-vū-LĔK-tō-mē
varices	VĂR-ĭ-sēz
vermiform	VĔR-mĭ-fŏrm
volvulus	VŎL-vū-lŭs

CHAPTER 6

ADDITIONAL SUFFIXES AND DIGESTIVE SYSTEM TERMINOLOGY

In this chapter you will:

- Define new suffixes and use them with digestive system combining forms;
- List and explain some laboratory tests, clinical procedures, and abbreviations common to the digestive system.

The chapter is divided into the following sections:

I. INTRODUCTION

This chapter will give you practice in word building, while not introducing a large number of new terms. It is designed to give you a breather after a long and difficult chapter.

Study the new suffixes in Section II first and complete the meanings of the terms in both Sections II and III. Checking the meanings of the terms with a dictionary may prove helpful and add additional understanding.

The information included in Section IV (Laboratory Tests, Clinical Procedures, and Abbreviations) should be useful to those of you who work in laboratory or clinical areas and also serve as a helpful reference.

Section V, Practical Applications, is designed to give you examples of medical language in context. Congratulate yourself as you decipher medical sentences, operation reports, case studies, and other material. You may also find this section useful in class as an oral reading exercise.

II. SUFFIXES

Suffix	*Meaning*	*Terminology*	*Meaning*
-clysis	irrigation, washing	enteroclysis	______
-ectasis, -ectasia	stretching, dilation	gastrectasia	______
		angiectasis	______
-emesis	vomiting	hyperemesis	______
		hematemesis	______
-lysis	destruction, breakdown	hemolysis	______
		Red blood cells are destroyed.	
-pepsia	digestion	dyspepsia	______
-phagia	eating, swallowing	polyphagia	______
		dysphagia	______
-plasty	surgical repair	palatoplasty	______
-ptysis	spitting	hemoptysis	______
-rrhagia, -rrhage	bursting forth of blood	gastrorrhagia	______
		hemorrhage	______
-rrhaphy	suture	glossorrhaphy	______
-rrhea	flow, discharge	rhinorrhea	______
-rrhexis	rupture	enterorrhexis	______
-spasm	sudden, violent, involuntary contraction of muscles	pylorospasm	______
-stalsis	contraction	peristalsis	______

-stasis	stopping, controlling	cholestasis	______
-stenosis	tightening, stricture	pyloric stenosis	______
-tresia	opening	esophageal atresia	______
		biliary atresia	______
		Bile ducts are affected.	

III. COMBINING FORMS AND TERMINOLOGY

Combining Form	*Meaning*	*Terminology*	*Meaning*
bucc/o	______	buccal	______
cec/o	______	cecopexy	______
celi/o	______	celiac artery	______
cheil/o	______	cheilostomatoplasty	______ ______
chol/e	______	cholelithotomy	______ ______
cholecyst/o	______	cholecystojejunostomy	______ ______
choledoch/o	______	choledochoduodenostomy	______ ______
col/o	______	colectomy	______
colon/o	______	colonoscopy	______
dent/i	______	dentalgia	______
duoden/o	______	duodenorrhaphy	______

enter/o	______	enteroanastomosis	______ ______
esophag/o	______	esophageal atresia	______
gastr/o	______	gastrospasm	______
gingiv/o	______	gingivectomy	______
gloss/o	______	glossopalatine	______
		-ine means pertaining to.	
glyc/o	______	hypoglycemia	______
hepat/o	______	hepatomegaly	______
herni/o	______	herniorrhaphy	______
ile/o	______	ileectomy	______
jejun/o	______	jejunojejunostomy	______ ______
labi/o	______	labioglossopharyngeal	______ ______
lingu/o	______	sublingual	______
lip/o	______	lipoid	______
lith/o	______	cholecystolithiasis	______ ______
odont/o	______	odontorrhagia	______
or/o	______	oropharynx	______
pancreat/o	______	pancreatogenic	______
proct/o	______	proctoclysis	______
pylor/o	______	pyloromyotomy	______
rect/o	______	rectostenosis	______

sial/o	________	sialodochoplasty	________
			________
splen/o	________	splenorrhagia	________
steat/o	________	steatorrhea	________
stomat/o	________	aphthous stomatitis	________

IV. LABORATORY TESTS, CLINICAL PROCEDURES, AND ABBREVIATIONS

Laboratory Tests

Liver Function Tests

SGOT (serum glutamic oxalacetic transaminase)
Also called **AST** (aspartic acid transaminase)

SGPT (serum glutamic pyruvic transaminase)
Also called **ALT** (alanine transaminase)

These tests reveal the levels of enzymes (transaminases) in the blood serum. Serum is the clear fluid that remains after blood has clotted. Enzyme levels are elevated when there is damage to liver cells because the enzymes leak out of liver cells into the blood. A high SGPT (ALT) level is especially indicative of liver disease.

ALP (alkaline phosphatase) — This is another enzyme test done on serum. An increased level of alkaline phosphatase is found in liver disease.

serum bilirubin — High levels of bilirubin in the blood produce a jaundiced condition in the patient. The test is also known as the icterus index.

Stool Analyses

stool culture — Feces are placed in a growth medium to test for the presence of microorganisms.

stool guaiac — Guaiac is added to a stool sample to reveal the presence of blood in the feces.

Clinical Procedures

abdominal ultrasonography — Sound waves are beamed into the abdomen and a record is made of the echoes as they bounce off the abdominal viscera.

barium enema — Barium sulfate, a substance that x-rays cannot penetrate, is injected, by enema, into the rectum and x-rays are taken of the rectum and colon.

barium swallow — Barium sulfate is swallowed and x-rays are taken of the esophagus, stomach, and small intestine. This procedure is also called an **upper GI series**.

computed tomography (CT scan, CAT scan) — X-ray beams are emitted from tubes positioned in or moved through, an arc directed through a plane of the patient's body. Information about the transmission of each beam is processed in a computer to produce a transverse picture of the abdominal organs. This is useful in detecting abdominal masses. (May also be called computerized tomography, computed axial tomography, computer-assisted tomography.) See Figure 6-1.

gastrointestinal endoscopy — A flexible fiberoptic tube is placed through the mouth or anus to visualize parts of the gastrointestinal tract.

nasogastric intubation — A nasogastric tube is passed through the nose into the stomach and upper area of the small intestine. The procedure is used to remove fluid postoperatively and to obtain gastric or intestinal contents for analysis.

intravenous cholangiography — Dye is injected into a vein and x-ray pictures of bile vessels are taken.

oral cholecystography — Dye that concentrates in the gallbladder is administered orally, and x-rays are taken.

endoscopic retrograde cholangiopancreatography — Dye is injected into the pancreatic and bile ducts via a tube (cannula) which is part of an endoscope, and x-ray pictures of the pancreas and bile ducts are taken. See Figure 6-2.

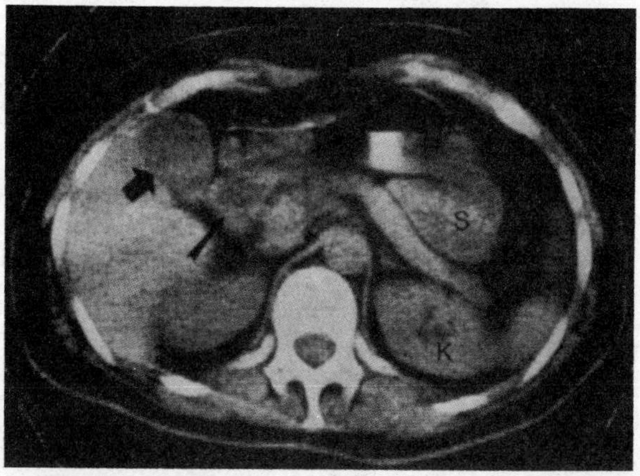

Figure 6-1 Normal computed tomogram. Transverse section is made at the level of the pancreas, and viewer is standing at the feet of a supine patient. A vertebra is visible inferiorly, and ribs outline the body. The aorta is superior to the vertebra, and branching arteries are visible. The kidneys (*K*) and stomach (*S*) are shown. The bile-filled gallbladder (thick arrow) lies in front of the liver. The second portion of the duodenum (thin arrow) is adjacent to the head of the pancreas. (From Berk, R.N.: Diagnostic imaging procedures in gastroenterology. In: Wyngaarden, J.B., and Smith, L.H., Jr.: Cecil Textbook of Medicine. 16th ed. Philadelphia, W.B. Saunders Co., 1982.)

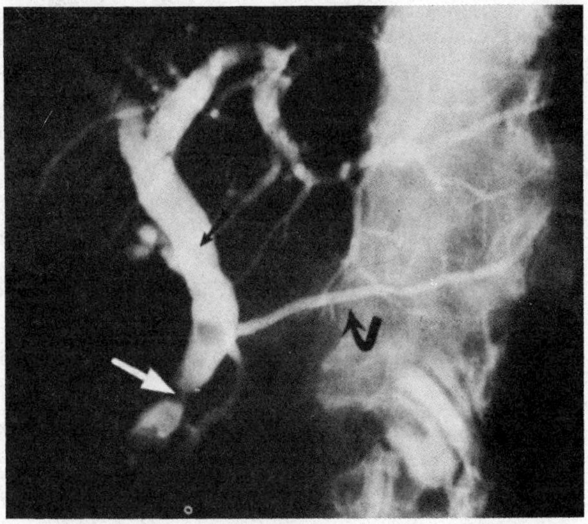

Figure 6-2 Endoscopic retrograde cholangiopancreatogram showing gallstones and a stricture (white arrow) of the common bile duct. The patient had a previous cholecystectomy. Note the cystic duct remnant (black arrow), mild dilatation of the common bile duct, and the normal pancreatic duct (curved arrow). The endoscope had been removed prior to the radiograph. (From Sherlock, P.: Gastrointestinal endoscopy. In: Wyngaarden, J.B., and Smith, L.H., Jr.: Cecil Textbook of Medicine. 16th ed. Philadelphia, W.B. Saunders Co., 1982.)

percutaneous transhepatic cholangiography — A needle is inserted through the skin into the liver and x-rays of the bile ducts are taken.

liver scan — Radioactive material is injected intravenously and taken up by the liver cells. An image of the liver called a scintiscan is made using a special scanner that records the uptake of radionuclide (radioactive material) by the liver cells. See Figure 6-3.

liver biopsy — A needle is inserted percutaneously into the liver and a sample of liver tissue is removed for microscopic examination. This procedure is useful in diagnosis of cirrhosis, chronic hepatitis, and carcinoma.

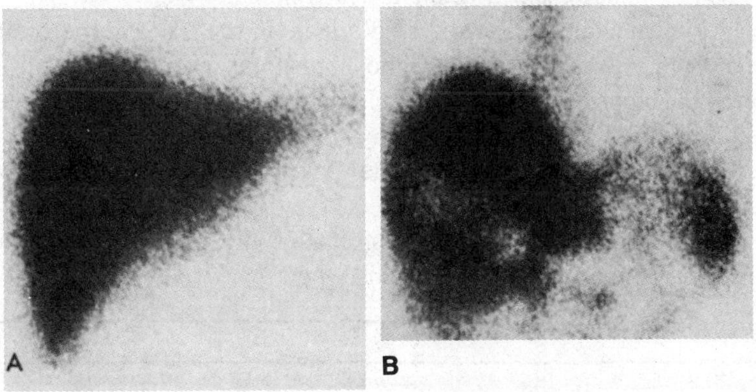

Figure 6-3 *A*, Normal liver scan in anterior view. *B*, Liver scan showing multiple metastases from carcinoma of the lung. Multiple "cold" areas (reduced radionuclide uptake) are visible in the liver. (From Berk, R.N.: Diagnostic imaging procedures in gastroenterology. In: Wyngaarden, J.B., and Smith, L.H., Jr.: Cecil Textbook of Medicine. 16th ed. Philadelphia, W.B. Saunders Co., 1982.)

Abbreviations

a.c.	Before meals (ante cibum)
ALP	Alkaline phosphatase
ALT AST	Enzyme tests of liver function
Ba	Barium
BaE	Barium enema
CT scan (CAT scan)	Computed tomography
GI	Gastrointestinal
IVC	Intravenous cholangiography
NG tube	Nasogastric tube
NPO	Nothing by mouth
OCG	Oral cholecystography
p.c.	After meals (post cibum)
p.o.	Given orally (per os)
PP	After meals (postprandial)
SBFT	Small-bowel follow-through (sequential x-rays of the small intestine as barium passes through).
SGOT SGPT	Enzyme tests of liver function
TPN	Total parenteral nutrition.
UGI	Upper gastrointestinal

V. PRACTICAL APPLICATIONS

Comments in brackets are added to help your understanding.

Case Report

The patient, a white male, 53 years old, had been well until 3 weeks before hospital admission. At that time he noted anorexia, malaise, and epigastric discomfort. His discomfort continued and was accompanied by hyperemesis on the day of admission. He had observed no sign of melena or change in bowel habit. He had previously undergone cholecystectomy for calculi and partial colectomy for diverticulitis.

Urine was normal. Hemoglobin was normal and leukocyte count was 16,800 [normal is 4,800 to 10,800], showing slight neutrophilia.

Physical examination revealed a mass in the LUQ. Laparotomy disclosed a tumor. Gastrojejunostomy and choledochojejunostomy were performed. Histological examination of the biopsied tumor revealed it to be a pancreatic adenocarcinoma. The patient was discharged to his home after 14 days in the hospital.

He returned to the hospital after 2 weeks and his condition progressively worsened. He died after 23 hospital days.

Autopsy revealed adenocarcinoma of the pancreas with metastatic hepatic and peritoneal carcinoma and peritonitis.

Surgical Report

Under adequate spinal anesthesia the patient was prepped and draped in the usual manner for a RLQ incision. An incision was made through the skin and carried down to the external oblique muscle bundle. Using blunt dissection [separating tissues along natural cleavage lines], the muscle bundle of the abdomen was opened down to the peritoneum. The peritoneum was grasped and carefully opened. The cecum and appendix were delivered through the incision. There was a small amount of free peritoneal fluid present when the peritoneum was opened and this was cultured. The appendix was noted to be edematous, with a fine fibrinous exudate [fluid with protein and cellular debris resulting from inflammation] over it. The mesoappendix [mesentery attached to the appendix] was incised down to the base of the appendix. Hemostasis was accomplished with #2-0 chromic catgut [chromic catgut indicates the type of suture material and #2-0 refers to the diameter of the suture material]. The base of the appendix was doubly ligated [tied] with silk suture. The appendix was grasped with a Pean clamp above the ligatures, and the appendix was excised. The appendiceal stump was closed over with #4-0 silk suture (#4-0 is thinner than #2-0]. The cecum was dropped back into the abdomen. The peritoneum was closed with a running suture and the muscle bundles were closed as well as the skin. Sterile dry dressing was applied and the patient was sent to the recovery room in satisfactory condition.

VI. EXERCISES

A. Build medical words:

1. Prolapse of the stomach ______________________
2. Process of recording (x-ray) the gallbladder ______________________
3. Irrigation of the rectum and anus ______________________
4. Vomiting blood ______________________
5. Dilation of the spleen ______________________
6. Hemorrhage from a tooth ______________________
7. Suture of a hernia ______________________
8. New opening between the cecum and colon ______________________
9. Spasm of the pylorus (region of the pyloric sphincter) ______________________

10. Spitting blood (from the respiratory tract) ____________________

11. Rupture of the colon ____________________

12. Removal of the pancreas ____________________

13. Process of visually examining the anus and rectum ____________________

14. Inability to swallow ____________________

15. Stone in the salivary gland ____________________

B. Give the meanings of the following medical terms:

1. enterotomy ____________________
2. cheilitis ____________________
3. nephropexy ____________________
4. celiocentesis ____________________
5. colonoscopy ____________________
6. anoplasty ____________________
7. buccal mucosa ____________________
8. linguodistal ____________________
9. choledochoduodenostomy ____________________
10. diarrhea ____________________
11. esophagostenosis ____________________
12. enteroclysis ____________________
13. gastric atrophy ____________________
14. gastrorrhaphy ____________________
15. steatorrhea ____________________

16. dyspepsia ____________________

17. jejunoileostomy ____________________

18. cholecystoptosis ____________________

19. pyorrhea ____________________

20. hyperemesis ____________________

C. *Select the medical term which suits the meaning:*

dysentery	deglutition
portal cirrhosis	dysphagia
anastomosis	anal fistula
pharyngitis	congenital bile duct atresia
peristalsis	colonic polyposis
diverticulosis	hiatal hernia

1. Difficult swallowing ____________________

2. Inflammation of the throat ____________________

3. Inflammation of the intestines with pain and diarrhea ____________________

4. Necrosis and atrophy of liver tissue and blood vessels ____________________

5. Normal wavelike contraction of tubes ____________________

6. Stomach slips through the esophageal opening in the diaphragm into the esophagus

____

7. Swallowing ____________________

8. Small growths in the large bowel ____________________

9. Closure of the bile duct at birth ____________________

10. Small outpouchings in the intestinal tract ____________________

11. Abnormal tubelike passageway near the anus ____________________

12. New opening between two previously unconnected tubes ____________________

D. Give the meanings for the following gastrointestinal symptoms:

1. melena ______________________
2. ascites ______________________
3. ileus ______________________
4. anorexia ______________________
5. icterus ______________________
6. achlorhydria ______________________
7. leukoplakia ______________________

E. Give the name of the laboratory test or clinical procedure described below:

1. Measurement of bile pigment in the blood ______________________
2. Dye is given orally and x-rays are taken of the gallbladder ______________________
3. Feces are placed in a growth medium for bacterial analysis ______________________
4. X-ray examination of the lower gastrointestinal tract ______________________
5. Sound waves make a picture of the abdominal organs ______________________
6. Test to reveal occult blood ______________________
7. Upper gastrointestinal series ______________________
8. Dye is injected through a vein and x-rays are taken of the bile vessels ______________________
9. Tube is inserted through the nose into the stomach ______________________
10. Transverse x-ray picture of the abdominal organs ______________________
11. Dye is injected through an endoscope and x-ray pictures of the pancreas and bile ducts are taken ______________________

12. Percutaneous removal of liver tissue followed by microscopic examination

____

13. Radioactive material is injected intravenously and an image is made of the material as it is taken up by liver cells _______________

14. Needle is inserted through the skin into the liver and x-rays are taken of bile ducts

____

F. *Match the abbreviation in Column I with its meaning in Column II:*

Column I		*Column II*
1. PP	______	A. Lower GI series
2. SGOT	______	B. Before meals
3. a.c.	______	C. Upper gastrointestinal
4. p.o.	______	D. After meals
5. BaE	______	E. Orally
6. OCG	______	F. Nothing by mouth
7. NPO	______	G. Liver function test
8. UGI	______	H. Gallbladder test

G. *Give the suffix for the following:*

1. rupture _______________
2. suture _______________
3. hemorrhage _______________
4. washing, irrigating _______________
5. breakdown _______________
6. stretching _______________
7. hardening _______________
8. narrowing _______________
9. prolapse _______________
10. digestion _______________
11. flow, discharge _______________
12. eating, swallowing _______________
13. spitting _______________

14. vomiting ____________

15. fixation ____________

16. surgical puncture ____________

17. contraction ____________

18. stop, control ____________

19. surgical repair ____________

20. opening ____________

ANSWERS

A.

1. gastroptosis
2. cholecystography
3. proctoclysis
4. hematemesis
5. splenectasia
6. odontorrhagia
7. herniorrhaphy
8. cecocolostomy; an anastomosis
9. pylorospasm
10. hemoptysis
11. colorrhexis
12. pancreatectomy
13. proctoscopy
14. aphagia
15. sialadenolithiasis

B.

1. Incision of the intestines.
2. Inflammation of the lips.
3. Fixation of the kidney.
4. Surgical puncture of the abdomen.
5. Visual examination of the colon.
6. Surgical repair of the anus.
7. Mucous membrane of the cheek.
8. Pertaining to the lingual and distal surfaces of a tooth.
9. New opening between the common bile duct and the duodenum.
10. "Flow through"–rapid movement of feces through the colon.
11. Narrowing of the esophagus.
12. Irrigation of the small intestine.
13. Wasting away of the stomach.
14. Suture of the stomach.
15. Fatty stools–"flow of fat."
16. Difficult digestion.
17. New opening between the jejunum and the ileum.
18. Prolapse of the gallbladder.
19. Discharge of pus (peridontal disease).
20. Excessive vomiting.

C.

1. dysphagia
2. pharyngitis
3. dysentery
4. portal cirrhosis
5. peristalsis
6. hiatal hernia
7. deglutition
8. colonic polyposis
9. congenital bile duct atresia
10. diverticulosis
11. anal fistula
12. anastomosis

D.

1. Black, blood-filled stools.
2. Fluid collection in the peritoneal cavity.
3. Intestinal obstruction.
4. Lack of appetite.
5. Jaundice.
6. Lack of hydrochloric acid.
7. White plaques.

E.

1. Serum bilirubin
2. Oral cholecystography
3. Stool culture
4. Barium enema
5. Abdominal ultrasonography
6. Stool guaiac
7. Barium swallow
8. Intravenous cholangiography
9. Nasogastric intubation
10. Abdominal CAT scan (CT scan)
11. Endoscopic retrograde cholangiopancreatography
12. Liver biopsy
13. Liver scan
14. Percutaneous transhepatic cholangiography

F.

1. D
2. G
3. B
4. E
5. A
6. H
7. F
8. C

G.

1. -rrhexis
2. -rrhaphy
3. -rrhagia, -rrhage
4. -clysis
5. -lysis
6. -ectasis, -ectasia
7. -sclerosis
8. -stenosis
9. -ptosis
10. -pepsia
11. -rrhea
12. -phagia
13. -ptysis
14. -emesis
15. -pexy
16. -centesis
17. -stalsis
18. -stasis
19. -plasty
20. -tresia

VII. PRONUNCIATION OF TERMS

angiectasis	ăn-jē-ĔK-tă-sĭs
atresia	ă-TRĒ-zē-ă
buccal	BŬK-ăl
cecopexy	SĒ-kō-pĕk-sē
cheilostomatoplasty	kī-lō-stō-MĂT-ō-plăs-tē
cholecystojejunostomy	kō-lē-sĭs-tō-jĕ-jo͞o-NŎS-tō-mē
cholecystolithiasis	kō-lē-sĭs-tō-lĭ-THĪ-ă-sĭs
choledochoduodenostomy	kō-lĕd-ō-kō-dū-ō-dĕ-NŎS-tō-mē
cholelithotomy	kō-lē-lĭ-THŎT-ō-mē
cholestasis	kō-lē-STĀ-sĭs
duodenorrhaphy	dū-ō-dĕ-NŎR-ă-fē
dyspepsia	dĭs-PĔP-sē-ă
dysphagia	dĭs-FĀ-jē-ă
enteroanastomosis	ĕn-tĕr-ō-ă-năs-tō-MŌ-sĭs
enteroclysis	ĕn-tĕr-ŎK-lĭ-sĭs
enterorrhexis	ĕn-tĕr-ō-RĔK-sis
gastrectasia	găs-trĕk-TĀ-zē-ă
gastrorrhagia	găs-trō-RĀ-jē-ă
gingivectomy	jĭn-jĭ-VĔK-tō-mē
glossopalatine	glŏs-ō-PĂL-ă-tīn
glossorrhaphy	glŏ-SŎR-ă-fē
hematemesis	hĕm-ă-TĔM-ĭ-sĭs
hemolysis	hē-MŎL-ĭ-sĭs
hemoptysis	hē-MŎP-tĭ-sĭs
hemorrhage	HĔM-ŏr-ĭj

hepatomegaly	hĕp-ă-tō-MĔG-ă-lē
herniorrhaphy	hĕr-nē-ŎR-ă-fē
hyperemesis	hī-pĕr-ĔM-ĕ-sĭs
ileectomy	ĭl-ē-ĔK-tō-mē
jejunojejunostomy	jĕ-joo-nō-jĕ-joo-NŎS-tō-mē
labioglossopharyngeal	lā-bē-ō-glŏs-ō-fă-RĬN-jē-ăl
lipoid	LĬP-ŏyd
odontorrhagia	ō-dŏn-tō-RĀ-jē-ă
oropharynx	ōr-ō-FĂR-ĭnks
palatoplasty	PĂL-ă-tō-plăs-tē
pancreatogenic	păn-krē-ă-tō-JĔN-ĭk
polyphagia	pŏl-ē-FĀ-jē-ă
proctoclysis	prŏk-TŎK-lĭ-sĭs
pyloromyotomy	pī-lōr-ō-mī-ŎT-ō-mē
pylorospasm	pī-LŌR-ō-spăzm
rectostenosis	rĕk-tō-stĕ-NŌ-sĭs
rhinorrhea	rī-nō-RĒ-ă
sialodochoplasty	sī-ă-lō-DŌ-kō-plăs-tē
splenorrhagia	splē-nō-RĀ-jē-ă
steatorrhea	stē-ă-tō-RĒ-ă
stenosis	stĕ-NŌ-sĭs
sublingual	sŭb-LĬNG-gwăl

REVIEW SHEET 5-6

Combining Forms

amyl/o	______	esophag/o	______
an/o	______	eti/o	______
appendic/o	______	gastr/o	______
bil/i	______	gingiv/o	______
bilirubin/o	______	gloss/o	______
bucc/o	______	gluc/o	______
cec/o	______	glyc/o	______
celi/o	______	glycogen/o	______
cervic/o	______	hepat/o	______
cheil/o	______	herni/o	______
chol/e	______	ile/o	______
cholecyst/o	______	jejun/o	______
choledoch/o	______	labi/o	______
cirrh/o	______	lingu/o	______
col/o	______	lip/o	______
colon/o	______	lith/o	______
dent/i	______	mandibul/o	______
diverticul/o	______	maxill/o	______
duoden/o	______	necr/o	______
enter/o	______	odont/o	______

or/o	______	sial/o	______
palat/o	______	sialaden/o	______
pancreat/o	______	sigmoid/o	______
peritone/o	______	splen/o	______
pharyng/o	______	steat/o	______
proct/o	______	stomat/o	______
pylor/o	______	tonsill/o	______
rect/o	______	uvul/o	______

Suffixes

-ase	______	-prandial	______
-centesis	______	-ptosis	______
-clysis	______	-ptysis	______
-ectasia	______	-rrhagia	______
-ectasis	______	-rrhaphy	______
-emesis	______	-rrhea	______
-iasis	______	-rrhexis	______
-lithiasis	______	-spasm	______
-lysis	______	-stalsis	______
-pepsia	______	-stasis	______
-pexy	______	-stenosis	______
-phagia	______	-tresia	______
-plasty	______		

Additional Terms

This is a list of many of the more difficult terms introduced in Chapters 5 and 6. These terms are not easily defined by simple word analysis. Use the list as a test of your knowledge by **checking off** the ones you can define and **circling** the terms you do not understand. Use the page references provided to find the definitions of the circled terms. Writing down the meanings of the terms you do not know will help you remember them.

achlorhydria (110)

anal fistula (114)

anastomosis (106)

anorexia (109)

antrum (101)

aphthous stomatitis (110)

ascites (113)

barium enema (131)

bile (101)

bilirubin (101)

borborygmus (114)

cirrhosis (110)

constipation (115)

Crohn's disease (111)

deglutition (103)

dental caries (110)

diverticula (112)

emulsification (103)

endoscopic retrograde cholangiopancreatography (132)

enzyme (103)

eructation (115)

etiology (103)

feces (103)

flatus (115)

fundus (103)

glucose (103)

glycogen (103)

hepatic portal system (103)

hiatal hernia (112)

icterus (111)

ileus (114)

intravenous cholangiography (132)

intussusception (114)

jaundice (111)

mastication (104)

melena (113)

mesentery (106)

nasogastric intubation (132)

oral cholecystography (132)

parotid gland (104)

peristalsis (104)

polyposis (114)

pylorus (104)

rugae (104)

sphincter (104)

stool culture (131)

stool guaiac (131)

ulcerative colitis (111)

varices (111)

villi (104)

volvulus (114)

CHAPTER 7

URINARY SYSTEM

In this chapter you will:

- Name the organs of the urinary system and describe their locations and functions;
- Give the meaning of various pathological conditions affecting the system;
- Recognize the use and interpretation of urinalysis as a diagnostic test;
- Detail the meanings of combining forms, prefixes, and suffixes of the system terminology; and
- List and explain some clinical procedures, laboratory tests, and abbreviations that pertain to the urinary system.

The chapter is divided into the following sections:

I. INTRODUCTION

You have just learned how food is brought into the bloodstream by the digestive system. In a future chapter you will learn how oxygen is brought into the bloodstream by the respiratory system. Food and oxygen are combined in the cells of the body to produce energy (catabolism). In the process, however, the substance of the food and oxygen is not destroyed. Instead, the small particles of which the food and oxygen are made are actually rearranged into new combinations. These are waste products. When foods like sugars and fats which contain particles of carbon, hydrogen, and oxygen combine with oxygen in cells, the wastes produced are gases called carbon dioxide (carbon and oxygen) and water (hydrogen and oxygen) in the form of vapor. These gases are removed from the body by exhalation through the lungs.

Protein foods are more complicated than sugars and fats. They contain carbon, hydrogen, and oxygen **plus** nitrogen and other elements. The waste that is produced when proteins combine with oxygen is called **nitrogenous waste**, and it is more difficult to excrete (to separate out) from the body than are gases like carbon dioxide and water vapor.

The body cannot efficiently put the nitrogenous waste into a gaseous form and exhale it, so it excretes it in the form of a soluble (dissolved in water) waste substance called **urea**. The major function of the urinary system is to remove urea from the bloodstream so that it does not accumulate in the body and become toxic.

Urea is formed in the liver from ammonia, which in turn is derived from the breakdown of simple proteins (amino acids) in the body cells. The urea is carried in the bloodstream to the kidneys, where it passes with water, salts, and acids out of the bloodstream and into the kidney tubules as **urine**. Urine then travels down the ureters into the bladder and out of the body.

Besides removing urea from the blood, another important function of the kidneys is to maintain the proper balance of water, salts, and acids in the body fluids. Salts, such as sodium and potassium, and some acids are known as **electrolytes** (small molecules which can conduct an electrical charge). Electrolytes are necessary for the proper functioning of muscle and nerve cells. The kidney adjusts the amounts of water and electrolytes by secreting some substances into the urine and holding back others in the bloodstream for use in the body.

In addition to forming urine and eliminating it from the body, the kidneys also act as endocrine organs, secreting into the bloodstream substances that act at some distant site in the body. Examples of the kidneys' endocrine function include the secretion of **renin**, a substance important in the control of blood pressure, and **erythropoietin**, a material that regulates the production of red blood cells. The kidneys also secrete an active form of vitamin D, necessary for the absorption of calcium from the intestine. In addition, hormones such as insulin and parathyroid hormone are degraded and extracted from the bloodstream by the kidney.

II. ANATOMY OF THE MAJOR ORGANS

The organs of the urinary system are: (See Figure 7-1)

1. Two **kidneys**—bean-shaped organs situated behind the abdominal cavity (retroperitoneal) on either side of the vertebral column in the lumbar region of the spine.

The kidneys are embedded in a cushion of adipose tissue and surrounded by fibrous connective tissue for protection. They are fist-sized and weigh about half a pound each.

The kidneys consist of an outer **cortex** region (cortex means outer portion or bark, as in bark of a tree) and an inner **medulla** region (medulla means marrow or inner portion). The depression on the medial border of the kidney, through which blood vessels and nerves pass, is called the **hilum**.

2. Two **ureters**—muscular tubes lined with mucous membrane. They convey urine in peristaltic waves from the kidney to the urinary bladder.
3. **Urinary bladder**—hollow, muscular, distensible sac in the pelvic cavity. It serves as a temporary reservoir for urine. The **trigone** is a triangular space at the base of the bladder where the ureters enter and the urethra leads out.
4. **Urethra**—membranous tube through which urine is discharged from the urinary bladder. The process of expelling (**voiding**) urine through the urethra is called **micturition**. The external opening of the urethra is called the urethral or urinary **meatus**.

III. HOW THE KIDNEYS PRODUCE URINE

Blood enters each kidney from the aorta by way of the right and left renal arteries. After the renal artery enters the kidney (at the hilum), the artery branches into smaller and smaller arteries. The smallest arteries are called **arterioles** and these are located throughout the cortex of the kidney. See Figure 7-2.

Since the arterioles are small, blood passes through them slowly, but constantly. Blood flow through the kidney is so essential that the kidneys have their own special device for maintaining blood flow. If blood pressure falls in the vessels of the kidney so that blood flow is diminished, the kidney produces a substance called **renin** and discharges it into the blood. Renin leads to the formation of a substance (angiotensin II) that stimulates the contraction of arterioles so that blood pressure is increased and blood flow in the kidneys is restored to normal.

Each arteriole in the cortex of the kidney leads into a mass of very tiny, coiled and intertwined smaller blood vessels called **capillaries**. The collection of capillaries, shaped in the

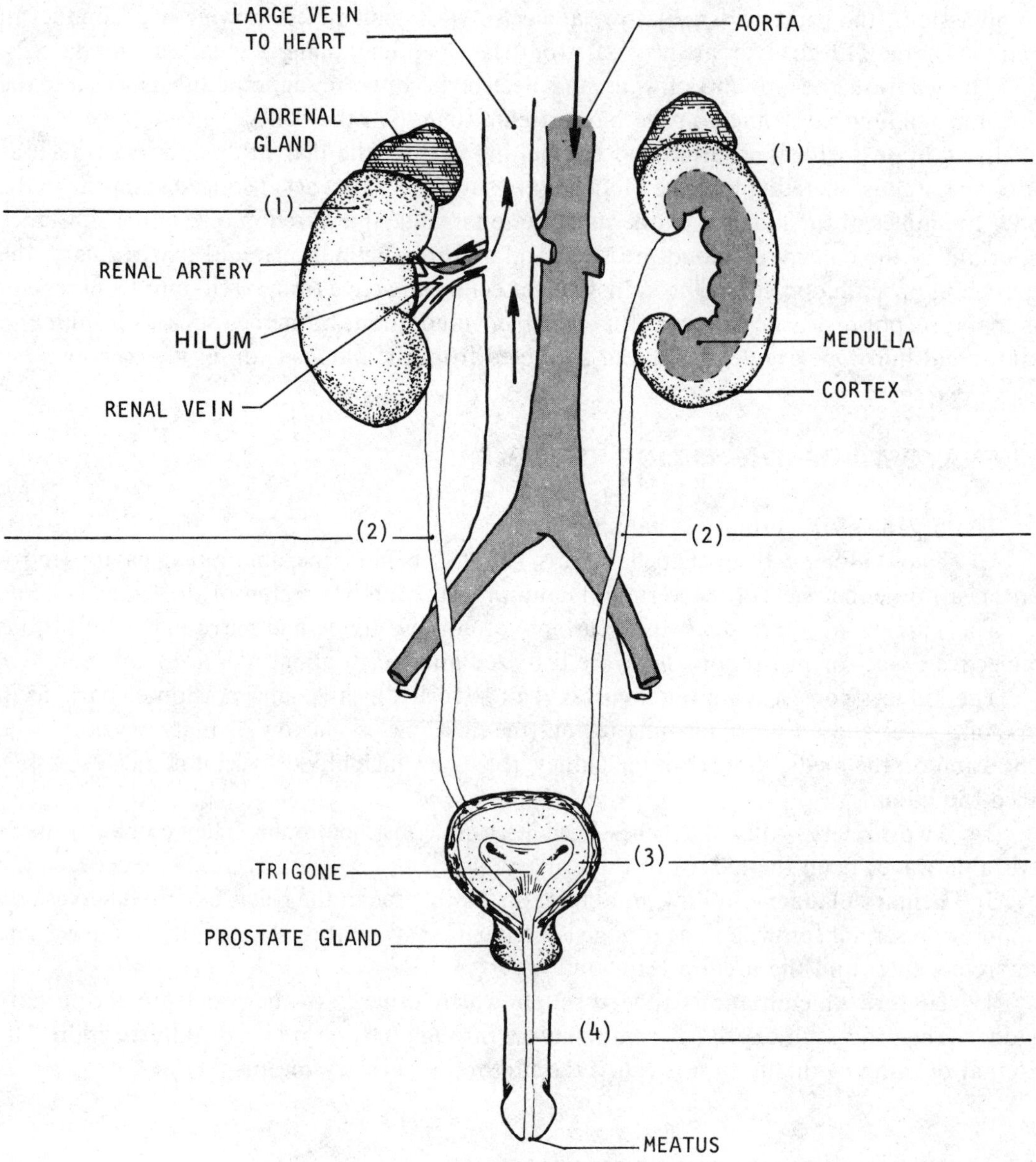

Figure 7-1 Organs of the urinary system.

form of a tiny ball, is called a **glomerulus**. There are thousands of glomeruli in the cortex region of each kidney.

As blood passes through the glomeruli, the process of forming urine begins. There are three steps to this process: **filtration**, **reabsorption**, and **secretion**. The walls of the glomeruli are thin enough to permit water, salts, sugar, and nitrogenous wastes such as **urea**, **creatinine**, and **uric acid** to filter out of the blood. Each glomerulus is surrounded by a cuplike structure which collects the substances filtering out of the blood. The cuplike structure is called **Bowman's capsule**. Large substances like proteins and blood cells cannot pass through the walls of the glomerulus into Bowman's capsule and thus, if the kidney is healthy, they remain in the blood. See Figure 7-3 for a picture of one glomerulus and its Bowman's capsule.

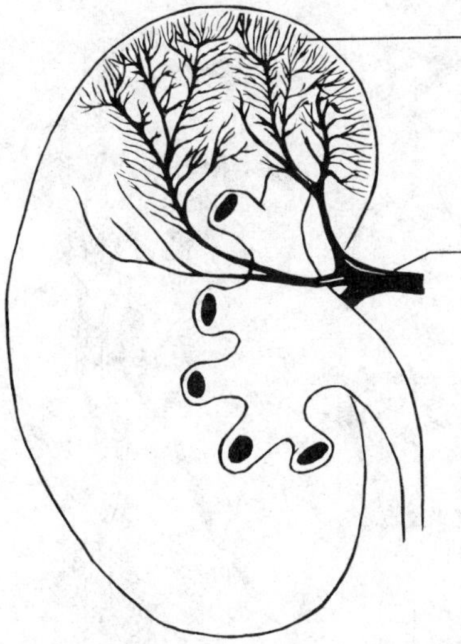

Figure 7-2 Renal artery branching to form smaller arteries and arterioles.

If the process of forming urine ended here, the body would lose a good deal of needed water, sugar, and salts that filtered out of the blood with the wastes. What happens next assures that those necessary substances remain in the body and not in the urine. Each Bowman's capsule is connected to a long, twisted tube called the **renal tubule**. As the water, salts, sugar, and wastes pass along the tubule, the materials that the body needs (most water, salts, and sugar) are able to reenter the bloodstream through tiny capillaries which lie close to each renal tubule. See Figure 7-4 for a picture of a renal tubule with its surrounding capillary network.

Thus, by the time the filtrated material reaches the end of the renal tubule, the materials that the body must keep have been **reabsorbed** into the bloodstream. Only the wastes, along with some water, some salts (electrolytes), and some acids (these are **secreted** into the tubule directly from the blood), pass from the renal tubule into the central collecting area of the kidney. Here, thousands of renal tubules deposit urine into the central **renal pelvis**, a space that fills most of the medulla of the kidney. Cuplike divisions of the renal pelvis which receive the urine

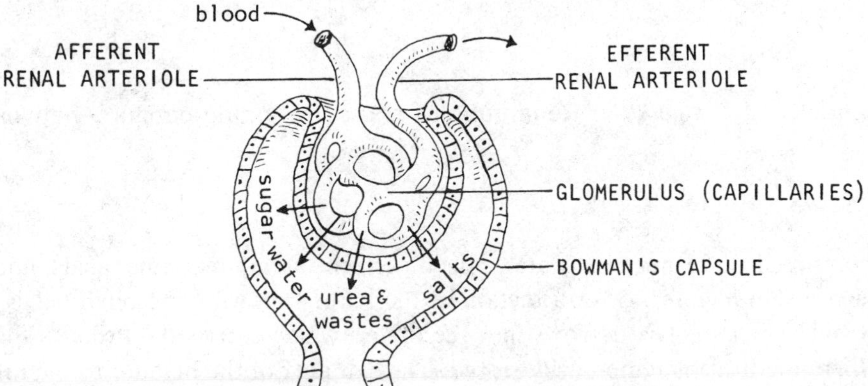

Figure 7-3 Glomerulus and Bowman's capsule.

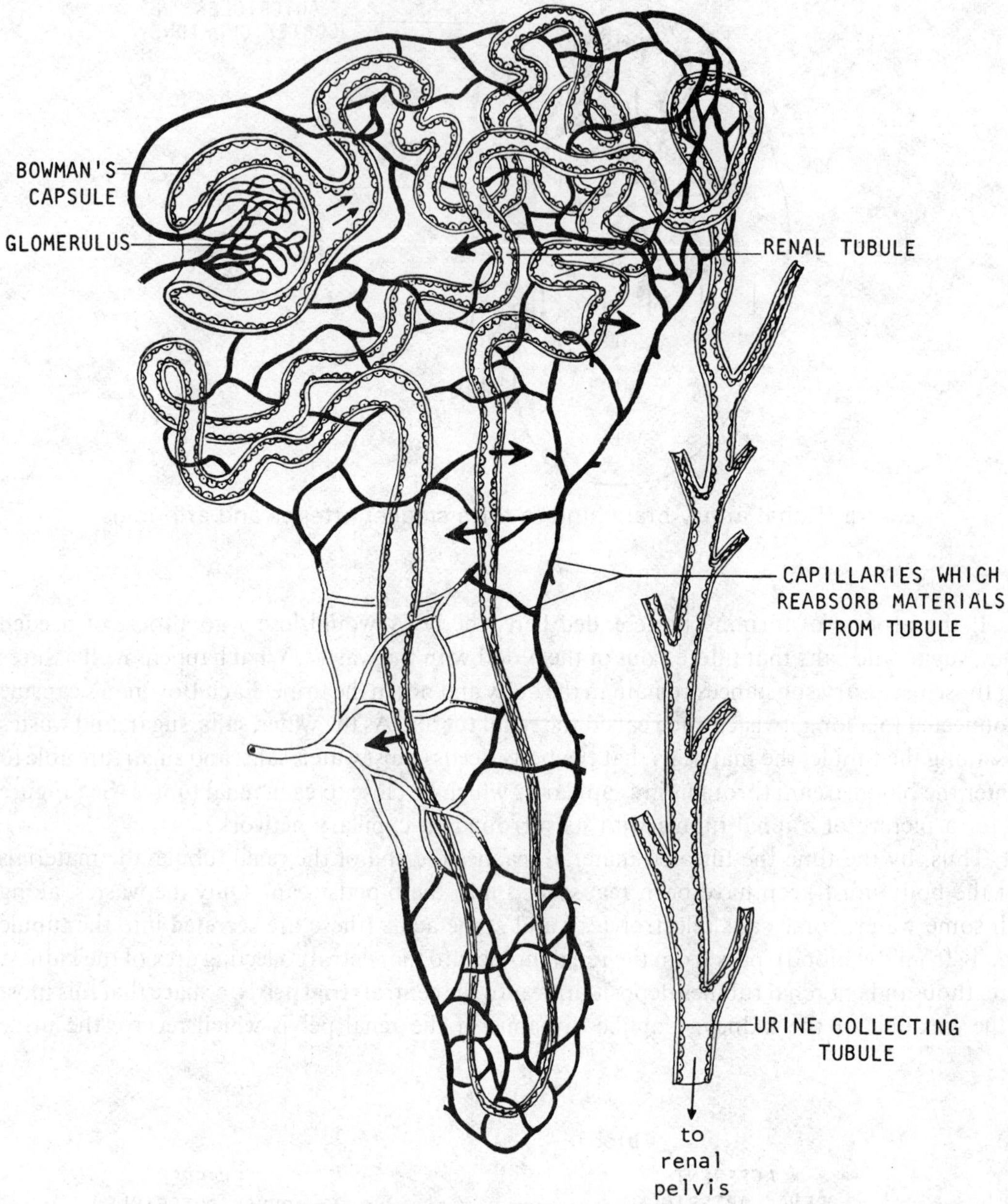

Figure 7-4 Renal tubules and surrounding capillary network.

(composed of 95 per cent water, plus 5 per cent urea, creatinine, acids, and salts) are called **calyces**. See Figure 7-5 for a section of the kidney showing the renal pelvis and calyces.

The renal pelvis narrows into the **ureter**, which carries the urine to the **urinary bladder** where the urine is temporarily stored. The exit area of the bladder to the **urethra** is closed by sphincters which do not permit urine to leave the bladder. As the bladder fills up, pressure is placed on the base of the urethra, which causes the desire to urinate.

Study the flow diagram in Figure 7-6 to trace the process of forming urine and expelling it from the body.

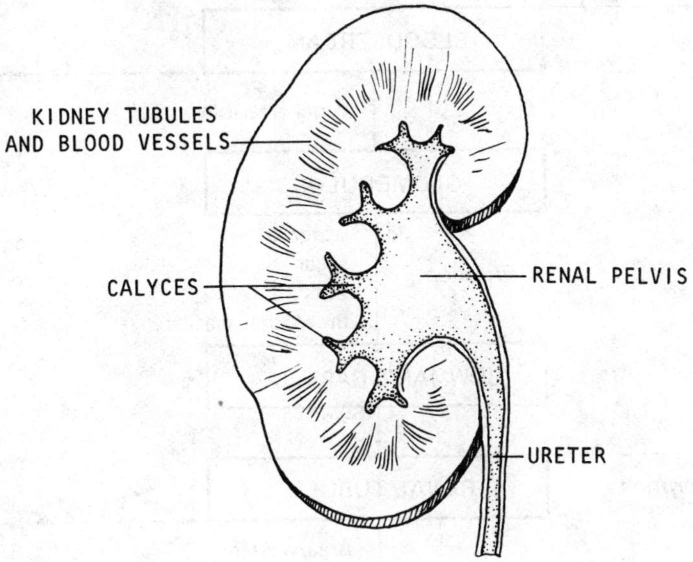

Figure 7-5 Section of kidney showing renal pelvis, calyces, and ureter.

IV. VOCABULARY

arteriole	A small artery.
Bowman's capsule	Cup-shaped capsule surrounding each glomerulus.
calyx; calyces	Cuplike collecting region of the renal pelvis.
cortex	Outer region; the renal cortex is the outer region of the kidney.
creatinine	Waste product of protein usage in cells; nitrogenous waste excreted in urine.
electrolyte	A small molecule that carries an electrical charge.
erythropoietin	Secreted by the kidney to regulate the production of red blood cells.
filtration	Process whereby some substances, but not all, pass through a filter or other material.
glomerulus	Tiny ball of capillaries (microscopic blood vessels) in cortex of kidney.
hilum	Notch on the medial surface of each kidney where blood vessels and nerves enter and leave.
meatus	Opening or canal.
medulla	Inner region; the renal medulla is the inner region of the kidney.
micturition	Urination; the act of voiding.

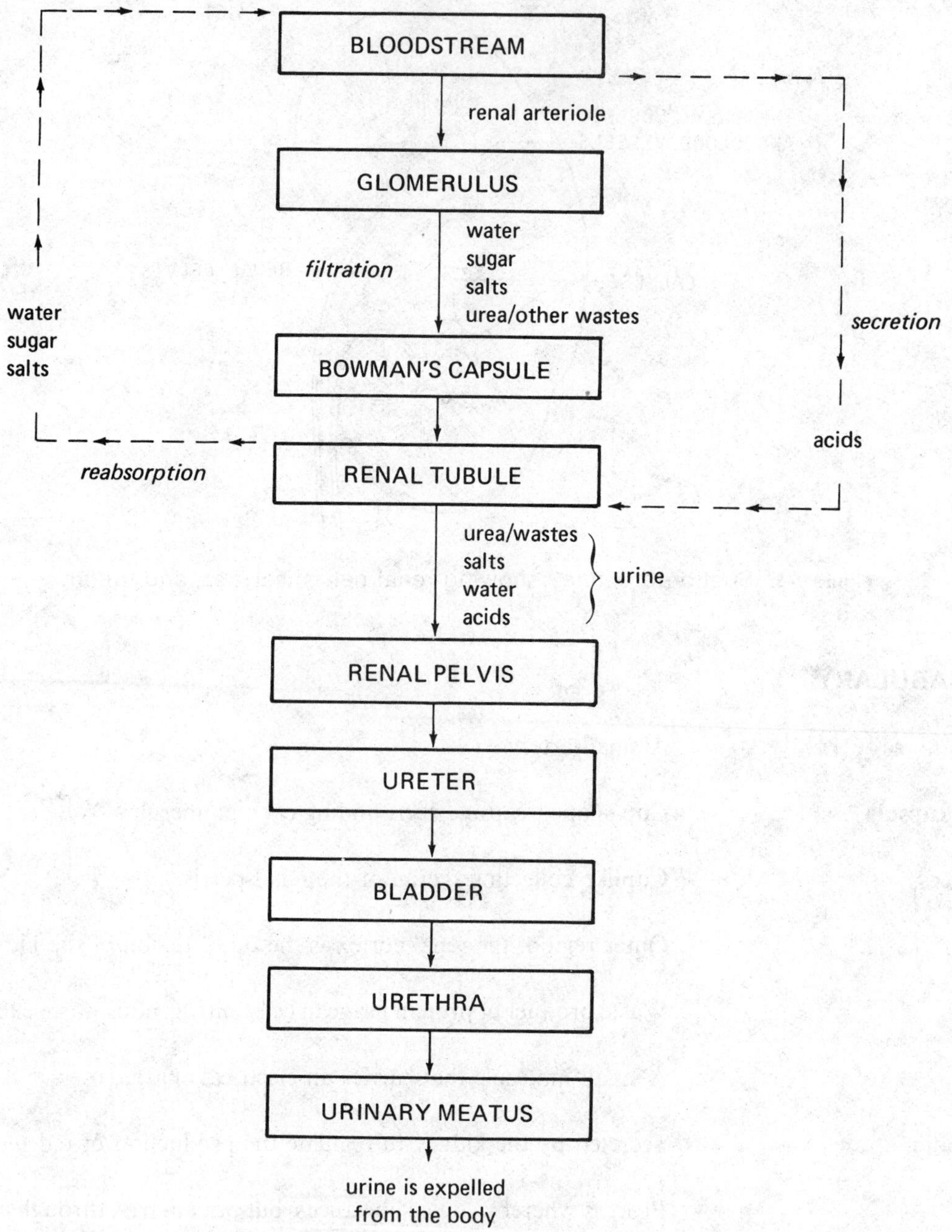

Figure 7-6 Flow diagram of the process of forming and expelling urine.

nitrogenous wastes Substances containing nitrogen and excreted in urine.

reabsorption The process of accepting again or taking back. Materials necessary to the body are reabsorbed into the blood from the renal tubules as urine is formed.

renal artery Carries blood to the kidney.

renal pelvis Central collecting region in the kidney.

renal tubules Microscopic tubes in the kidney where urine is formed as water, sugar, and salts are reabsorbed into the bloodstream.

renal vein Carries blood away from the kidney.

renin Substance, made in the kidney, that increases blood pressure by causing the formation of angiotensin II.

trigone Triangular area in the bladder where the ureters enter and the urethra exits.

urea Major nitrogenous waste product excreted in urine.

ureter One of two tubes leading from the kidney to the bladder.

urethra Tube leading from the bladder to the outside of the body.

uric acid Nitrogenous waste excreted in the urine.

urinary bladder Sac which holds urine.

urinary catheter A tube for injecting fluids into or removing fluids from the urinary tract.

voiding Expelling urine.

V. COMBINING FORMS AND TERMINOLOGY

Combining Form	*Meaning*	*Terminology*	*Meaning*
cortic/o	cortex; the renal cortex is the outer section of the kidney.	cortical	____________________
glomerul/o	glomerulus *(collection of capillaries)*	glomerular	____________________
medull/o	medulla; the renal medulla is the inner section of the kidney.	medullary	____________________
nephr/o	kidney	paranephric	____________________
		nephroptosis	____________________

		nephrohypertrophy ________________
		nephrectomy ________________
		nephrolithotomy ________________
		-tomy is used with lith/o to mean an incision to remove a stone.
		nephrosclerosis ________________
		nephropexy ________________
		nephrotomography ________________
		________________
		Tomography is an x-ray process whereby different x-ray pictures of an organ are taken to show it in varying depths. Tom/o means to cut; hence, the many x-rays give different views or "cuts" of the organ.
ren/o	kidney	renal ischemia ________________
		renal transplantation ________________
		________________
		See clinical procedures.
		renal calculus ________________
		renal dialysis ________________
		________________
		See clinical procedures.
pyel/o	renal pelvis	intravenous pyelogram (IVP) ________________
		________________
		See clinical procedures.
		retrograde pyelogram (RP) ________________
		________________
		Retrograde means that the dye travels in reverse direction.
		pyelolithotomy ________________

cali/o	calyx, calyces	caliectasis ______
ur/o	urine (urea), urinary tract	uremia ______ *Higher than normal levels of urea in the blood.*
		excretory urogram ______ *An IVP.*
		diuresis ______ *di- (dia-) means complete. Caffeine, alcohol, and urea can act as diuretics.*
		enuresis ______ *Bedwetting; literally, a condition of being "in urine."*
		antidiuretic hormone ______ ______ *Also called vasopressin.*
azot/o	urea, nitrogen	azotemia ______
ureter/o	ureter	ureteral ______
		ureterolithotomy ______
		ureteroileostomy ______ *A segment of the ileum is used in place of the bladder to carry urine from the ureters out of the body.* ______
cyst/o	urinary bladder	cystitis ______
		cystourethrogram ______ ______
		cystoscopy ______
		cystocele ______
vesic/o	urinary bladder	perivesical ______

		vesicorectal fistula ______________
trigon/o	trigone	trigonitis ______________
urethr/o	urethra	urethritis ______________
		urethroplasty ______________
meat/o	meatus	meatotomy ______________
		meatal stenosis ______________
dips/o	thirst	polydipsia ______________
-uria	urination, urine	dysuria ______________
		anuria ______________
		hematuria ______________
		glycosuria ______________ *A symptom of diabetes mellitus. See pathological terminology section.*
		polyuria ______________ *A symptom of diabetes insipidus as well as diabetes mellitus.*
		phenylketonuria ______________ *See urinalysis section.* ______________
albumin/o	albumin, a protein in the blood	albuminuria (proteinuria) ______________
py/o	pus	pyuria ______________
noct/i	night	nocturia ______________
olig/o	scanty	oliguria ______________
bacteri/o	bacteria	bacteriuria ______________
keton/o	ketones, acetones	ketonuria ______________

ket/o	ketones, acetones	<u>ket</u>osis ______________________
		Ketones collect in the blood and body fluids, causing acidosis.

VI. URINALYSIS

Urinalysis is an examination of urine to determine the presence of abnormal elements which may indicate various pathological conditions.

The following are some of the tests made in a urinalysis:

1. **Color**—Normal urine color is yellow (amber) or straw colored. A colorless, pale urine indicates a large amount of water in the urine while a smoky red or brown color of urine is due to the presence of large amounts of blood. Foods, such as beets, and certain drugs can also produce red hues in urine.

2. **pH**—This is a test of the chemical nature of urine. The pH test indicates to what degree a solution (such as urine or blood) is acid or alkaline (basic). The pH range is from 0 (very acid) to 14 (very alkaline). Normal urine is slightly acid (6.5). However, in infections of the bladder, the urine pH may be alkaline owing to the actions of bacteria in the urine which break down the urea and release an alkaline substance called ammonia.

3. **Protein**—Small amounts of protein are normally found in the urine but not in sufficient quantity to produce a positive result by ordinary methods of testing. When urinary tests for protein become positive, **albumin** is usually responsible. Albumin is the major protein in blood plasma. If it is detected in urine (**albuminuria**) it may indicate a leak in the glomerular membrane which allows albumin to enter the renal tubule and pass into the urine.

4. **Glucose**—Sugar is not normally found in the urine. In most cases, when it does appear (**glycosuria**), it indicates **diabetes mellitus**. In diabetes mellitus, there is an excess of sugar in the bloodstream (hyperglycemia), which leads to "spilling over" of sugar into the urine. The renal tubules are unable to reabsorb all the sugar that filters out through the glomerular membrane.

5. **Specific gravity**—The specific gravity of urine reflects the amount of wastes, minerals, and solids in the urine. It is a comparison of the density of urine with that of water. The urine of patients with diabetes mellitus has a higher than normal specific gravity because of the presence of sugar. In kidney diseases such as nephritis, the specific gravity of urine is low because the urine is diluted by large quantities of water which cannot be reabsorbed into the blood.

6. **Ketone bodies**—Ketones (sometimes referred to as **acetones**, which are a type of ketone body) are breakdown products from fat catabolism in cells. Ketones accumulate in large quantities in blood and urine when fat, instead of sugar, is used as fuel for energy in cells. This happens, for example, in diabetes mellitus when cells which are deprived of sugar must use up their available fat for energy. Also, in starvation, when sugar is not available, ketonuria and ketosis (ketones in the blood) occur as fat is abnormally catabolized.

   The presence of ketones in the blood is quite dangerous since they increase the acidity of the blood (**acidosis**). This can lead to coma (unconsciousness) and death.

7. **Casts**—These are substances which appear in the urine as a sign of various pathological conditions. Casts, composed of materials such as red blood cells, pus, fat globules, and granules, accumulate in the renal tubules and are formed into a mold or shape of the tubule in which they collect. Figure 7-7 shows some of the various types of casts which are observed under a microscope.

8. **Pus**—**Pyuria** gives a **turbid** (cloudy) appearance to urine. Large numbers of leukocytes (polymorphonuclears) are present because of infection or inflammation in the kidney or bladder.

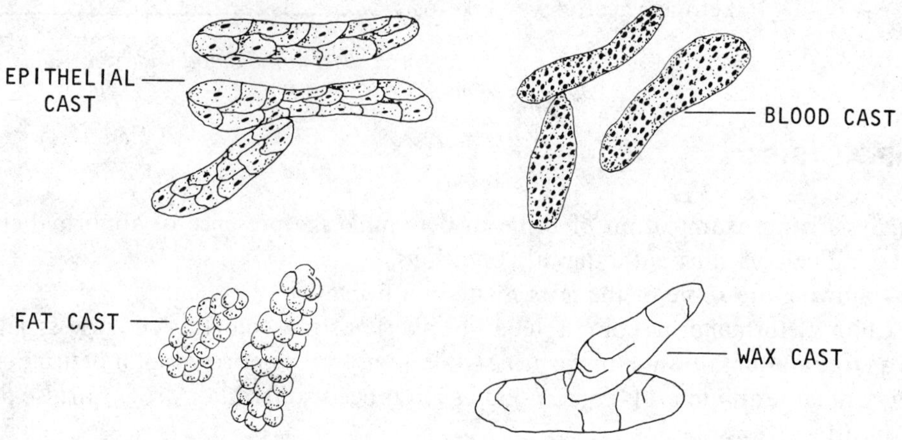

Figure 7-7 Urinary casts.

9. **Phenylketonuria (PKU)**—Phenylketones are substances which accumulate in the urine of infants born with a special congenital problem. These infants are born lacking an important enzyme. The enzyme (phenylalanine hydroxylase) is necessary in cells to change one amino acid (phenylalanine) to another amino acid (tyrosine). Lack of the enzyme causes phenylalanine to reach high levels in the infant's bloodstream, and this will eventually lead to mental retardation. The PKU test, done just after birth, can detect the phenylketonuria or phenylalanine in the blood. When it is detected, the infant is fed a low-protein diet that excludes phenylalanine so that mental retardation is prevented. This strict diet is necessary until the child is an adult.

10. **Bilirubin**—This pigment substance from hemoglobin breakdown may appear in the urine, darkening it, as an indication of liver or gallbladder disease. The diseased liver has difficulty removing bilirubin from the blood (**hyperbilirubinemia**) which causes excessive bilirubin to appear in the urine (**bilirubinuria**).

VII. PATHOLOGICAL TERMINOLOGY

glomerulonephritis Inflammation of the kidney glomerulus (**Bright's disease**).

Acute glomerulonephritis may develop after an acute infection, as part of a systemic disorder (affecting many organs in the body) such as systemic lupus erythematosus, or without apparent cause. A well known form, post-streptococcal glomerulonephritis, appears 10 to 14 days after an infection with certain strains of beta-hemolytic streptococcus. No bacteria are found in the kidney, but it is thought that inflammation results from the deposition of circulating complexes of antigen (streptococcus) and antibody in the glomerulus. Most patients recover spontaneously, but in some cases the disease becomes chronic. Chronic glomerulonephritis can result in hypertension (high blood pressure), albuminuria (protein seeps through damaged glomerular walls), renal failure (loss of kidney function), and uremia. Drugs may be useful in some cases to control inflammation, and dialysis or transplant may be necessary if uremia occurs.

pyelonephritis

Inflammation of the renal pelvis.

This common type of renal disease is caused by bacterial infection. Many small **abscesses** (collections of pus) form in the renal pelvis. Pyuria is found on urinalysis. Treatment consists of antibiotics and surgical correction of any obstruction to urine flow.

nephrotic syndrome

A condition caused by excessive protein loss in the urine; nephrosis.

In addition to marked proteinuria, symptoms include **edema** (swelling due to fluid in tissue spaces), hypoalbuminemia, and susceptibility to infections. Nephrotic syndrome may follow acute glomerulonephritis, exposure to toxins or drugs, and other pathological conditions, such as diabetes mellitus, malignant disease, and syphilis. Drugs may be useful to heal the leaky glomerulus.

interstitial nephritis

Inflammation of the renal interstitium (connective tissue that lies between the renal tubules)

Acute interstitial nephritis is an increasingly frequent disorder that may develop after the administration of drugs. It is characterized by fever, skin rash, eosinophils in the blood and urine, and poor renal function. Recovery may be anticipated when the offending agent is discontinued and may be hastened by the use of corticosteroids.

essential hypertension

High blood pressure without an apparent cause.

Many factors, such as heredity and environmental and neurogenic influences, may predispose a person to essential hypertension but there is no known cause. Over many years, the hypertension may cause arteriole walls in the kidney to become narrow and thickened (nephrosclerosis). This leads to glomerular ischemia, atrophy, and scarring of kidney tissue.

secondary hypertension

High blood pressure due to kidney disease or other ailment.

Secondary hypertension is often directly related to renal disease such as renal artery stenosis or glomerulonephritis or to other disorders (adrenal gland problems). It may also be associated with the use of oral contraceptives. **Renal hypertension** is high blood pressure resulting from kidney disease.

nephrolithiasis

Kidney stones.

Renal calculi are usually composed of uric acid or calcium salts. Although the etiology is unknown in many cases, conditions associated with an increase in the concentration of calcium (parathyroid gland tumors) or uric acid (gout) in the blood or urine may contribute to the formation of calculi. Stones often lodge in the ureter or bladder as well as in the renal pelvis and may require surgical removal to prevent kidney damage or infection.

hydronephrosis Abnormal condition of water (fluid) in the kidney.

The kidney becomes enlarged and distended as urine flow is obstructed. Obstruction may be caused by renal calculi, **stricture** (narrowing), tumor of the ureter, or hypertrophy of the prostate gland (at the base of the bladder in males).

polycystic kidney Multiple fluid-filled sacs (cysts) within and upon the kidney.

This is a hereditary condition that usually remains asymptomatic until adult life. Cysts progressively develop in both kidneys, leading to kidney enlargement, hematuria, urinary tract infection, hypertension, and uremia.

hypernephroma Renal carcinoma occurring in adulthood.

This cancerous tumor (also called a renal cell carcinoma) often metastasizes to the bone and lungs. Its name ("tumor above the kidney") refers to the observation that the tumor tissue, to the naked eye, resembles adrenal gland tissue.

Wilms' tumor Malignant tumor of the kidney occurring in childhood.

This tumor may be treated with surgery, radiation, and chemotherapy. There is a high percentage of cure if it is treated before metastasis has occurred.

urinary retention Blockage in passage of urine from the bladder.

urinary incontinence Inability to hold urine in the bladder.

Urinary stress incontinence is the inability to prevent escape of urine brought on by laughing, coughing, sneezing, and so forth.

diabetes insipidus Inadequate secretion of antidiuretic hormone (ADH), leading to polyuria and polydipsia.

Lack of ADH prevents water from being reabsorbed into the blood through the renal tubules. Insipidus means "tasteless," reflecting that the urine is very dilute and watery, not sweet as in diabetes mellitus. The term diabetes is taken from a Greek term meaning "siphon." It was recognized that diabetes leads to an inability to retain ingested water, which instead runs through the body as through a siphon.

diabetes mellitus Inadequate secretion or improper utilization of insulin leads to glycosuria, hyperglycemia, and other symptoms.

Sugar is prevented from leaving the bloodstream and cannot be used by body cells in the production of energy. Sugar thus remains in the blood (hyperglycemia) and spills over into the urine (glycosuria). Other symptoms are ketonuria, polyuria, and polydipsia. Mellitus means "sweet." The term diabetes, when used by itself, usually refers to diabetes mellitus.

VIII. LABORATORY TESTS, CLINICAL PROCEDURES, AND ABBREVIATIONS

Laboratory Tests

blood urea nitrogen (BUN) This test measures the amount of urea in the blood. Normally the urea level is low since urea is excreted in the urine continuously. When the kidney is diseased or fails, however, urea accumulates in the blood (a condition known as uremia) and this can lead to unconsciousness and death.

creatinine clearance test This test measures the ability of the kidney to remove creatinine from the blood. A blood sample is drawn and the amount of creatinine concentration is compared with the amount of creatinine excreted in the urine during a 24-hour period. If the kidney is not functioning well in its job of clearing creatinine from the blood, there will be a disproportionate amount of creatinine in the blood, compared with the urine.

Clinical Procedures

kidney, ureter, and bladder (KUB) This x-ray test (no dye is used) demonstrates the size and location of the kidneys in relationship to other organs in the abdominopelvic region.

intravenous pyelogram (IVP) Contrast material is injected within a vein and travels to the kidney where it is filtered into the urine. X-rays are then taken that show the dye filling the kidneys, ureters, bladder, and urethra. Cysts, tumors, infections, hydronephrosis, and calculi can be detected.

retrograde pyelogram (RP) Contrast material is introduced directly into the bladder and ureters through a cystoscope and x-rays are taken to determine the presence of stones or obstruction of these organs. This x-ray technique may be indicated when poor renal function makes it impossible to visualize the kidneys, ureters, and bladder by use of intravenous dye as in IVP. It may also be used as a substitute for an IVP when a patient is allergic to intravenous dye.

voiding cystourethrogram (VCU) The bladder is filled with contrast material, as in a retrograde pyelogram, and x-rays are taken of the bladder and urethra as a patient is expelling urine. See Figure 7-8.

ultrasonography Kidney size, tumors, hydronephrosis, polycystic kidney, and ureteral and bladder obstruction are some of the many conditions which can be diagnosed using sound waves.

renal biopsy Biopsy of the kidney may be performed at the time of surgery (open) or through the skin (percutaneous or closed). When the latter technique is used the patient lies in the prone position and, following local anesthesia of the overlying skin and muscles of the back, a biopsy needle is inserted with the aid of fluoroscopy or ultrasonography, and tissue is obtained.

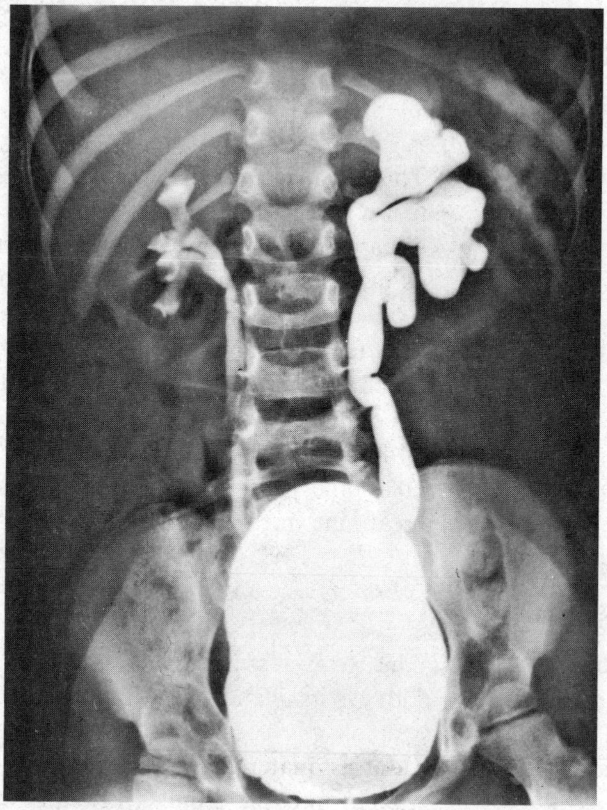

Figure 7-8 Voiding cystourethrogram. The urethra is not shown but note the swollen bladder and ureter (hydroureter), and hydronephrosis. This condition is due to an abnormality of the bladder causing vesicoureteral reflux of urine. (From James, A.E. Jr., and Squire, L.F.: Nuclear Radiology. Philadelphia, W.B. Saunders Co., 1973.)

angiography

Contrast material injected into the circulation fills arteries or veins of the kidney. Pictures of the filled blood vessels may then be taken by x-ray. Narrowing of the vessels, blood clots, cysts, and tumors can be detected.

CT scans

Transverse x-ray views of the kidney are taken and are useful in the diagnosis of tumors, cysts, abscesses, and hydronephrosis. Studies may be obtained in renal failure when contrast material should not be given.

radioisotope studies

Any one of various radioactive substances (isotopes) is injected into the bloodstream in small amounts and is taken up by the kidneys. Pictures show the size and shape of the kidney (**renal scan**), and its function (**renogram**). These studies can show size of kidney blood vessels, diagnose obstruction, and determine the separate function of each kidney.

renal transplantation

A kidney is transplanted into a patient with renal failure from an identical twin (isograft) or other individual (allograft). The kidney may come from a living related donor or a cadaver. Except in the case of identical twins, treatment with drugs to prevent rejection of the graft is necessary. See Figure 7-9.

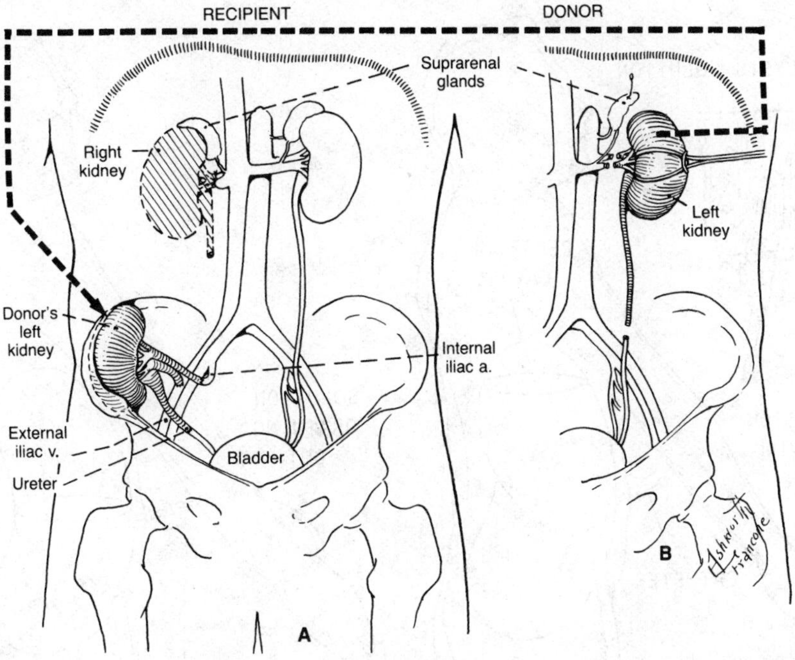

Figure 7-9 *A*, Kidney transplanted to right renal pelvis. *B*, Kidney of donor. (From Jacob, S.W., Francone, C.A., and Lossow, W.J.: Structure and Function in Man. 5th ed. Philadelphia, W.B. Saunders Co., 1982.)

dialysis

This procedure separates waste materials such as urea from the bloodstream when the kidneys can no longer function. There are two kinds of dialysis:

hemodialysis (HD)—using an artificial kidney machine which filters wastes from the patient's bloodstream.

peritoneal dialysis (PD)—using a peritoneal **catheter** (tube), fluid is introduced into the abdominal cavity. The presence of this fluid causes wastes circulating in the peritoneal blood vessels to pass out of the bloodstream and into the fluid. The fluid is then removed, and with it the wastes are removed as well. Peritoneal dialysis may be performed intermittently (IPD) with the aid of a mechanical apparatus or continuously by the patient without artificial support. The latter technique is known as continuous ambulatory peritoneal dialysis (CAPD). See Figure 7-10.

Abbreviations

ADH	Antidiuretic hormone; vasopressin
BUN	Blood urea nitrogen
CAPD	Continuous ambulatory peritoneal dialysis
CRF	Chronic renal failure
Cl^-	Chloride; an electrolyte excreted by the kidney
CMG	Cystometrogram; study of the ability of the bladder to contract
Cysto	Cystoscopic examination
IVP	Intravenous pyelogram
HCO_3^-	Bicarbonate; an electrolyte conserved by the kidney
HD	Hemodialysis
K^+	Potassium; an electrolyte
KUB	Kidney, ureter, and bladder

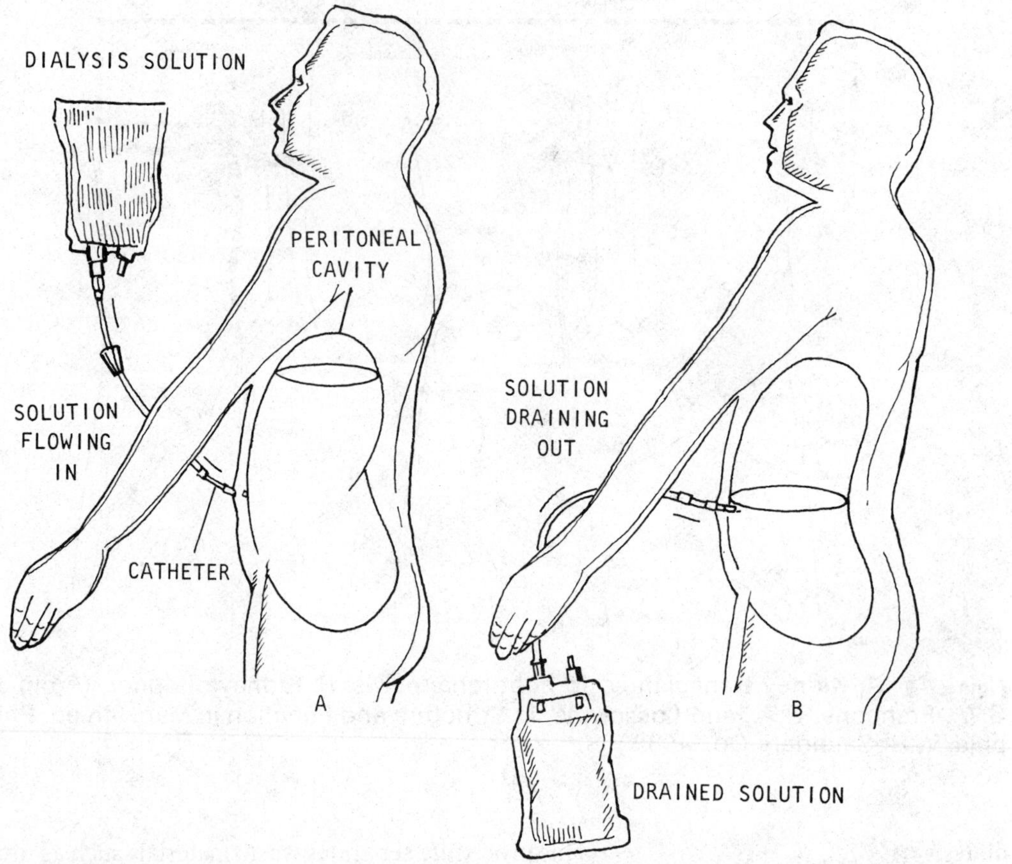

Figure 7-10 Continuous ambulatory peritoneal dialysis (CAPD). *A*, The dialysis solution (dialysate) flows from a collapsible plastic bag through a catheter into the patient's peritoneal cavity. The empty bag is folded and inserted into undergarments. *B*, After 4 to 8 hours, the bag is unfolded, and the fluid is allowed to drain into it by gravity. The full bag is discarded and a new bag of fresh dialysate is attached.

Na^+	Sodium; an electrolyte	RP	Retrograde pyelogram
PD	Peritoneal dialysis	U/A	Urinalysis
pH	Symbol for degree of acidity or alkalinity	UTI	Urinary tract infection
PKU	Phenylketonuria	VCU	Voiding cystourethrogram

XI. PRACTICAL APPLICATIONS

Diagnostic Radiology Report: Urethrogram

Retrograde urethrogram: A scout [first-look film before dye is injected] and single postinjection film of the pelvis demonstrate no significant soft-tissue abnormalities on the preliminary examination and there is no evidence of prostatic [the prostate gland is at the base of the bladder on either side of the urethra] calculi. After injection, there is good distention [stretching out] of the membranous urethra [the male urethra has three sections:

prostatic, membranous, and penile], with marked attenuation [narrowing] of the prostatic urethra and significant irregular elevation of the vesical floor.

Summary of a Clinical Medical Paper: Percutaneous Removal of Kidney Stones*

We have performed percutaneous extractions of renal pelvic stones in 15 patients with the use of the Wolf percutaneous universal nephroscope. At one session, with the patient under general anesthesia, a percutaneous tract is dilated to 24 F [indicates the size of the catheter used to dilate the tract], and the stone is immediately removed. Fifteen stones have been removed successfully by ultrasonic lithotripsy [crushing of stones], basket retrieval, use of a forceps [two-bladed instrument with handle, used for grasping or clamping], or a combination of these techniques. Average operating time has been 1 hour and the mean [average] hospitalization time 4 days. The advantages of this technique are that a skin incision of only 1 or 2 cm is required to remove the stone, hospital days are fewer than with open procedures, and postoperative morbidity [condition of being diseased or sick] is minimal. In selected situations, this method represents a significant advance over standard open surgical procedures for removal of renal pelvic stones.

*by Segura, J.W., et al. Mayo Clinic Proceedings, *57*:615–619, 1982. Used with permission.

X. EXERCISES

A. Give the meaning of the following:

1. nephrorrhaphy ____________________
2. glomerulonephritis ____________________
3. nephrosis ____________________
4. renal ectopia ____________________
5. nephrolithiasis ____________________
6. pyeloplasty ____________________
7. nephrectomy ____________________
8. bilateral cortical renal necrosis ____________________

   ____
9. renal hyperplasia ____________________

10. ureterosigmoidostomy ______________________________

____

B. Build medical terms:

1. Condition (abnormal) of water in the kidney ______________________________
2. Bursting forth of blood from the kidney ______________________________
3. Incision of the urinary bladder ______________________________
4. Enlargement of the kidney ______________________________
5. Painful urination ______________________________
6. Pus in the urine ______________________________
7. Dilation of the renal pelvis ______________________________
8. Condition of hardening (or arteries) in the kidney ______________________________
9. Fixation of the kidney ______________________________
10. Removal of the urethra ______________________________
11. Inflammation of the trigone ______________________________
12. Incision of the meatus ______________________________

C. Give the meaning of the following terms:

1. hypoproteinemia ______________________________
2. albuminuria ______________________________
3. renal calculi ______________________________
4. essential hypertension ______________________________
5. uremia ______________________________
6. hematuria ______________________________
7. pyelonephritis ______________________________

8. micturition ______

9. Wilms' tumor ______

10. caliectasis ______

11. polydipsia ______

12. phenylketonuria ______

13. casts ______

14. ketonuria ______

15. Bowman's capsule ______

16. dialysis ______

______

17. renal ischemia ______

18. oliguria ______

19. specific gravity of urine ______

______

D. *Give the names of the major structures that are involved in the urinary process from the point at which blood enters the glomerulus from the renal arterioles in the cortex of the kidney:*

1. *glomerulus*
2. ______
3. ______
4. ______
5. ______
6. ______
7. ______
8. ______

E. *Give the meaning of the following combining forms:*

1. noct/i ______
2. albumin/o ______
3. vesic/o ______
4. cortic/o ______

5. cali/o ____________ 8. azot/o ____________

6. pyel/o ____________ 9. olig/o ____________

7. py/o ____________ 10. cyst/o ____________

F. *Match the following pathological conditions with their descriptions below:*

hypernephroma	glomerulonephritis
nephrotic syndrome	hydronephrosis
diabetes mellitus	diabetes insipidus
renal calculi	urinary incontinence
secondary hypertension	urinary retention

1. Inflammation of tiny balls of capillaries in cortex of kidney ____________
2. Excessive amount of protein in the urine; edema; associated with kidney disease or other conditions ____________
3. Kidney stones ____________
4. Disorder characterized by inadequate secretion of insulin; hyperglycemia; glycosuria ____________
5. Excess fluid build-up in kidney ____________
6. High blood pressure due to kidney ailment ____________
7. Inadequate secretion of ADH; polyuria; polydipsia ____________
8. Inability to hold urine in the body ____________
9. Renal carcinoma in adults ____________
10. Blockage of passage of urine from the bladder ____________

G. *Tell what the following tests or procedures mean:*

1. KUB ____________
2. RP ____________
3. BUN ____________

4. VCU ______________________________

5. IVP ______________________________

6. Renal biopsy ______________________________

7. Creatinine clearance test ______________________________

8. Renal ultrasonogram ______________________________

9. Cysto ______________________________

10. pH ______________________________

11. CAPD ______________________________

12. Renal scan ______________________________

H. *What is the difference between hemodialysis and peritoneal dialysis?*

____

____

____

ANSWERS

A.

1. Suture of the kidney.
2. Inflammation of the glomerulus of the kidney.
3. Abnormal condition of the kidney; characterized by degeneration of renal tubules, edema, and albuminuria.
4. Displacement of the kidney.
5. Kidney stones.
6. Surgical repair of the renal pelvis.
7. Removal of the kidney.
8. Death of the cortex region in both kidneys.
9. Excessive development, or growth, of the kidney(s).
10. New opening (anastomosis) between the ureter and the sigmoid colon.

B.

1. hydronephrosis
2. nephrorrhagia
3. cystotomy
4. nephromegaly
5. dysuria
6. pyuria
7. pyelectasis
8. nephrosclerosis
9. nephropexy
10. urethrectomy
11. trigonitis
12. meatotomy

C.

1. Deficient protein in the blood; common in glomerulonephritis.
2. Albumin (protein) in the urine.
3. Stones in the kidney.
4. High blood pressure due to no apparent cause.
5. Higher than normal levels of urea in the blood.
6. Blood in the urine.
7. Inflammation of the renal pelvis.
8. Urination.
9. Malignant tumor of the kidney, occurring in childhood.
10. Dilation of the calyces of the renal pelvis.
11. Excessive thirst.
12. Phenylketones in the urine.
13. Molds of the renal tubules; they are found in the urine and named for the substance of which they are composed.
14. Acetone or ketone bodies in the urine.
15. Capsule under each glomerulus; collects filtered materials from the blood.
16. Literally means "complete separation"—it is a method of removing the toxic materials from the blood, must commonly done in renal failure.
17. Deficiency of blood flow to renal cells; isch- means to hold back.
18. Scanty urine flow.
19. A comparison of the density of urine with that of water.

D.

1. glomerulus
2. Bowman's capsule
3. renal tubules
4. renal pelvis
5. ureter
6. urinary bladder
7. urethra
8. urinary meatus

E.

1. night
2. albumin; a blood protein
3. urinary bladder
4. cortex (outer section)
5. calyces
6. renal pelvis
7. pus
8. urea, nitrogen
9. scanty
10. urinary bladder

F.

1. glomerulonephritis
2. nephrotic syndrome
3. renal calculi
4. diabetes mellitus
5. hydronephrosis
6. secondary hypertension
7. diabetes insipidus
8. urinary incontinence
9. hypernephroma
10. urinary retention

G.

1. X-ray of the kidneys, ureters, and bladder; no dye used.
2. Retrograde pyelogram; dye is injected via catheter into ureters and x-rays are taken of the urinary tract.
3. Blood urea nitrogen; blood test to measure the amount of urea in the blood.
4. Voiding cystourethrogram; x-ray of the bladder and urethra is taken while the patient is voiding.
5. Intravenous pyelogram; dye is injected into a vein and x-rays are taken of the kidney.
6. Living tissue is removed from the kidney and the microscopic examination is made.
7. Measurement of the amount of creatinine in blood and urine.
8. Record of sound waves as they bounce off the kidneys.
9. Visual examination of the urinary bladder with cystoscope.
10. Symbol for degree of the acidity or alkalinity of the urine.
11. Continuous ambulatory peritoneal dialysis.
12. Radioactive substance is injected and picture shows size and shape of the kidney.

H.

Hemodialysis is the use of a kidney machine to filter wastes from the bloodstream. Peritoneal dialysis involves filling the peritoneal cavity with a special fluid (using an abdominal catheter), which, when removed, carries with it nitrogenous wastes that the kidney would normally excrete in the urine.

XI. PRONUNCIATION OF TERMS

abscess	ĂB-sĕs
albuminuria	ăl-bū-mĭ-NŪ-rē-ă
anuria	ă-NŪ-rē-ă
bacteriuria	băk-tē-rē-Ū-rē-ă
calculus	KĂL-kū-lŭs
caliectasis	kā-lē-ĔK-tă-sĭs
calyx; calyces	KĀ-lĭks; KĂL-ĭ-sēz
cortical	KŎR-tĭ-kăl
creatinine	krē-ĂT-ĭ-nēn
cystoscopy	sĭs-TŎS-kō-pē
cystourethrogram	sĭs-tō-ū-RĒ-thrō-grăm
diuresis	dī-ū-RĒ-sĭs
dysuria	dĭs-Ū-rē-ă
edema	ĕ-DĒ-mă
electrolyte	ē-LĔK-trō-līt
enuresis	ĕn-ū-RĒ-sĭs
glomerular	glō-MĔR-ū-lăr
glomerulonephritis	glō-mĕr-ū-lō-nĕ-FRĪ-tĭs
glomerulus	glō-MĔR-ū-lŭs
glycosuria	glī-kō-SŪ-rē-ă
hematuria	hĕm-ă-TŪ-rē-ă
hilum	HĪ-lŭm
hydronephrosis	hī-drō-nĕ-FRŌ-sĭs
hypernephroma	hī-pĕr-nĕ-FRŌ-mă
incontinence	ĭn-KŎN-tĭ-nĕns
insipidus	ĭn-SĬP-ĭ-dŭs
interstitial nephritis	ĭn-tĕr-STĬ-shŭl nĕ-FRĪ-tĭs
ischemia	ĭs-KĒ-mē-ă
ketonuria	kē-tō-NŪ-rē-ă
meatal	mē-Ā-tăl

meatotomy	mē-ă-TŎT-ō-mē
meatus	mē-Ā-tŭs
medulla	mĕ-DŬL-ă or mĕ-DŪL-ă
medullary	MĔD-ū-lăr-ē
mellitus	MĔL-ĭ-tŭs or mĕl-LĒ-tŭs
micturition	mĭk-tū-RĬSH-ŭn
nephrohypertrophy	nĕf-tō-hī-PER-trō-fē
nephrolithiasis	nĕf-rō-lĭ-THĪ-ă-sĭs
nephrolithotomy	nĕf-rō-lĭ-THŎT-ō-mē
nephroptosis	nĕf-rŏp-TŌ-sĭs
nephrorrhaphy	nĕf-RŎR-ă-fē
nephrosclerosis	nĕf-rō-sklĕ-RŌ-sĭs
nephrotic	nĕ-FRŎT-ĭk
nephrotomography	nĕf-rō-tō-MŎG-ră-fē
nitrogenous	nī-TRŎJ-ĕ-nŭs
nocturia	nŏk-TŪ-rē-ă
oliguria	ŏl-ĭ-GŪ-rē-ă
perivesical	pĕ-rē-VĔS-ĭ-kăl
phenylketonuria	fē-nĭl-kē-tō-NŪ-rē-ă or fĕn-ĭl-kē-tō-NŪ-rē-ă
polydipsia	pŏl-ē-DĬP-sē-ă
polyuria	pŏl-ē-Ū-rē-ă
pyelogram	PĪ-ĕ-lō-grăm
pyelonephritis	pī-ĕ-lō-nĕ-FRĪ-tĭs
pyeloplasty	PĪ-ĕ-lō-plăs-tē
pyelostomy	pī-ĕ-LŎS-tō-mē
pyuria	pī-Ū-rē-ă
renin	RĒ-nĭn
trigone	TRĪ-gōn
trigonitis	trī-gō-NĪ-tĭs
urea	ū-RĒ-ă
uremia	ū-RĒ-mē-ă
ureter	ū-RĒ-tĕr

ureteral	ū-RĒ-tĕr-ăl
ureterectomy	ū-rē-tĕr-ĔK-tō-mē
ureterocele	ū-RĒ-tĕr-ō-sēl
ureteroileostomy	ū-rē-tĕr-ō-ĭl-ē-ŎS-tō-mē
urethra	ū-RĒ-thră
urethroscopy	ū-rē-THRŎS-kō-pē
vesicorectal	vĕs-ĭ-kō-RĔK-tăl

REVIEW SHEET 7

Combining Forms

albumin/o	______________	necr/o	______________
azot/o	______________	nephr/o	______________
bacteri/o	______________	noct/i	______________
cali/o	______________	olig/o	______________
cortic/o	______________	py/o	______________
cyst/o	______________	pyel/o	______________
dips/o	______________	ren/o	______________
glomerul/o	______________	tox/o	______________
glyc/o	______________	ur/o	______________
glycos/o	______________	ureter/o	______________
hydr/o	______________	urethr/o	______________
medull/o	______________	vesic/o	______________

Suffixes

-cele ____________________

-ectasis ____________________

-lithiasis ____________________

-lithotomy ____________________

-lysis ____________________

-megaly ____________________

-ole ____________________

-pexy ____________________

-ptosis ____________________

-rrhaphy ____________________

-rrhea ____________________

-rrhexis ____________________

-sclerosis ____________________

-spasm ____________________

-stomy ____________________

-tomy ____________________

-ule ____________________

-uria ____________________

Prefixes

a-, an- ____________________

anti- ____________________

dia- ____________________

dys- ____________________

en- ____________________

poly- ____________________

retro- ____________________

Match the urinary system structure in Column I with its location or function in Column II:

Column I

1. urethra
2. cortex
3. Bowman's capsule
4. calyces
5. renal pelvis
6. glomerulus
7. medulla
8. renal tubules
9. urinary bladder
10. ureters

Column II

______ Tiny structure surrounding each glomerulus; receives filtered materials from blood.

______ Tubes carrying urine from kidney to urinary bladder.

______ Tubules leading from Bowman's capsule. Urine is formed there as water, sugar, and salts are reabsorbed into the bloodstream.

______ Inner (middle) region of the kidney.

______ Muscular sac which serves as a reservoir for urine.

______ Cuplike divisions of the renal pelvis which receive urine from the renal tubules.

______ Tube carrying urine from the bladder to the outside of the body.

______ Central urine-collecting basin in the kidney which narrows into the ureter.

______ Collection of capillaries through which materials from the blood are filtered into Bowman's capsule.

______ Outer region of the kidney.

Additional Terms

Use this list of terms as a test of your knowledge by **checking off** the ones you can define and **circling** the ones you do not understand. Use the page references provided to find the definitions of the circled terms. Writing down the meanings of the terms you do not know will help you remember them.

acetone (157)

albumin (157)

antidiuretic hormone (155)

BUN (161)

cast (157)

creatinine (151)

creatinine clearance test (161)

diabetes insipidus (160)

diabetes mellitus (160)

edema (159)

electrolyte (151)

enuresis (155)

essential hypertension (159)

hemodialysis (163)

hilum (151)

hypernephroma (160)

interstitial nephritis (159)

intravenous pyelogram (161)

ketone bodies (157)

KUB (161)

meatus (151)

micturition (151)

nephrotic syndrome (159)

nitrogenous waste (152)

peritoneal dialysis (163)

pH (157)

phenylketonuria (158)

polycystic kidney (160)

renal hypertension (159)

renal scan (162)

renal transplantation (162)

renin (153)

renogram (162)

retrograde pyelogram (161)

secondary hypertension (159)

specific gravity of urine (157)

stricture (160)

trigone (153)

urea (153)

uric acid (153)

urinary catheter (153)

urinary incontinence (160)

urinary retention (160)

voiding (153)

Wilms' tumor (160)

CHAPTER 8

FEMALE REPRODUCTIVE SYSTEM

In this chapter you will:

- Name the organs of the female reproductive system, their locations, and combining forms;
- Explain how these organs and their hormones function in the processes of menstruation and pregnancy;
- Identify abnormal conditions of the female reproductive system and of the newborn child; and
- Explain some important laboratory tests, clinical procedures, and abbreviations related to gynecology and obstetrics.

The chapter is divided into the following sections:

I. INTRODUCTION

Sexual reproduction is the union of the female sex cell (**ovum**) and the male sex cell (**sperm**) which results in the creation of a new individual. The ovum and sperm cell are specialized cells differing primarily from normal body cells in one important way. Each sex cell (also called a **gamete**) contains exactly half the number of chromosomes that a normal body cell contains. When the ovum and sperm cell unite, the cell produced receives half of its genetic material from its female parent, and half from its male parent; thus it contains a full, normal complement of hereditary material.

Gametes are produced in special organs called **gonads** in the male and female. The female gonads are the **ovaries**, and the male gonads are the **testes**. An ovum, after leaving the ovary, travels down a duct (**uterine** or **fallopian tube**) leading to the **uterus** (womb). If **coitus** (copulation, sexual intercourse) has occurred, and sperm cells are present in the uterine tube, union of the ovum and sperm may take place. This union is called **fertilization**. The **embryo** (called the **fetus** after the second month) then begins a 9-month period of development (**gestation, pregnancy**) within the uterus.

The female reproductive system consists of organs that produce **ova** and provide a place for the growth of the embryo. In addition, the female reproductive organs supply important hormones that contribute to the development of female secondary sex characteristics (body hair, breast development, structural changes in bones and fat).

Ova are produced by the ovary from the onset of **puberty** (beginning of the fertile period when secondary sex characteristics develop) to **menopause** (cessation of fertility and diminishing of hormone production). If fertilization occurs at any time during the years between puberty and menopause, the fertilized egg may grow and develop within the uterus. Various hormones are secreted from the ovary and from a blood-vessel-filled organ (**placenta**) that grows in the wall of the uterus during pregnancy. If fertilization does not occur, hormone changes result in the shedding of the uterine lining, and bleeding, or **menstruation**, occurs.

The names of the hormones from the ovaries that play important roles in the processes of menstruation and pregnancy, and in the development of secondary sex characteristics, are **estrogen** and **progesterone**. Other hormones that govern the functions of the ovary, breast, and uterus are secreted by the **pituitary gland**, which is located behind the bridge of the nose in the anterior portion of the brain.

Gynecology is the study of the female reproductive system (organs, hormones, and diseases); **obstetrics** (obstetrix means midwife) is a specialty concerned with pregnancy and delivery of the fetus; and **neonatology** is the study and treatment of the newborn child.

II. MAJOR ORGANS OF THE FEMALE REPRODUCTIVE SYSTEM

Uterus, Ovaries, and Associated Organs

Figures 8-1 and 8-3 should be labeled as you read and study the following paragraphs.

Figure 8-1 is a lateral view of the female reproductive organs and shows their relationship to the other organs in the pelvic cavity. The **ovaries** (1) (only one ovary is shown in this lateral view) are a pair of small almond-shaped organs located in the lower abdomen. The **uterine tubes** (2) (only one is shown in this view) lead from each ovary to the **uterus** (3), which is a muscular organ situated between the urinary bladder and the rectum. The uterus is normally in a position of **anteflexion** (bent forward). Midway between the uterus and the rectum is a region in the abdominal cavity known as the **cul-de-sac** (4). This region is often examined for the presence of cancerous growths.

The **vagina** (5) is a muscular tube extending from the uterus to the exterior of the body. **Bartholin's glands** (6) are two small, rounded glands on either side of the vaginal orifice. These glands produce a mucous secretion which lubricates the vagina. The **clitoris** (7) is an organ of sensitive, erectile tissue located anterior to the vaginal orifice and in front of the urethral meatus. The clitoris is similar in structure to the penis in the male.

The region between the vaginal orifice and the anus is called the **perineum** (8). This region, at the floor of the pelvic cavity, may be torn in childbirth, resulting in damage to the urinary meatus and the anus. To avoid a perineal tear, the obstetrician often cuts the perineum before delivery. This incision is called an **episiotomy**.

The external genitalia (organs of reproduction) of the female are collectively called the **vulva**. Figure 8-2 shows the various structures that are part of the vulva. The **labia majora** are the outer lips of the vagina and the **labia minora** are the smaller, inner lips. The **hymen** is a mucous membrane which normally partially covers the entrance to the vagina. The clitoris and Bartholin's glands are also parts of the vulva.

Figure 8-3 is an anterior view of the female reproductive system. The **ovaries** (1) are held in place on either side of the uterus by **ligaments** (2) and are protected by a surrounding mass of fat.

Within each ovary are thousands of small sacs called **graafian follicles** (3). Each graafian follicle contains an **ovum** (4). When an ovum is mature, the graafian follicle ruptures to the surface and the ovum leaves the ovary. The release of the ovum from the ovary is called

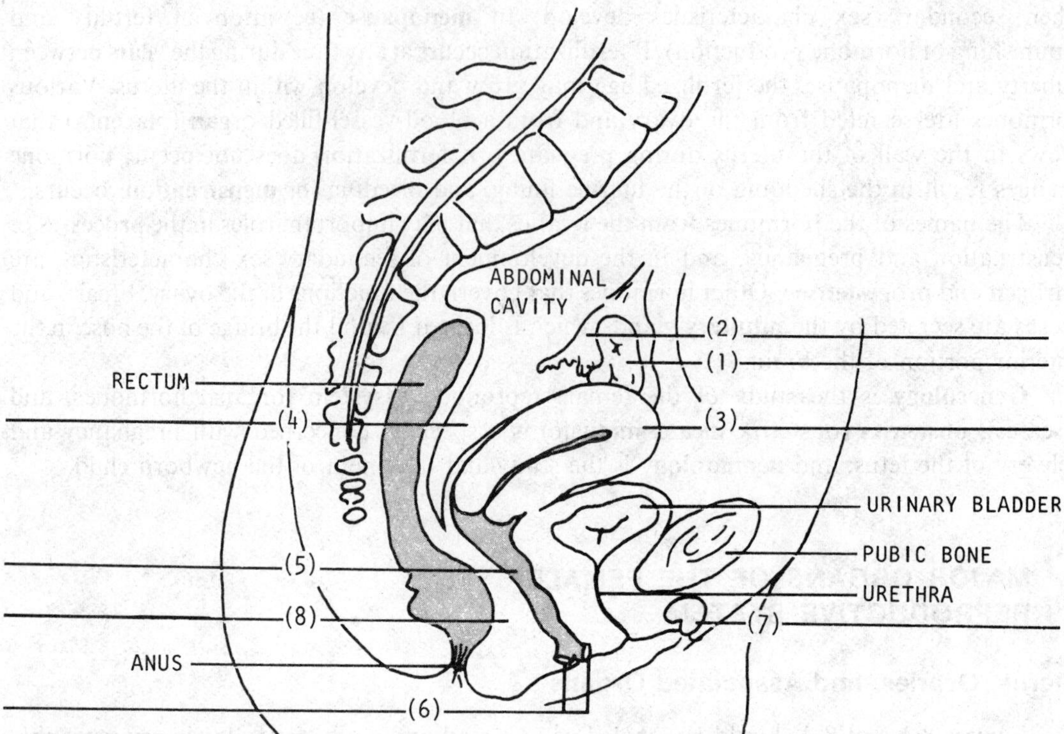

Figure 8-1 Organs of the female reproductive system, lateral view.

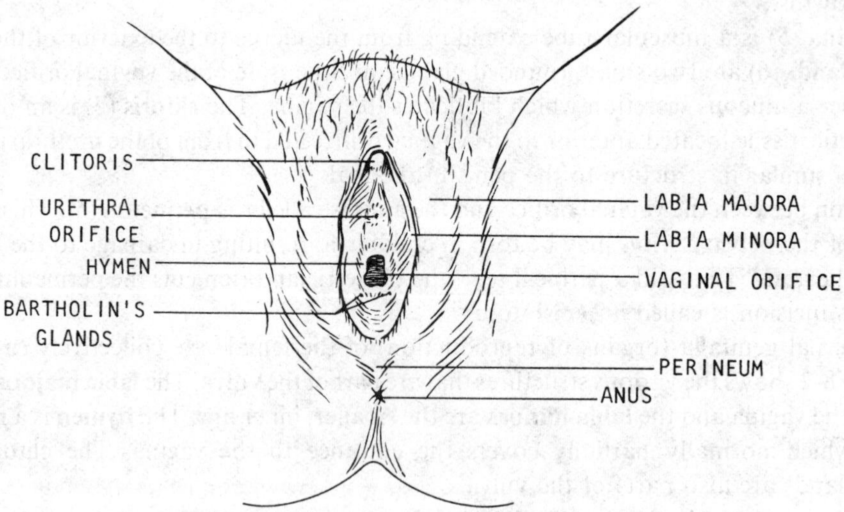

Figure 8-2 External female genitalia (vulva).

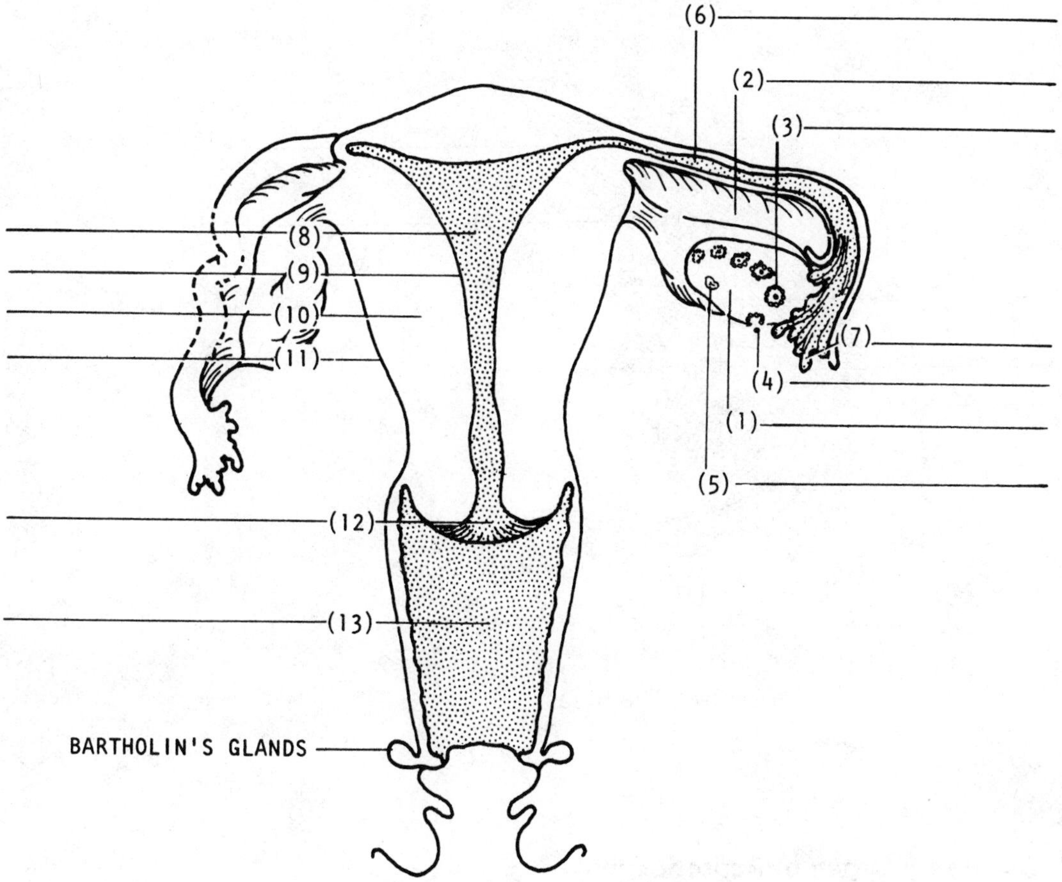

Figure 8–3 Organs of the female reproductive system, anterior view.

ovulation. The ruptured follicle fills first with blood, and then with a yellow fatlike material. It is then called the **corpus luteum** (5) (meaning "yellow body").

Near each ovary is a duct, about 5½ inches long, called a **uterine** or **fallopian tube** (6). Collectively, the uterine tubes and ovaries are called the **adnexa** (accessory structures) of the uterus. The egg, after its release from the ovary, is caught up by the finger-like ends of the uterine tube. These ends are called **fimbriae** (7). The tube itself is lined with small hairs which, through their motion, sweep the ovum along. It usually takes the ovum about 5 days to pass through the uterine tube.

It is within the uterine tube that fertilization takes place if any sperm cells are present. If coitus takes place near the time of ovulation and no contraception is used, there is a likelihood that sperm cells will be in the uterine tube when the egg cell is passing through. If coitus has not taken place, the ovum remains unfertilized and, after a day or two, disintegrates.

The uterine tubes, one on either side, lead into the **uterus** (8), a pear-shaped organ with muscular walls and a mucous membrane lining filled with a rich supply of blood vessels. The rounded upper portion of the uterus is called the **fundus**, while the larger, central section is the **corpus** (body of the organ). The specialized epithelial mucosa of the uterus is called the **endometrium** (9); the middle, muscular layer is the **myometrium** (10); and the outer, membranous tissue layer is the **perimetrium** (11).

The narrow, lower portion of the uterus is called the **cervix** (12) (meaning "neck"). The cervical opening leads into a 3-inch-long tube called the **vagina** (13), which opens to the outside of the body.

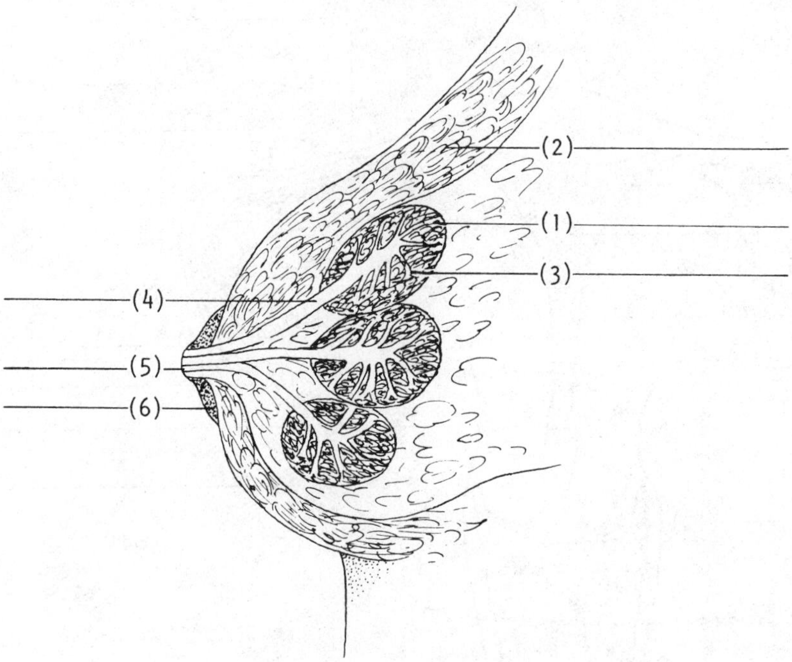

Figure 8-4 The breast.

The Breast (Accessory Organ of Reproduction)

Label Figure 8-4 as you read the following description of breast structures.

The breasts are two **mammary** (milk-producing) **glands** located in the upper anterior region of the chest. They are composed of **glandular tissue** (1) which develops in response to hormones from the ovaries during puberty. The breasts also contain **fatty tissue** (2), special **lactiferous** (milk-carrying) **ducts** (3), and **sinuses** (cavities) (4) which carry milk to the opening, or nipple. The breast nipple is called the **mammary papilla** (5), and the dark-pigmented area around the mammary papilla is called the **areola** (6).

During pregnancy, the hormones from the ovaries and the placenta stimulate glandular tissue in the breasts to their full development. After **parturition** (giving birth), hormones from the pituitary gland stimulate the production of milk (**lactation**).

III. TERMINOLOGY OF MENSTRUATION AND PREGNANCY

Menstrual Cycle

The beginning of menstruation at the time of puberty is called **menarche**. Each menstrual cycle is divided into 28 days. These days can be grouped into four time periods, which are useful in describing the events of the cycle. The time periods are:

Days 1–5 (Menstrual Period) These are the days during which bloody fluid containing disintegrated endometrial cells, glandular secretions, and blood cells is discharged through the vagina.

Days 6–13 (Postmenstrual Period)

After the menstrual period is ended, the lining of the uterus begins to repair itself as the hormone estrogen is released by the maturing graafian follicle in the ovaries. This is also the period of the growth of the ovum in the graafian follicle.

Days 13–14 (Ovulatory Period)

On about the 14th day of the cycle, the graafian follicle ruptures (**ovulation**) and the egg leaves the ovary to travel slowly down the uterine tube.

Days 15–28 (Premenstrual Period)

The empty graafian follicle fills with a yellow material and becomes known as the **corpus luteum**. The corpus luteum functions as an endocrine organ and secretes two hormones, **estrogen** and **progesterone**, into the bloodstream. These hormones stimulate the building up of the lining of the uterus in anticipation of fertilization of the egg and pregnancy.

If fertilization does **not** occur, the corpus luteum in the ovary stops producing progesterone and estrogen and regresses. The fall in levels of progesterone and estrogen leads to the breakdown of the uterine endometrium and a new menstrual cycle begins (days 1–5).

Figure 8-5 illustrates the menstrual cycle.

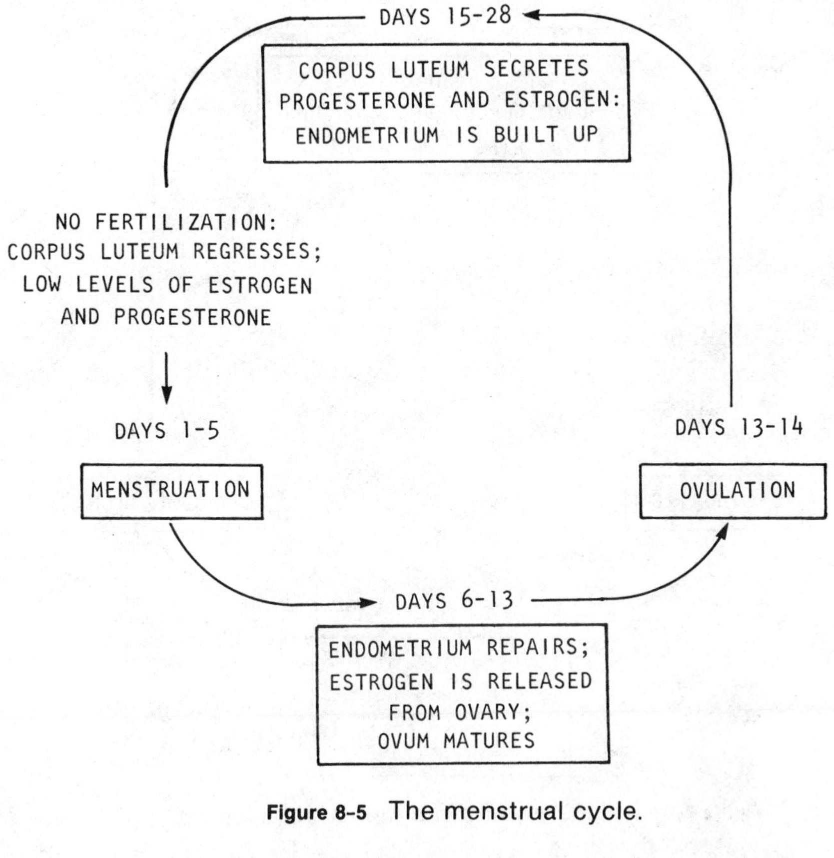

Figure 8-5 The menstrual cycle.

Pregnancy

If fertilization does occur in the uterine tube, the fertilized egg travels to the uterus and implants in the uterine endometrium. The corpus luteum in the ovary continues to produce progesterone and estrogen, which support the vascular and muscular development of the uterine lining.

The **placenta**, which is the organ of communication between the mother and embryo, now forms within the uterine wall. The placenta is derived from maternal endometrium and partly from the **chorion**, the outermost membrane which surrounds the developing embryo. The **amnion** is the innermost of the embryonic membranes, and it holds the fetus suspended in an amniotic cavity surrounded by a fluid called the **amniotic fluid**. The amnion and fluid are sometimes known as the "bag of water" which breaks to signal the onset of labor.

At no time during gestation do the maternal blood and fetal blood mix, but important nutrients, oxygen, and wastes are exchanged as the blood vessels of the baby (coming from the umbilical cord) lie side by side with the mother's blood vessels in the placenta.

The placenta, also known as the "after-birth" because it becomes detached from the uterus

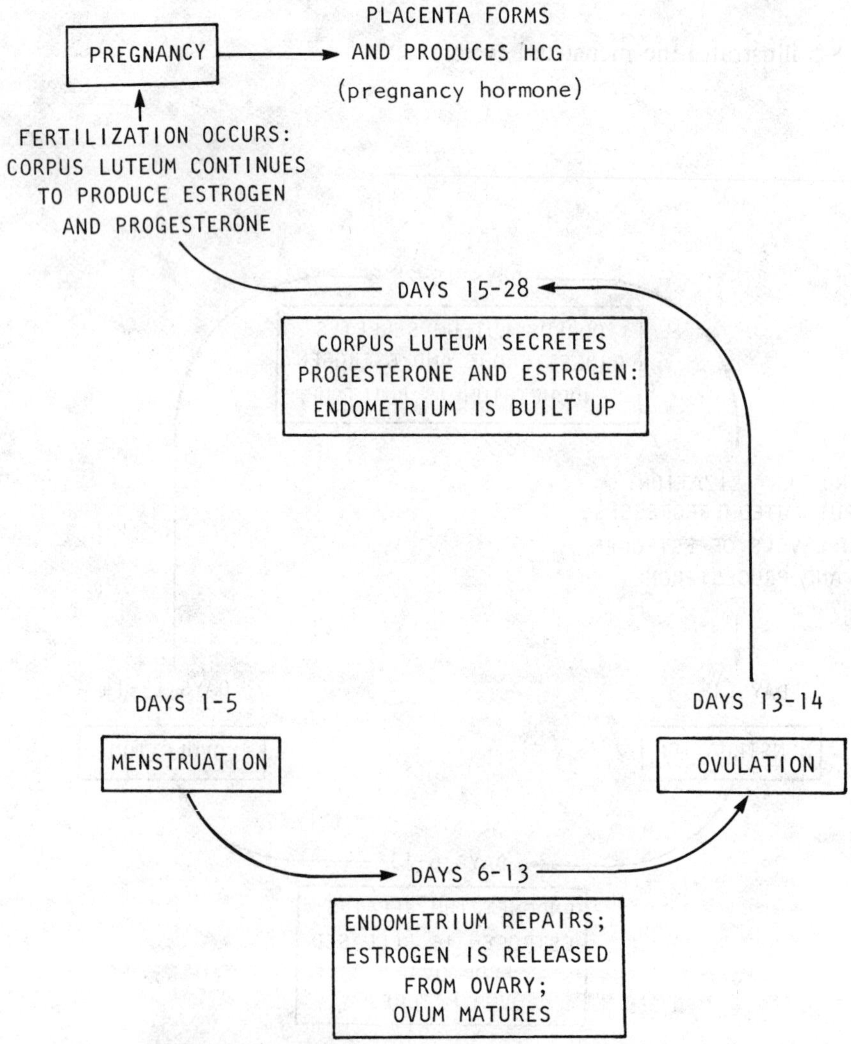

Figure 8-6 Pregnancy and the menstrual cycle.

after delivery, produces its own hormone as it develops in the uterus. This hormone is called **human chorionic gonadotropin (HCG)**. HCG stimulates the corpus luteum to continue producing hormones until about the third month of pregnancy, when the placenta itself takes over the endocrine function and releases estrogen and progesterone. HCG is the hormone tested for in the urine of women who suspect that they are pregnant. Figure 8-6 reviews the events that occur if the menstrual cycle is interrupted by pregnancy.

Figure 8-7 shows the embryo, its placenta, and the membranes that surround it as it develops in the uterus.

IV. HORMONAL INTERACTIONS

The events of menstruation and pregnancy are dependent not only upon hormones from the ovary (estrogen and progesterone) but also on hormones from the pituitary gland. These pituitary gland hormones are **follicle-stimulating hormone (FSH)** and **luteinizing hormone (LH)**. After the onset of menstruation, the pituitary gland begins to secrete FSH and LH, so that

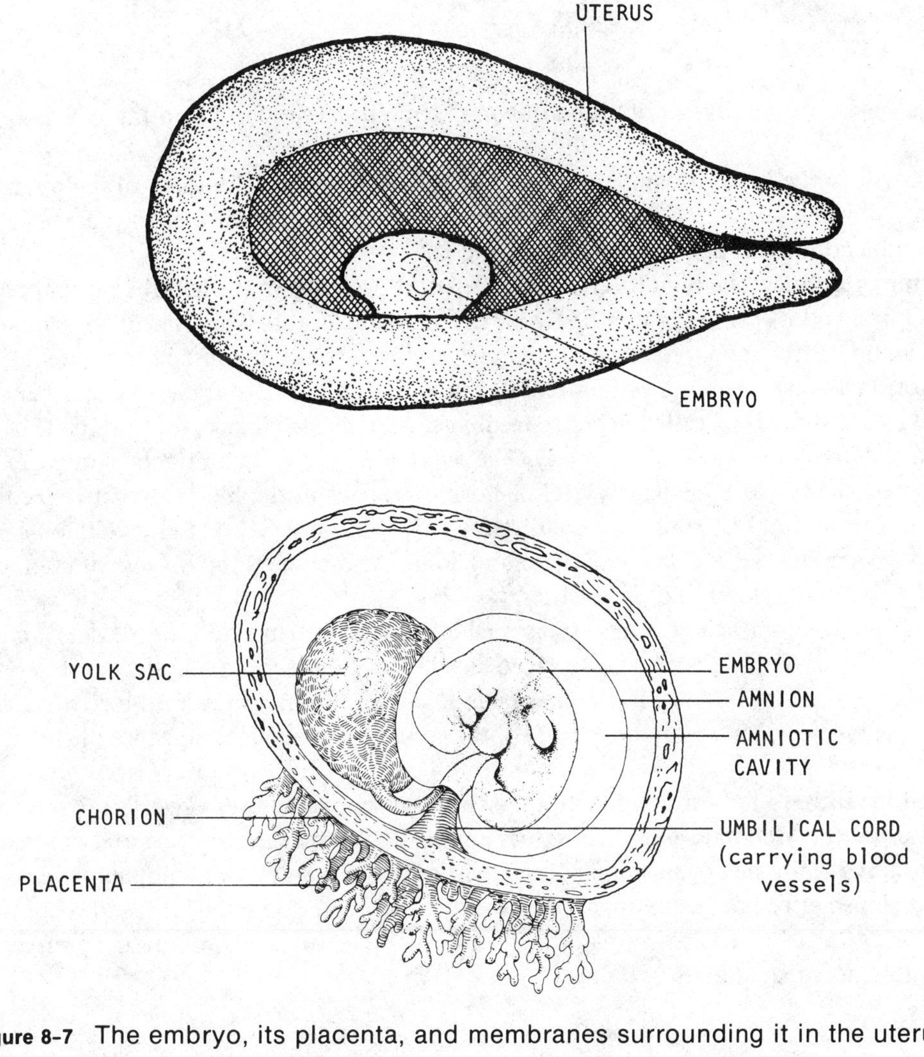

Figure 8-7 The embryo, its placenta, and membranes surrounding it in the uterus.

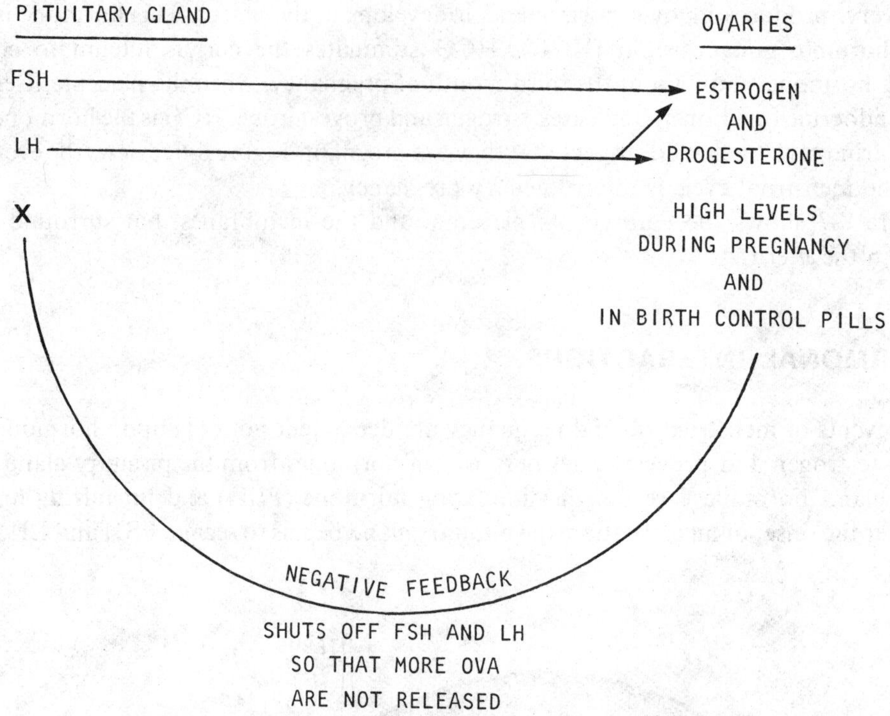

Figure 8-8 Hormonal interactions between the pituitary gland and the ovaries.

their levels rise in the bloodstream. FSH and LH stimulate the development of the ovum and ovulation. After ovulation, LH in particular influences the maintenance of the corpus luteum and its production of estrogen and progesterone.

During pregnancy, the high levels of estrogen and progesterone affect the pituitary gland itself by shutting off its production of FSH and LH. This means that while a woman is pregnant, new eggs do not mature and ovulation cannot occur. This hormonal interaction wherein a high level of hormones (estrogen and progesterone) acts to **shut off** the production of another set of hormones (FSH and LH) is called **negative feedback**. Negative feedback is the principle behind the action of birth control pills on the body. The pills contain varying amounts of estrogen and progesterone. As they are taken, the level of hormones rises in the blood. Negative feedback occurs, and the pituitary does not release FSH or LH. Without FSH or LH, ovulation cannot occur and a woman does not become pregnant. Figure 8-8 reviews the hormonal interaction between the pituitary gland and the ovaries.

Other female contraceptive measures include the **IUD** (intrauterine device) and the **diaphragm**. The IUD is a small coil placed inside the uterus by a physician. It prevents implantation of the fertilized egg in the uterine lining. The diaphragm is a rubber, cup-shaped device inserted, before coitus, on the outside of the cervix to prevent the entrance of sperm into the uterus.

When the secretion of estrogen from the ovaries lessens and fewer egg cells are produced, menopause begins. **Menopause** is the gradual ending of the menstrual cycle and is a natural process resulting from the normal aging of the ovaries. Other names for menopause are change of life and climacteric. Premature menopause occurs before age 35, while delayed menopause occurs after age 58. Artificial menopause can occur if the ovaries are removed by surgery or made nonfunctional by radiation therapy.

V. VOCABULARY

adnexa	Accessory parts of an organ. The adnexa uteri (ovaries and uterine tubes) are the accessory parts of the uterus.
amnion	Innermost membrane around the developing embryo.
areola	Dark-pigmented area around the breast nipple.
anteflexion	Bending forward; the uterus is normally anteflexed.
Bartholin's glands	Small exocrine glands at the vaginal orifice.
cervix	Lower, necklike portion of the uterus.
chorion	Outermost layer of the two membranes surrounding the embryo.
clitoris	Organ of sensitive erectile tissue anterior to the urinary meatus.
coitus	Sexual intercourse; copulation.
corpus luteum	Empty graafian follicle, after release of the egg cell.
cul-de-sac	Region of the abdomen, midway between the rectum and the uterus.
embryo	Stage in development from fertilization of the ovum through the second month of pregnancy.
endometrium	The inner mucous membrane lining the uterus.
estrogen	Hormone produced by the ovaries; responsible for female secondary sex characteristics and buildup of the uterine lining during the menstrual cycle.
fallopian tubes	Uterine tubes.
fertilization	Union of the sperm and ovum.
fetus	The embryo from the third month to birth.
fimbriae	Finger-like ends of the fallopian tubes.
follicle-stimulating hormone (FSH)	Hormone produced by the pituitary gland; stimulates maturation of the ovum.
gamete	Sex cell; sperm or ovum.
genitalia	Reproductive organs; also called genitals.

gestation	Pregnancy.
gonads	Organs in the male and female that produce gametes; ovaries and testes.
graafian follicle	Sac within the ovary; contains the ovum.
human chorionic gonadotropin (HCG)	Hormone produced by the placenta to sustain pregnancy.
hymen	Mucous membrane partially or completely covering the vaginal orifice.
labia	Lips of the vagina; labia majora are the larger, outermost lips and labia minora are the smaller, innermost lips.
luteinizing hormone (LH)	Hormone produced by the pituitary gland; promotes ovulation.
menarche	The beginning of the first menstrual period during puberty.
menopause	The gradual ending of menstrual function.
menstruation	The monthly shedding of the uterine lining; menses means month.
myometrium	The muscle layer lining the uterus.
orifice	An opening.
ovaries	Organs in the female lower abdomen that produce ova and hormones; female gonads.
ovulation	Release of the ovum from the ovary.
ovum; ova	Egg cell; female gamete.
papilla	Nipple.
parturition	Act of giving birth.
perimetrium	The membrane surrounding the uterus.
perineum	In females, the area between the anus and vagina.
placenta	Vascular organ that develops during pregnancy in the uterine wall and serves as a communication between the maternal and fetal blood streams.
progesterone	Hormone produced by the corpus luteum in the ovary.
puberty	Beginning of the fertile period when gametes are produced and secondary sex characteristics appear.

uterine tubes — Ducts through which the egg travels into the uterus from the ovary; also called fallopian tubes or oviducts.

uterus — Womb; muscular organ in which the embryo develops. The upper portion is the fundus; the middle portion is the corpus; and the lower, neck portion is the cervix.

vagina — A tube extending from the uterus to the exterior of the body.

vulva — External genitalia of the female; includes the labia, perineum, hymen, and clitoris.

VI. COMBINING FORMS AND TERMINOLOGY

Combining Form	*Meaning*	*Terminology*	*Meaning*
oophor/o	ovary	oophorectomy	________
		oophoropexy	________
oo/o	egg	oocyte	________
ovari/o	ovary	ovarian	________
ov/o	egg	ovulate	________
		ovum	________
salping/o	uterine tubes, oviducts, fallopian tubes	salpingo-oophorectomy	________
-salpinx *(as a suffix)*	uterine tubes	pyosalpinx	________
		hematosalpinx	________
		hydrosalpinx	________
hyster/o	uterus, womb	hysterectomy *Abdominal: removal through abdominal wall; vaginal: removal through vagina.*	________
		hysterosalpingo-oophorectomy	________

		panhysterectomy ________
		Cervix is removed as well; total hysterectomy.
uter/o	uterus	uterovesical ________
metr/o, metri/o	uterus	metrorrhagia ________
		Intermenstrual.
		endometriosis ________
		See pathological conditions.
		parametrium ________
		Connective tissue around the uterus.
my/o	muscle	myometrium ________
myom/o	muscle tumor	myomectomy ________
cervic/o	cervix, neck	cervicitis ________
bartholin/o	Bartholin's glands	bartholinitis ________
vagin/o	vagina	vaginal ________
		vaginitis ________
colp/o	vagina	colporrhaphy ________
		colposcope ________
culd/o	cul-de-sac	culdoscopy ________
perine/o	perineum	colpoperineoplasty ________
		________
episi/o	vulva	episiotomy ________
vulv/o	vulva, external genitalia	vulvectomy ________
		vulvovaginitis ________
men/o	menses, menstruation	amenorrhea ________
		dysmenorrhea ________

		menorrhagia ______________________
		Hypermenorrhea.
		oligomenorrhea ______________________
		polymenorrhea ______________________
		Menstrual periods occur more frequently than normal.
chori/o	chorion	choriogenesis ______________________
amni/o	amnion	amniocentesis ______________________
		amniotic fluid ______________________
mamm/o	breast	mammary ______________________
		mammoplasty ______________________
		Reduction and augmentation operations.
mast/o	breast	mastectomy ______________________
gynec/o	woman, female	gynecomastia ______________________
		This condition is found in males.
lact/o	milk	lactation ______________________
galact/o	milk	galactorrhea ______________________
nat/i	birth	neonatal ______________________
gravid/o	pregnancy	gravida ______________________
		primigravida ______________________
		Gravida I; primi means first.
-para	to bear, bring forth, live births	primipara ______________________
		Para I.
-tocia	labor, birth	dystocia ______________________
		eutocia ______________________
-cyesis	pregnancy	pseudocyesis ______________________

-version	to turn	cephalic version ______________
		The change in position of the fetus may occur naturally or may be done mechanically by the physician during delivery.
		Presentation is the manner in which the fetus appears to the examiner during delivery. A breech presentation is buttocks first; cephalic presentation is head first.
-arche	beginning	menarche ______________
dys-	painful	dyspareunia ______________
		Pareunia means sexual intercourse.
in-	into, inward	involution of the uterus ______________
		Retrograde changes occur in the uterus so that it shrinks to its former nonpregnant size. Vol- means to roll.
intra-	within	intrauterine ______________
nulli-	none	nulliparous ______________
		Para 0. Figure 8-9 shows the cervix of a nulliparous woman and the cervix of a parous woman.
multi-	many	multipara ______________
		Para II, III, IV, etc.
		multigravida ______________
		Grav. II, III, IV, etc.

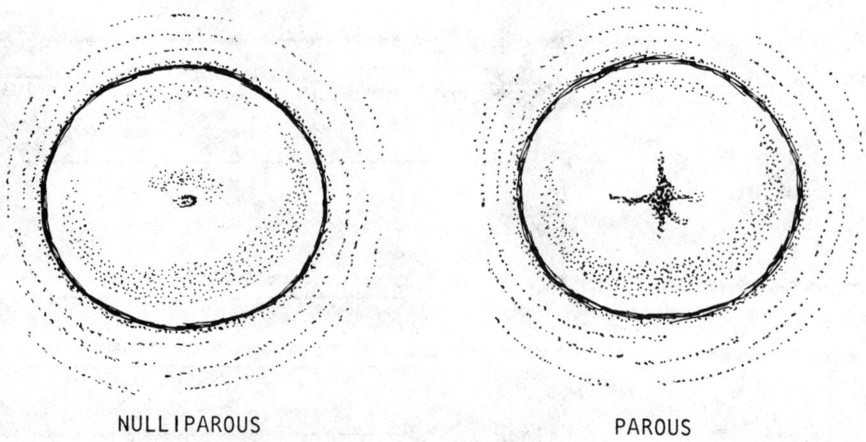

Figure 8-9 The cervix of a nulliparous woman and the cervix of a parous woman.

VII. PATHOLOGICAL CONDITIONS

Gynecological and Obstetrical

endocervicitis Inflammation of the inner lining of the cervix.

The lining of the cervix is not renewed each month as is the uterine lining during menstruation. **Cervical erosions**, or ulcers, appear as raw, red patches on the cervical mucosa. **Leukorrhea** (discharge of white or yellow mucoid substance) is a symptom of cervical erosion.

After excluding the presence of malignancy (by cervical biopsy or cytological test), **cryocauterization** (destroying tissue by freezing) of the eroded area and treatment with antibiotics may be indicated.

endometriosis Endometrial tissue in abnormal locations, including the ovaries, cul-de-sac, pelvic peritoneum, and small intestine.

Endometriosis can be associated with dysmenorrhea, pelvic pain, infertility (inability to become pregnant), and dyspareunia. Most cases of endometriosis probably develop as a result of retrograde passage of bits of menstrual endometrium through the lumen (opening) of the uterine tube into the peritoneal cavity. Treatment ranges from symptomatic relief of pain to surgical removal of endometrial implants.

ectopic pregnancy Pregnancy which is not in the uterus.

Ninety-five per cent of ectopic pregnancies occur in the uterine tubes, in which case the condition is called **tubal pregnancy**. Rupture of the placenta and its detachment from the wall of the tube, with massive hematosalpinx, may occur. Surgery is indicated to remove the implant and preserve the uterine tube before rupture occurs.

choriocarcinoma Malignant tumor of the pregnant uterus.

The tumor may appear following pregnancy or abortion. Cure is possible with surgery and chemotherapy.

eclampsia Disorder during pregnancy or shortly after; marked by high blood pressure, proteinuria, edema, convulsions, and coma. Also called **toxemia**.

abruptio placentae Premature separation of the normally implanted placenta.

placenta previa Displaced placenta; implanted in the lower region of the uterine wall.

ovarian cysts Collections of fluid within a sac (cyst) in the ovary.

Cystadenoma and **cystadenocarcinoma** are both types of cystic tumors of the ovary. Resection of such cysts is advisable because it is difficult to distinguish between benign and malignant tumors without pathological examination.

ovarian carcinoma

Malignant tumor of the ovary (**adenocarcinoma**). It may be cystic (see above) or solid in consistency.

About 18 per cent of gynecologic neoplasms are ovarian carcinomas, most often occurring in women over 50 years of age. The tumor is usually discovered in an advanced stage as an abdominal mass; it may produce few symptoms in its early stages. In most patients, the disease metastasizes within or beyond the pelvic region before diagnosis. Surgery (oophorectomy and salpingectomy), radiotherapy, and, more important, chemotherapy are used as therapeutic measures.

fibrocystic disease of the breast

Small sacs of tissue and fluid in the breast; **chronic cystic mastitis**.

This is a benign condition and a common disease condition of the female breast. The patient notices a nodular (lumpy) consistency of the breast, often associated with premenstrual tenderness and engorgement, or fullness. At times, mammography and then surgical biopsy may be indicated to differentiate fibrocystic disease from carcinoma of the breast.

breast carcinoma

Malignant tumor of the breast.

This tumor may spread to the skin, chest wall, and commonly to the lymph nodes located in the axilla (armpit) adjacent to the affected breast. From the lymph nodes it may spread to any of the other body organs, including bone, liver, lung, or brain. The tumor is usually removed for purposes of diagnosis and as a primary means of treatment.

There are two objectives in the surgical treatment of breast cancer: first, to remove the tumor, and second, to sample the axillary lymph nodes to determine if the tumor has spread beyond the breast. Various operations may be performed to accomplish these objectives. For small primary tumors the lump may be removed (**lumpectomy**), with the remainder of the breast left intact. This operation is usually followed by radiation therapy to the breast to kill remaining tumor cells. Alternatively, the surgeon may remove the entire breast (**simple** or **total mastectomy**). With either of these operations a separate incision is made to remove axillary lymph nodes to determine whether spread beyond the breast has taken place. Another surgical procedure is removal of the breast, lymph nodes, and adjacent chest wall muscles (pectorals) in a single procedure called a **radical mastectomy**. It is important to sample lymph nodes to determine if metastasis is present. If additional tumor is found in the axillary nodes, the patient can then be treated with drugs (chemotherapy) and cure is possible.

It is also important to test the tumor for the presence of **estrogen receptors**. These receptors are proteins that indicate that the tumor will respond to hormone therapy. If metastases should subsequently develop, this information will be valuable in selecting further treatment.

pelvic inflammatory disease (PID)

Inflammation in the pelvic region.

This general condition is usually used to refer to **salpingitis**, but many physicians use it to include other problems, such as cervicitis, endometritis, and oophoritis. Symptoms are vaginal discharge, pain in the abdomen (LLQ and RLQ) in early stages, and dysmenorrhea, metrorrhagia, and severe tenderness on **palpation** (examining by touch) of the cervix and adnexa. Etiology is commonly gonococcal infection, although nongonococcal PID occurs as well. An intrauterine device is the most common iatrogenic cause of PID. Antibiotics are used in treatment.

fibroids — Benign tumors in the uterus.

Fibroids (also called leiomyomas or leiomyomata) are composed of fibrous tissue and muscle. If they grow too large and cause symptoms such as metrorrhagia, pelvic pain, or menorrhagia, hysterectomy or myomectomy is indicated.

carcinoma of the cervix — Malignant tumor of the cervix.

Carcinoma of the cervix ranks third in frequency (after breast and skin cancers) of the malignant diseases affecting women. Neoplastic changes in the cervix vary from **minimal cervical dysplasia** (abnormal cell growth in the lower third of the cervical epithelium) to **carcinoma in situ** (localized cancer growth). The tumor can metastasize to lymph nodes and other pelvic organs. The Papanicolaou test (**Pap test**) detects early cervical neoplasia by microscopic examination of cells scraped off the cervical epithelium. Cold-knife **conization** (biopsy is taken by excising a cone of tissue) is used to diagnose and treat **in situ** disease.

endometrial carcinoma — Malignant tumor of the uterus.

The major symptom of adenocarcinoma of the uterus is postmenopausal bleeding. **Dilation** (opening the cervical canal) and **curettage** (scraping off the lining of the uterus) is the best method for diagnosing the disease. Invasive tumors of the uterus are treated either by surgical removal or by irradiation.

Neonatal

The following terms describe a few of the conditions or symptoms which may affect the newborn. The **Apgar score** is a system of scoring an infant's physical condition 1 minute after birth. Heart rate, respiration, color, muscle tone, and response to stimuli are rated 0, 1, or 2. Maximal total score is 10. Infants with low Apgar scores require prompt medical attention.

erythroblastosis fetalis — Hemolytic disease due to Rh incompatibility between the mother and fetus.

kernicterus — Serious condition involving jaundice, brain damage, and mental retardation.

Bilirubin accumulates in the blood as a result of excessive hemolysis of red blood cells.

hydrocephalus — Accumulation of fluid in the spaces of the brain.

In an infant the entire head can enlarge because the bones of the skull are never completely fused together at birth. The soft spot, normally present between the cranial bones of the fetus, is called a **fontanelle**.

hyaline membrane disease — Respiratory problem primarily in the premature newborn; lack of protein in the air sacs of the lungs causes collapse of the lungs.

This condition is also called respiratory distress syndrome.

pylorospasm — Contractions of the muscle at the opening between the stomach and the duodenum.

Surgical repair of the pyloric orifice may be necessary.

meconium — First feces of the newborn; greenish black to light brown.

The Greek word "mekonion" means poppy juice.

Down's syndrome — Chromosomal abnormality which leads to mental retardation, Oriental appearance of the eyes, low-set ears, and generally dwarfed physique.

VIII. CLINICAL TESTS, PROCEDURES, AND ABBREVIATIONS

Clinical Tests

Pap test — The physician, after inserting a vaginal speculum (instrument to hold apart the vaginal walls), uses a spatula to scrape the cervix. See Figure 8-10. Microscopic analysis of the cell smear (spread on a glass slide) can detect the presence of cervical or vaginal carcinoma.

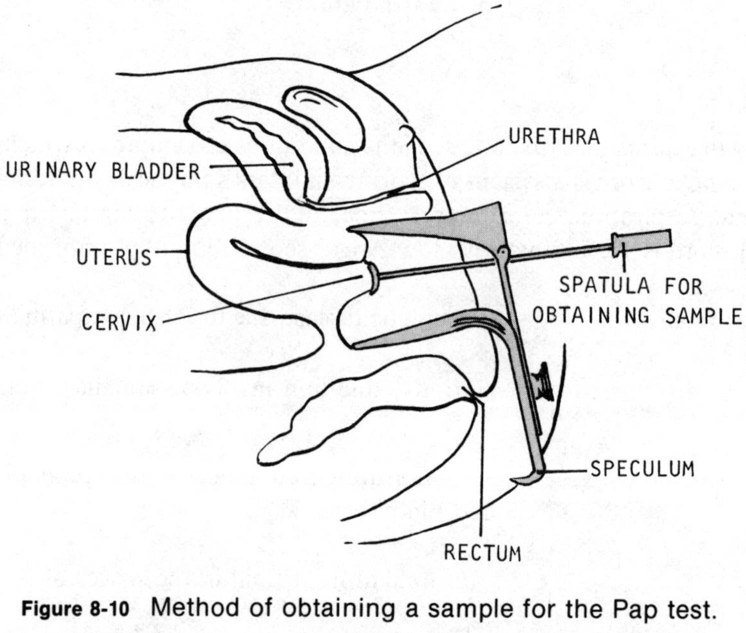

Figure 8-10 Method of obtaining a sample for the Pap test.

pregnancy test — This test detects the presence of **HCG** in the urine or blood. The slide test is done with a sample of the patient's urine which reacts with a prepared substance on a glass slide. Animal tests involve injecting a patient's urine or blood into female mice or rabbits and noting changes in the animal's ovaries.

Procedures

abortion — This is the premature termination of pregnancy before the embryo or fetus is able to exist on its own. Three major methods for abortion are used: (1) vaginal evacuation by **D & C** (dilation and curettage) or vacuum aspiration (suction); (2) stimulation of uterine contractions by saline (salt) injected into the amniotic cavity (second trimester); and (3) hysterotomy.

amniocentesis — Surgical puncture (transabdominal) of the amniotic sac to withdraw amniotic fluid for analysis. The cells of the fetus, found in the fluid, are cultured (grown) and cytological and biochemical studies are made.

aspiration — Fluid is withdrawn from a cavity or sac by means of a needle. Aspiration cytology is a valuable technique for the evaluation of a patient with breast disease.

cesarean section — Removal of the fetus by abdominal incision into the uterus. Julius Caesar is said to have been born in this way.

chorion villus biopsy — A new test to detect birth defects. It can be done earlier than amniocentesis (8 weeks into the pregnancy rather than the 16th week). Cells removed from the chorion by a tube inserted into the cervix under the guidance of ultrasound are tested for chromosomal abnormalities and biochemical disorders.

conization — Removal of a cone of tissue from the mouth of the cervix.

cryosurgery (cryocauterization) — Using cold temperatures to destroy tissue. The cold is usually produced by a probe containing liquid nitrogen.

dilation (dilatation) and curettage — **Dilation** (widening) of the cervical opening is accomplished by inserting a series of probes of increasing size. **Curettage** (scraping) is accomplished by using a curette (metal loop at the end of a long, thin handle) to remove the lining of the uterus. See Figure 8-11.

exenteration — Removal of internal organs. Pelvic exenteration is the removal of the uterus, ovaries, uterine tubes, vagina, bladder, rectum, and lymph nodes.

fetal monitoring — Recording of the fetal heart rate from an electrode placed on the fetal head (through the maternal vagina) and monitoring uterine contractions by an intrauterine catheter placed across the cervix.

pelvimetry — Clinical and x-ray measurements of the proportions and dimensions of the hip (pelvic bone) to help determine whether or not it will be possible to deliver a fetus through the normal route.

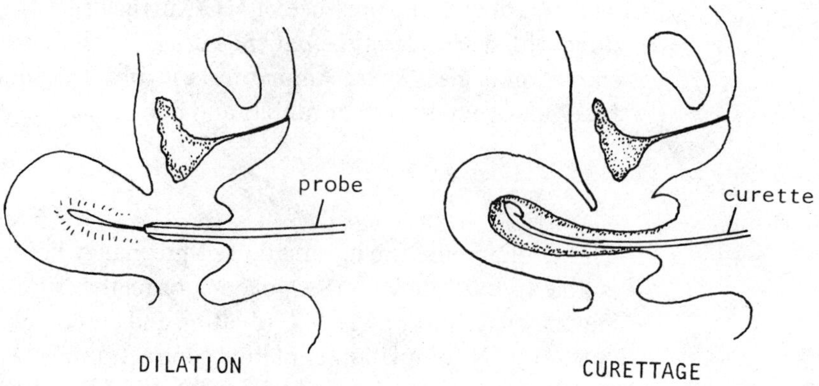

Figure 8-11 Dilation and curettage.

tubal ligation

This sterilization procedure involves cutting and ligating (tying off) the uterine tubes so that ova and sperm cannot unite. A laparoscope is inserted through the abdominal wall and the uterine tubes can be sealed off by means of high-frequency sparks (fulguration).

Abbreviations

C-section	Cesarean section
CS	Cesarean section
D & C	Dilation and curettage
DES	Diethylstilbestrol; an estrogen compound used in the treatment of menopausal problems involving estrogen deficiency. If administered during pregnancy, it has been found to be related to subsequent tumors in the daughters (rarely in sons) of mothers so treated
DUB	Dysfunctional uterine bleeding
FHT	Fetal heart tones
FSH	Follicle-stimulating hormone
Gyn	Gynecology
HCG	Human chorionic gonadotropin
HSG	Hysterosalpingography
IUD	Intrauterine device
LH	Luteinizing hormone
LMP	Last menstrual period
MH	Marital history
NB	Newborn
OB	Obstetrics
Path	Pathology
PID	Pelvic inflammatory disease
PU	Pregnancy urine
UC	Uterine contractions

IX. PRACTICAL APPLICATIONS

Operating Schedule: General Hospital

Operation	*Anesthesia*
Right breast biopsy—possible right simple mastectomy	General
D and C, cold conization of the cervix	General
Total vaginal hysterectomy	General
D and C, laparoscopy with possible laparotomy	General
Total abdominal hysterectomy and left salpingo-oophorectomy	General
Exploratory laparotomy for uterine myomectomy	General
Excision two breast tumors, right, frozen sections, no mastectomy	General

Operative Report. Preoperative Diagnosis: Menorrhagia, Leiomyomata

Anesthetic: General

Material forwarded to laboratory for examination:

A. endocervical curettings

B. endometrial curettings

Operation performed: Dilation and curettage of the uterus

With the patient in the dorsal lithotomy position [legs are flexed on the thighs, thighs flexed on the abdomen and abducted] and sterilely prepped and draped, manual examination of the uterus revealed it to be 6 to 8 week size, retroflexed; no adnexal masses noted. The anterior lip of the cervix was then grasped with a tenaculum [hooklike surgical instrument for grasping and holding parts]. The cervix was dilated up to a #20 Hank's dilator. The uterus was sounded [widened] up to 4 inches. A sharp curettage of the endocervix showed only a scant amount of tissue. Using a sharp curettage the uterus was curetted in a clockwise fashion with an irregularity noted in the posterior floor. A large amount of hyperplastic endometrial tissue was removed. The patient tolerated the procedure well.

Operative diagnosis: leiomyomata uteri

Sentences Using Medical Terminology

1. Tubal patency [patent means open] may be evaluated by a hysterosalpingogram or direct instillation [drop-by-drop administration] of dye at laparoscopy.

2. Persistent vaginal bleeding during the second half of pregnancy indicates the need for placental localization by ultrasonography. Clinically, it is not always easy to differentiate placenta previa from abruptio placentae, but when a woman has massive uterine bleeding, clinical judgment alone dictates immediate cesarean section or vaginal delivery.

3. There is no question that exogenous estrogens can cause endometrial hyperplasia, which may be a premalignant lesion.

X. EXERCISES

A. Build medical words:

1. Muscular layer of the uterus ______________________
2. Rupture of the uterus ______________________
3. Fixation of an ovary ______________________
4. Suture of the area between the anus and vagina ______________________
5. Excessive bleeding during menses ______________________
6. Presence of endometrial tissue in nonuterine sites ______________________
7. Inflammation of uterine tubes (both sides) ______________________
8. Pus in the uterine tubes ______________________
9. Removal of the uterus through the vagina ______________________
10. Suture of the vagina and the vulva ______________________
11. Incision of the cervix ______________________
12. Normal delivery or labor ______________________
13. Inflammation of the breast ______________________
14. Pertaining to producing milk ______________________
15. False pregnancy ______________________
16. Beginning of the first menstrual period during puberty ______________________
17. Inflammation of the inner lining of the cervix ______________________
18. Scanty menstrual flow ______________________
19. Egg cell ______________________
20. New opening in the fallopian tubes ______________________

B. Give the meaning of the following:

1. D & C ______________________

2. graafian follicle ______________________________

3. para II ______________________________

4. PID ______________________________

5. fibroids ______________________________

6. LH ______________________________

7. grav. III ______________________________

8. panhysterectomy ______________________________

9. ectopic pregnancy ______________________________

10. FSH ______________________________

11. placenta ______________________________

12. estrogen ______________________________

13. HCG ______________________________

14. culdocentesis ______________________________

15. gonads ______________________________

16. radical mastectomy ______________________________

17. anteflexion ______________________________

18. areola ______________________________

19. gamete ______________________________

20. clitoris ______________________________

C. *Match the process with its correct meaning:*

1. parturition	______	Release of egg from ovary
2. micturition	______	Sexual intercourse
3. menopause	______	Monthly discharge of blood
4. fertilization	______	Prevention of pregnancy

5. ovulation	______	Urination
6. menstruation	______	Giving birth
7. lactation	______	Pregnancy
8. gestation	______	Producing milk
9. coitus	______	Gradual ending of menstrual function
10. contraception	______	Union of egg and sperm cells

D. *Match the structure with its location or description:*

1. fimbriae	______	Membrane covering vaginal orifice
2. Bartholin's glands	______	Innermost embryonic membrane
3. chorion	______	Lips of the vagina
4. corpus luteum	______	Fringelike processes surrounding the abdominal opening of each uterine tube
5. myometrium	______	Middle layer of uterine tissue
6. amnion	______	Region between rectum and uterus
7. perineum	______	Outermost embryonic membrane
8. cul-de-sac	______	Empty egg sac
9. hymen	______	Near the vaginal meatus; exocrine
10. labia	______	Area between the vulva and anus

E. *Supply the correct word part:*

1. Suture of the vagina: colp/o/ ______________.
2. Inflammation of the uterus with pus: ______________ /o/ ______________ itis.
3. Water in the fallopian tube: hydr/o/ ______________.
4. Inflammation of an ovary: ______________ itis.
5. Difficult labor: dys ______________.

6. Excessive growth of the uterine inner lining: endo ____________ al hyper ____________.

7. Removal of a muscle tumor: ____________ ectomy.

8. Woman who has borne no children: ____________ parous.

9. Woman who is undergoing first pregnancy: ____________ gravida.

10. Excessive bleeding between menstrual periods: ____________ /o/ ________.

F. *Supply the missing words. These are easy! Just spell them correctly!*

1. Doctor who delivers babies is called an ____________________________.
2. One who cares for newborns is called a ____________________________.
3. General term for reproductive organs is ____________________________.
4. Beginning of the fertile period in males and females is ____________________.
5. Another name for the womb is the ____________________________.
6. The embryo from the beginning of the third month on is called ____________.
7. Medical term for nipple is ____________________________.
8. Two ovarian hormones are ____________________ and ____________.
9. Two pituitary hormones which influence the ovaries and pregnancy are ____________________________ and ____________________.
10. High blood levels of ____________________ and ____________ cause the ____________________ gland to stop producing ____________ and ____________________. This negative feedback situation prevents the development of ova and ____________________ does not occur.
11. Accessory parts of the uterus are called ____________________________.
12. The external female genitalia are called the ____________________________.

G. *Match the pathological condition in Column I with a closely associated term in Column II:*

Column I		*Column II*
1. salpingitis	______	A. localized cancer growth
2. fibroids	______	B. nodular tissue; mastitis
3. cystadenoma	______	C. uterine tube inflammation
4. fibrocystic disease	______	D. leukorrhea; cervical erosions
5. endocervicitis	______	E. malignant ovarian neoplasm
6. endometrial carcinoma	______	F. adenocarcinoma of the uterus
7. carcinoma in situ	______	G. benign ovarian growth
8. cystadenocarcinoma	______	H. benign uterine growth

H. *Give the name of the test or procedure described below:*

1. Widening of the cervical opening and scraping the uterine lining ______________
2. Cells are taken from the cervix for microscopic examination ______________
3. Premature termination of pregnancy ______________
4. HCG is measured in the urine or blood ______________
5. Oviducts are cut and tied off ______________
6. Withdrawal of fluid from breast mass ______________
7. Fetus is delivered through an abdominal incision ______________
8. Surgical puncture to remove fluid from the sac around the fetus ______________
9. Using cold temperatures to kill tissue ______________
10. Removal of a segment of tissue from the cervix ______________
11. Removal of internal organs in hip region ______________

I. Give the meaning for the following abbreviations:

1. DUB ______________________________

2. HSG ______________________________

3. DES ______________________________

4. LMP ______________________________

J. Complete the following with the proper obstetrical or neonatal term:

1. Turning the fetus from one position to another is called ______________.

2. ______________ means excessive fluid in the head.

3. Measurements of the pelvic bone are called ______________.

4. ______________ is the manner in which the fetus appears to the examiner during delivery. ______________ indicates that the head appears first; ______________ indicates that the buttocks appears first.

5. Malignant tumor of the pregnant uterus ______________.

6. Soft spot between the newborn's cranial bones is the ______________.

7. When the placenta is misplanted in the lower portion of the uterus, the condition is called ______________.

8. The evaluation of the newborn's physical condition is called the ______________.

9. Toxemia of pregnancy involving proteinuria, hypertension, and edema is called ______________.

10. The first feces of the newborn are called ______________.

11. A serious respiratory condition involving collapse of air sacs in the newborn, premature infant is ______________.

12. Premature separation of the normally implanted placenta is called ________________________________.

ANSWERS

A.

1. myometrium
2. hysterorrhexis
3. oophoropexy
4. perineorrhaphy
5. menorrhagia
6. endometriosis
7. bilateral salpingitis
8. pyosalpinx
9. vaginal hysterectomy
10. colpoepisiorrhaphy
11. cervicotomy
12. eutocia
13. mastitis
14. lactogenic
15. pseudocyesis
16. menarche
17. endocervicitis
18. oligomenorrhea
19. oocyte; ovum
20. salpingostomy

B.

1. Dilation and curettage (scraping).
2. Sac in the ovary in which the ovum grows and matures.
3. Woman who has given birth to two live infants.
4. Pelvic inflammatory disease.
5. Benign tumors of the uterus (literally, resembling fibers).
6. **Luteinizing hormone**; produced by the pituitary gland; stimulates the graafian follicle (in the ovary) to rupture, which results in ovulation. (Also, this hormone stimulates the formation and continuation of the corpus luteum in the ovary.)
7. Woman who has had three pregnancies.
8. Removal of the uterus including the cervix.
9. Implantation of the embryo in a place other than uterine wall, e.g., uterine tubes, ovary, ligaments.
10. **Follicle-stimulating hormone**; produced by the pituitary gland; stimulates the ovaries to produce estrogen and the ovum to mature in the graafian follicle.
11. Vascular tissue in the uterus which provides the necessary communication between mother and fetus.
12. Hormone produced by the ovaries which is responsible for secondary sex characteristics and sustaining of the endometrium during pregnancy.
13. **Human chorionic gonadotropin**; a hormone produced by the placenta during pregnancy.
14. Surgical puncture of the cul-de-sac (the space between the rectum and the uterus).
15. Organs in the male and female which produce sex cells; ovaries and testes.
16. Removal of breast, pectoral muscles, and contents of the axilla for breast carcinoma.
17. Forward bending; the normal position of the uterus in the pelvic cavity.
18. Dark-pigmented area around the nipple of the breast.
19. Sperm or egg cell.
20. Sensitive, erectile tissue of the external female genitalia.

C.

5	1
9	8
6	7
10	3
2	4

D.

9	8
6	3
10	4
1	2
5	7

E.

1. colporrhaphy
2. pyometritis
3. hydrosalpinx
4. oophoritis
5. dystocia
6. endometrial hyperplasia
7. myomectomy
8. nulliparous
9. primigravida
10. metrorrhagia

F.

1. obstetrician
2. neonatologist or perinatologist
3. genitalia
4. puberty
5. uterus
6. fetus
7. papilla
8. estrogen and progesterone
9. follicle-stimulating hormone (FSH) and luteinizing hormone (LH)
10. estrogen and progesterone; pituitary; FSH and LH; ovulation or pregnancy
11. uterine adnexa
12. vulva

G.

1. C
2. H
3. G
4. B
5. D
6. F
7. A
8. E

H.

1. dilation and curettage
2. Pap test
3. abortion
4. pregnancy test
5. tubal ligation
6. aspiration cytology
7. cesarean section
8. amniocentesis
9. cryosurgery
10. conization
11. pelvic exenteration

I.

1. dysfunctional uterine bleeding
2. hysterosalpingogram
3. diethylstilbestrol
4. last menstrual period

J.

1. version
2. hydrocephalus
3. pelvimetry
4. presentation; cephalic; breech
5. choriocarcinoma
6. fontanelle
7. placenta previa
8. Apgar score
9. eclampsia
10. meconium
11. hyaline membrane disease
12. abruptio placentae

XI. PRONUNCIATION OF TERMS

abruptio placentae	ă-BRŬP-shē-ō plă-SĔN-tē
adnexa	ăd-NĔK-să
amenorrhea	ā-mĕn-ō-RĒ-ă
amnion	ĂM-nē-ŏn
areola	ă-RĒ-ō-lă
bartholinitis	băr-thō-lĭ-NĪ-tĭs
carcinoma in situ	kăr-sĭ-NŌ-mă ĭn-SĪ-tū
cervicitis	sĕr-vĭ-SĪ-tĭs
cesarean	sĕ-SĀ-rē-ăn
choriocarcinoma	kōr-ē-ō-kăr-sĭ-NŌ-mă

chorion	KŌ-rē-ŏn
clitoris	KLĬ-tō-rĭs
coitus	KŌ-ĭ-tŭs
colpoperineoplasty	kŏl-pō-pĕ-rĭ-NĒ-ō-plăs-tē
colporrhaphy	kŏl-PŎR-ă-fē
colposcope	KŎL-pō-skōp
conization	kō-nĭ-ZĀ-shŭn
corpus luteum	KŎR-pŭs LŪ-tē-ŭm
cryocauterization	krī-ō-kăw-tĕr-ĭ-ZĀ-shŭn
culdoscopy	kŭl-DŎS-kō-pē
curettage	kū-rĕ-TAZH
cystadenocarcinoma	sĭs-tăd-ē-nō-kăr-sĭ-NŌ-mă
cystadenoma	sĭs-tăd-ĕ-NŌ-mă
dilation	dĭ-LĀ-shŭn
dysmenorrhea	dĭs-mĕn-ō-RĒ-ă
dyspareunia	dĭs-pă-ROO-nē-ă
dystocia	dĭs-TŌ-sē-ă
eclampsia	ĕ-KLĂMP-sē-ă
endometriosis	ĕn-dō-mē-trē-Ō-sĭs
episiotomy	ĕ-pĭ-zē-ŎT-ō-mē
erythroblastosis fetalis	ĕ-rĭth-rō-blăs-TŌ-sis fē-TĂ-lĭs
eutocia	ū-TŌ-sē-ă
exenteration	ĕks-ĕn-tĕ-RĀ-shŭn
fibroids	FĪ-broydz
fimbriae	FĬM-brē-ē
fontanelle	fŏn-tă-NĔL
galactorrhea	gă-lăk-tō-RĒ-ă
gamete	GĂM-ēt
genitalia	jĕn-ĭ-TĀ-lē-ă
gestation	jĕs-TĀ-shŭn
gonad	GŌ-năd
gonadotropin	gō-năd-ō-TRŌ-pĭn

graafian follicle	GRĂF-ē-ăn FŎL-lĭ-k'l
gravida	GRĂV-ĭ-dă
gynecomastia	gī-nĕ-kō-MĂS-tē-ă or jĭ-nĕ-kō-MĂS-tē-ă
hematosalpinx	hĕm-ă-tō-SĂL-pĭnks
hydrocephalus	hī-drō-SĔF-ă-lŭs
hydrosalpinx	hī-drō-SĂL-pĭnks
hysterectomy	hĭs-tĕr-ĔK-tō-mē
hysterosalpingo-oophorectomy	hĭs-tĕr-ō-săl-pĭng-gō-ō-ŏf-ō-RĔK-tō-mē or hĭs-tĕr-ō-săl-pĭng-gō-ō-ō-fō-RĔK-tō-mē
kernicterus	kĕr-NĬK-tĕr-ŭs
labia	LĀ-bē-ă
lactation	lăk-TĀ-shŭn
leukorrhea	lo͞o-kō-RĒ-ă
luteinizing	LŪ-tē-ĭ-nī-zing
mammoplasty	MĂM-ō-plăs-tē
meconium	mĕ-KŌ-nē-ŭm
menarche	mĕ-NĂR-kē
menorrhagia	mĕn-ō-RĂ-jă
menstruation	mĕn-stro͞o-Ā-shŭn
metrorrhagia	mĕt-rō-RĂ-ja
multigravida	mŭl-tē-GRĂV-ĭ-dă
multipara	mŭl-TĬP-ă-ră
myomectomy	mī-ō-MĔK-tō-mē
myometrium	mī-ō-MĒ-trē-ŭm
nulliparous	nŭ-LĬP-ă-rŭs
oligomenorrhea	ŏl-ĭ-gō-mĕn-ō-RĒ-ă
oocyte	Ō-ō-sīt
oophorectomy	ō-ŏf-ō-RĔK-tō-mē or oo-fō-RĔK-tō-mē or ō-ō-fō-RĔK-tō-mē
oophoropexy	ō-ŎF-ō-rō-pĕk-sē
orifice	ŎR-ĭ-fĭs
ovarian	ō-VĀ-rē-ăn
ovulate	Ō-vū-lāt
palpation	păl-PĀ-shŭn

papilla	pă-PĬL-ă
parturition	păr-tū-RĬSH-ŭn
pelvimetry	pĕl-VĬM-ĕ-trē
perimetrium	pĕ-rĭ-MĒ-trē-ŭm
perineum	pĕ-rĭ-NĒ-ŭm
placenta	plă-SĔN-tă
placenta previa	plă-SĔN-tă PRĒ-vē-ă
primigravida	prī-mĭ-GRĂV-ĭ-dă
primipara	prī-MĬP-ă-ră
progesterone	prō-JĔS-tĕ-rōn
pseudocyesis	soo͞-dō-sī-Ē-sĭs
pyosalpinx	pī-ō-SĂL-pĭnks
salpingitis	săl-pĭn-JĪ-tĭs
salpingo-oophorectomy	săl-pĭng-gō-ō-ŏf-ō-RĔK-tō-mē or săl-pĭng-gō-ō-ō-fō-RĔK-tō-mē
vaginitis	vă-jĭ-NĪ-tĭs
vulva	VŬL-vă
vulvectomy	vŭl-VĔK-tō-mē
vulvovaginitis	vŭl-vō-vă-jĭ-NĪ-tĭs

REVIEW SHEET 8

Combining Forms

amni/o	______	metri/o	______
bartholin/o	______	my/o	______
cervic/o	______	myom/o	______
chori/o	______	nat/i	______
colp/o	______	olig/o	______
culd/o	______	oo/o	______
episi/o	______	oophor/o	______
fibr/o	______	ov/o	______
galact/o	______	ovari/o	______
gravid/o	______	perine/o	______
gynec/o	______	peritone/o	______
hyster/o	______	py/o	______
lact/o	______	salping/o	______
mamm/o	______	uter/o	______
mast/o	______	vagin/o	______
men/o	______	vulv/o	______
metr/o	______		

Suffixes

excessive bleeding	______	suture	______
surgical repair	______	flow, discharge	______

rupture	______________	narrowing, tightening	______________
incision	______________	hernia	______________
new opening	______________	to bear, to bring forth	______________
fixation, put in place	______________	labor, birth	______________
prolapse	______________	pregnancy	______________
dilation, dilatation	______________	fallopian tube	______________

Prefixes

bi	____________________	endo	____________________
brady	____________________	eu	____________________
dys	____________________	pan	____________________
multi	____________________	peri	____________________
nulli	____________________	pseudo	____________________

Additional Terms

Use this list of terms as a test of your knowledge by **checking off** the ones you can define and **circling** the ones you do not understand. Use the page references provided to find the definitions of the circled terms. Writing down the meanings of the terms you do not know will help you remember them.

abruptio placentae (195)

adnexa (189)

amnion (189)

Apgar score (197)

areola (189)

aspiration (199)

carcinoma in situ (197)

cervix (189)

chorion (189)

coitus (189)

conization (199)

corpus luteum (189)

cryosurgery (199)

cul-de-sac (189)

curettage (199)

dilation (dilatation) (199)

Down's syndrome (198)

eclampsia (195)

endometriosis (195)

erythroblastosis fetalis (197)

estrogen (189)

estrogen receptor (196)

exenteration (199)

fertilization (189)

fetal monitoring (199)

fibroids (197)

fimbriae (189)

follicle-stimulating hormone (189)

fontanelle (198)

gamete (189)

genitalia (189)

gestation (190)

gonad (190)

graafian follicle (190)

gravida (193)

human chorionic gonadotropin (190)

hyaline membrane disease (198)

hydrocephalus (197)

involution (194)

kernicterus (197)

lumpectomy (196)

luteinizing hormone (190)

meconium (198)

menarche (190)

menopause (190)

menstruation (190)

palpation (197)

papilla (190)

Pap test (198)

parturition (190)

perineum (190)

placenta previa (195)

presentation (194)

primipara (193)

progesterone (190)

puberty (190)

pylorospasm (198)

radical mastectomy (196)

version (194)

vulva (191)

CHAPTER 9

MALE REPRODUCTIVE SYSTEM

In this chapter you will:

- Name, locate, and describe the functions of the organs of the male reproductive system;
- Define some abnormal and pathological conditions which affect the male system;
- Differentiate between several types of sexually transmitted diseases;
- Define many combining forms used to describe the structures of this system; and
- Explain various laboratory tests, clinical procedures, and abbreviations which are pertinent to the system.

The chapter is divided into the following sections:

I. INTRODUCTION

The male sex cell, the **spermatozoon** (sperm cell), is microscopic—in volume, only one-third the size of an erythrocyte, and less than 1/100,000th the size of the female ovum. It is a relatively uncomplicated cell, composed of a head region, which contains nuclear hereditary material (chromosomes), and a tail region, consisting of a **flagellum** (hairlike process) that makes the sperm motile, somewhat resembling a tadpole. The sperm cell contains relatively little food and cytoplasm, for it need live only long enough to travel from its point of release from the male to where the egg cell lies within the female (uterine tube). Only one spermatozoon of approximately 100 million sperm cells which may be released during a single **ejaculation** (ejection of sperm and fluid from the male urethra) can penetrate a single ovum and produce fertilization of the ovum.

If more than one egg is passing down the uterine tube when sperm are present, multiple fertilizations are possible, and twins, triplets, quadruplets, and so forth, may occur. Twins resulting from the fertilization of separate ova by separate sperm cells are called **fraternal twins**. Fraternal twins, developing "in utero" with separate placentas, have individual patterns of inheritance and resemble each other no more than ordinary brothers and sisters.

Identical twins are formed from the fertilization of a single egg cell by a single sperm. As the fertilized egg cell divides and forms many cells, it somehow comes apart and each part continues separately to undergo further division, each producing an embryo. Both embryos share the same placenta. Identical twins are always of the same sex and very similar in form and feature.

The organs of the male reproductive system are designed to produce and release billions of spermatozoa throughout the lifetime of a male from puberty onward. In addition, the male reproductive system secretes a hormone called **testosterone**. Testosterone is responsible for the production of bodily characteristics of the male (such as beard, pubic hair, voice deepening) and also for the proper development of male gonads (**testes**) and accessory organs (**prostate gland** and **seminal vesicles**) which secrete fluids to insure the lubrication and viability of sperm.

II. ANATOMY OF THE MALE REPRODUCTIVE SYSTEM

Label Figure 9-1 as you study the following description of the anatomy of the male reproductive system.

The male gonads consist of a pair of **testes** (singular; testis), also called **testicles** (1), which develop in the kidney region of the body before descending during embryonic development into the **scrotum** (2), a sac enclosing the testes on the outside of the body.

The scrotum, lying between the thighs, exposes the testes to a lower temperature than they would have to endure if they were enclosed within the body. This lower temperature is necessary for the adequate maturation and development of sperm. Lying between the anus and the scrotum, at the floor of the pelvic cavity in the male, is the **perineum** (3), which is analogous to the perineal region in the female.

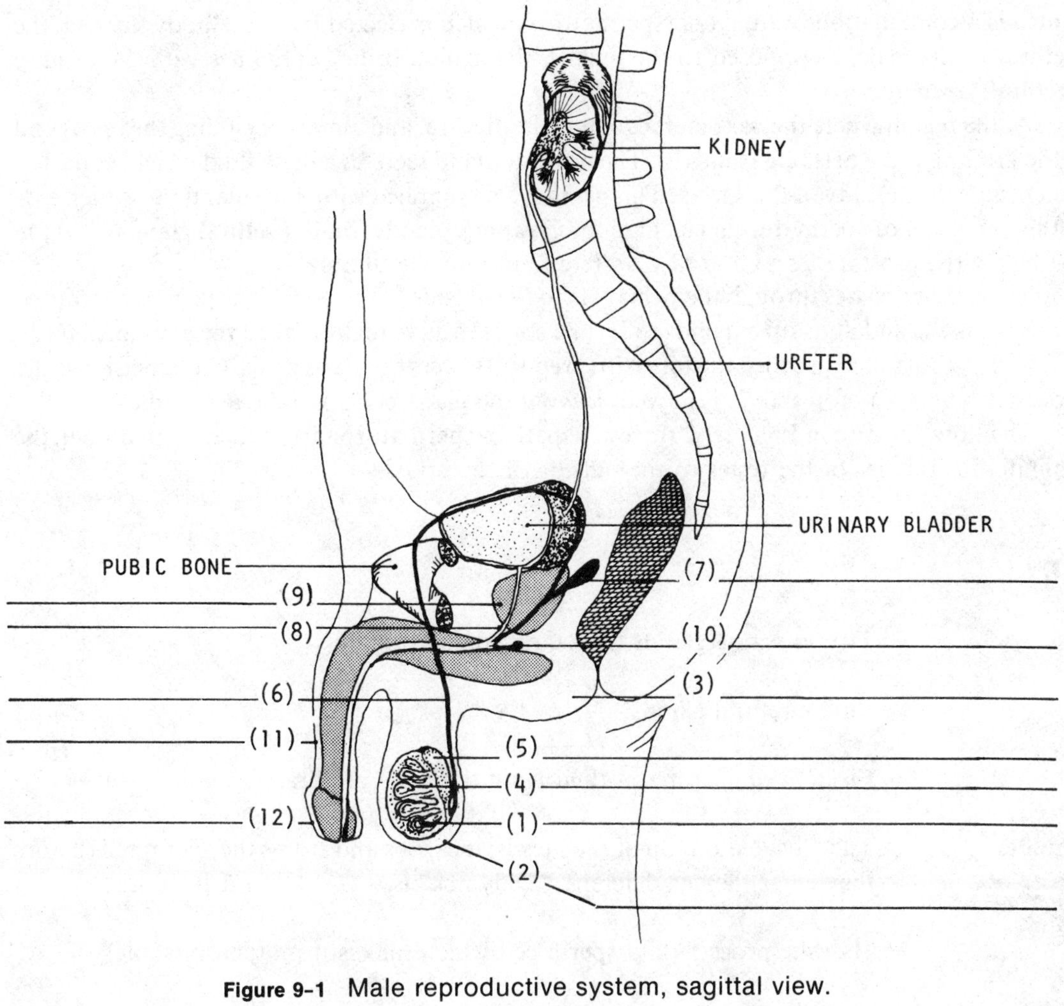

Figure 9-1 Male reproductive system, sagittal view.

The interior of a testis is composed of a large mass of narrow, coiled tubules called the **seminiferous tubules** (4). These tubules contain cells which manufacture spermatozoa. The seminiferous tubules are the **parenchymal tissue** of the testis, which means that they perform the essential work of the organ. Other cells in the testis, called **interstitial cells**, manufacture an important male hormone, **testosterone**.

All body organs contain **parenchyma** (parenchymal cells or tissue) which perform the essential functions of the organ. Organs also contain supportive, connective, and framework tissue, such as blood vessels, connective tissues, and sometimes muscle as well. This supportive tissue is called **stroma** (stromal tissue).

As soon as they are formed, sperm cells move through the seminiferous tubules and are collected in ducts which lead to a large tube at the upper part of each testis. This is the **epididymis** (5). The spermatozoa become motile in the epididymis and are temporarily stored there. The epididymis runs down the length of the testicle and then turns upward again and becomes a narrow, straight tube called the **vas deferens** (6). The vas deferens is about 2 feet long and carries the sperm up into the pelvic region, around the urinary bladder, and then into a duct leading toward the urethra. It is the vas deferens that is cut or tied off when a **sterilization** procedure called a **vasectomy** is performed.

The **seminal vesicles** (7) are glands which are located at the base of the bladder and open into the vas deferens as it joins the **urethra** (8). The seminal vesicles secrete a thick, yellowish substance that nourishes the sperm cells and forms much of the volume of ejaculated semen. **Semen** is a combination of fluid and spermatozoa which is ejected from the body through the urethra. In the male, as opposed to the female, the genital orifice combines with the urinary (urethral) opening.

At the region where the vas deferens enters the urethra, and almost encircling the upper end of the urethra, is the **prostate gland** (9). The prostate gland secretes a thick fluid which, as part of semen, aids the motility of the sperm. This gland is also supplied with muscular tissue which aids in the expulsion of sperm during ejaculation. **Cowper's glands (bulbourethral glands)** (10) are just below the prostate gland and also secrete fluid into the urethra.

The urethra passes through the **penis** (11) to the outside of the body. The penis is composed of erectile tissue and at its tip expands to form a soft, sensitive region called the **glans penis** (12). Ordinarily, a fold of skin called the **foreskin (prepuce)** covers the glans penis. Circumcision is the process whereby the foreskin is removed, leaving the glans penis visible at all times.

The flow diagram in Figure 9-2 traces the path of spermatozoa from their formation in the seminiferous tubules of the testes to the outside of the body.

III. VOCABULARY

bulbourethral glands	Two exocrine glands near the male urethra.
Cowper's glands	Bulbourethral glands.
ejaculation	Ejection of sperm and fluid from the male urethra.
epididymis; epididymides	Tube located on top of each testis; it carries and stores the sperm cells before they enter the vas deferens. "Didymos" is a Greek word for testis.
flagellum	Hairlike process on a sperm cell which makes it motile (movable).

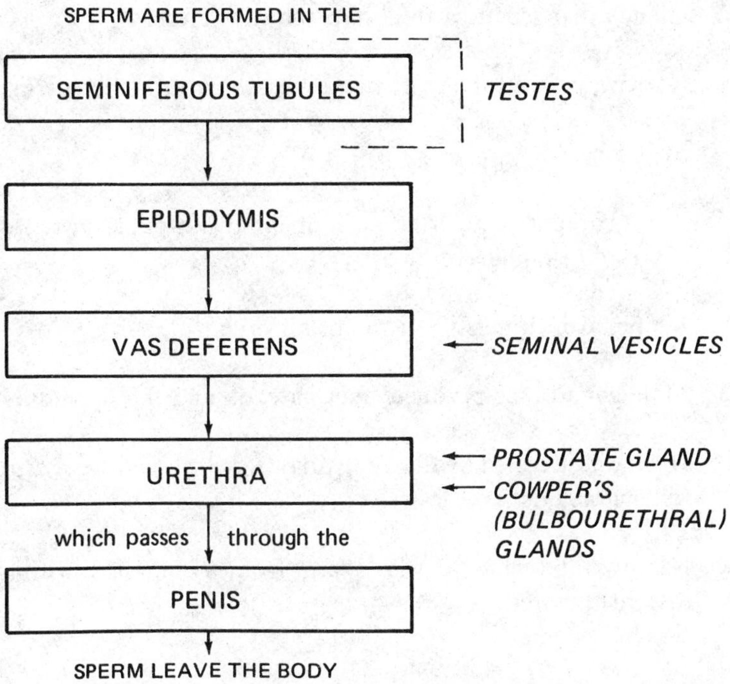

Figure 9-2 The passage of sperm from the seminiferous tubules in the testes to the outside of the body.

foreskin	Skin covering the tip of the penis.
fraternal twins	Twins resulting from two separate, concurrent fertilizations.
glans penis	Sensitive tip of the penis.
identical twins	Twins resulting from the separation of one fertilized egg into two distinct embryos.
interstitial cells of the testis	Cells that produce the hormone testosterone.
parenchymal tissue (parenchyma)	Essential cells of an organ. In the testes these are the seminiferous tubules which produce sperm.
perineum	Area between the anus and scrotum in the male.
prepuce	Foreskin.
prostate gland	Gland at the base of the urinary bladder which secretes a fluid into the urethra during ejaculation.
scrotum	External sac (double pouch) which contains the testes.
semen	Spermatozoa and fluid.

seminal vesicles	Glands that secrete a fluid into the vas deferens.
seminiferous tubules	Narrow, coiled tubules in the testes which produce sperm.
spermatozoon; spermatozoa	Sperm cell.
sterilization	Any procedure rendering an individual incapable of reproduction; vasectomy and salpingectomy are examples.
stroma	Supportive, connective tissue of an organ.
testis; testes (testicle)	Male gonad that produces spermatozoa and the hormone testosterone.
testosterone	Hormone secreted by the interstitial tissue of the testes; responsible for male sex characteristics.
vas deferens	Narrow tube which carries sperm from the epididymis into the body and toward the urethra.

IV. COMBINING FORMS AND TERMINOLOGY

Combining Form	*Meaning*	*Terminology*	*Meaning*
test/o	testis, testicle	testicular	________________
orch/o, orchi/o, orchid/o	testis, testicle	orchitis	________________
	the botanical name for orchid, the flower, is derived from the Greek word "orchis," meaning testicle; this name tries to describe the fleshy tubers on the rootstocks of the plant)	orchiectomy	________________
		Castration in males.	
		orchotomy	________________
		cryptorchism	________________
		Crypt means hidden, in this case, in the abdominal cavity.	
		orchiopexy	________________
		anorchism	________________
vas/o	vessel, duct	vasectomy	________________
	(referring to the vas deferens)	*See Clinical Procedures.*	
prostat/o	prostate gland	prostatitis	________________

		prostatectomy ____________
balan/o	glans penis	balanitis ____________
vesicul/o	seminal vesicles	vesiculectomy ____________
epididym/o	epididymis	epididymitis ____________
		epididymectomy ____________
sperm/o spermat/o	spermatozoa	aspermatogenesis ____________
		oligospermia ____________
		spermolytic ____________ *Noun suffixes ending in -sis, like -lysis, form adjectives by dropping the -sis and adding -tic.*
zo/o	animal life	azoospermia ____________ *Also called aspermia.*
andr/o	male	androgen ____________
cry/o	cold	cryogenic ____________

V. PATHOLOGICAL CONDITIONS; SEXUALLY TRANSMITTED DISEASES

Pathological Conditions

cryptorchism Undescended testicles.

Normally, 2 months before birth the testes leave the abdomen and descend into the scrotal sac. If this does not occur, the condition is known as cryptorchism. Orchiopexy is performed to bring the testes into the scrotum if they do not descend on their own by age 6 or 7 years. The condition can be unilateral (uni = one) or bilateral.

phimosis Narrowing of the opening of the foreskin over the glans penis.

This condition can interfere with urination and cause secretions to accumulate under the prepuce, leading to infection. Treatment is circumcision.

hypospadias; hypospadia Congenital opening of the male urethra on the undersurface of the penis.

epispadias; epispadia Congenital opening of the male urethra on the upper surface of the penis.

Both hypospadias and epispadias can be corrected surgically.

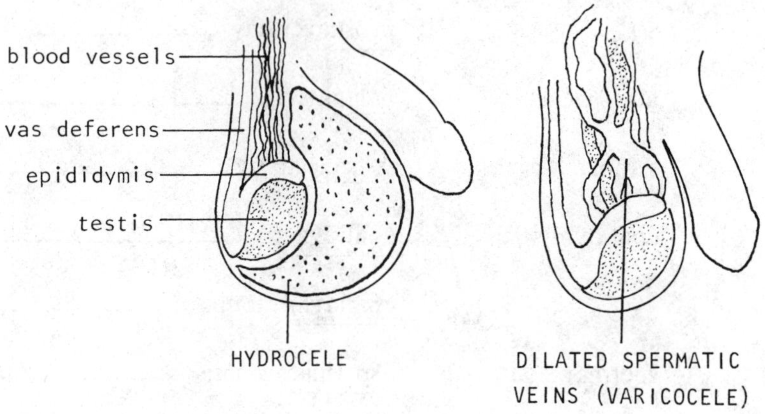

Figure 9-3 Hydrocele and varicocele.

hydrocele

Hernia (sac) of fluid in the testes or in the tubes leading from the testes.

Hydroceles occurring in infancy often resolve during the first year of life. In an older child or adult, surgery (hydrocelectomy) may be necessary.

varicocele

Enlarged, herniated, swollen veins near the testicle.

This condition is often associated with oligospermia and infertility. Oligospermic men with varicoceles and scrotal pain should have a varicocelectomy. In this procedure, the internal spermatic vein is ligated (piece is cut out and ends are tied off), leading to a marked increase in fertility. Figure 9-3 shows a hydrocele and a varicocele.

benign prostatic hyperplasia

Overgrowth of the glandular tissue of the prostate.

This is a common occurrence in men over 60 years old. Urinary obstruction and inability to empty the bladder completely are symptoms. Surgical treatment is prostatectomy, and it can be accomplished in several ways. An endoscope can be passed through the urethra and prostate tissue removed by cauterization or cryogenic devices. This is called **transurethral resection** (**TUR** or **TURP**). The gland may also be removed through the perineum or from an opening in the bladder.

adenocarcinoma of the prostate

Malignant tumor of the prostate.

This is the most common cause of cancer in men over 50 years of age (not including skin cancer). Radical (complete) prostatectomy, along with radiotherapy and chemotherapy to treat metastases, is a common method of treatment.

testicular carcinoma

Malignant tumor of the testes.

These tumors are classified according to the type of tissue that is involved in disease. Examples of testicular carcinomas are **seminoma**, **embryonal carcinoma**, **choriocarcinoma**, and **teratocarcinoma** (malignant teratoma). The last tumor is composed of embryonic tissue such as bone, hair, cartilage, and skin cells and has an unpleasant or monster-like appearance (terat/o means monster). **Mature teratomas** are benign tumors commonly found in the testes and ovaries.

Tumors of the testes are commonly treated with surgery (orchiectomy), radiotherapy, and chemotherapy.

Sexually Transmitted Diseases (STD, Venereal Diseases)

The following conditions, occurring in both men and women, are the most communicable diseases in the world and are transmitted by sexual intercourse (vener/o means sexual intercourse).

gonorrhea

Inflammation of the genital tract mucous membranes; caused by infection with gonococcus.

Other areas of the body such as eye, oral mucosa, rectum, and joints may be affected as well. Symptoms include dysuria and a yellow, mucopurulent (purulent means pus-filled) discharge from the urethra. Many women carry the disease asymptomatically, while others have pain, vaginal and urethral discharge, and salpingitis. Penicillin is the method of treatment.

syphilis

Chronic infectious disease affecting any organ of the body; caused by a spirochete (spiral-shaped) bacterium.

A **chancre** (hard ulcer) usually appears a few weeks after infection with the bacteria. It most often appears on external genitalia, but may also appear on the lip, tongue, eyelid, or anus. Lymphadenopathy follows, as the infection spreads to internal organs. Later stages include damage to the brain, spinal cord, and heart. Syphilis (named after a shepherd in an Italian poem) can be congenital in the fetus if transmitted from the mother during pregnancy. Penicillin is the method of treatment.

genital herpes

Infection of the skin and mucosa of the genitals; caused by the herpes virus.

Symptoms are reddening of the skin with small, fluid-filled blisters and ulcers. Remission and relapse periods occur; no drug is known to be effective as a cure.

trichomoniasis

Infection of the genitourinary tract of either sex; caused by Trichomonas, a one-celled organism.

This condition is more commonly found in women and causes vaginitis, urethritis, and cystitis. In men, it causes prostatitis, cystitis, and urethritis, but most infected males are asymptomatic carriers who are infectious to their partners. Metronidazole (Flagyl) is the most effective treatment.

VI. LABORATORY TESTS, CLINICAL PROCEDURES, AND ABBREVIATIONS

Laboratory Tests

semen analysis
This test is done as a part of fertility studies and is also required to establish the effectiveness of vasectomy. The semen specimen is collected in a sterile container and is analyzed microscopically. Sperm cells are counted and examined for motility and shape.

VDRL (Venereal Disease Research Laboratory) test
This is a test for syphilis. The patient's blood (serum) is placed with the syphilis antigen (spirochete). If the patient has syphilis, the antibodies in his or her blood will react with the antigen and produce a positive VDRL test.

FTA-ABS test
This is a more specific test for syphilis. The syphilis bacterium is actually searched for under the microscope.

Clinical Procedures

castration
Orchiectomy in the male, and oophorectomy in the female.

cauterization
Destruction of tissue by burning.

vasectomy
The vas deferens on each side is cut, a piece is removed, and the free ends are either **ligated** (tied) with sutures, fulgurated, or occluded with metal clips. The procedure is done through an incision in the scrotal sac. Vasectomy sterilizes the male so that sperm are not released with the semen. It does not interfere with nerves or blood vessel supply to the testes or penis, so hormone secretion, sex drive, and potency (ability to have an erection) are not impaired.

circumcision
A surgical procedure to remove the end of the prepuce.

transurethral resection of the prostate (TUR or TURP)
A special endoscope is inserted through a catheter into the urethra and pieces of the prostate gland are removed by electrocautery (heating) or cryogenic (freezing) techniques.

Abbreviations

BPH	Benign prostatic hyperplasia	TUR, TURP	Transurethral resection of the prostate
FTA-ABS	Fluorescent treponemal antibody absorption test	VDRL	Venereal Disease Research Laboratory
GU	Genitourinary		

VII. PRACTICAL APPLICATIONS

Case Report

A 22-year-old white male presents with a scrotal mass that does not transilluminate. An orchiectomy reveals embryonal carcinoma with teratoma. Chest x-rays and lung tomograms are normal. Serum levels of AFP [alpha-fetoprotein, a protein secreted by tumor cells] and beta HCG [a hormone secreted by testicular tumor cells] are elevated. Abdominal CAT scan reveals minimal retroperitoneal lymphadenopathy. A retroperitoneal lymphadenectomy is performed which reveals 4 of 42 nodes positive for embryonal carcinoma.

One month post-op, AFP and beta HCG are normal. The patient is followed up with monthly AFP and beta HCG determinations, plus chest x-rays. Six months after his node dissection, the patient remains asymptomatic but his chest x-ray reveals pulmonary metastases. His AFP and beta HCG levels are slightly elevated. Chemotherapy with cisplatin (Platinol), vinblastine (Velban), and bleomycin (Blenoxane) is given over 12 weeks. AFP and beta HCG return to normal, but residual abnormality remains on his chest x-ray. One month after completion of chemotherapy, a thoracotomy is done and these residual lesions are removed. Pathologically, they are mature teratomas [a tumor that is not malignant]. After surgery, no further chemotherapy is given but the patient is followed with serial markers [levels of AFP and beta HCG are taken routinely] and chest x-rays for a 2 year period. He remains free of disease 32 months after the start of chemotherapy.

Operative Report. Preoperative Diagnosis: Cryptorchid Left Testis

Operation performed:
1. Right vasectomy
2. Left orchiectomy

Anesthesia: Spinal

Postoperative diagnosis: same as above

The patient was prepped and draped in the routine manner as for a left inguinal herniorrhaphy. The right vas deferens was identified through the scrotal skin, isolated, and by sharp dissection was freed from the surrounding cord structures. A 1.5 cm section was resected and the severed ends were suture-ligated with #3-0 chromic catgut suture. The incision was closed and attention was turned to the left inguinal canal, which was entered with an incision paralleling the inguinal ligament. Dissection was carried down until an atrophic left testicle was delivered into the operative field. The vas deferens and other cord structures were suture-ligated and the left testicle was excised. After satisfactory hemostasis was obtained the incision was closed. Patient tolerated the procedure well and was left in the OR in excellent condition.

VIII. EXERCISES

A. Build medical words:

1. Inflammation of the testes ______
2. Removal of the tubules that carry the spermatozoa to the vas deferens

   ______
3. Excessive development of the prostate gland ______
4. Inflammation of the prostate gland ______
5. The process of producing (formation of) sperm cells ______
6. Fixation of undescended testicle ______
7. Excision of the prostate and seminal vesicles ______
8. Condition of scanty sperm ______
9. Discharge from the glans penis ______
10. Sperm in the urine ______

B. Give the meaning of the following:

1. hypospadias ______
2. parenchymal ______
3. seminiferous tubules ______
4. cryogenic ______
5. interstitial cells of the testes ______
6. testosterone ______
7. phimosis ______
8. azoospermia ______
9. androgen ______
10. teratocarcinoma of the testes ______

11. stroma ______________________________

C. *From the description below, give the medical term:*

1. Tube above each testis; carries and stores sperm ______________
2. Gland surrounding the urethra at the base of the urinary bladder ______________

   ____
3. Parenchymal tissue of the testes; produces spermatozoa ______________
4. Sperm cell ______________________________
5. Foreskin ______________________________
6. Male gonad; produces hormone and sperm cells ______________
7. Pair of sacs; secrete fluid into ducts leading to the urethra ______________
8. Sac on outside of the body enclosing the testes ______________
9. Tube carrying sperm from the epididymis into the body toward the urethra

   ____
10. Pair of glands near the urethra; secrete fluid into the urethra; Cowper's glands

    ____

D. *Match the term in Column I with its meaning in Column II:*

Column I		*Column II*
1. castration	____	A. to tie off or bind
2. semen analysis	____	B. removal of a piece of the vas deferens
3. ejaculation	____	C. orchiectomy
4. purulent	____	D. removal of the prepuce
5. vasectomy	____	E. destruction of tissue by burning
6. circumcision	____	F. pus-filled

7. ligation ______ G. test of fertility (reproductive ability)

8. cauterization ______ H. ejection of sperm and fluid from the urethra

E. *Give the names of the following abnormal conditions:*

1. Prostatic enlargement; nonmalignant ____________________
2. Opening of the urethra on the upper surface of the penis ____________________
3. Sexually transmitted disease; infection with herpes virus ____________________
4. Malignant tumor of the prostate gland ____________________
5. Hernia of swollen veins in and near the testes ____________________
6. Sexually transmitted disease; primary stage marked by chancre ____________________
7. Malignant tumor of the testes (3 types) ____________________

   ____________________, ____________________
8. Venereal disease marked by inflammation of genital mucosa and mucopurulent discharge ____________________
9. Venereal disease caused by infection with Trichomonas ____________________
10. Undescended testicles ____________________

F. *Give the meanings for the following abbreviations:*

1. VDRL ____________________
2. TUR ____________________
3. GU ____________________
4. D & C ____________________

G. *Review exercise. Give the meaning of the following:*

1. -stasis ____________________ 3. -stenosis ____________________

2. -sclerosis ____________________ 4. -rrhexis ____________________

5. -rrhagia ____________
6. -ptosis ____________
7. -plasia ____________
8. -phagia ____________
9. -rrhaphy ____________
10. -pexy ____________
11. -ectasis ____________
12. -centesis ____________
13. -genesis ____________
14. culd/o ____________
15. oophor/o ____________
16. salping/o ____________
17. hyster/o ____________
18. metr/o ____________
19. colp/o ____________
20. mast/o ____________

ANSWERS

A.

1. orchitis
2. epididymectomy
3. prostatic hyperplasia
4. prostatitis
5. spermatogenesis
6. orchiopexy
7. prostatovesiculectomy
8. oligospermia
9. balanorrhea
10. spermaturia

B.

1. Congenital anomaly in which the urethra opens on the underside of the penis.
2. The distinctive tissue or cells of an organ, as for example, glomerulus and tubules of the kidney, seminiferous tubules and interstitial cells of the testis.
3. The tubules in the testes that produce sperm cells.
4. Pertaining to producing cold or low temperatures.
5. The cells that produce the hormone testosterone.
6. A hormone made by the interstitial cells of the testes; responsible for secondary sex characteristics.
7. A narrowing, or stenosis, of the foreskin on the glans penis.
8. Lack of spermatozoa in the semen.
9. Hormone producing male characteristics.
10. Malignant tumor of the testes composed of differentiated tissue such as bone, hair, skin, teeth, cartilage.
11. Supportive, connective tissue of an organ.

C.

1. epididymis
2. prostate gland
3. seminiferous tubules
4. spermatozoon
5. prepuce
6. testis; testicle
7. seminal vesicles
8. scrotum; scrotal sac
9. vas deferens
10. bulbourethral glands

D.

1. C
2. G
3. H
4. F
5. B
6. D
7. A
8. E

E.

1. benign prostatic hyperplasia
2. epispadias
3. genital herpes
4. adenocarcinoma of the prostate
5. varicocele
6. syphilis
7. malignant teratoma; choriocarcinoma; seminoma
8. gonorrhea
9. trichomoniasis
10. cryptorchism

F.

1. Venereal Disease Research Laboratory; test for syphilis
2. transurethral resection of the prostate gland
3. genitourinary
4. dilation and curettage

G.

1. stopping, controlling
2. hardening
3. narrowing
4. rupture
5. hemorrhage
6. prolapse
7. formation
8. eating, swallowing
9. suture
10. fixation
11. widening
12. surgical puncture
13. beginning, producing
14. cul-de-sac
15. ovary
16. uterine tube
17. uterus
18. uterus
19. vagina
20. breast

IX. PRONUNCIATION OF TERMS

androgen	ĂN-drō-jĕn
anorchism	ăn-ŎR-kĭzm
aspermatogenesis	ā-spĕr-mă-tō-JĔN-ĕ-sĭs
azoospermia	ā-zō-ō-SPĔR-mē-ă
balanitis	băl-ă-NĪ-tĭs
bulbourethral	bŭl-bō-ū-RĒ-thrăl
castration	kăs-TRĀ-shŭn
cauterization	kăw-tĕr-ĭ-ZĀ-shŭn
chancre	SHĂNG-kĕr
circumcision	sĕr-kŭm-SĬZH-ŭn
cryptorchism	krĭp-TŎR-kĭzm
ejaculation	ē-jăk-ū-LĀ-shŭn
epididymectomy	ĕp-ĭ-dĭd-ĭ-MĔK-tō-mē
epididymis	ĕp-ĭ-DĬD-ĭ-mĭs
epididymitis	ĕp-ĭ-dĭd-ĭ-MĪ-tĭs
epispadias	ĕp-ĭ-SPĀ-dē-ăs
flagellum	flă-JĔL-ŭm
genital herpes	JĔN-ĭ-tăl HĔR-pēz
gonorrhea	gŏn-ō-RĒ-ă
hydrocele	HĪ-drō-sēl
hypospadias	hī-pō-SPĀ-dē-ăs
interstitial cells	ĭn-tĕr-STĬSH-ăl sĕlz
oligospermia	ŏl-ĭ-gō-SPĔR-mē-ă
orchiectomy	ŏr-kē-ĔK-tō-mē
orchiopexy	ŏr-kē-ō-PĔK-sē
orchitis	ŏr-KĪ-tĭs

orchotomy	ŏr-KŎT-ō-mē
parenchymal	pă-RĔNG-kĭ-măl
perineum	pĕr-ĭ-NĒ-ŭm
phimosis	fi-MŌ-sĭs
prepuce	PRĒ-pūs
prostate	PRŎS-tāt
prostatectomy	prŏs-tă-TĔK-tō-mē
prostatic hyperplasia	prŏs-TĂT-ĭk hī-pĕr-PLĀ-zē-ă
prostatitis	prŏs-tă-TĪ-tĭs
purulent	PŪR-ōō-lĕnt
scrotum	SKRŌ-tŭm
semen	SĒ-mĕn
seminal vesicles	SĔM-ĭnăl VĔS-ĭ-k'lz
seminiferous	sĕ-mĭ-NĬF-ĕr-ŭs
seminoma	sĕ-mĭ-NŌ-mă
spermatozoon	spĕr-mă-tō-ZŌ-ōn
spermolytic	spĕr-mō-LĬT-ĭk
sterilization	stĕr-ĭ-lĭ-ZĀ-shŭn
stroma	STRŌ-mă
syphilis	SĬF-ĭ-lĭs
teratoma	tĕr-ă-TŌ-mă
testicular	tĕs-TĬK-ū-lăr
testis	TĔS-tĭs
testosterone	tĕs-TŎS-tĕ-rōn
trichomoniasis	trĭk-ō-mō-NĪ-ă-sĭs
varicocele	VĂR-ĭ-kō-sēl
vas deferens	văs DĔF-ĕr-ĕnz
vasectomy	vă-SĔK-tō-mē
venereal	vĕ-NĒ-rē-ăl
vesiculectomy	vĕ-sĭk-ū-LĔK-tō-mē

REVIEW SHEET 9

Combining Forms

andr/o	______________	prostat/o	______________
balan/o	______________	sperm/o	______________
cry/o	______________	spermat/o	______________
epididym/o	______________	test/o	______________
orchid/o	______________	vas/o	______________
orchi/o	______________	vesicul/o	______________
orch/o	______________	zo/o	______________

Suffixes

-ectomy	______________	-pexy	______________
-genic	______________	-tomy	______________
-lysis	______________	-trophy	______________

Additional Terms

Use this list of terms as a test of your knowledge by **checking off** the ones you can define and **circling** the ones you do not understand. Use the page references provided to find the definitions of the circled terms. Writing down the meanings of the terms you do not know will help you remember them.

adenocarcinoma of the prostate (222)	ejaculation (218)
benign prostatic hyperplasia (222)	epispadias (221)
bulbourethral glands (218)	flagellum (218)
castration (224)	fraternal twins (219)
circumcision (224)	genital herpes (223)
cryptorchism (221)	glans penis (219)

gonorrhea (223)

hydrocele (222)

hypospadias (221)

identical twins (219)

interstitial cells (219)

parenchymal tissue (219)

perineum (219)

phimosis (221)

prepuce (219)

prostate gland (219)

scrotum (219)

semen (219)

seminal vesicles (220)

seminiferous tubules (220)

seminoma (222)

sterilization (220)

stroma (220)

teratocarcinoma (222)

testosterone (220)

trichomoniasis (223)

varicocele (222)

vas deferens (220)

CHAPTER 10

NERVOUS SYSTEM

In this chapter you will:

- Name, locate, and describe the functions of the major organs and parts of the nervous system;
- Recognize nervous system combining forms and make terms using them with new and familiar suffixes;
- Define several pathological conditions affecting the nervous system; and
- Describe some laboratory tests, clinical procedures, and abbreviations which pertain to the system.

The chapter is divided into the following sections:

I. INTRODUCTION

The nervous system is one of the most complex of all human body systems. More than 10 billion nerve cells are operating constantly all over the body to coordinate the activities we do consciously and voluntarily, as well as those that occur unconsciously or involuntarily. We speak, we move muscles, we hear, we taste, we see, we think, our glands secrete hormones, we respond to danger, pain, temperature, touch, we have memory, association, discrimination—all of these composing a small number of the many activities controlled by our nervous system.

Microscopic **nerve cells** collected into macroscopic bundles called **nerves** carry electrical messages all over the body. External stimuli, as well as internal chemicals such as **acetylcholine**, activate the cell membranes of nerve cells so as to release stored electrical energy within the cells. This energy when released and passed through the length of the nerve cell is called the **nervous impulse**. External receptors, like sense organs, as well as internal receptors in muscles and blood vessels receive and transmit these impulses to the complex network of nerve cells in the brain and spinal cord. Within this central part of the nervous system, impulses are recognized, interpreted, and finally relayed to other nerve cells which extend out to all parts of the body, such as muscles, glands, and internal organs.

II. GENERAL STRUCTURE OF THE NERVOUS SYSTEM

The nervous system can be classified into two major divisions: the **central nervous system (CNS)** and the **peripheral nervous system**. The central nervous system consists of the **brain** and **spinal cord**. The peripheral nervous system consists of 12 pairs of **cranial nerves** and 31 pairs of

spinal nerves. The cranial nerves carry impulses between the brain and the head and neck. The tenth cranial nerve is called the vagus nerve; it carries messages to and from the chest and abdomen, as well as the head and neck regions. The spinal nerves carry messages between the spinal cord and the chest, abdomen, and extremities. Figure 10-1 illustrates these parts of the central and peripheral nervous systems.

In addition to the spinal and cranial nerves (whose functions are mainly voluntary and involved with sensations of smell, taste, sight, hearing, and muscle movements), the peripheral nervous system consists of a large group of nerves that function involuntarily or automatically without conscious control. These peripheral nerves are those of the **autonomic nervous system**. This system of nerve fibers carries impulses **from** the central nervous system to the glands, heart, blood vessels, and the involuntary muscles found in the walls of tubes like the intestines and hollow organs like the stomach and urinary bladder. These nerves are called **efferent**, since they carry impulses away from the central nervous system.

Some of the autonomic nerves are called **sympathetic** nerves and others are called **parasympathetic** nerves. The sympathetic nerves stimulate the body in times of stress and crisis,

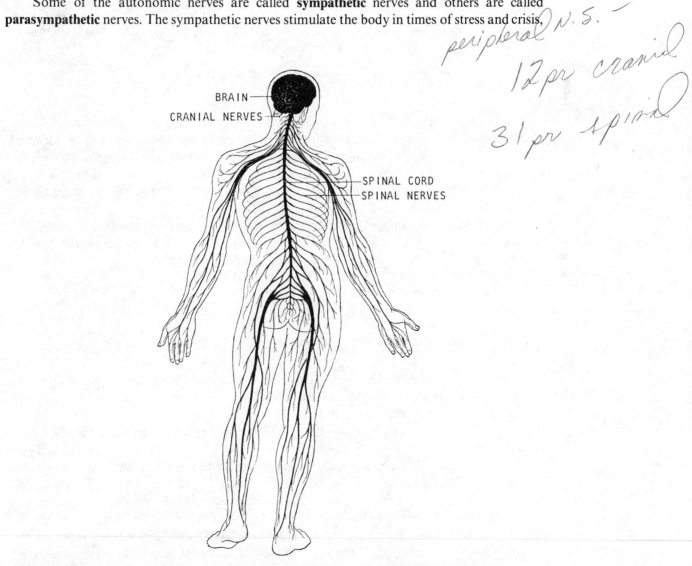

peripheral N.S. —
12 pr cranial
31 pr spinal

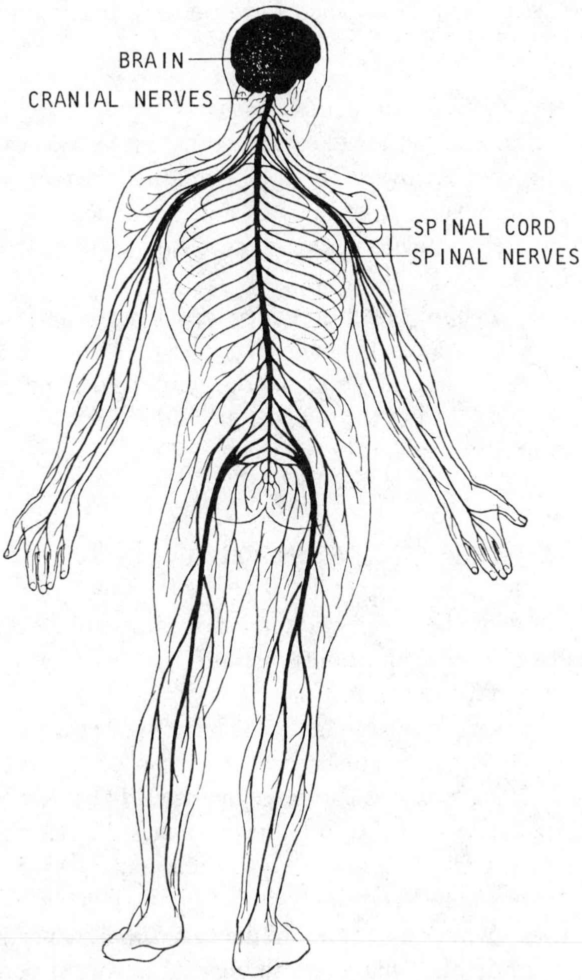

Figure 10-1 The central nervous system, consisting of the brain and the spinal cord. Cranial and spinal nerves (part of the peripheral nervous system) carry impulses to and from the brain and spinal cord.

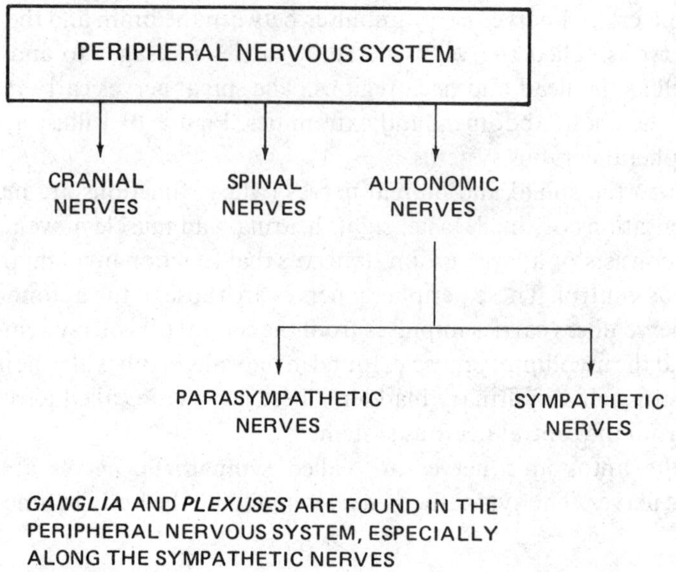

Figure 10-2 Divisions of the peripheral nervous system.

i.e., increase heart rate and forcefulness, dilate airways so more oxygen can enter, increase blood pressure, stimulate the adrenal glands to secrete epinephrine (adrenalin), and inhibit intestinal contractions so that digestion is slower. The parasympathetic nerves normally act as a balance for the sympathetic nerves. Parasympathetic nerves slow down heart rate, contract the pupils of the eye, lower blood pressure, stimulate peristalsis to clear the rectum, and increase the quantity of secretions like saliva.

Ganglia (singular: **ganglion**), which are collections of nerve tissue outside the brain and spinal cord, and **plexuses** (singular: **plexus**), which are larger networks of nerves, are prevalent in the automatic nervous system. Consult your dictionary and note the numerous and widespread distribution of ganglia and plexuses throughout the body.

Figure 10-2 summarizes the divisions of the peripheral nervous system.

III. NEURONS, NERVES, AND NEUROGLIA

A **neuron** is an individual nerve cell, a microscopic structure. Impulses are passed along the parts of a nerve cell in a definite manner and direction. The parts of a neuron are pictured in Figure 10-3; label it as you study the following.

A **stimulus** begins a wave of excitability in the receptive branching fibers of the neuron which are called **dendrites** (1). A change in the electrical charge of the dendrite membranes is thus begun and the nervous impulse wave moves along the dendrites like the movement of falling tenpins. The impulse, traveling in only one direction, next reaches the **cell body** (2) which contains the **cell nucleus** (3). Extending from the cell body is the **axon** (4) which carries the impulse away from the cell body. Axons may be covered with a fatty tissue sheath called a **myelin sheath** (5). The myelin sheath gives a white appearance to the nerve fiber; hence the term "white matter," as in parts of the spinal cord, white matter of the brain, and most peripheral nerves. The "gray matter" of the brain and spinal cord refers to the collections of cell bodies and dendrites which appear gray because they are not covered by a myelin sheath.

Another axon covering, called the **neurilemma** (6), is a membranous sheath outside the

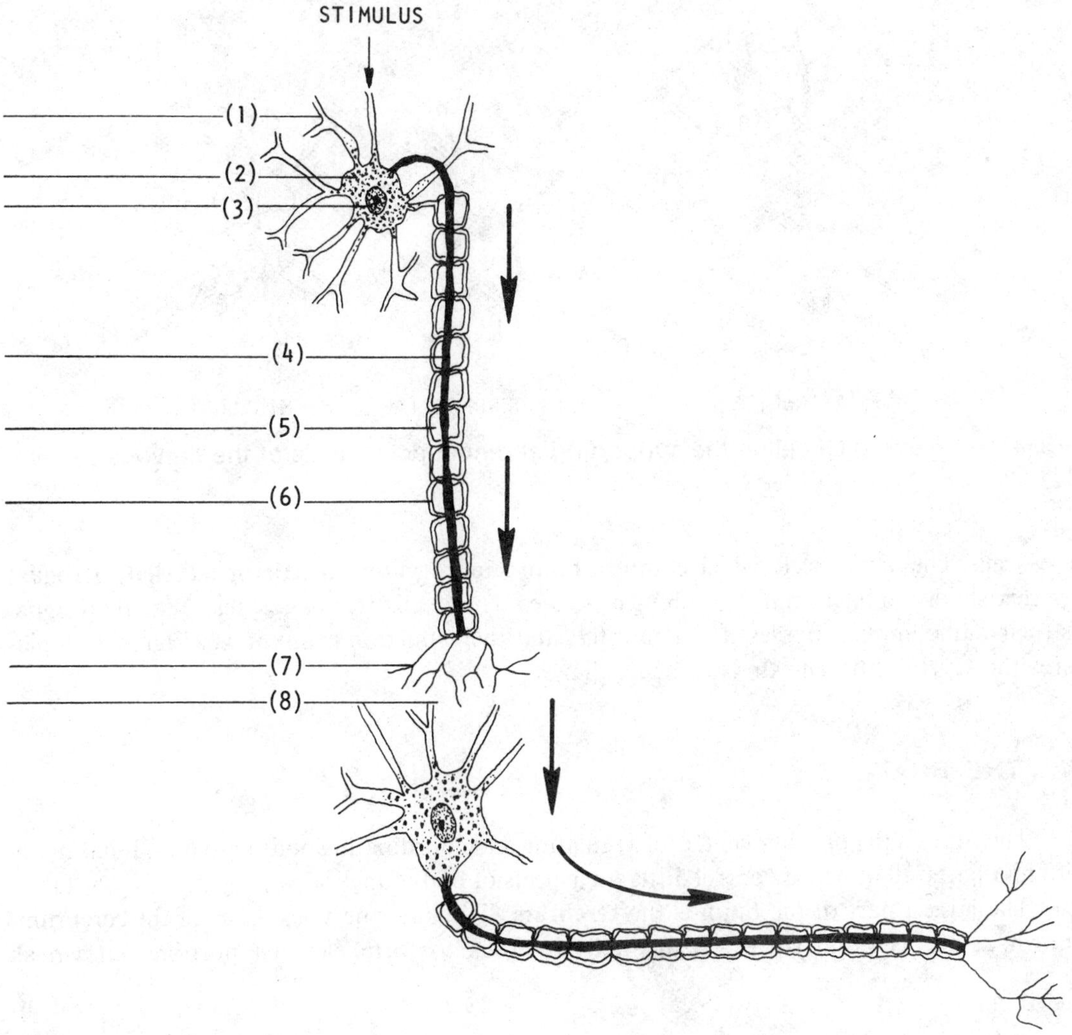

Figure 10-3 Parts of a neuron and the pathway of a nervous impulse.

myelin sheath on the nerve cells of peripheral nerves. The nervous impulse passes through the axon to leave the cell via the **terminal end fibers** (7) of the neuron. The space where the nervous impulse jumps from one neuron to another is called the **synapse** (8).

While a neuron is a microscopic structure within the nervous system, a **nerve** is macroscopic, able to be seen with the naked eye. A nerve consists of a bundle of dendrites and axons which travel together like strands of rope. Peripheral nerves that carry impulses to the brain and spinal cord from stimulus receptors like the skin, eye, ear, and nose are called **afferent nerves**; those which carry impulses **from** the CNS to organs that produce responses, for example, muscles and glands, are called **efferent nerves**.

Neurons and nerves are the parenchymal tissue of the nervous system; that is, they do the essential work of the system by conducting impulses throughout the body. The stromal tissue of the nervous system consists of other cells called **neuroglia**. Neuroglial cells are supportive and connective in function, as well as phagocytic, and are able to help the nervous system ward off infection and injury. Neuroglial cells do not transmit impulses.

There are three types of neuroglial cells. **Astrocytes (astroglia)**, as their name suggests, are starlike, and are believed to be responsible for transporting water and salts between capillaries and

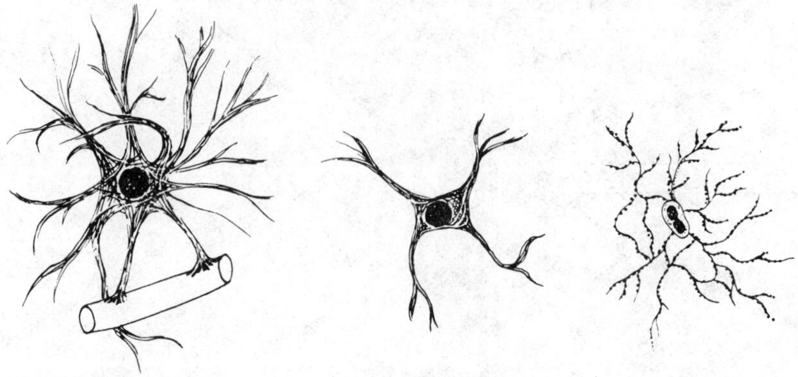

Figure 10-4 Neuroglial cells—the supporting and connective cells of the nervous system.

nerve cells. They are the cells which compose brain tumors (gliomas). **Microglial cells (microglia)** are very small and have many branching processes. These cells are phagocytes. **Oligodendroglia**, as their name implies, possess few dendrites, and their function is unknown. Figure 10-4 pictures the several different kinds of neuroglia.

IV. THE BRAIN

The brain is the primary center for regulating and coordinating body activities. It has many different parts, all of which control different aspects of body functions.

The largest part of the brain is the **cerebrum**. The outer nervous tissue of the cerebrum, known as the **cerebral cortex**, is arranged in folds to form elevated portions known as

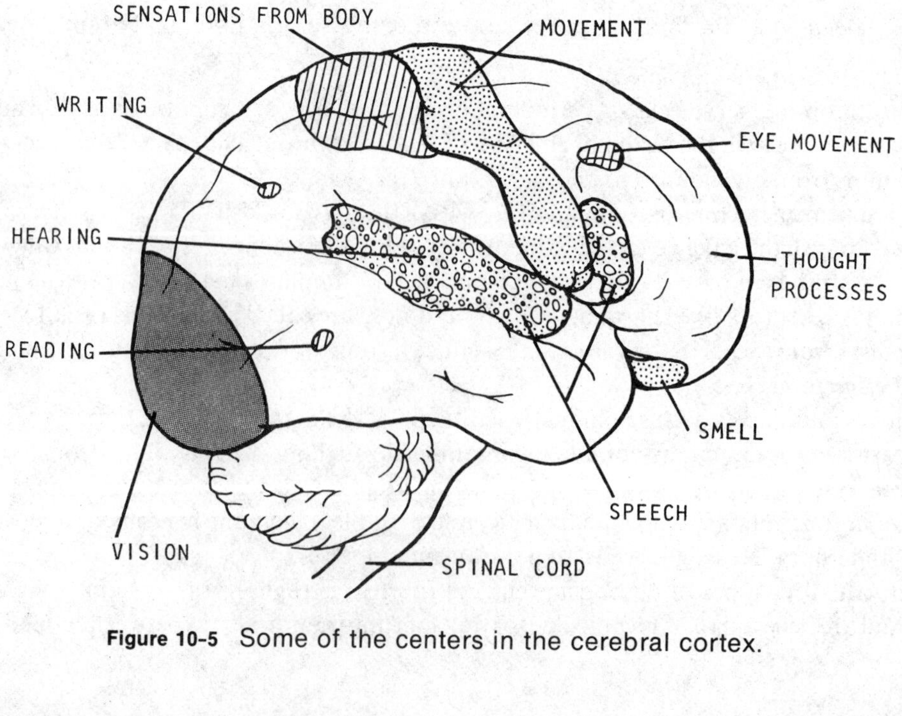

Figure 10-5 Some of the centers in the cerebral cortex.

convolutions (also called **gyri**) and depressions or grooves known as **fissures** (also called **sulci**). The **cerebral hemispheres** are the paired halves of the cerebrum.

The cerebrum has many functions. All thought, judgment, memory, association, and discrimination take place within it. In addition, sensory impulses are received through afferent cranial nerves, and when registered in the cortex are the basis for perception. Efferent cranial nerves carry motor impulses from the cerebrum to muscles and glands, and these produce movement and activity. Figure 10-5 shows the location of some of the centers in the cerebral cortex which control speech, vision, smell, movement, hearing, thought processes, and so forth.

Within the middle region of the cerebrum are spaces, or canals, called **ventricles** (pictured in Figure 10-6). They contain a watery fluid which flows throughout the brain and around the spinal cord. This fluid is called **cerebrospinal fluid (CSF)** and protects the brain and spinal cord from shock as might a cushion. It is usually clear and colorless, and contains lymphocytes, sugar, chlorides, and some protein. Spinal fluid can be withdrawn for diagnosis or relief of pressure on the brain; this is called a **spinal puncture** or **lumbar puncture (LP)**. A hollow needle is inserted in the lumbar region of the spinal column below the region where the nervous tissue of the spinal cord ends, and fluid is withdrawn.

Two other important parts of the brain, the **thalamus** and **hypothalamus**, are below the cerebrum in an area called the diencephalon. The thalamus is a large mass of gray matter that acts as a relay center for impulses that travel from receptors such as the eye, ear, and skin through the thalamus to the cerebrum. Thus, the thalamus integrates and monitors these sensory impulses, suppressing some and magnifying others. Perception of pain is controlled by this area of the brain. The hypothalamus (below the thalamus) contains neurons which control body temperature, sleep, appetite, sexual desire, and emotions such as fear and pleasure. The hypothalamus also

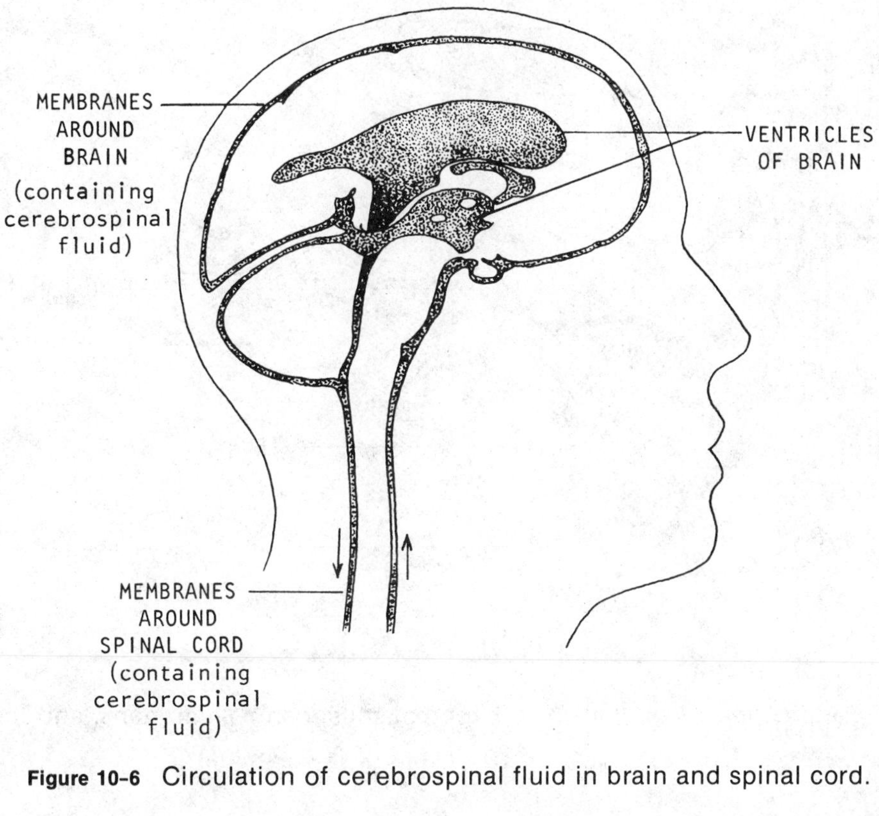

Figure 10-6 Circulation of cerebrospinal fluid in brain and spinal cord.

regulates the release of hormones from the pituitary gland at the base of the brain and integrates the activities of the sympathetic and parasympathetic nervous systems.

The following structures within the brain lie below the posterior portion of the cerebrum and connect the cerebrum with the spinal cord: the cerebellum, pons, and medulla oblongata. These structures are collectively called the **brain stem**.

The **cerebellum** is located beneath the posterior part of the cerebrum. Its function is to aid in the coordination of voluntary movements and to maintain balance, posture, and muscular tone.

The **pons** is a part of the brain which literally means "bridge." It contains nerve fiber tracts which connect the cerebellum and cerebrum with the rest of the brain.

The **medulla oblongata**, located at the base of the brain, connects the spinal cord with the rest of the brain. Nerve tracts cross over in the medulla oblongata. For example, nerve cells that control the movement of the left side of the body are found in the right half of the cerebrum. These cells send out axons that cross over (decussate) to the opposite side of the brain in the medulla oblongata and then travel down the spinal cord.

In addition, the medulla oblongata contains important vital centers that regulate internal activities of the body. These are:

1. Respiratory center, which controls muscles of respiration in response to chemicals or other stimuli;
2. Cardiac center, which slows the heart rate when the heart is beating too rapidly; and
3. Vasomotor center, which affects (constricts or dilates) the muscles in the walls of blood vessels, thus influencing blood pressure.

Figure 10-7 shows the locations of the thalamus, hypothalamus, cerebellum, pons, and medulla oblongata. Table 10-1 reviews the functions of the parts of the brain.

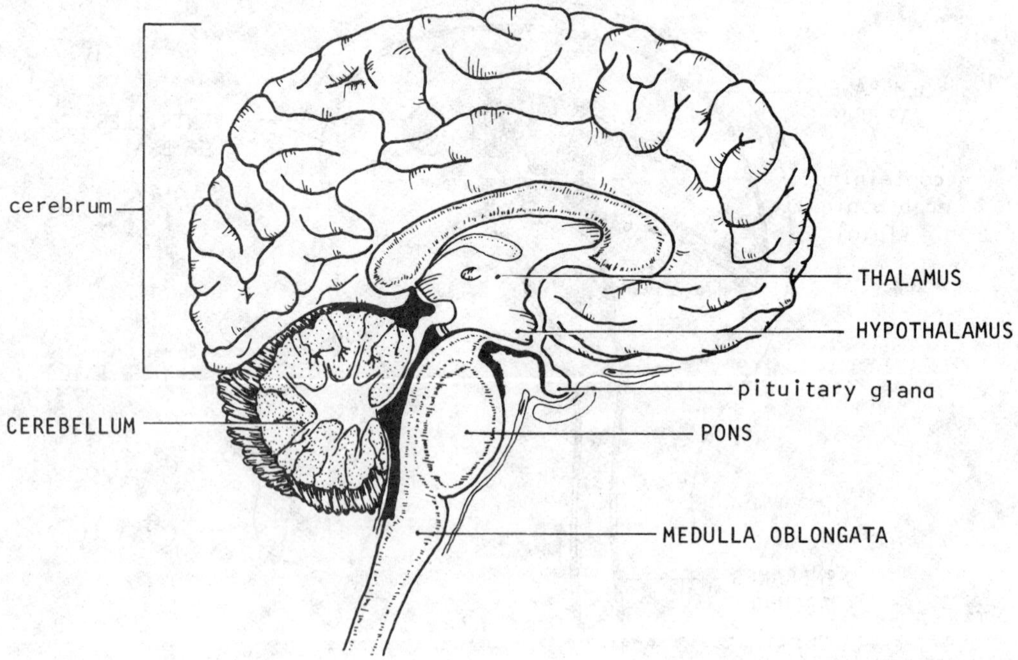

Figure 10-7 Parts of the brain: thalamus, hypothalamus, cerebellum, pons, and medulla oblongata.

Table 10-1 FUNCTIONS OF THE PARTS OF THE BRAIN

Part of the Brain	Functions
Cerebrum	Thinking, reasoning, sensations, movements, memory
Thalamus	Relay station for body sensations; pain
Hypothalamus	Body temperature, sleep, appetite, emotions, control of the pituitary gland
Cerebellum	Coordination of voluntary movements
Pons	Connection of nerve fiber tracts
Medulla oblongata	Nerve fibers cross over, left to right and right to left; centers to regulate heart, blood vessels, and respiratory system

V. THE SPINAL CORD AND MENINGES

Spinal Cord

The **spinal cord** is a column of nervous tissue extending from the medulla oblongata to the second lumbar vertebra within the vertebral column. It ends as the **cauda equina** (horse tail), a fan of nerve fibers found below the second lumbar vertebra of the spinal column (see Figure 10-8). It carries all the nerves which affect the limbs and lower part of the body, and is the pathway for impulses going to and from the brain. A cross-section of the spinal cord (shown in Figure 10-9) reveals an inner section of gray matter (containing cell bodies and dendrites of peripheral nerves) and an outer region of white matter (containing the nerve fiber tracts with myelin sheaths) conducting impulses to and from the brain.

Meninges

The **meninges** are three layers of connective tissue membranes that surround the brain and spinal cord. Label Figure 10-10 as you study the following description of the meninges.

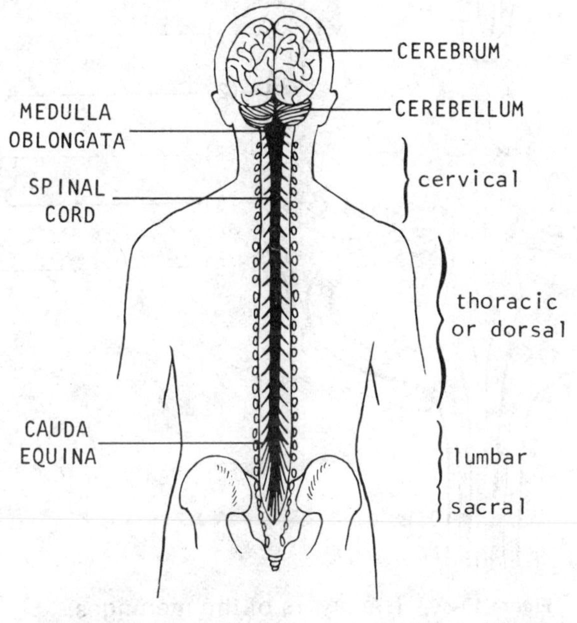

Figure 10-8 Dorsal view of the spinal cord and the brain. Note the cauda equina.

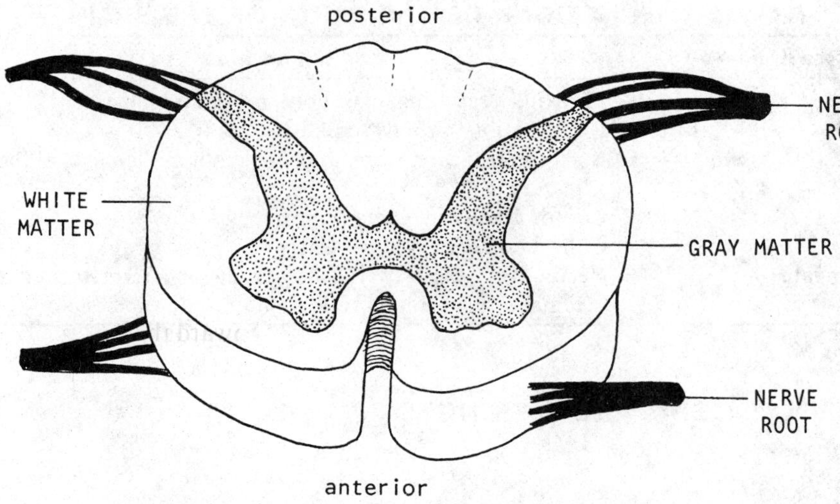

Figure 10-9 Transverse section of the spinal cord.

The outermost membrane of the meninges is called the **dura mater** (1). It is a thick and tough membrane and contains channels for blood to come into the brain tissue. The **subdural space** (2) is a space below the dura membrane and contains many blood vessels. The second layer around the brain and spinal cord is called the **arachnoid membrane** (3). The arachnoid ("spider-like") membrane is loosely attached to the other meninges by weblike fibers so there is a space for fluid between the fibers and the third membrane. This space is called the **subarachnoid space** (4), and it contains the cerebrospinal fluid. The third layer of the meninges, closest to the brain and spinal

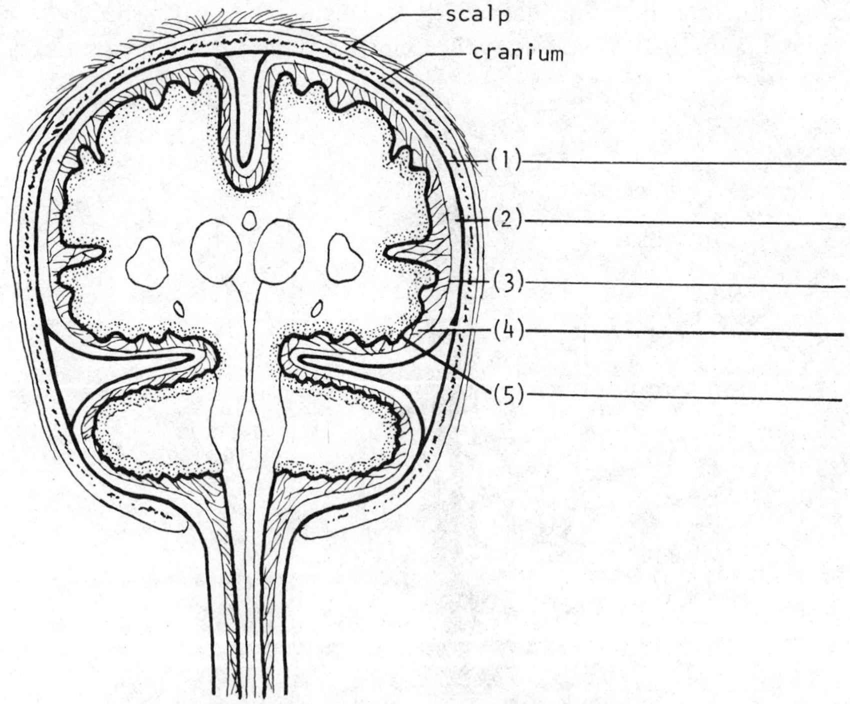

Figure 10-10 The layers of the meninges.

cord, is called the **pia mater** (5). It is made of delicate ("pia") connective tissue with a rich supply of blood vessels.

VI. VOCABULARY

acetylcholine	Chemical released at the ends of nerve cells. Acetylcholine aids in the transmission of nerve impulses.
afferent nerves	Nerves that carry impulses toward the brain and spinal cord.
arachnoid membrane	Middle layer of the three membranes (meninges) which surround the brain and spinal cord.
astrocyte	A type of neuroglial cell; connective, supporting cell of the nervous system.
autonomic nervous system	Nerves that control involuntary body functions; automatically carry impulses from the brain and spinal cord to muscles, glands, and internal organs.
axon	Microscopic fiber that carries the nervous impulse along a nerve cell.
cauda equina	"Horse tail"—a fan of nerve fibers formed below the second lumbar vertebra in the spinal column.
cell body	Part of a nerve cell which contains the cell nucleus.
central nervous system (CNS)	The brain and the spinal cord.
cerebellum	Posterior part of the brain. It is responsible for coordinating voluntary muscle movements and maintaining balance.
cerebral cortex	Outer region of the cerebrum; also called the "gray matter" of the brain.
cerebrospinal fluid (CSF)	Liquid that circulates throughout the brain and spinal cord.
cerebrum	Largest part of the brain; responsible for voluntary muscular activity, vision, speech, taste, hearing, thought, memory, and many other functions.
convolution	Elevated portion of the cerebral cortex; gyrus.
dendrite	Microscopic branching fiber of a nerve cell which is the first part to receive the nervous impulse.
dura mater	Outermost layer of the meninges surrounding the brain and spinal cord.
efferent nerves	Nerves that carry impulses away from the brain and spinal cord to the muscles, glands, and organs.

fissure	Depression, or groove, in the surface of the cerebral cortex; sulcus.
ganglion; ganglia	"Knot"—collection of many nerve cell bodies outside the brain and spinal cord. This term also describes a cystic (saclike) enlargement of a tendon on the back of the wrist.
gyrus; gyri	Elevation in the surface of the cerebral cortex; convolution.
hypothalamus	Portion of the brain beneath the thalamus; controls sleep, appetite, body temperature, and the secretions from the pituitary gland.
medulla oblongata	Part of the brain just above the spinal cord; controls breathing, heartbeat, and the size of blood vessels; nerve fibers cross over here.
meninges	Three protective membranes that surround the brain and spinal cord.
microglial cell	One type of neuroglial cell.
motor	Pertaining to movement. Motor nerves carry messages from the brain and spinal cord to muscles and organs throughout the body.
myelin sheath	Tissue that surrounds the axon of some nerve fibers.
nerve	Macroscopic structure consisting of axons and dendrites in bundles like strands of rope.
neurilemma	Membranous covering around the myelin sheath of nerve cells.
neuroglia	Nerve cells that do not carry impulses but are supportive and connective in function. Examples are astrocytes, microglial cells, and oligodendroglia.
neuron	A nerve cell; carries impulses throughout the body.
parasympathetic nerves	Involuntary, autonomic nerves which help regulate body functions like heart rate and respiration.
peripheral nervous system	Nerves outside the brain and spinal cord; cranial and spinal nerves and autonomic nerves.
pia mater	Thin, delicate, inner membrane of the meninges.
plexus; plexuses	A large network of nerves.
pons	"Bridge"—part of the brain anterior to the cerebellum and between the medulla and the rest of the brain.
receptor	An organ that receives a nervous stimulation and passes it on to nerves within the body. The skin, ears, eyes, and taste buds are receptors.

sensory — Pertaining to sensation, feeling. Sensory nerves carry messages from a receptor to the brain and spinal cord.

stimulus; stimuli — An agent capable of initiating a response from a living tissue.

sulcus; sulci — Depression in the surface of the cerebral cortex; fissure.

sympathetic nerves — Autonomic nerves that influence body functions involuntarily in times of stress.

synapse — The space between neurons through which the nervous impulse "jumps" from one nerve cell to another.

thalamus — Portion of the brain that relays impulses from sense organs to the cerebrum.

ventricles of the brain — Canals in the interior of the brain which are filled with cerebrospinal fluid.

VII. COMBINING FORMS AND TERMINOLOGY

Combining Form	*Meaning*	*Terminology*	*Meaning*
neur/o	nerve	neurotomy	incision of nerve
		neuralgia	pain in nerves
		polyneuritis	inflammation of many nerves
		neurorrhaphy	to suture nerves
		neurogenic	formation of nerves
		neuropathy	disease of nerves
gangli/o ganglion/o	ganglion *("knot" of nerve cell bodies)*	ganglionectomy	excision (removal) of ganglion
plex/o	network, especially of nerves	cervical plexus	network of cervical nerves
		lumbosacral plexus	network of lumbar/sacral nerves
cerebr/o	brain, cerebrum	cerebromalacia	softening of the cerebrum
		cerebrospinal	pertaining to the brain/spinal cord
encephal/o	brain	encephalitis	inflammation of the brain

		encephalopathy disease of the brain
		anencephaly w/out the brain
cerebell/o	cerebellum	cerebellar pertaining to the cerebellum
		cerebellospinal pertaining to the cerebellar & spine
pont/o	pons	cerebellopontine ______
thalam/o	thalamus	thalamic pertaining to thalamus
ventricul/o	ventricles of the brain	ventriculography study (test) of ... brain *Cerebrospinal fluid is removed and replaced by contrast medium which outlines the ventricles on an x-ray film.*
myel/o	spinal cord	myelogram record of spinal cord
	(means bone marrow in other contexts)	myelitis inflammation of s. cord
		myelodysplasia underdeveloped s. cord
radicul/o	nerve root	radiculitis inflammation of nerve roots
	(of spinal nerves)	
mening/o meningi/o	membranes, meninges	meningioma tumor of meninges
		meningococcus bacteria in meninges
		meningeal pertaining to meninges
		meningomyelocele opening in the meninges
thec/o	sheath	intrathecal pertaining to the inner sheath of the meninges
	(meninges)	
dur/o	dura mater	subdural hematoma blood tumor under the dura mater *Figure 10-11 shows a subdural hematoma and an epidural hematoma.*
lept/o	thin, slender	leptomeningitis inflammation of thin meninges *The pia and arachnoid membranes are known as the leptomeninges because of their thinner, more delicate structure.*

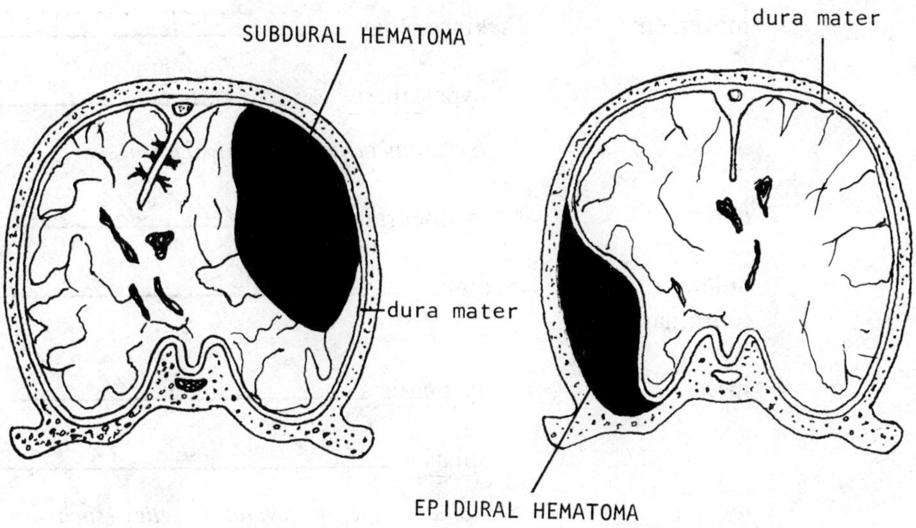

Figure 10-11 Subdural and epidural hematomas.

algesi/o	excessive sensitivity to pain	analgesia no sensitivity to pain
atel/o	incomplete	atelomyelia incomplete spinal cord
brachi/o	arm	brachial plexus plexus in the arm
esthesi/o	feeling, nervous sensation	anesthesia no feeling *This term applies to a lack of nervous sensation—for example, absence of sense of touch or pain.* dysesthesia painful feelings hypesthesia lack of feeling hyperesthesia excess of feeling paresthesia partial feeling *Para- means abnormal.*
gli/o	"glue," parts of the nervous system that support and connect	neuroglial pertaining to the glio in the nervous glioma tumor in the glio of N.S.
blephar/o	eyelid	blepharoptosis condition of the eyes & eyelids

kinesi/o	movement	kinesiology study of movement
		hyperkinesis excessive movement
		Hyperkinetic is the adjectival form.
my/o	muscle	myoneural pertaining to nerves & muscles
tax/o	order, coordination	ataxia incomplete coordination
phas/o	speech	dysphasia poor speech
		aphasia without speech
		Aphasias are of several varieties, such as: motor (ability to formulate but not execute or coordinate the muscles which are necessary for speech); and sensory (ability to see and hear and execute speech, but inability to understand speech or read language).
polio-	gray matter of the brain and spinal cord	poliomyelitis inflammation of brain matter
extra-	outside	extradural outside the dura
-asthenia	lack of strength	neurasthenia lack of nerves
		Nervous exhaustion; weakness and irritability.
-lexia	speech, word, phrase	dyslexia ____________
		Variety of reading, writing, and learning disorders.
-praxia	action	apraxia ____________
		Movements and behavior are not purposeful.
-paresis	slight paralysis	hemiparesis ____________
		Affects either right or left side (half) of the body.
-plegia	paralysis, palsy	hemiplegia ____________
	(loss or impairment of the ability to move parts of the body)	*Affects right or left half of the body.*
		paraplegia ____________
		Affects the lower extremities.
		quadriplegia ____________
		Affects all four extremities.

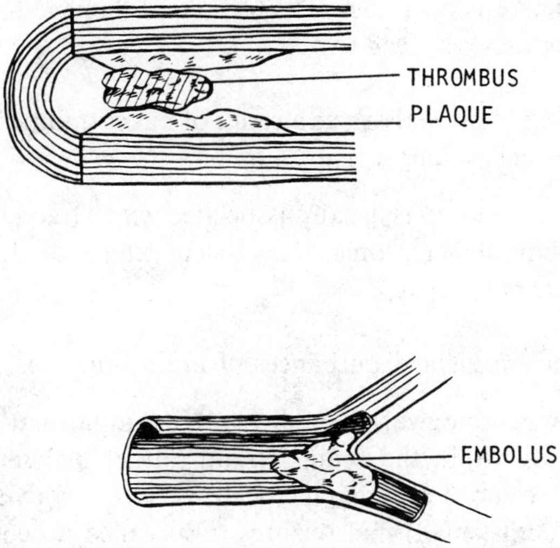

Figure 10-12 Top, A thrombus (blood clot) in a cerebral artery can lead to occlusion of the vessel and ischemia of brain tissue (stroke). Bottom, An embolus is brought by the blood from another vessel and is forced into a smaller area, thus blocking the circulation of blood.

VIII. PATHOLOGICAL CONDITIONS

cerebrovascular accident (CVA) Damage to the brain caused by a disorder within the blood vessels of the cerebrum.

This condition, also known as a **stroke** or **apoplexy**, is the result of a localized area of ischemia in the brain. This may be caused by:

1. **Thrombosis**—blood clot (thrombus) in the arteries leading to the brain, resulting in **occlusion** (blocking) of the vessel. This is the most common type of stroke, and may lead to paralysis.
2. **Embolism**—a piece of clot (embolus) breaks off from its place or origin and occludes a cerebral artery. This type of stroke occurs very suddenly. See Figure 10-12.
3. **Hemorrhage**—bursting forth of blood from a cerebral artery. This can be caused by advancing age, arteriosclerosis, or high blood pressure, all of which result in degeneration of cerebral blood vessels. If the hemorrhage is small, the blood is reabsorbed and the patient can make a good recovery with only slight disability. In a younger patient cerebral hemorrhage is usually due to mechanical injury associated with skull fracture or bursting of an arterial **aneurysm** (a weakness in the vessel wall which balloons and eventually bursts).

coma A state of unconsciousness from which the patient cannot be aroused.

An irreversible coma is one in which there is complete unresponsivity to stimuli, no spontaneous breathing or movement, and a flat electroencephalogram. This is also called brain death.

concussion of the brain Temporary brain dysfunction after injury, usually clearing within 24 hours.

There is no evidence of structural damage to the brain tissue. Severe concussions may lead to coma.

cerebral contusion

Bruising of brain tissue as a result of direct trauma to the head; neurological deficits persist longer than 24 hours.

A contusion is usually associated with a fracture of the skull. Extradural or subdural hematomas may occur and may lead to permanent brain damage or epilepsy.

epilepsy

Sudden transient disturbances of brain function.

A neurological disorder involving abnormal recurrent firing of nerve impulses within the brain. **Grand** (large) **mal** seizures (also called tonic-clonic seizures) are characterized by severe convulsions and unconsciousness. **Petit** (small) **mal** seizures (also called absence seizures) consist of a momentary lapse of consciousness.

Huntington's chorea (disease)

Hereditary nervous disorder involving bizarre, abrupt, involuntary movements.

This condition begins in adulthood and results in mental decline with choreic movements (twitching of the limbs and facial muscles).

hydrocephalus

Abnormal accumulation of fluid in the brain.

If circulation of cerebrospinal fluid in the brain or spinal cord is impaired, fluid may accumulate under pressure in the ventricles of the brain. Characteristic features, in infants, are enlarged head and small face. To relieve pressure on the brain, a catheter (shunt) is placed from the ventricle of the brain to the venous blood in the chest or heart so that the CSF is continually drained away from the brain.

meningitis

Inflammation of the meninges.

This condition may be caused by bacterial (meningococcus) or viral infection of the subarachnoid spaces. Treatment is with antibiotics.

multiple sclerosis

Destruction of the myelin sheath and its replacement by scar tissue.

Demyelination and replacement by neurological scar tissue prevents the conduction of nerve impulses through the axon and this causes muscle weakness and paralysis.

myasthenia gravis

Muscle weakness marked by progressive paralysis.

Loss of muscle strength due to lack of a chemical in the myoneural region. Nerve impulses fail to induce normal muscle contraction. It may affect any muscle of the body, but especially those of the face, lips, tongue, throat, and neck. Blepharoptosis may be a symptom. Drugs, such as neostigmine, are helpful in reversing the chemical disorder at the myoneural space, and removal of the thymus gland may even be curative.

palsy

Paralysis

Cerebral palsy is partial paralysis and lack of muscular coordination due to damage to the cerebrum during gestation or in the perinatal period. **Bell's palsy** involves unilateral facial paralysis, which is due to a disorder of the facial nerve. Etiology is unknown, but complete recovery is possible.

Parkinson's disease

Degeneration of nerves in the brain, occurring in later life, leading to tremors, weakness of muscles, and slowness of movement.

This slowly progressive condition leads to muscle stiffness, shuffling **gait** (manner of walking), and forward-leaning posture. Damage is to small areas of the midbrain which may be the result of viral infection or cerebral arteriosclerosis. Some drugs are useful in controlling symptoms, and surgery may be **palliative** (relieving) as well.

shingles

Viral disease affecting peripheral nerves.

Blisters and pain spread, in a bandlike pattern, over the skin, following the peripheral nerves which are affected. Shingles is also called **herpes zoster**.

spina bifida

Congenital defect of the spinal column due to imperfect union of the vertebral parts.

Spina bifida usually occurs in the lumbar region and there are several forms:

Spina bifida occulta—The vertebral lesion is covered over with skin and evident only on x-ray examination.

Spina bifida with meningocele—The meninges protrude through the vertebral defect. See Figure 10-13.

Spina bifida with meningomyelocele—The spinal cord and meninges herniate through the vertebral lesion.

Spina bifida may involve hydrocephalus, paraplegia, and lack of control of bladder and rectum. Surgery may be indicated to remove the herniated tissue.

syncope

Fainting; sudden loss of consciousness.

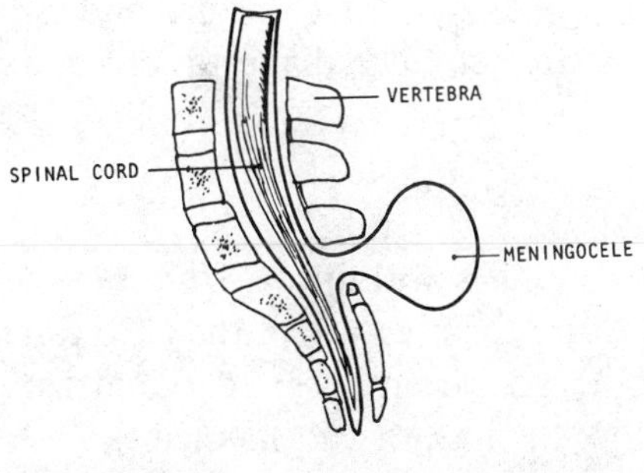

Figure 10-13 Spina bifida with meningocele.

tumors of the brain

Abnormal growths of brain tissue and meninges.

Most of the primary intracranial tumors arise from neuroglial cells (**gliomas**) or the meninges (**meningiomas**).

Gliomas are highly malignant tumors which, however, almost never metastasize. An example of a glioma is an **astrocytoma** (tumor composed of astrocytes). There are several types of astrocytomas, classified in order of degree of malignancy. One of the benign lesions is a cystic cerebellar astrocytoma; a highly malignant form is the glioblastoma multiforme. Oligodendrogliomas, medulloblastomas, and ependymomas are other types of gliomas. Gliomas are usually removed surgically. Radiotherapy is used for tumors that cannot be removed surgically and those that are incompletely resected.

Meningiomas are usually benign and surrounded by a capsule but may cause compression and distortion of the brain.

neuroblastoma

Malignant tumor arising from primitive nerve cells (neuroblasts).

Neuroblastomas may be inherited in some cases, and they occur most frequently in the adrenal gland. The tumor often occurs in childhood and is effectively treated with combined surgery and chemotherapy.

Alzheimer's disease

Brain disorder marked by deterioration of mental capacity beginning at middle age.

This disorder develops gradually, and early signs are loss of memory for recent events followed by impairment of judgment, comprehension, and intellect. Anxiety, depression, and other emotional disturbances can occur as well. Abnormal protein surrounded by bits of degenerated nerve fibers are commonly found at autopsy in the brains of patients who had Alzheimer's disease. There is as yet no effective treatment.

IX. LABORATORY TESTS, CLINICAL PROCEDURES, AND ABBREVIATIONS

Laboratory Tests

cerebrospinal fluid analysis

Cell counts, bacterial smears, and cultures of samples of CSF are done when disease of the meninges or brain is suspected. Normal constituents of CSF are water, glucose, sodium chloride, and protein, and changes in their concentrations are helpful in diagnosis of brain disease.

Clinical Procedures

lumbar (spinal) puncture

Cerebrospinal fluid is withdrawn from between two lumbar vertebrae. A device to measure the pressure of the CSF can be attached to the end of the needle after it has been inserted. Contrast medium for x-ray studies (myelography) or intrathecal medicines may be administered through lumbar puncture as well.

myelography
Contrast medium is injected into the cerebrospinal fluid and x-rays are taken of the spinal cord.

pneumoencephalography
Small amounts of air are injected intrathecally by lumbar puncture. The air travels through the spinal cord to the ventricles of the brain, and x-rays are taken of the entire brain. A method of visualizing only the ventricles is called **ventriculography**. In this technique, contrast medium is injected directly into the ventricles of the brain.

cerebral angiography
Contrast medium is injected into an artery and x-rays are taken of the blood vessel system of the brain. Also called **arteriography**.

electroencephalography
Recording of the electrical activity in the brain.

echoencephalography
Ultasonic waves are beamed through the head and echoes coming from brain structures are recorded as a picture. This is useful in detecting head injuries, brain tumors, and hydrocephalus.

computed tomography
X-rays are used to compose a computerized cross-sectional picture of the brain. Contrast medium may also be injected to see abnormalities. The contrast medium leaks through the **blood-brain barrier** from blood vessels into the brain tissue. Normally, the blood-brain barrier serves to slow the passage of drugs and fluids from the blood into the brain tissue. (May also be called computerized tomography or computed axial tomography.)

positron emission tomography (PET)
An isotope (radioactive chemical) that gives off particles called positrons is injected intravenously combined with a form of glucose. The uptake of the radioactive material is then recorded on a television screen. The cross-sectional images show how the brain metabolizes glucose and give information about brain function. Thus far, PET has yielded information in patients with epilepsy, stroke, schizophrenia, and Alzheimer's disease, as well normal subjects.

radioactive brain scan
Radioactive chemicals are given and are absorbed into the body. Special machines then record the passage and absorption of the chemicals into brain tissue. If there is a brain lesion, the radioactive molecules "leak" across the blood-brain barrier and concentrate in abnormal sites.

stereotaxic neurosurgery
Use of a stereotaxic instrument which, when fixed onto the skull, can locate a neurosurgical target by three-dimensional measurement. A probe containing an electrical, chemical, or cryogenic agent can then be introduced into the brain.

trephination
Cutting a circular opening into the skull (**craniotomy**).

Abbreviations

ACh	Acetylcholine
AFP	Alpha-fetoprotein (elevated levels in amniotic fluid and maternal blood are associated with congenital malformations of the nervous system, such as anencephaly and spina bifida)
CNS	Central nervous system
CSF	Cerebrospinal fluid
CT	Computed tomography (also CAT—computed axial tomography)
CVA	Cerebrovascular accident
EEG	Electroencephalogram
LP	Lumbar puncture
MS	Multiple sclerosis
PEG	Pneumoencephalography
PET	Positron emission tomography
TIA	Transient ischemic attack (temporary interference with the blood supply to the brain)

X. PRACTICAL APPLICATIONS

Autopsy Report: Brain and Meninges

Meninges were clear and adherent to underlying brain. The brain was grossly without evidence of metastases. There was questionable evidence of herniation bilaterally over the sphenoid ridge [the sphenoid bone is at the base of the brain] and herniation of the cerebellum. The brain was edematous. On the lateral surface of the pons there is a small (less than 1 cm), brownish red lesion located below the arachnoid thought to be hemorrhage vs. metastasis. Microscopically, the cerebral cortex over the sphenoid ridge did not demonstrate evidence of herniation; however, the grossly nonpigmented area of necrosis in the cerebellum revealed metastatic melanoma [malignant tumor of pigmented skin cells]. On the right lateral surface of the pons, the grossly pigmented lesion was on microscopic examination metastatic melanoma.

Diagnosis: 1. Brain, edema.
2. Metastatic melanoma, pons, cerebellum.

Case Report

This patient was admitted on January 14 with a history of progressive right hemiparesis for the previous 1 to 2 months, fluctuating numbness of the right arm, thorax, and buttocks, jerking of the right leg, periods of speech arrest, diminished comprehension in reading, and recent development of a spastic hemiplegic gait [partial hemiplegia with spasmodic contractions of muscles when walking]. He is suspected of having a left parietal tumor [the parietal lobes of the cerebrum are on either side under the roof of the skull].

Examinations done prior to hospitalization included skull films, EEG, brain scan, and CSF analysis, which were all normal. Following admission the brain scan was abnormal in the left parietal region, as was the EEG.

Left percutaneous common carotid angiography [the carotid arteries are in the neck and supply the brain with blood] was attempted, but the patient became progressively more restless and agitated after receiving the sedation, so that it was impossible to do the procedure. During the recovery phase from the sedation the patient was alternately somnolent [sleepy] and violent, but it was later apparent that he had developed almost a complete aphasia and right hemiplegia.

In the next few days be became more alert although he remained dysarthric [from arthroun—to utter distinctly] and hemiplegic.

Bilateral carotid angiograms under general anesthesia on January 19 showed complete occlusion of the left internal carotid artery with cross-filling of the left anterior and middle cerebral arteries from the right internal carotid circulation.

Final diagnosis: Left cerebral infarction due to left internal carotid artery occlusion.

[Figure 10-14 shows the common carotid arteries and their branches within the head and brain.]

XI. EXERCISES

A. Identify:

1. middle meningeal membrane arachoid membrane
2. sulci fissures of the cerebrum

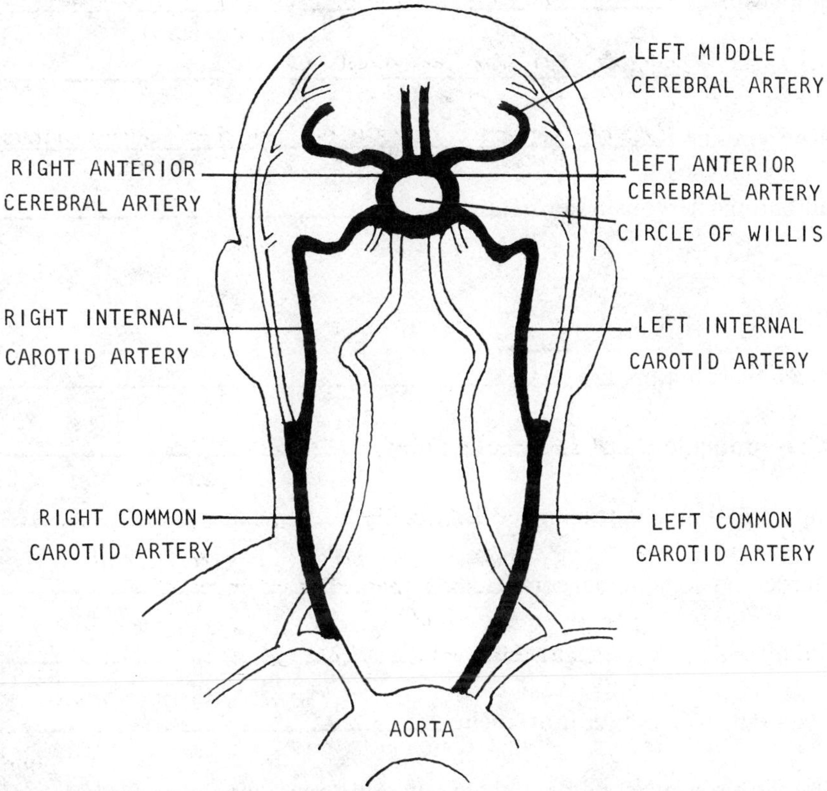

Figure 10-14 Common carotid arteries and their branches.

3. ganglion nerve cell bodies outside brain knotted

4. dendrites neuron fibers

5. pons bridge bet. medulla & brain

6. plexus networks of nerves pertaining to A.N.S.

7. medulla oblongata brain stem, nerve fibers cross here

8. efferent neuron takes messages away from brain to body

9. cerebellum posterior in brain, coordinates movement

10. dura mater outer most meninge

11. synapse space that impulse travels across

12. peripheral nervous system cranial, spinal nerves & auto. N.S.

13. neuroglia supportive & connective cells

14. axon carries nerve impulse from the cell body

15. embolism piece of clot breaks off & clogs artery

16. astrocyte type of neuroglial cell

17. acetylcholine chemical which aids in nerve transmission

18. autonomic nervous system involemtary movements

B. Build medical words:

1. Incomplete brain atelencephalia

2. No coordination atataxia

3. Inflammation of the meninges meningitis

4. Hardening of the spinal cord myeloscrelosis

5. Suture of a nerve neurorraphy

6. Pertaining to excessive movement ____________

7. One who specializes in the study of rendering one feelingless anethesiologist

8. Pertaining to the network of nerves in the arm ______

9. No strength in muscles ______

10. Difficult speech dysphagia ______

11. Slight paralysis hemiparalysis (pareses) ______

12. Incision into the thalamus thalamotomy ______

13. Tumor of the membranes surrounding the brain and spinal cord ______

14. Hernia of the spinal cord ______

15. Pertaining to the cerebellum and pons ______

C. *Give the meaning of the following:*

1. hyperesthesia ______

2. gyri ______

3. paraplegia ______

4. sympathectomy ______

5. glioma ______

6. hypothalamus ______

7. myelogram ______

8. lumbar puncture ______

9. subdural hematoma ______

10. apoplexy ______

11. multiple sclerosis ______

12. analgesia ______

13. polioencephalitis ______

14. spina bifida ______

15. syncope ______

16. hypesthesia ______________________________

17. concussion ______________________________

18. myoneural ______________________________

19. coma ______________________________

20. aphasia ______________________________

21. cerebral contusion ______________________________

D. *Select the medical term from those listed below to complete the following sentences:*

cerebral cortex	neurilemma
gait	leptomeningitis
radiculitis	intrathecal
occlusion	parenchymal
thalamus	stromal

1. Inflammation of the inner two membranes surrounding the brain and spinal cord is called ______________________________.

2. A manner of walking is known as ______________________________.

3. The neuron is the ______________________ tissue of the nervous system.

4. Neuroglial cells are the ______________________ tissue of the nervous system.

5. The ______________________________ is the outer region of the brain.

6. Inflammation of a nerve root near the spinal cord is called ____________________.

7. Blockage of a tube or vessel is called ______________________________.

8. An outer covering surrounding part of a nerve cell is the ____________________.

9. A term meaning "within the membranes" around the spinal cord is ______________________________.

10. An important relay center in the diencephalon is the ____________________.

E. Name the nervous system symptom:

1. Excessive sensitivity (nervous feeling) ethesia
2. Slight paralysis in lower limbs paraplegia
3. Abnormal sensations (tingling, numbness) ____________
4. Movements which are not purposeful ____________
5. Lack of muscular coordination ____________
6. Difficult speech dysphagia
7. Fainting ____________
8. Paralysis of half (right or left side) of the body ____________
9. Nervous exhaustion, weakness ____________
10. Inability to understand the meaning of a written word ____________

F. What's your diagnosis?

1. Grand mal seizures; "electrical storm" in the brain ____________
2. Muscle weakness; defect at the myoneural junction ____________
3. Demyelination of nerve fibers occurs; hard scar tissue forms ____________
4. Viral disease affects peripheral nerves; blisters and pain ____________
5. Unilateral facial paralysis ____________
6. Congenital defect of vertebral column resulting in herniation of the meninges and spinal cord ____________
7. Hereditary nervous disorder marked by bizarre muscle movements and mental deterioration ____________
8. Tremors, rigidity, shuffling gait in later life ____________
9. Intracranial malignant neuroglial mass ____________

10. Partial paralysis, poor muscular coordination caused by cerebral damage at birth ____________________

G. *Name the procedure or test:*

1. Record of the electricity in the brain ____________________
2. Radioactive chemicals are traced throughout the brain ____________________
3. Air is injected by lumbar puncture and x-rays are taken of the brain ____________________
4. Contrast medium is injected into an artery and x-rays are taken of the brain ____________________
5. Process of cutting out a piece of skull bone with a trephine ____________________
6. Location of a neurosurgical target using a special three-dimensional instrument ____________________
7. Fluid is taken from the subarachnoid space and examined ____________________
8. X-ray record of the spinal cord ____________________

H. *Give the meaning of the following medical abbreviations:*

1. LP ____________________
2. EKG ____________________
3. CVA ____________________
4. CNS ____________________
5. CSF ____________________
6. EEG ____________________
7. TIA ____________________
8. PEG ____________________

ANSWERS

A.

1. Arachnoid membrane.
2. Depressions or grooves in the cerebral cortex.
3. Mass or knot of nerve cells.
4. Branching fibers that conduct impulses to the cell body of a neuron.
5. Portion of the brain that connects the cerebellum and medulla oblongata to the cerebrum.
6. Nerve network.
7. Posterior part of the brain; contains vital centers of regulation.
8. Nerve cell that conducts impulse away from CNS.
9. Portion of the brain which controls balance and coordination.
10. Tough outer membrane surrounding the brain and spinal cord.
11. Connection between two neurons for passage of impulse.
12. Part of the nervous system that consists of nerves outside the brain and spinal cord.
13. "Nerve glue," i.e., interstitial nerve cells which are supportive; aid in nourishment and fighting disease.
14. Part of a neuron which conducts impulse away from cell body.
15. Floating clot or other material occluding a blood vessel.
16. Type of neuroglial cell; aids in nourishment of neurons. They are frequently gliomas.
17. Body chemical released at the synapse which aids in the transmission of nerve impulse.
18. Involuntary, peripheral nerves which direct functions not under conscious control.

B.

1. atelencephalia
2. ataxia
3. meningitis
4. myelosclerosis
5. neurorrhaphy
6. hyperkinetic
7. anesthesiologist
8. brachial plexus
9. myasthenia
10. dysphasia
11. paresis
12. thalamotomy
13. meningioma
14. myelocele
15. cerebellopontine

C.

1. Excessive feeling.
2. Elevations in the cerebral cortex.
3. Paralysis—lower half of the body.
4. Removal of a sympathetic nerve.
5. A tumor of neuroglial cells.
6. Part of brain under the thalamus; controls sleep, temperature, and pituitary gland.
7. Record (x-ray) of the spinal cord.
8. Puncture into the lumbar spinal cord to remove cerebrospinal fluid.
9. Collection of blood in the subdural space.
10. Cerebrovascular accident—a stroke.
11. Destruction of the myelin sheath and its replacement by scar tissue.
12. Lack of excessive sensitivity to pain.
13. Inflammation of the gray matter of the brain.
14. Congenital defect of imperfect closure of spinal column.
15. Fainting.
16. Diminished pain sensation.
17. Temporary brain dysfunction after injury.
18. Pertaining to muscles and nerves.
19. State of unconsciousness from which the patient cannot be aroused.
20. Inability to speak.
21. Bruising of brain tissue as a result of head trauma.

D.

1. leptomeningitis
2. gait
3. parenchymal
4. stromal
5. cerebral cortex
6. radiculitis
7. occlusion
8. neurilemma
9. intrathecal
10. thalamus

E.

1. hyperesthesia
2. paraparesis
3. paresthesias
4. apraxia
5. ataxia
6. dysphasia
7. syncope
8. hemiplegia
9. neurasthenia
10. dyslexia

F.

1. epilepsy
2. myasthenia gravis
3. multiple sclerosis
4. shingles; herpes zoster
5. Bell's palsy
6. spina bifida with meningomyelocele
7. Huntington's chorea (disease)
8. Parkinson's disease
9. glioma; astrocytoma, glioblastoma
10. cerebral palsy

G.

1. electroencephalogram
2. brain scan
3. pneumoencephalography
4. cerebral angiography; arteriography
5. trephination
6. stereotaxic neurosurgery
7. cerebrospinal fluid analysis
8. myelogram

H.

1. lumbar puncture
2. electrocardiogram
3. cerebrovascular accident
4. central nervous system
5. cerebrospinal fluid
6. electroencephalogram
7. transient ischemic attack
8. pneumoencephalography

XII. PRONUNCIATION OF TERMS

acetylcholine	ăs-ĕ-tĭl-KŌ-lēn
afferent	ĂF-ĕr-ĕnt
analgesia	ăn-ăl-JĒ-zē-ă
anencephaly	ăn-ĕn-SĔF-ă-lē
anesthesia	ăn-ĕs-THĒ-zē-ă
aneurysm	ĂN-ū-rĭzm
angiography	ăn-jē-ŎG-ră-fē
aphasia	ă-FĀ-zē-ă
apoplexy	ĂP-ō-plĕk-sē
apraxia	ā-PRĂK-sē-ă
arachnoid	ă-RĂK-noyd
astrocyte	ĂS-trō-sīt
astrocytoma	ăs-trō-sī-TŌ-mă
ataxia	ă-TĂK-sē-ă
atelomyelia	ăt-ĕl-ō-mī-Ē-lē-ă
autonomic	ăw-tō-NŎM-ĭk
axon	ĂK-sŏn
blepharoptosis	blĕf-ă-rŏp-TŌ-sĭs
brachial plexus	BRĀ-kē-ăl PLĔK-sŭs
cauda equina	KĂW-dă ē-QUĪ-nă
cerebellar	sĕr-ĕ-BĔL-ăr
cerebellopontine	sĕr-ĕ-bĕl-ō-PŎN-tēn
cerebellum	sĕr-ĕ-BĔL-ŭm

cerebral cortex	sĕ-RĒ-brăl (or SĔR-ĕ-brăl) KŎR-tĕks
cerebromalacia	sĕ-rē-brō-mă-LĀ-shă or sĕr-eĕ-brō-mă-LĀ-shă
cerebrospinal	sĕ-rē-brō-SPĪ-năl or sĕr-ĕ-brō-SPĪ-năl
cerebrovascular	sĕ-rē-brō-VĂS-kū-lăr or sĕr-ĕ-brō-VĂS-kū-lăr
cerebrum	sĕ-RĒ-brŭm or SĔR-ĕ-brŭm
cervical plexus	SĔR-vĭ-kăl PLĔK-sŭs
chorea	kō-RĒ-ă
concussion	kŏn-KŬSH-ŭn
contusion	kon-TŪ-zhŭn
convolution	kŏn-vō-LŪ-shŭn
dendrite	DĔN-drīt
dura mater	DŪ-ră MĀ-tĕr
dysesthesia	dĭs-ĕs-THĒ-zē-ă
dyslexia	dĭs-LĔK-sē-ă
dysphasia	dĭs-FĀ-zē-ă
echoencephalography	ĕk-ō-ĕn-sĕf-ă-LŎG-ră-fē
efferent	ĔF-ĕr-ĕnt
electroencephalography	ē-lĕk-trō-ĕn-sĕf-ă-LŎG-ră-fē
embolism	ĔM-bō-lĭzm
encephalitis	ĕn-sĕf-ă-LĪ-tĭs
encephalopathy	ĕn-sĕf-ă-LŎP-ă-thē
epilepsy	ĔP-ĭ-lĕp-sē
extradural	ĕks-trĕ-DŪ-răl
fissure	FĬSH-ūr
gait	gāt
ganglion; ganglia	GĂNG-glē-ŏn; GĂNG-glē-ă
ganglionectomy	găng-glē-ō-NĔK-tō-mē
glioma	glī-Ō-mă
grand mal	grăhn măl
gyrus; gyri	JĪ-rŭs; JĪ-rē
hemiparesis	hĕm-ē-pă-RĒ-sĭs or hĕm-ē-PĂR-ĕ-sĭs
hemiplegia	hĕm-ē-PLĒ-jă

herpes zoster	HĔR-pēz ZŎS-tĕr
hyperesthesia	hī-pĕr-ĕs-THĒ-zē-ă
hyperkinetic	hī-pĕr-kĭ-NĔT-ĭk
hypesthesia	hīp-ĕs-THĒ-zē-ă or hĭp-ĕs-THĒ-zē-ă
hypothalamus	hī-pō-THĂL-ă-mŭs
intrathecal	ĭn-tră-THĒ-kăl
kinesiology	kĭ-nē-sē-ŎL-ō-jē
leptomeningitis	lĕp-tō-mĕn-ĭn-JĪ-tĭs
lumbosacral plexus	lŭm-bō-SĀ-krăl PLĔK-sŭs
medulla oblongata	mĕ-DŪL-ă (or mĕ-DŬL-ă) ŏb-lŏng-GĂ-tă
meningeal	mĕ-NIN-jē-ăl or mĕ-nĭn-JĒ-ăl
meninges	mĕ-NĬN-jēz
meningioma	mĕ-nĭn-jē-Ō-mă
meningitis	mĕn-ĭn-JĪ-tĭs
meningococcus	mĕ-nĭng-go-KŎK-ŭs
meningomyelocele	mĕ-nĭng-gō-MĪ-ĕ-lō-sēl
microglial	mī-krō-GLĒ-ăl or mī-KRŎG-lē-ăl
myasthenia gravis	mī-ăs-THĒ-nē-ă GRĂ-vĭs
myelin sheath	MĪ-ĕ-lĭn shēth
myelitis	mī-ĕ-LĪ-tĭs
myelodysplasia	mī-ĕ-lō-dĭs-PLĀ-zē-ă
myelogram	MĪ-ĕ-lō-grăm
myoneural	mī-ō-NŪ-răl
neuralgia	nū-RĂL-jă
neurasthenia	nū-răs-THĒ-nē-ă
neurilemma	nū-rĭ-LĔM-mă
neuroblastoma	nū-rō-blăs-TŌ-mă
neurogenic	nū-rō-JĔN-ĭk
neuroglial	nū-RŎG-lē-ăl
neuron	NŪ-rŏn
neuropathy	nū-RŎP-ă-thē
neurorrhaphy	nū-RŎR-ă-fē

neurotomy	nū-RŎT-tō-mē
oligodendroglioma	ŏl-ĭ-gō-dĕn-drō-glī-Ō-mă
palsy	PAWL-zē
paraplegia	păr-ă-PLĒ-jă
parasympathetic	păr-ă-sĭm-pă-THĔT-ĭk
paresthesia	păr-ĕs-THĒ-zē-ă
petit mal	pĕ-TĒ măl
pia mater	PĒ-ă MĀ-tĕr
plexus	PLĔK-sŭs
pneumoencephalography	nū-mō-ĕn-sĕf-ă-LŎG-ră-fē
poliomyelitis	pō-lē-ō-mī-ĕ-LĪ-tĭs
polyneuritis	pŏl-ē-nū-RĪ-tĭs
pons	pŏnz
quadriplegia	kwŏd-rĭ-PLĒ-jă
radiculitis	ră-dĭk-ū-LĪ-tĭs
spina bifida	SPĪ-nă BĬF-ĭ-dă
stereotaxic	stĕ-rē-ō-TĂK-sĭk
sulcus; sulci	SŬL-kŭs; SŬL-sī
sympathetic	sĭm-pă-THĔT-ĭk
synapse	SĬN-ăps
syncope	SĬN-kō-pē
thalamic	THĂL-ă-mĭk or thă-LĂM-ĭk
thalamus	THĂL-ă-mŭs
trephination	trĕf-ĭ-NĀ-shŭn
ventricles	VĔN-trĭ-k'lz
ventriculography	vĕn-trĭk-ū-LŎG-ră-fē

REVIEW SHEET 10

Combining Forms

algesi/o	________	hydr/o	________
angi/o	________	kinesi/o	________
atel/o	________	lept/o	________
blephar/o	________	mening/o	________
brachi/o	________	meningi/o	________
cerebell/o	________	my/o	________
cerebr/o	________	myel/o	________
crani/o	________	neur/o	________
cry/o	________	plex/o	________
dur/o	________	pont/o	________
encephal/o	________	radicul/o	________
esthesi/o	________	tax/o	________
gangli/o	________	thalam/o	________
ganglion/o	________	thec/o	________
gli/o	________	ventricul/o	________

Prefixes

a-, an-	________	extra-	________
dys-	________	hemi-	________
hyper-	________	micro-	________
hypo-	________	polio-	________
macro-	________	quadri-	________

Suffixes

Give the suffix:		*Give the meaning:*	
____________	embryonic	-phasia	____________
____________	hernia	-phagia	____________
____________	hardening	-plasia	____________
____________	suture	-praxia	____________
____________	paralysis	-malacia	____________
____________	slight paralysis	-lexia	____________
____________	lack of strength	-ptosis	____________
____________	pain	-kinesia	____________
____________	berry-shaped (bacteria)	-algesia	____________
		-taxia	____________
		-esthesia	____________

Additional Terms

Use this list of terms as a test of your knowledge by **checking off** the ones you can define and **circling** the ones you do not understand. Use the page references provided to find the definitions of the circled terms. Writing down the meanings of the terms you do not know will help you remember them.

acetylcholine (243)

afferent nerves (243)

arachnoid membrane (243)

astrocyte (243)

astrocytoma (252)

autonomic nervous system (243)

axon (243)

cauda equina (243)

cerebellum (243)

cerebral angiography (253)

cerebral cortex (243)

cerebrospinal fluid (243)

cerebrovascular accident (249)

cerebrum (243)

coma (249)

computed tomography (CT) (253)

concussion (249)

contusion (250)

convolutions (gyri) (243)

dendrites (243)

dura mater (243)

echoencephalography (253)

efferent nerves (243)

epilespy (250)

fissures (sulci) (244)

ganglion (244)

glioma (252)

herpes zoster (251)

Huntington's chorea (250)

hydrocephalus (250)

hypothalamus (244)

leptomeninges (246)

lumbar puncture (252)

medulla oblongata (244)

meninges (244)

microglial cells (244)

multiple sclerosis (250)

myasthenia gravis (250)

myelin sheath (244)

myelography (253)

neurilemma (244)

neuroblastoma (252)

neuroglia (244)

neuron (244)

palliative (251)

palsy (251)

parasympathetic nerves (244)

Parkinson's disease (251)

pia mater (244)

plexus (244)

pons (244)

positron emission tomography (PET) (253)

pneumoencephalography (253)

radioactive brain scan (253)

receptor (244)

shingles (251)

spina bifida (251)

stereotaxic neurosurgery (253)

stimulus (245)

sympathetic nerves (245)

synapse (245)

syncope (251)

thalamus (245)

trephination (253)

ventricles of the brain (245)

ventriculography (253)

CHAPTER 11

CARDIOVASCULAR SYSTEM

In this chapter you will:

- Name the parts of the heart, and associated blood vessels, and their functions in the circulation of blood;
- Trace the pathway of blood through the heart;
- List the meanings of major pathological conditions affecting the heart and blood vessels;
- Define combining forms which relate to the cardiovascular system; and
- Recognize the meaning of many laboratory tests, clinical procedures, and abbreviations pertaining to the circulatory system.

This chapter is divided into the following sections:

I. INTRODUCTION

In previous chapters we have discussed the diverse and important functions of many organs of the body. These functions include conduction of nerve impulses, production of hormones and reproductive cells, excretion of waste materials, and digestion and absorption of food substances into the bloodstream. In order to perform these functions reliably and efficiently, the body organs are powered by a unique energy source. The cells of each organ receive energy from the food substances which reach them after being taken into the body. Food contains stored energy which can be converted into the energy of movement and work. This conversion of stored energy into the active energy of work occurs when food and oxygen combine in cells during the chemical process of catabolism. It is obvious then that each cell of each organ is dependent on a constant supply of food and oxygen in order to receive sufficient energy to work well.

How does the body assure that oxygen and food will be delivered to all its cells? The cardiovascular system, consisting of a fluid called blood, vessels to carry the blood, and a hollow, muscular pump called the heart, transports food and oxygen to all organs and cells of the body. Blood vessels in the lungs absorb the oxygen that has been inhaled from the air, and blood vessels in the small intestine absorb food substances from the digestive tract. In addition, blood vessels carry cellular waste materials such as carbon dioxide and urea, and transport these substances to the lungs and kidneys, respectively, where they can be eliminated from the body.

The heart and blood vessels and the terminology related to their anatomy, physiology, and disease conditions will be explored in this chapter. The nature of blood and another body fluid called lymph will be discussed in a later chapter.

II. BLOOD VESSELS AND THE CIRCULATION OF BLOOD

Blood Vessels

There are three major types of blood vessels in the body. These are called arteries, veins, and capillaries.

Arteries are the large blood vessels that lead blood away from the heart. Their walls are made of connective tissue, elastic fibers, and an innermost layer of epithelial cells. Because arteries carry blood away from the heart, they must be strong enough to withstand the high pressure of the pumping action of the heart. Their elastic walls allow them to expand as the heartbeat forces blood into the arterial system throughout the body. Smaller branches of arteries are called **arterioles**. Arterioles are thinner than arteries and carry the blood to the tiniest of blood vessels, the capillaries.

Capillaries have walls which are only one epithelial cell in thickness. These delicate, microscopic vessels carry nutrient-rich, oxygenated blood from the arteries and arterioles to the body cells. Their walls are thin enough to allow passage of oxygen and nutrients out of the bloodstream and into the tissue fluid surrounding the cells. Once inside the cells, the nutrients are burned in the presence of oxygen (catabolism) to release needed energy within the cell. At the same time, waste products such as carbon dioxide and water pass out of the cells and into the thin-walled capillaries. The waste-filled blood then flows back to the heart in small veins called **venules,** which branch to form larger vessels called veins.

Veins are thinner-walled than arteries. They conduct waste-filled blood toward the heart from the tissues. Veins have little elastic tissue and less connective tissue than arteries, and blood pressure in veins is extremely low as compared to pressure in arteries. In order to keep blood moving back toward the heart, veins have valves that prevent the backflow of blood and keep the blood moving in one direction. Muscular action also helps the movement of blood in veins. Figure 11-1 illustrates the differences in blood vessels.

Circulation of Blood

Arteries, arterioles, veins, venules, and capillaries, together with the heart, form a circulatory system for the flow of blood. Figure 11-2 is a schematic representation of this circulatory system. Refer to it as you read the following paragraphs.

Blood deficient in oxygen flows through two large veins, the **venae cavae** (1), on its way from the tissue capillaries to the heart. The blood became oxygen-poor at the tissue capillaries when oxygen left the blood and entered the body cells.

Oxygen-poor blood enters the **right side of the heart** (2) and travels through the side and into the **pulmonary artery** (3), a vessel which divides in two, one branch leading to the left lung, the other to the right lung. The arteries continue dividing and subdividing within the **lungs** (4), forming smaller and smaller vessels (arterioles) and finally reaching the lung capillaries. The pulmonary artery is unusual in that it is the only artery in the body that carries blood deficient in oxygen.

While passing through the lung (pulmonary) capillaries, blood absorbs the oxygen which entered the body during inhalation. The newly oxygenated blood next immediately returns to

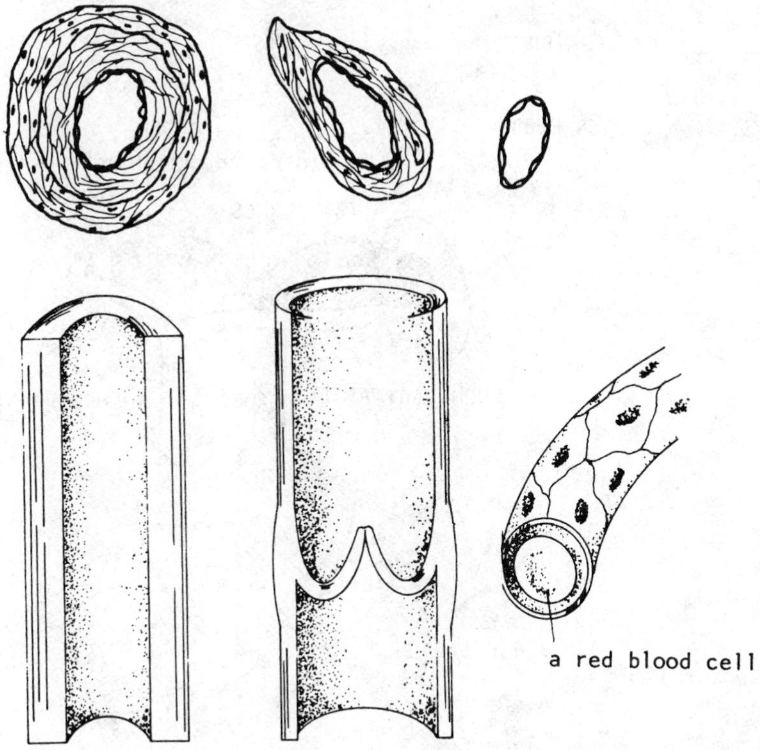

Figure 11-1 Blood vessels.

the heart through the **pulmonary vein** (5). The pulmonary vein is unusual in that it is the only vein in the body that carries oxygen-rich (**oxygenated**) blood. The circulation of blood through the vessels from the heart to the lungs and then back to the heart again is known as the **pulmonary circulation**.

Oxygen-rich blood enters the **left side of the heart** (6) from the pulmonary veins. The muscles in the left side of the heart pump the blood out of the heart through the largest single artery in the body, the **aorta** (7). The aorta moves up at first (ascending aorta) but then arches over dorsally and runs downward (descending aorta) just in front of the vertebral column. The aorta divides into numerous branches called **arteries** (8) which carry the oxygenated blood to all parts of the body. The names of some of these arterial branches will be familiar to you: brachiocephalic, intercostal, esophageal, celiac, renal, and iliac arteries. The **carotid** arteries supply blood to the head and neck.

The relatively large arterial vessels branch further to form the smaller **arterioles** (9). The arterioles, still containing oxygenated blood, branch into smaller tissue **capillaries** (10), which are near the body cells. Oxygen leaves the blood and passes through the thin capillary walls to enter the body cells. There, involved in complicated chemical (metabolic) processes, it combines with food to release needed energy.

One metabolic product of these chemical processes is **carbon dioxide** (CO_2). CO_2 is produced in the cell but is harmful to the cell if it remains. It must thus pass out of the cells and into the capillary bloodstream, at the same time that oxygen is entering the cell. As the blood makes it way back from the tissue capillaries toward the heart in **venules** (11) and **veins** (12), it is full of CO_2 and is oxygen-poor.

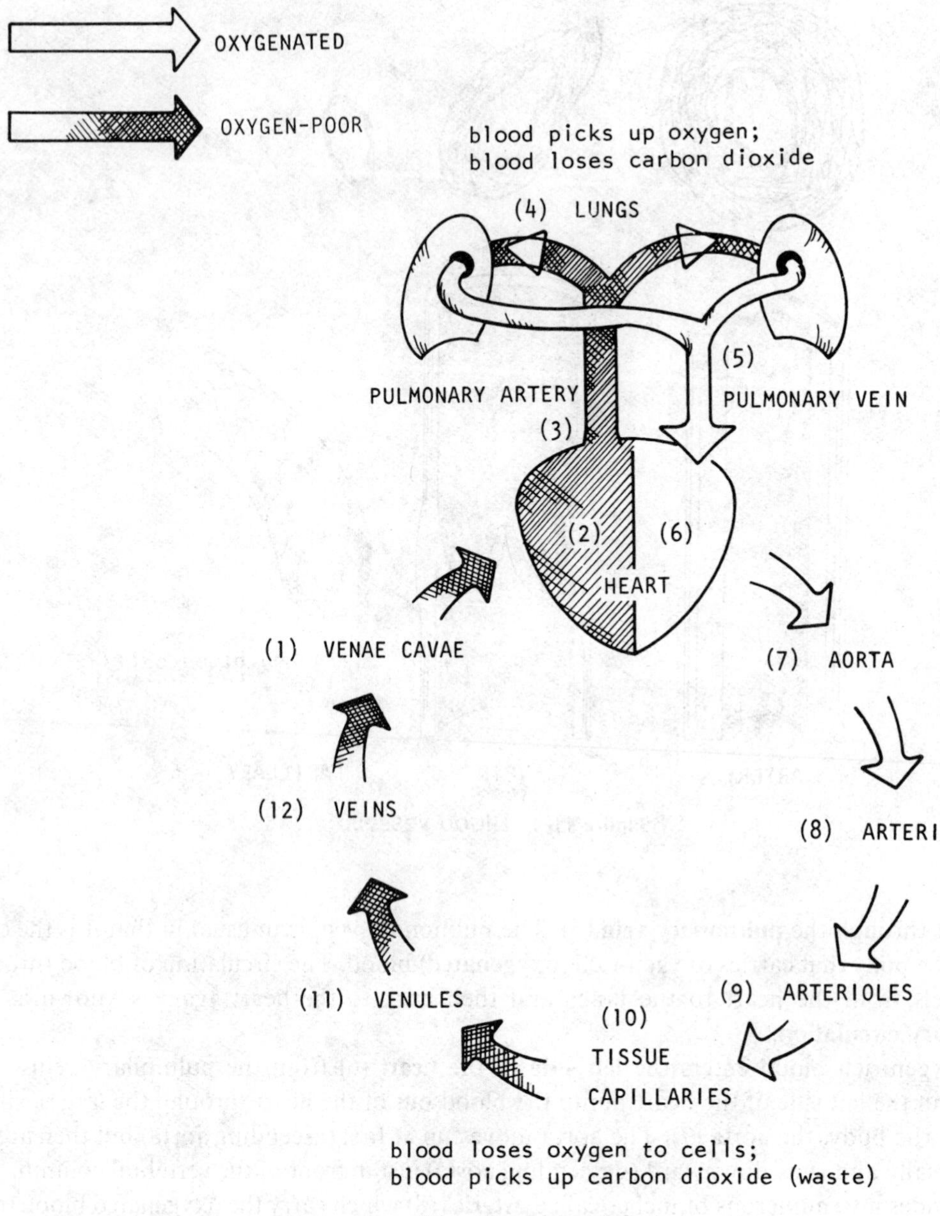

Figure 11-2 Circuit of blood flow.

The circuit is thus completed when oxygen-poor blood enters the heart from the venae cavae. This circulation of blood from the body organs (except the lungs) to the heart and back again is called the **systemic circulation**.

III. ANATOMY OF THE HEART

The human heart weighs less than a pound, is roughly the size of the human fist, and lies in the thoracic cavity, just behind the breastbone and between the lungs.

The heart is a pump, consisting of four chambers: two upper chambers called **atria** (singular: atrium), and two lower chambers called **ventricles**. It is actually a double pump, bound into one organ and synchronized very carefully. Blood passes through each pump in a definite pattern. Pump station number one, on the right side of the heart, sends oxygen-deficient blood to the lungs, where the blood picks up oxygen and releases its carbon dioxide. The newly oxygenated blood returns to the left side of the heart to pump station number two and does not mix with the oxygen-poor blood in pump station number one. Pump station number two then forces the oxygenated blood out to all parts of the body. At the body tissues, the blood loses its oxygen and upon returning to the heart, to pump station number one, blood poor in oxygen (rich in carbon dioxide) is sent out to the lungs to begin the cycle anew.

Label Figure 11-3 as you learn the names of the parts of the heart and the vessels that carry blood to and from it.

Oxygen-poor blood enters the heart through the two largest veins in the body, the **venae cavae**. The **superior vena cava** (1) drains blood from the upper portion of the body, while the **inferior vena cava** (2) carries blood from the lower part of the body.

The venae cavae bring oxygen-poor blood that has passed through all of the body to the **right atrium** (3), the thin-walled upper right chamber of the heart. The right atrium contracts to force blood through the **tricuspid valve** (4) (cusps are the flaps of the valves) into the **right ventricle** (5), which is the lower right chamber of the heart. The cusps of the tricuspid valve form a one-way passageway designed to keep the blood flowing in only one direction. As the right ventricle contracts to pump oxygen-poor blood through the **pulmonary valve** (6) into the

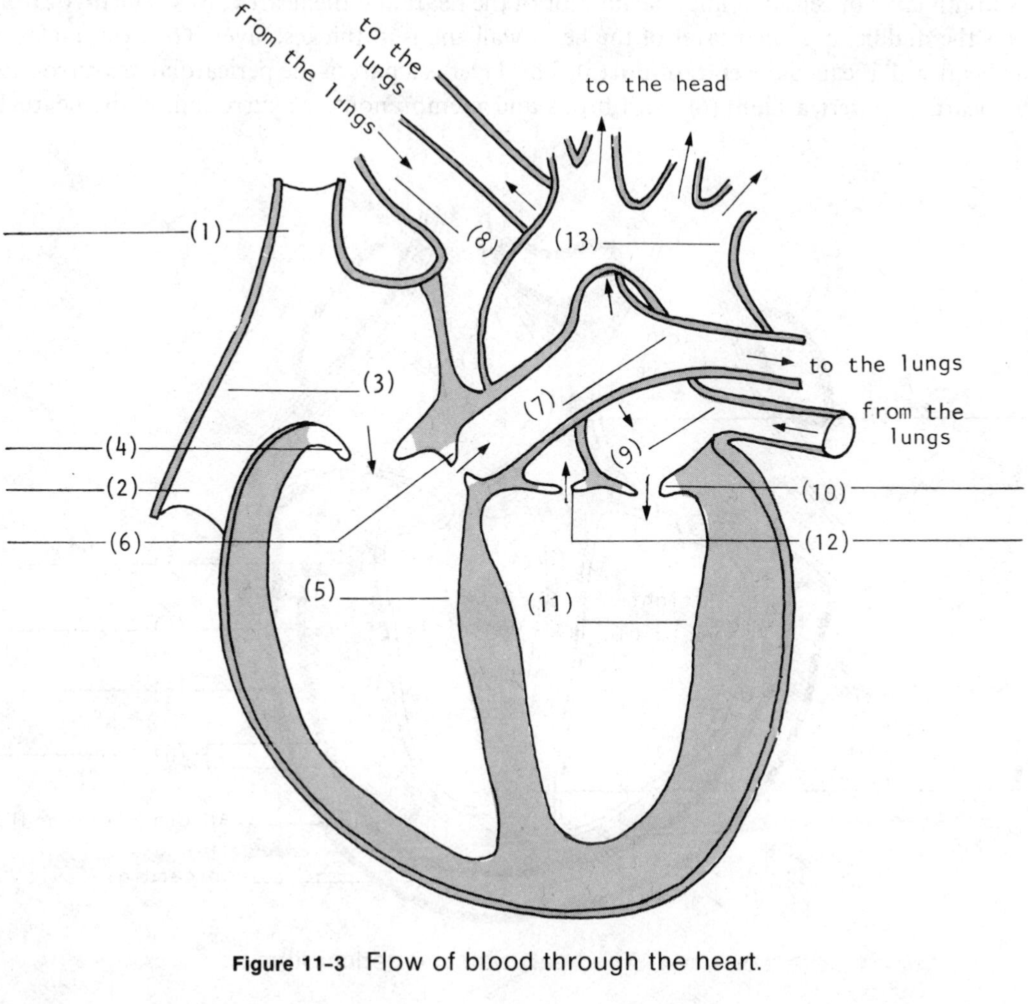

Figure 11-3 Flow of blood through the heart.

pulmonary artery (7), the tricuspid valve stays shut, thus preventing blood from pushing back into the right atrium. The pulmonary artery then branches to carry oxygen-deficient blood to each lung.

The blood that enters the lung capillaries from the pulmonary artery soon loses it large quantity of carbon dioxide into the lung tissue and the carbon dioxide is expelled. At the same time, oxygen enters the capillaries of the lungs and is brought back to the heart within the **pulmonary vein** (8). There are several pulmonary veins that transport oxygen-rich blood back to the left side of the heart from both lungs. The newly oxygenated blood enters the **left atrium** (9) of the heart from the pulmonary veins. The walls of the left atrium contract to force blood through the **mitral valve** (10) into the **left ventricle** (11).

The left ventricle has the thickest walls of all four heart chambers (three times the thickness of the right ventricle). It must pump blood with great force so that the blood travels through arteries to all parts of the body. The blood is pumped out of the left ventricle through the **aortic valve** (12) and into the **aorta** (13), which branches to carry blood all over the body. The aortic valve prevents the return of aortic blood to the left ventricle once it has been pumped out.

In Figure 11-4 it can be seen that the four chambers of the heart are separated by partitions called **septa** (singular: septum). The **interatrial septum** (1) separates the two upper chambers (atria), and the **interventricular septum** (2) is a muscular wall which comes between the two lower chambers (ventricles).

The heart wall is composed of three layers as shown in Figure 11-4. The **endocardium** (3) is a smooth layer of cells that lines the interior of the heart and the heart valves. The **myocardium** (4) is the middle, muscular layer of the heart wall and is its thickest layer. The external layer of the heart wall is called the **epicardium** (5). This layer is a part of the pericardial sac surrounding the heart. The **pericardium** (6) is a fibrous and membranous sac surrounding the heart. It is

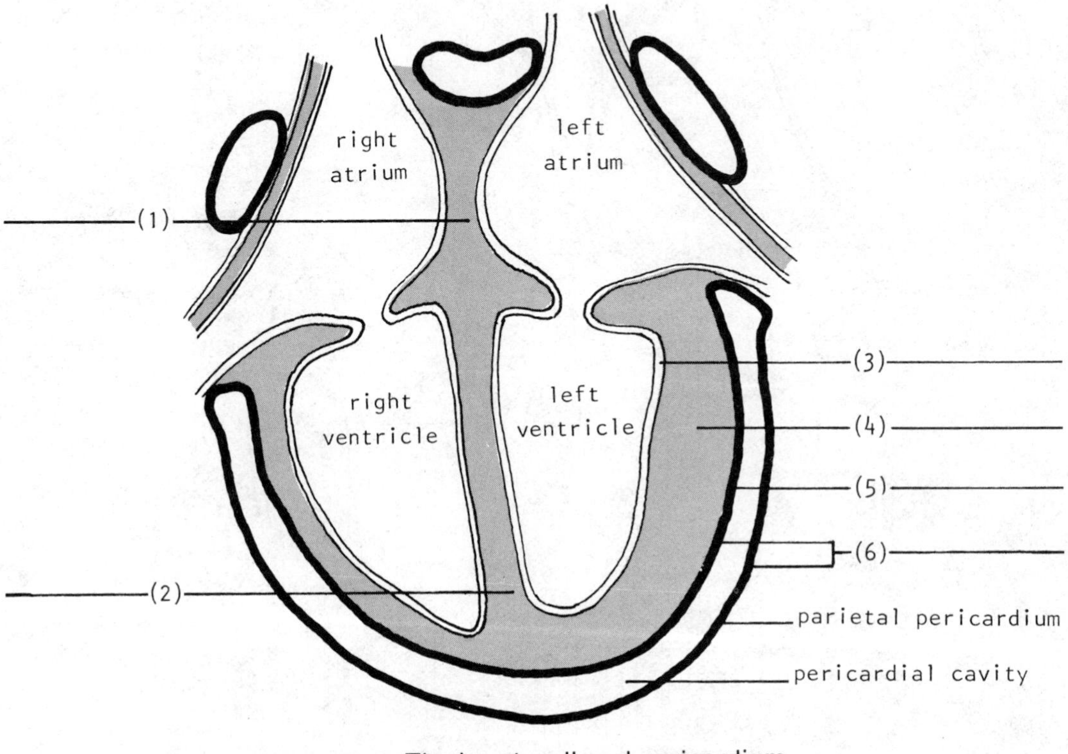

Figure 11-4 The heart wall and pericardium.

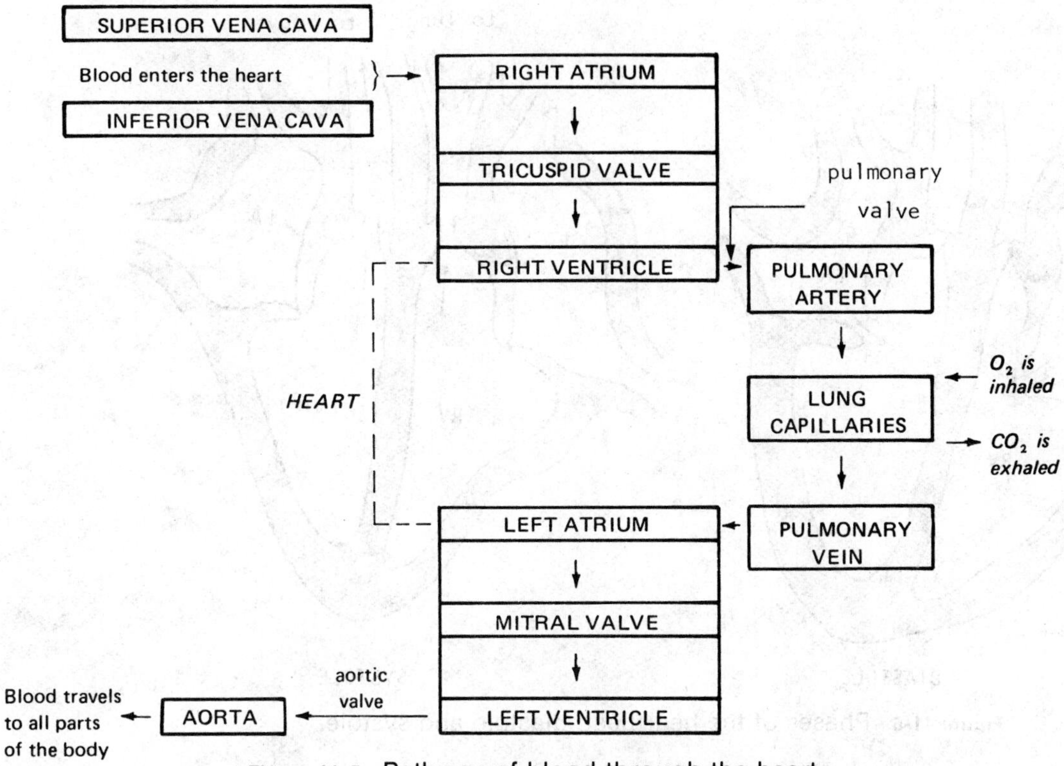

Figure 11-5 Pathway of blood through the heart.

composed of two layers, the epicardium (visceral pericardium), which adheres to the heart, and the parietal (parietal means wall) pericardium, which lines the outer fibrous coat. The pericardial cavity (between the visceral and parietal pericardium) normally contains 10 to 15 ml of fluid which lubricates the membranes as the heart beats.

Figure 11-5 traces the flow of blood through the heart.

IV. PHYSIOLOGY OF THE HEART

Heartbeat

There are two phases of the heartbeat. These phases are called **diastole** (relaxation) and **systole** (contraction). Diastole occurs when the ventricle walls relax and blood flows into the heart from the venae cavae and the pulmonary veins. The tricuspid and mitral valves are open in diastole, as blood passes from the right and left atria into the ventricles. The pulmonary and aortic valves are closed during diastole. See Figure 11-6.

Systole occurs next, as the walls of the right and left ventricles contract to pump blood into the pulmonary artery and the aorta. Both the tricuspid and mitral valves are closed during systole, thus preventing the flow of blood back into the atria. See Figure 11-6.

This diastole-systole cardiac cycle (relaxation-filling, then contraction-pumping) lasts about 0.9 second and occurs between 70 and 80 times per minute (100,000 times a day). The heart pumps about 2½ ounces of blood with each contraction. This means that about 5 quarts of blood are pumped by the heart in 1 minute (75 gallons an hour)!

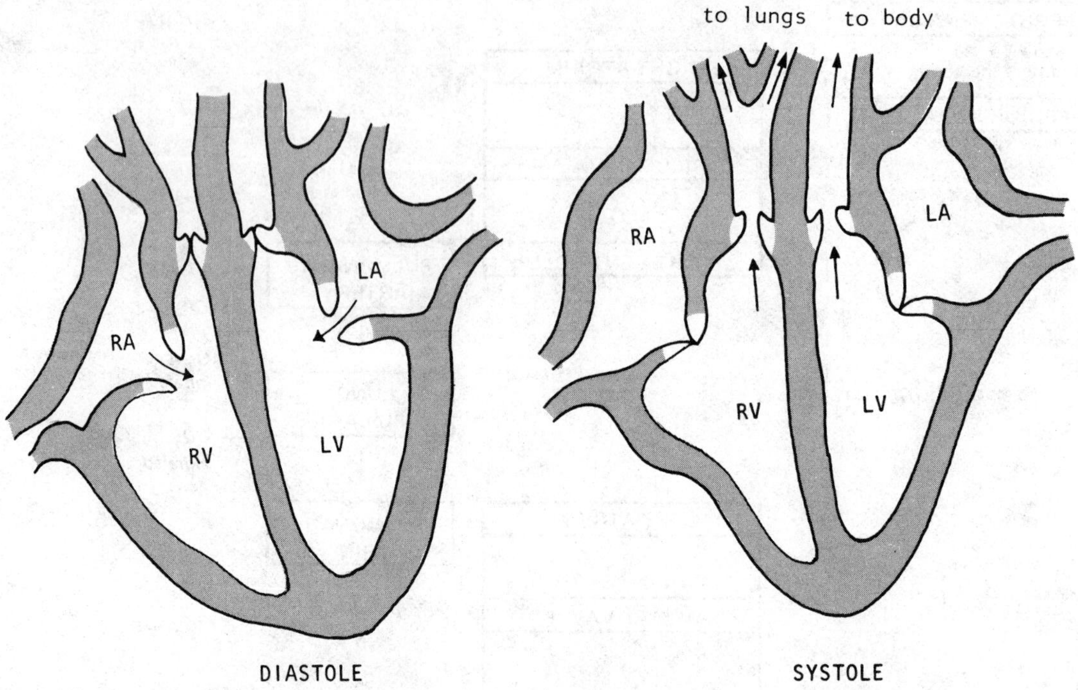

Figure 11-6 Phases of the heartbeat: diastole and systole.

Conduction System of the Heart

What keeps the heart at its perfect rhythm? Although the heart does have nerves that can affect its rate, they are not primarily responsible for its beat. It is known that the heart starts beating in the embryo before it is supplied with nerves, and it will continue to beat in experimental animals even when the nerve supply is cut.

Primary responsibility for initiating the heartbeat rests with a small region of specialized muscle tissue in the posterior portion of the right atrium, where an electrical impulse originates. This region of the right atrium is called the **sinoatrial node (S-A node)**. The S-A node is also called the **pacemaker** of the heart. The current of electricity generated by the pacemaker causes the walls of the atria to contract and force blood into the ventricles (ending diastole).

Almost like ripples in a pond of water when a stone is thrown, the wave of electricity passes from the pacemaker to another region of the myocardium. This region is at the posterior portion of the interatrial septum and is called the **atrioventricular node (A-V node)**. The A-V node immediately sends the excitation wave to a bundle of specialized muscle fibers called the **bundle of His** (pronounced hiss). Within the interventricular septum, the bundle of His divides into right and left bundle branches, which carry the impulse to the right and left ventricles, causing them to contract. Thus, systole occurs and blood is pumped away from the heart. A short rest period follows, and then the pacemaker begins the wave of excitation across the heart again. Figure 11-7 shows the location of the S-A node, the A-V node, and the bundle of His.

The record used to detect these electrical changes in heart muscle as the heart beats is called an **electrocardiogram** (ECG or EKG, from the Greek root kardia). The normal EKG shows five waves, or deflections, which represent the electrical changes as a wave of excitation spreads through the heart. The deflections are called P, Q, R, S, and T waves. The P wave occurs as the electrical impulse passes from the S-A node to the A-V node. The Q, R, and S waves represent the spread of excitation through the bundle of His and the ventricle wall (during systole). The T

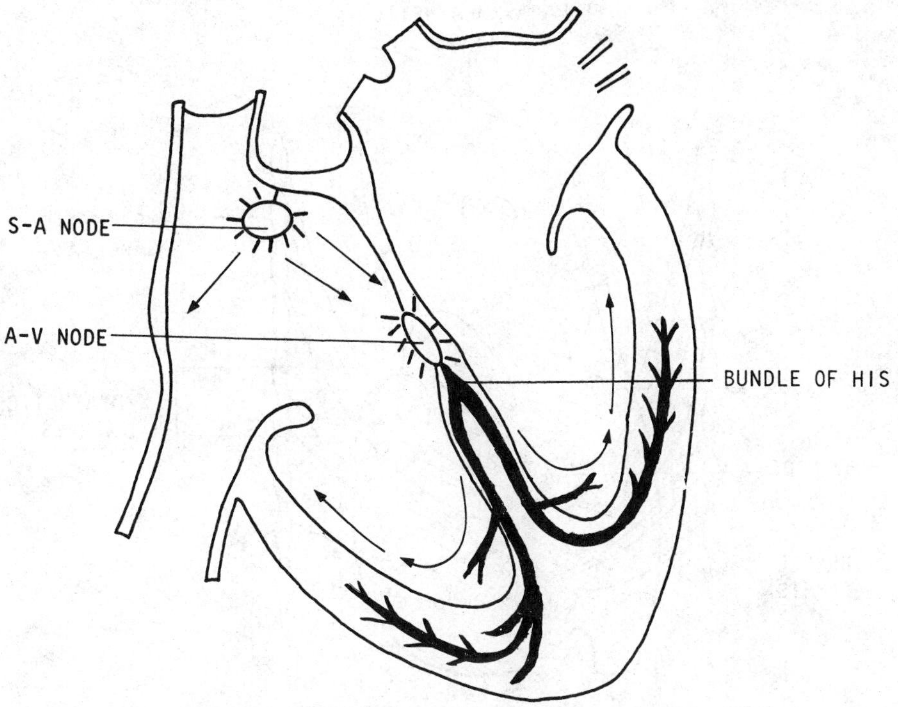

Figure 11-7 Conduction system of the heart.

wave represents the electrical recovery and relaxation of the ventricles. Figure 11-8 illustrates P, Q, R, S, and T waves in a normal electrocardiogram.

Nervous Control of the Heart

The heartbeat can be regulated by nervous impulses from the autonomic nervous system (parasympathetic and sympathetic nerves). The parasympathetic nerve supply to the heart is distributed mainly to the S-A and A-V nodes and causes a fall in the heart rate. Massive

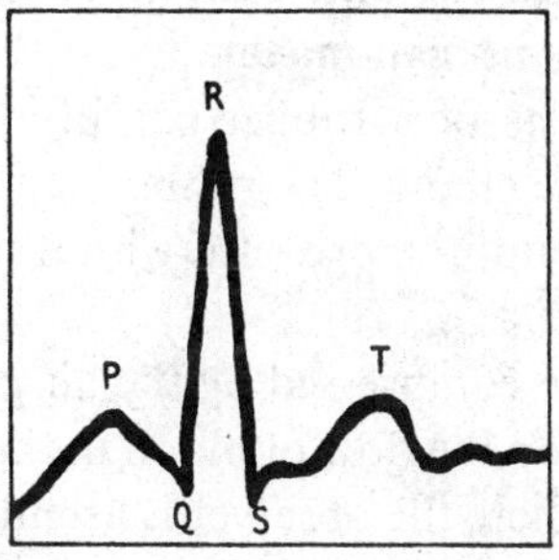

Figure 11-8 An electrocardiogram.

P wave = spread of excitation wave over the atria

QRS wave = spread of excitation wave over the ventricle

T wave = electrical recovery and relaxation of the ventricles

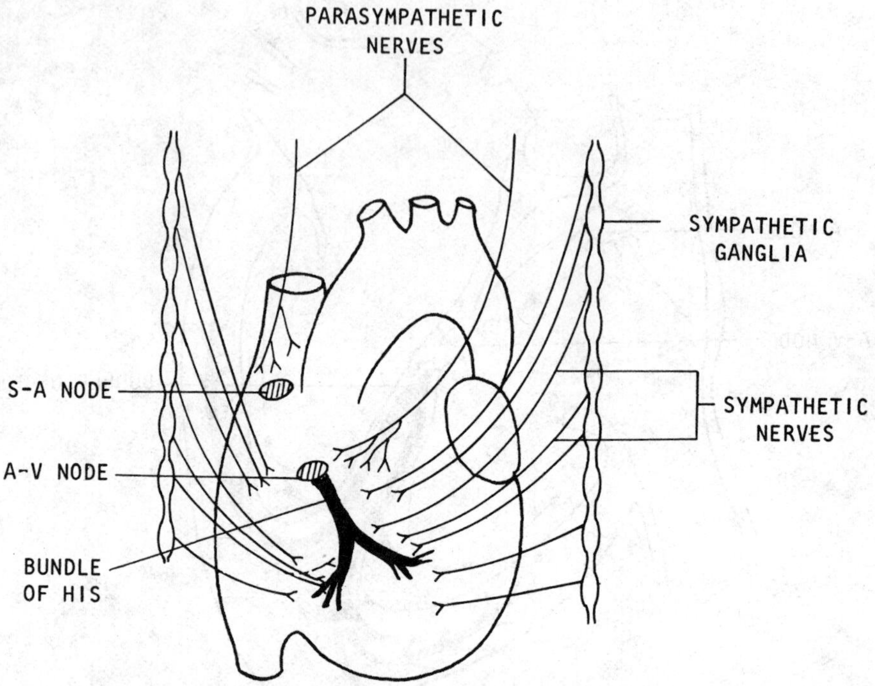

Figure 11-9 The parasympathetic and sympathetic nerve supply to the heart.

parasympathetic stimulation (the vagus nerve is the major nerve involved) can stop the heart for several seconds.

Sympathetic nerves lead to all areas of the heart, but especially to the ventricular muscle. Sympathetic stimulation increases heart rate and can even strengthen the force of the ventricular contraction. This is felt, for example, during exercise and periods of emotional distress.

Figure 11-9 shows the parasympathetic and sympathetic nerve supply to the heart.

V. BLOOD PRESSURE

Blood pressure is the force which the blood exerts on the arterial walls. This pressure is measured by a device called a **sphygmomanometer**.

The sphygmomanometer consists of a rubber bag inside a cloth cuff which is wrapped around the upper arm, just above the elbow. The rubber bag is inflated with air by means of a rubber bulb. As the bag is pumped up, the pressure within it increases and is measured on a recording device attached to the cuff.

The vessels in the upper arm are compressed by the air pressure in the bag. When there is sufficient air pressure in the bag to stop the flow of blood in the main artery of the arm (brachial artery), the pulse in the lower arm (where the observer is listening with a stethoscope) obviously drops.

Air is then allowed to escape from the bag and the pressure is lowered slowly, allowing the blood to begin to make its way through the gradually opening artery. At the point when the person listening with the stethoscope first hears the sounds of the pulse beats, the reading on the device attached to the cuff shows the higher, systolic, blood pressure (pressure in the artery when the ventricles are contracting).

As air continues to escape, the sounds become progressively louder. Finally, when a change in sound from loud to soft occurs, the observer makes note of the pressure on the recording device. This is called the diastolic blood pressure (pressure in the artery when the ventricles are relaxing).

Blood pressure is usually expressed as a fraction: for example, 120/80, in which 120 represents the systolic pressure and 80 the diastolic pressure.

VI. VOCABULARY

aorta	Largest artery in the body.
artery	Largest type of blood vessel; carries oxygenated blood away from the heart to all parts of the body.
atrioventricular node (A-V node)	Specialized tissue at the base of the wall between the two upper heart chambers. Electrical impulses pass from the pacemaker (S-A node) through the A-V node to the bundle of His.
atrium; atria	Upper chamber of the heart.
bundle of His	Specialized muscle fibers in the wall between the ventricles that carry the electric impulse to the ventricles.
capillary	Smallest blood vessel. Materials pass to and from the bloodstream through the thin capillary walls.
carbon dioxide (CO_2)	A gas released as a metabolic product of catabolism in body cells.
coronary arteries	The blood vessels that branch from the aorta and carry oxygen-rich blood to the heart muscle.
diastole	Relaxation phase of the heartbeat.
endocardium	Inner lining of the heart.
epicardium	Inner layer of the pericardium, adhering to the outside of the heart (visceral pericardium).
mitral valve	Valve found between the left atrium and ventricle of the heart.
pacemaker	Sensitive tissue in the right atrium which begins the heartbeat; also called the sinoatrial node.
pericardium	Saclike membrane surrounding the heart.
pulmonary artery	An artery carrying oxygen-poor blood from the heart to the lungs.
pulmonary circulation	The flow of blood from the heart to the lungs and back to the heart.

pulmonary valve	Valve between the right ventricle and the pulmonary artery.
pulmonary vein	A vein carrying oxygenated blood from the lungs to the heart.
septum; septa	A partition; in the cardiovascular system, a partition between the right and left sides of the heart.
sinoatrial node (S-A node)	The pacemaker of the heart.
sphygmomanometer	Instrument to measure blood pressure.
systemic circulation	The flow of blood from the body cells to the heart and then back out from the heart to the cells.
systole	The contraceptive phase of the heartbeat.
tricuspid valve	Valve located between the right atrium and ventricle; it has three (tri) leaflets, or cusps.
valve	A structure in veins or in the heart that temporarily closes an opening so that blood flows in only one direction.
vein	Thin-walled blood vessel that carries oxygen-poor blood from the body tissues to the heart.
vena cava; venae cavae	Largest vein in the body. The superior and inferior venae cavae bring blood into the right atrium of the heart.
ventricle	Lower and larger chamber of the heart.

VII. COMBINING FORMS AND TERMINOLOGY

Combining Forms	*Meaning*	*Terminology*	*Meaning*
cardi/o	heart	bradycardia	______________
		Slower than 60 beats per minute.	
		tachycardia	______________
		Faster than 100 beats per minute.	
		cardiomegaly	______________
		cardiomyopathy	______________
		Toxic or infectious agents may be the cause, but often the cause is unknown (idiopathic).	

coron/o	heart	coronary arteries ______
		These arteries come down over the top of the heart like a crown ("corona"). See Figure 11-10.
aort/o	aorta	aortic stenosis ______
angi/o	vessel	angiogram ______
		angiospasm ______
		hemangioma ______
vas/o	vessel	vasoconstriction ______
		vasodilation ______
arteri/o	artery	arteriosclerosis ______
		arterial anastomosis ______
		arteriorrhaphy ______
arteriol/o	arteriole, small artery	arteriolitis ______
phleb/o	vein	phlebitis ______
		phlebotomy ______
ven/o	vein	venotomy ______
		venous ______
venul/o	venule, small vein	venulitis ______
atri/o	atrium	atrioventricular ______
ventricul/o	ventricle	ventriculotomy ______
		ventricular ______
valv/o valvul/o	valve	valvulotomy ______
steth/o	chest	stethoscope ______
		A misnomer since the examination is by ear, not by eye.

sphygm/o	pulse	sphygmomanometer ________
ox/o	oxygen	hypoxia ________
cyan/o	blue	cyanosis ________
ather/o	yellowish plaque, fatty substance	atherosclerosis ________ *A form of arteriosclerosis (hardening and inflexibility of arteries).*
		atheroma ________
cholesterol/o	cholesterol (a fatlike substance)	hypercholesterolemia ________
aneurysm/o	aneurysm	aneurysmectomy ________
de-	lack of	deoxygenation ________

VIII. PATHOLOGICAL CONDITIONS OF THE HEART AND BLOOD VESSELS

coronary artery disease Disease of the arteries surrounding the heart.

The coronary arteries are two large vessels that arise from the aorta and supply oxygenated blood to the heart. It is interesting that the blood that constantly flows through the four hollow chambers of the heart does not itself nourish the myocardial tissue. Instead, after blood leaves the heart via the aorta, a portion is at once led back over the surface of the heart through the coronary arteries so that the heart feeds itself before any other organ. This seems logical since the energy requirements of the heart are greater than those of any other organ. Figure 11-10 shows the right and left coronary arteries as they branch from the aorta.

Coronary artery disease is usually the result of **atherosclerosis**. This is the deposition of fatty compounds on the inner lining of the coronary arteries (any other artery in the body can be similarly affected). The ordinarily smooth lining of the artery becomes roughened as the atherosclerotic plaque collects in the artery.

Atherosclerosis is dangerous for two important reasons. First, the roughened lining of the artery can cause abnormal clotting of blood in the coronary arteries leading to a **thrombotic occlusion** (blocking of the artery by a clot). Second, narrowing of the vessel due to atherosclerotic deposits may itself lead to inflexibility and plugging up of the vessel. In both cases, blood flow is decreased (**ischemia**) or stopped entirely, leading to death of a part of the myocardium. The area of dead myocardial tissue is known as an **infarction**. The infarcted area is eventually replaced by scar tissue.

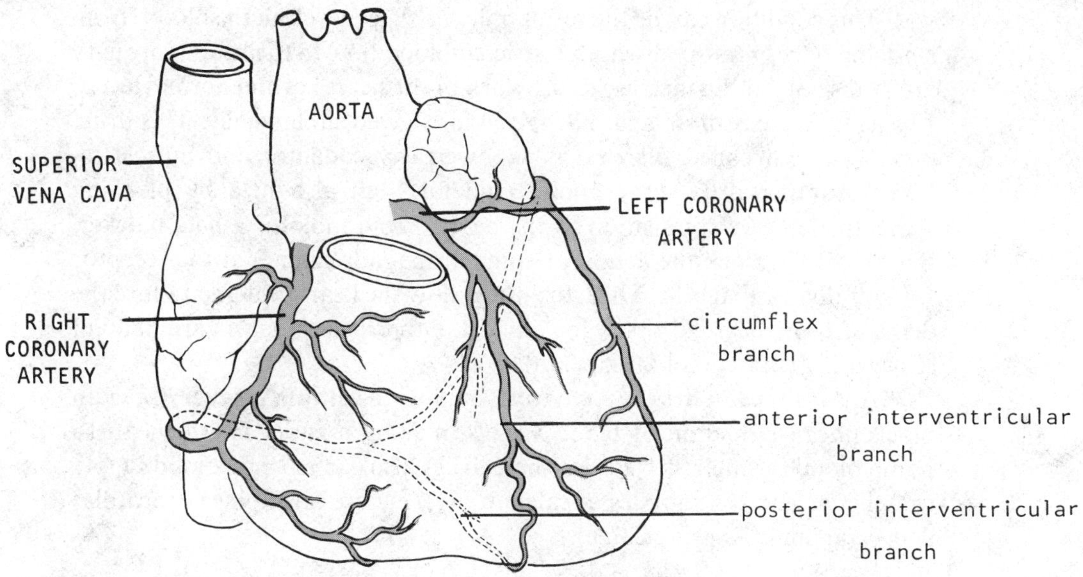

Figure 11-10 Coronary arteries supplying the heart.

Figure 11-11 shows how coronary artery occlusion leads to ischemia and infarction of heart muscle.

The severity of a **myocardial infarction** (also known as a **heart attack**) depends on the size of the artery which is blocked and the extent of the blockage. If the blocked artery is small enough the result may be death of only a small portion of the heart immediately fed by the artery. After scar tissue forms, the patient may be able to resume completely normal activity.

angina pectoris

An episode of chest pain due to a temporary difference between the supply and demand of oxygen to the heart muscle.

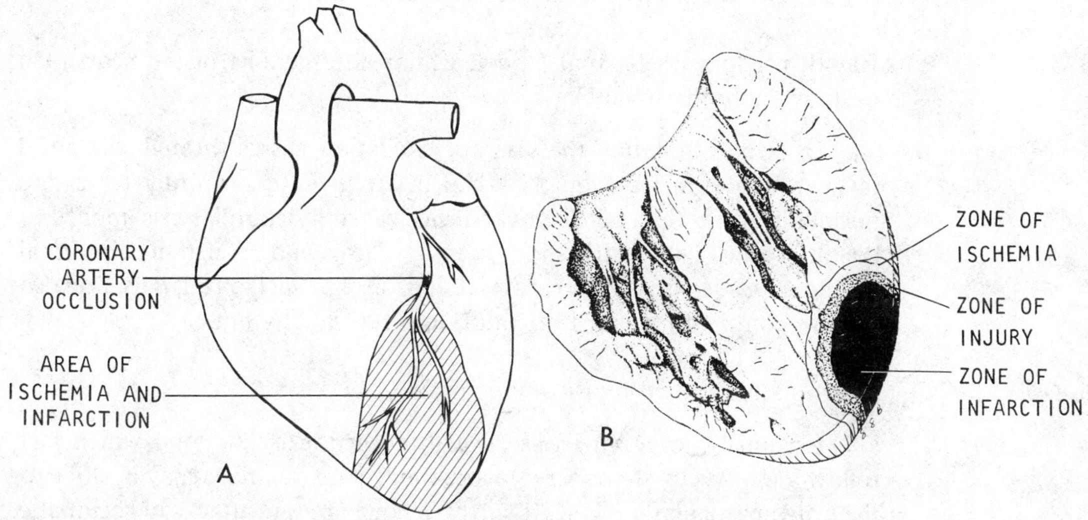

Figure 11-11 *A,* Ischemia and infarction produced by coronary artery occlusion. *B,* Myocardial infarction shown in cross-section of heart (ventricles only).

This condition can be the result of low oxygen levels in the blood (from smoking or respiratory disease), restricted blood flow to the heart (coronary artery disease), or an increase in the work of the heart beyond normal levels. For acute attacks of angina, **nitroglycerin** is given sublingually. This drug, one of several called **nitrates**, is a powerful vasodilator and muscle relaxer. Another drug, **propranolol** (Inderal), can also help by blocking sympathetic nerve stimulation to the heart. Propranolol is a **beta blocker.** Beta blockers block the action of epinephrine (adrenaline) at the receptor sites on myocardial cells. Thus, the drugs slow the heart beat and reduce the demand of myocardial tissue for oxygen. Other beta blockers are nadolol (Corgard) and atenolol (Tenormin).

A third type of drug used to treat angina is a **calcium blocker**. Calcium blockers cause dilation of blood vessels, making it easier for the heart to pump blood through the vessels. These drugs also can increase blood supply to ischemic areas. Examples of calcium blockers are nifedipine (Procardia) and verapamil (Isoptin, Calan).

arrhythmias

Abnormal heart rhythms.

Some examples of cardiac arrhythmias are:

1. **heart block (atrioventricular block)**

Failure of proper conduction of impulses through the A-V node to the bundle of His.

The implantation of an electric pacemaker can overcome heart block and establish a new rate for the heart by serving as an artificial source of excitation for the heart.

2. **flutter**

Rapid but regular contractions of atria or ventricles.

This condition occurs mainly in patients with heart disease. The heart rhythm can reach up to 240 to 260 beats per minute.

3. **fibrillation**

Rapid, random, ineffectual, and irregular contractions of the heart (350 beats or more per minute).

In atrial fibrillation the wave of excitation passes through the atrial myocardium even more quickly than in atrial flutter. In order to restore normal heart rhythm, an electrical device called a **defibrillator** is applied to the chest wall. The electric shock stops the heart and reverses its abnormal rhythm. This is also called **cardioversion**. Drugs, such as **digitalis**, are also used to convert flutter or fibrillation into regular rhythm.

rheumatic heart disease

Heart disease caused by rheumatic fever.

Rheumatic fever is a disease, usually occurring in childhood, which may follow a few weeks after a streptococcal infection. Damage may be done to the heart, particularly the heart valves, by one or more attacks of rheumatic fever. The valves, especially the mitral valve, become inflamed and scarred so that they do not open and close normally. **Mitral stenosis**, atrial fibrillation, and heart failure due to weakening of the myocardium can occur. Treatment consists of reduced activity, drugs to control arrhythmia, surgery to repair a damaged valve, and anticoagulant therapy to prevent emboli from forming. Teflon valve implants are also used to replace deteriorated heart valves. Figure 11-12 shows artificial valves implanted in a patient's heart.

bacterial endocarditis Inflammation of the inner lining of the heart caused by bacteria.

This condition may be a complication of another infectious disease, an operation, or an injury. Damage to the heart valves can produce lesions called **vegetations**, which may break off into the bloodstream as **emboli** (floating clots). When the emboli lodge in the small vessels of the skin, multiple pinpoint hemorrhages known as **petechiae** form. Antibiotics are effective in curing bacterial endocarditis.

heart murmur An extra heart sound, heard between normal heart sounds.

Murmurs are usually heard with the aid of a stethoscope, and are usually caused by a valvular defect or disease which disrupts the smooth flow of blood in the heart. They can also be heard in cases of interseptal defects where blood is abnormally flowing between chambers through holes in the septa. A functional murmur is one that is not caused by a valve or septal defect and is not a serious danger to the patient's health.

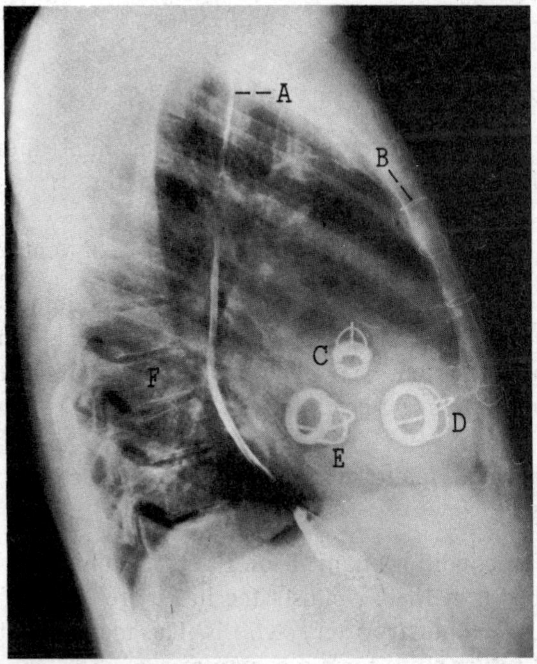

Figure 11-12 Three artificial valves implanted in a patient's heart by Dr. A. Starr of the University of Oregon Medical School: *A*, esophagus; *B*, wire sutures in sternum; *C*, aortic valve; *D*, tricuspid valve; *E*, mitral valve; *F*, vertebral column. (From Jacob, S.W., Francone, C.A., and Lossow, W.J.: Structure and Function in Man. 5th ed. Philadelphia, W.B. Saunders Co., 1982.)

mitral valve prolapse (MVP)

Improper closure of the mitral valve when the heart is pumping blood.

This condition, found most frequently in otherwise healthy young women, is known as the "click-murmur syndrome," which describes what the physician might hear through a stethoscope. It is also known as **Barlow's syndrome** after the doctor who first described it. Most people with MVP live normal lives, but because prolapsed valves can on rare occasions become infected, persons with MVP are usually advised to have preventive antibiotics at the time of dental procedures.

hypertensive heart disease

High blood pressure affecting the heart.

This disease is caused by the contracting of the arterioles of the body leading to increased pressure in arteries. The heart itself is affected because it has to pump more vigorously to overcome the increased resistance in the arteries. The vessels lose their elasticity, become like solid pipes, and place increased burden on the heart to pump blood through the body.

congestive heart failure

A condition in which the heart is unable to pump its required amount of blood. Blood accumulates in the lungs and liver.

In severe cases, fluid accumulates in the abdomen and legs or in the pulmonary air sacs (pulmonary edema). Congestive heart failure often develops gradually over several years, although it can be acute. It is treated with drugs, such as digitalis, to strengthen the heart, and diuretics to promote loss of fluid.

congenital heart disease

Abnormalities in the heart at birth.

The following conditions are congenital anomalies resulting from some failure in the development of the fetus.

1. septal defects

Small holes in the septa between the atria or ventricles.

Septal defects can be closed while maintaining a general circulation by means of a **heart-lung machine**. This machine is connected to the patient's circulatory system and relieves the heart and lungs of pumping and oxygenation during heart surgery.

2. tetralogy of Fallot

A congenital malformation of the heart involving **four** (tetra) distinct defects.

The condition, named for Etienne Fallot, the French physician who described it in 1888, is illustrated in Figure 11-13. The four defects are:

1. Pulmonary artery stenosis. This means that blood is not adequately passed to the lungs for oxygenation.
2. Ventricular septal defect. The gap in the septum allows deoxygenated blood to pass into the left ventricle, and from there to the aorta.
3. Shift of the aorta to the right, so that the aorta overrides the interventricular septum. Oxygen-poor blood passes even more easily from the right ventricle to the aorta.

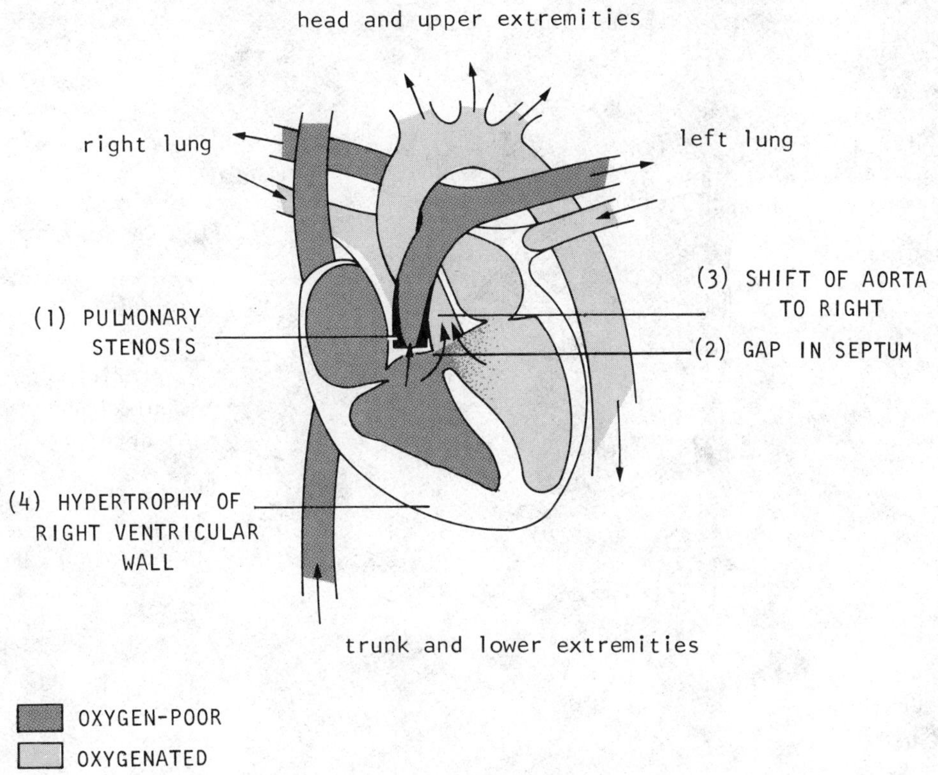

Figure 11-13 Tetralogy of Fallot.

4. Hypertrophy of the right ventricle.

An infant with this condition is described as a "**blue baby**" because of the extreme degree of **cyanosis** present at birth (other congenital conditions can lead to "blue baby" as well). Surgery is required to repair the various heart defects.

3. patent ductus arteriosus

A congenital heart defect in which a small duct between the aorta and pulmonary artery, which normally closes soon after birth, remains open.

This condition, illustrated in Figure 11-14, means that oxygenated blood flows from the aorta to the pulmonary artery. **Patent** means open. Treatment is surgery to close the ductus arteriosus.

4. coarctation of the aorta

Narrowing of the aorta.

Surgical treatment consists of removal of the constricted region and end-to-end anastomosis of the aortic segments.

arterial hypertension

High blood pressure in arteries.

There are two kinds of high blood pressure, or hypertension: **essential** and **secondary**. In essential hypertension, the cause of the increased pressure is **idiopathic** (unknown). In secondary hypertension, there is always some associated lesion, such as glomerulonephritis, pyelonephritis, or adenoma of the adrenal cortex, which is responsible for the elevated blood pressure.

In adults, a blood pressure equal to or greater than 140/90 mm Hg is

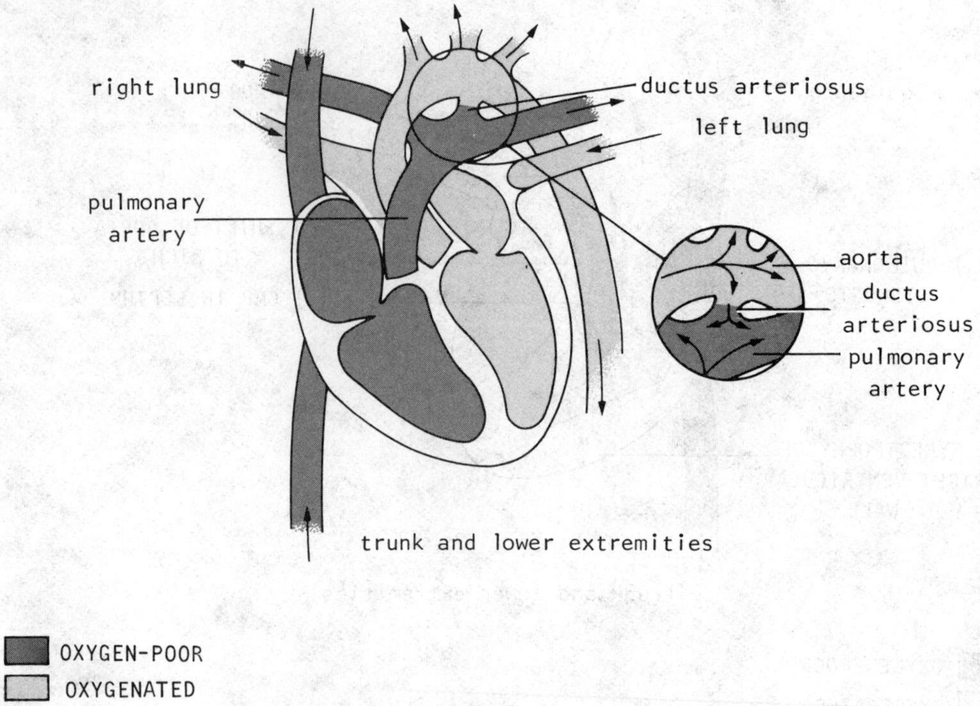

Figure 11-14 Patent ductus arteriosus.

considered abnormally high. Diuretics, beta blockers, and other drugs such as reserpine and guanethidine sulfate are used as treatment for essential hypertension. Weight loss, limiting sodium (salt) intake, stopping smoking, and reducing fat in the diet are also important in therapy.

aneurysm Local widening of an artery.

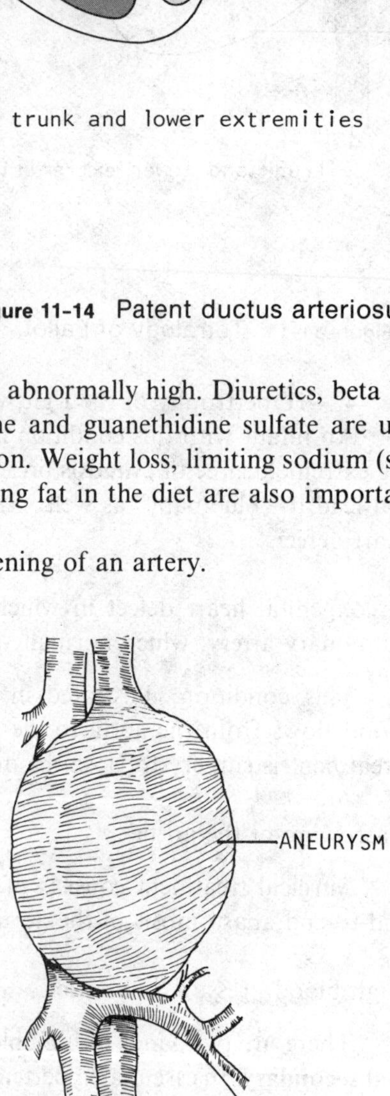

Figure 11-15 Aneurysm of the aorta.

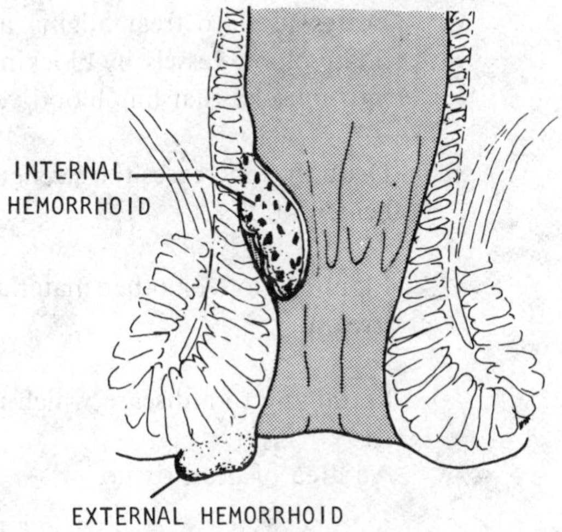

Figure 11-16 Hemorrhoids (internal and external).

Aneurysms may be due to a weakness in the arterial wall or breakdown of the wall due to atherosclerosis. The weak part of the wall bellies out with each beat of the heart. Figure 11-15 shows an aneurysm of the aorta. An **aneurysmectomy** is a surgical procedure which removes an aneurysm. After removal, a bypass arterial segment is necessary.

varicose veins Abnormally swollen veins, usually occurring in the legs.

This condition is due to damaged valves which fail to prevent the backflow of blood. The blood then collects in the veins, which distend to many times their normal size. Because of the slow flow of blood in the varicose veins and frequent injury to the vein, thrombosis may occur as well. **Hemorrhoids** (piles) are varicose veins near the anus. See Figure 11-16.

Treatment of varicose veins includes wearing elastic or supportive stockings, elevation of the legs if edema occurs, and surgery to ligate (tie off) and strip (remove) the twisted swollen veins. The surgical procedure is called vein stripping.

Raynaud's phenomenon Short episodes of pallor and numbness in the fingers and toes due to temporary constriction of arterioles in the skin.

This condition is usually idiopathic, but also may be secondary to some other more serious disorder. The episodes may be triggered by cold temperatures, emotional stress, or cigarette smoking. Protecting the body from cold and use of vasodilators are effective treatment.

The following terms were used for the first time in this section and are reviewed for you with their definitions:

beta blockers Drugs used to treat angina, hypertension, and arrhythmias. They block the action of epinephrine (adrenaline) at receptor sites on cells.

calcium blockers	Drugs used to treat angina and arrhythmias. They dilate blood vessels by blocking the influx of calcium into muscles that line blood vessels.
digitalis	Drug that increases the strength and regularity of the heartbeat.
emboli	Floating clots or other material carried in the bloodstream.
idiopathic	Pertaining to a disease which is of unknown cause.
infarction	An area of dead tissue.
nitrates	Drugs used in the treatment of angina pectoris.
nitroglycerin	A nitrate drug used in the treatment of angina pectoris to relieve pain.
occlusion	Closure of a blood vessel.
patent	Open.
petechiae	Small, pinpoint hemorrhages.
propranolol	A beta blocker used in the treatment of angina, hypertension, and cardiac arrhythmias.
vegetations	A collection of platelets, clotting proteins, red blood cells, and organisms that attaches to the endocardium in conditions such as bacterial endocarditis and rheumatic heart disease.

IX. LABORATORY TESTS, CLINICAL PROCEDURES, AND ABBREVIATIONS

Laboratory Tests

Serum enzyme tests During a myocardial infarction, enzymes are released into the bloodstream from the dying heart muscle. These enzymes can be measured and are useful as evidence of an infarction. The enzymes tested for are: **creatine kinase** (CK), **lactic dehydrogenase** (LD), and **aspartate aminotransferase** (AST). The latter enzyme is also known as serum glutamic-oxaloacetic transaminase (SGOT).

Lipid tests Lipids are fatty substances found in foods and in the body. Examples of lipids are **cholesterol** and **triglycerides**. Lipid tests measure the amounts of these substances in a blood sample. High levels of triglycerides and cholesterol in the blood may be associated with a greater risk of coronary atherosclerosis. A diet high in **saturated fat** (solid fats of animal origin, such as in milk, butter, and meats) tends to increase the amount of cholesterol in the blood. **Polyunsaturated fats** (such as corn oil and safflower oil) are chemically able to absorb hydrogen and tend to lower blood cholesterol.

Lipoprotein electrophoresis Lipoproteins are fat (lipid) and protein molecules bound together. Protein electrophoresis is the process of physically separating lipoproteins from a blood sample. High levels of **low density lipoproteins** (LDL) and **very low density lipoproteins** (VLDL) are associated with cholesterol and triglyceride deposits in arteries (atherosclerosis). High levels of **high density lipoproteins** (HDL), which contain less lipid, are found in persons who have less evidence of atherosclerosis.

Clinical Procedures

Electrocardiography The record of the electricity flowing through the heart.

Echocardiography A diagnostic procedure in which pulses of high-frequency sound waves (ultrasound) are transmitted into the chest and echoes returning from the surfaces of the heart are electronically plotted and recorded. This can show the structure and movement of the heart over time and may be useful in determining structural defects in the heart.

Angiocardiography A diagnostic procedure involving injection of an x-ray dye into the bloodstream, followed by chest x-rays to show the dimensions of the heart and large blood vessels.

Digital subtraction angiography Video equipment and a computer are used to produce x-ray pictures of blood vessels. First, an x-ray is taken of the area to be studied, and the results are stored in a computer. Next, contrast material is injected into a vein and a second image is produced which is also recorded (digitized) in the computer. The computer then compares the two images and subtracts the first image from the second (removing parts not being studied such as bone, muscle, and fat), leaving nothing but an image of the contrast medium in the vessels.

Cardiac catheterization A thin, flexible tube (catheter) is introduced into a vein or artery and is guided into the heart for purposes of detecting pressures and patterns of blood flow. Dye can also be injected and x-rays taken. Figure 11-17 shows right heart catheterization.

Cardiac scan A radioactive substance is injected intravenously and its accumulation in heart muscle is measured with a special detection device (scanner). The presence of areas of ischemia and myocardial infarction can be demonstrated on the scan.

Stress test This diagnostic procedure determines the body's response to physical

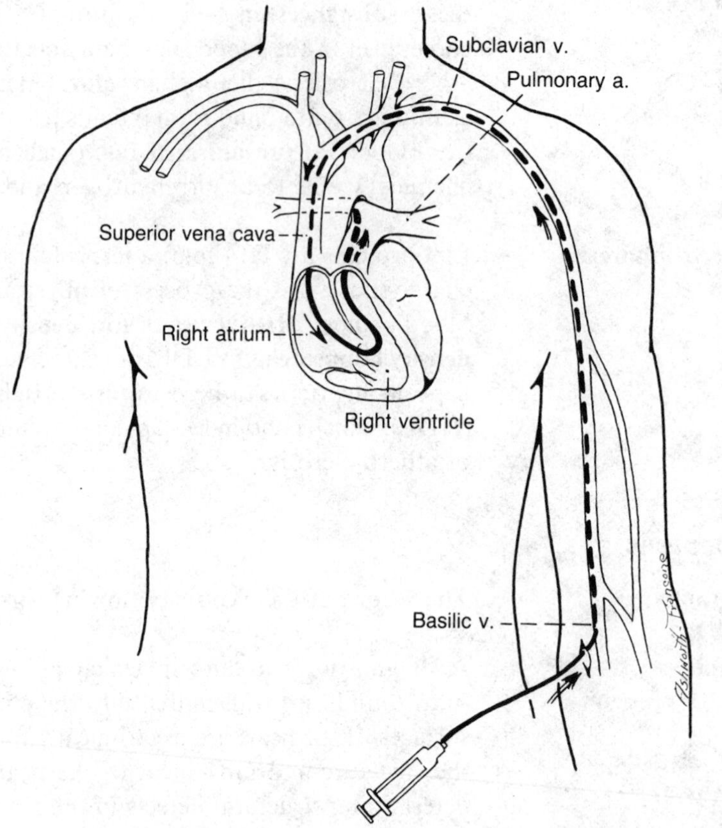

Figure 11-17 Right heart catheterization. (From Jacob, S.W., Francone, C.A., and Lossow, W.J.: Structure and Function in Man. 5th ed. Philadelphia, W.B. Saunders Co., 1982.)

exertion (stress). An electrocardiogram and other measurements (blood pressure and breathing rate) are taken while the patient is exercising, usually jogging on a treadmill.

Cardioversion (defibrillation) This is a treatment procedure whereby very brief discharges of electricity are applied across the chest to stop a cardiac arrhythmia and to allow a more normal rhythm to begin.

Coronary bypass surgery This surgical treatment procedure is used to improve the blood supply to the heart muscle when narrowed coronary arteries reduce the flow of blood. Detours, using veins and arteries taken from other parts of the body, are anastomosed to existing coronary arteries to keep the myocardium supplied with oxygenated blood.

Endarterectomy This procedure involves surgical removal of the innermost lining of an artery when it is thickened by fatty deposits (atheromas) and thromboses.

Heart-lung machine This machine is used during open-heart surgery to do the work of the lungs and heart while the heart is being repaired. Blood leaves the body, enters the heart-lung machine, where it is oxygenated, and then returns into a blood vessel to circulate throughout the system. This is known as extracorporeal (outside the body) circulation.

Intracoronary thrombolytic therapy A drug, streptokinase, that dissolves clots is injected directly into the coronary vessel blocked by a clot. This technique, which restores blood flow to the heart and limits irreversible damage to heart muscle, is undertaken within a few hours after the onset of a heart attack.

Percutaneous transluminal coronary angioplasty In this procedure, also called balloon catheter dilation, a catheter equipped with a small balloon on the end is inserted via the femoral (thigh) artery into a coronary artery. The balloon is then carefully inflated, compressing fatty deposits or plaque against the side of the artery and opening it to allow for the passage of blood.

Abbreviations

AI	Aortic insufficiency
AS	Aortic stenosis
ASD	Atrial septal defect
ASH	Asymmetrical septal hypertrophy
ASHD	Arteriosclerotic heart disease
AST	Aspartate aminotransferase
A-V	Atrioventricular
BP	Blood pressure
CAD	Coronary artery disease
CCU	Coronary care unit
CK	Creatine kinase
ECC	Extracorporal circulation
ECG	Electrocardiogram
EKG	Electrocardiogram
HDL	High density lipoproteins
IHSS	Idiopathic hypertrophic subaortic stenosis (wall of left ventricle enlarges, impairing outflow of blood into aorta)
LA	Left atrium
LD	Lactic dehydrogenase
LDL	Low density lipoproteins
LV	Left ventricle
MI	Myocardial infarction
MS	Mitral stenosis
MVP	Mitral valve prolapse
PAT	Paroxysmal (sudden, violent) atrial tachycardia
PTCA	Percutaneous transluminal coronary angioplasty
PVC	Premature ventricular contractions
RA	Right atrium
RV	Right ventricle
S-A	Sinoatrial
SCD	Sudden cardiac death
SGOT	Serum glutamic-oxaloacetic transaminase
VLDL	Very low density lipoproteins
VSD	Ventricular septal defect

X. PRACTICAL APPLICATIONS

Operating Schedule: General Hospital

Operation	Anesthesia
Aortic valve replacement, coronary artery bypass with ECC	General
Left carotid endarterectomy	General
Left thoracotomy w/insertion of epicardial pacemaker	General
Varicose vein bil. lig. and stripping	General

Medical Language as Written

1. The main determinants of death after acute MI are the extent of left ventricular damage and occurrence of arrhythmias.
2. Evaluation of risk factors for sudden cardiac death is important in patients with coronary artery disease. Risk factors include a family history of sudden cardiac death and early MI (before age 50), hypertension and left ventricular hypertrophy, smoking, diabetes mellitus, and markedly elevated serum cholesterol levels.
3. A 24-year-old woman with a history of palpitations [heartbeat is unusually strong, rapid, or irregular so that patient is aware of it] and vague chest pains enters the hospital. With the patient supine, you hear a mid-systolic click which is followed by a grade 3/6 [moderately loud—6/6 is loud and 1/6 is quiet] honking murmur. Your diagnosis: mitral valve prolapse (click murmur syndrome).
4. A 47-year-old man had a myocardial infarction in November, 1984. On March 3, 1985, he was readmitted to the hospital with an acute inferior myocardial infarction, documented by electrocardiograms and blood enzyme elevations. On April 8, the patient developed a loud systolic murmur and his blood pressure fell sharply. A diagnosis of rupture of the ventricular septum was made and he was transferred to the surgical service. Right cardiac catheterization confirmed the presence of a left-to-right shunt [of blood] at the ventricular level. Emergency surgery was attempted but the patient died suddenly. Autopsy diagnosis: ruptured ventricular septum secondary to myocardial infarction.

XI. EXERCISES

A. Match the following terms with their definitions below:

arteriole	superior vena cava
aorta	inferior vena cava
mitral valve	tricuspid valve
capillary	pulmonary artery
venule	pulmonary vein
atrium	ventricle

1. Lies between the right atrium and right ventricle ______________________

2. Smallest blood vessel ______________________

3. Carries oxygenated blood from the lungs to the heart ______________________

4. Largest artery in the body ______________________

5. Brings oxygen-poor blood into the heart from the upper parts of the body

____

6. Upper chamber of the heart ______________________

7. Carries oxygen-deficient blood to the lungs from the heart ______________________

8. Small artery ______________________

9. Lies between the left atrium and the left ventricle ______________________

10. Brings blood from the lower half of the body to the heart ______________________

11. A small vein ______________________

12. Lower chamber of the heart ______________________

B. *Trace the path of blood through the heart. Begin as the blood enters the right atrium from the venae cavae (include the valves within the heart):*

1. ______________________
2. ______________________
3. ______________________
4. ______________________
5. ______________________
6. capillaries of the lung
7. ______________________
8. ______________________
9. ______________________
10. ______________________
11. ______________________
12. aorta

C. *Complete the following sentences:*

1. The pacemaker of the heart is called the ______________________

2. The saclike membrane surrounding the heart is called the ______________________

3. The wall of the heart between the right and left atria is called the ______________________

4. The relaxation phase of the heartbeat is called ______________________

5. Specialized conductive tissue in the wall between the ventricles is called the

____

6. The inner lining of the heart is called the ______________________

7. The contractive phase of the heartbeat is called ______________________

8. A gas released as a metabolic product of catabolism is called ______________

9. Specialized conductive tissue at the base of the wall between the two upper heart chambers is called ______________________________

10. The inner lining of the pericardium, adhering to the outside of the heart, is called the

____

D. Complete the following medical terms:

1. Connection between two arteries: arterial ______________________
2. Instrument to measure blood pressure: ______________________ manometer
3. Suture of a vein: ______________________ rrhaphy
4. Slow heartbeat: ______________________ cardia
5. Inflammation of small arteries: ______________________ itis
6. Disease of heart muscle: cardio______________________
7. Hardening of arteries: arterio ______________________
8. Mass of yellowish plaque: ______________________ oma
9. Rapid heartbeat: ______________________ cardia
10. Removal of a dilated blood vessel: ______________________ ectomy
11. Narrowing of the mitral valve: mitral ______________________
12. Process of recording vessels and the heart: ______________________ graphy

E. Give meanings for the following medical terms:

1. cardiomegaly ______________________________
2. hemangioma ______________________________
3. coronary arteries ______________________________
4. phlebotomy ______________________________
5. vasoconstriction ______________________________
6. hypoxia ______________________________
7. cyanosis ______________________________
8. hypercholesterolemia ______________________________
9. atrioventricular ______________________________
10. atherosclerosis ______________________________

F. Match the following pathological conditions with their meanings below:

myocardial infarction
angina pectoris
heart block
atrial flutter
atrial fibrillation
rheumatic heart disease
bacterial endocarditis
heart murmur
mitral valve prolapse
hypertensive heart disease
congestive heart failure
aneurysm

1. An extra heart sound ______________________________
2. An episode of chest pain due to a temporary difference between the supply and demand of oxygen to heart muscle ______________________________
3. Inflammation of the inner lining of the heart ______________________________
4. Rapid but regular contractions of the upper heart chambers ______________________________
5. Local widening of an artery ______________________________
6. High blood pressure affecting the heart ______________________________
7. Heart attack ______________________________

8. Rapid, random, irregular contractions of the upper heart chambers ____________

____

9. Click-murmur syndrome ____

10. Heart is unable to pump its required amount of blood ____________

11. The valves of the heart are damaged secondary to a streptococcal infection

____

12. Failure of proper conduction of impulses through the A-V node to the bundle of His

____

G. *Give meanings for the following medical terms:*

1. thrombotic occlusion ____
2. emboli ____
3. nitroglycerin ____
4. beta blocker ____
5. digitalis ____
6. defibrillator ____
7. cardioversion ____
8. petechiae ____
9. vegetations ____
10. congenital heart defects ____

H. *Name the medical condition described below:*

1. Small holes in the walls between the atria or ventricles ____________

2. Abnormally swollen, twisted veins ______________________

3. Narrowing of the aorta at birth ______________________

4. High blood pressure in arteries of idiopathic origin ______________________

5. Congenital heart defect in which a small duct is open between the aorta and the pulmonary artery ______________________

6. Varicose veins located near the anus ______________________

7. Short episodes of pallor and numbness in the fingers and toes ______________________

8. Congenital malformation of the heart consisting of four distinct defects ______________________

I. Supply short answers for the following:

1. What are creatine kinase, lactic dehydrogenase, and aspartate aminotransferase? ______________________

2. What are propranolol, nadolol, and atenolol? ______________________

3. What are calcium blockers? ______________________

4. What is lipoprotein electrophoresis? ______________________

5. What is the difference between electrocardiography and echocardiography? ______________________

J. *Match the following terms with their descriptions below:*

cardiac scan	stress test
coronary bypass surgery	digital subtraction angiography
extracorporeal circulation	intracoronary thrombolytic therapy
endarterectomy	lipid tests
serum enzyme tests	cardiac catheterization

percutaneous transluminal coronary angioplasty

1. A test to determine the body's response to physical exertion ______
2. A thin, flexible tube is introduced into the heart to detect patterns of blood flow, pressures, and heart defects ______
3. Veins and arteries are anastomosed to coronary arteries to keep them supplied with oxygenated blood ______
4. Video equipment and a computer are used to produce x-ray pictures of blood vessels by subtracting one image from another ______
5. A radioactive substance is injected intravenously and a scanner detects its presence in heart muscle ______
6. Heart-lung machine ______
7. Surgical removal of the innermost lining of an artery ______
8. Blood levels of cholesterol and triglycerides are measured ______
9. A drug called streptokinase is injected into a coronary artery blocked by a clot ______
10. A catheter equipped with a small balloon is inserted into a coronary artery and inflated ______
11. Levels of substances released from dying heart muscle are detected in the blood ______

K. Give meanings for the following abbreviations:

1. CAD ____________________
2. CCU ____________________
3. BP ____________________
4. VSD ____________________
5. MVP ____________________
6. S-A ____________________
7. MI ____________________
8. ASD ____________________
9. ECG ____________________
10. PVC ____________________

ANSWERS

A.

1. tricuspid valve
2. capillary
3. pulmonary vein
4. aorta
5. superior vena cava
6. atrium
7. pulmonary artery
8. arteriole
9. mitral valve
10. inferior vena cava
11. venule
12. ventricle

B.

1. right atrium
2. tricuspid valve
3. right ventricle
4. pulmonary valve
5. pulmonary artery
7. pulmonary veins
8. left atrium
9. mitral valve
10. left ventricle
11. aortic valve

C.

1. sinoatrial (S-A) node
2. pericardium
3. interatrial septum
4. diastole
5. bundle of His
6. endocardium
7. systole
8. carbon dioxide (CO_2)
9. atrioventricular (A-V) node
10. epicardium (visceral pericardium)

D.

1. anastomosis
2. sphygmo
3. phlebo
4. brady
5. arteriol
6. myopathy
7. sclerosis
8. ather
9. tachy
10. aneurysm
11. stenosis
12. angiocardio

E.

1. enlargement of the heart
2. tumor of blood vessels
3. blood vessels that carry oxygenated blood to the heart muscle
4. incision of a vein
5. narrowing of a vessel
6. deficiency of oxygen
7. bluish discoloration of the skin
8. excessive cholesterol in the blood
9. pertaining to the atrium and ventricle
10. hardening of arteries due to collection of fatty material

F.

1. heart murmur
2. angina pectoris
3. bacterial endocarditis
4. atrial flutter
5. aneurysm
6. hypertensive heart disease
7. myocardial infarction
8. atrial fibrillation
9. mitral valve prolapse
10. congestive heart failure
11. rheumatic heart disease
12. heart block

G.

1. closure of a blood vessel due to clot formation
2. floating clots or other material carried through the bloodstream
3. a drug used in the treatment of angina pectoris
4. a type of drug used to treat angina, hypertension, and arrhythmias
5. a drug that increases the strength and regularity of the heartbeat
6. an apparatus used to terminate fibrillation by applying brief electroshock to the heart
7. delivering electric shock to the heart muscle to end rapid and irregular heartbeats
8. small, pinpoint hemorrhages
9. collection of material that attaches to the endocardium in conditions such as bacterial endocarditis and rheumatic heart disease
10. abnormalities of the heart present at birth

H.

1. septal defects
2. varicose veins
3. coarctation of the aorta
4. essential hypertension
5. patent ductus arteriosus
6. hemorrhoids
7. Raynaud's phenomenon
8. tetralogy of Fallot

I.

1. Enzymes released from injured heart muscle.
2. Beta blocker drugs used to treat angina pectoris.
3. Drugs used to treat angina pectoris by dilating blood vessels.
4. Separation of lipoproteins from a blood sample. They are separated into high density lipoproteins, and very low density lipoproteins.
5. Electrocardiography is recording the electricity flowing through the heart. Echocardiography is the use of ultrasound to form an image of heart structures.

J.

1. stress test
2. cardiac catheterization
3. coronary bypass surgery
4. digital subtraction angiography
5. cardiac scan
6. extracorporeal circulation
7. endarterectomy
8. lipid tests
9. intracoronary thrombolytic therapy
10. percutaneous transluminal coronary angioplasty
11. serum enzyme tests

K.

1. coronary artery disease
2. coronary care unit
3. blood pressure
4. ventricular septal defect
5. mitral valve prolapse
6. sino-atrial
7. myocardial infarction
8. atrial septal defect
9. electrocardiogram
10. premature ventricular contractions

XII. PRONUNCIATION OF TERMS

anastomosis	ă-năs-tō-MŌ-sĭs
aneurysm	ĂN-ū-rĭzm
aneurysmectomy	ăn-ū-rĭz-MĔK-tō-mē
angina pectoris	ăn-JĪ-nă PĔK-tō-rĭs; ĂN-jĭ-nă PĔK-tō-rĭs
angiocardiography	ăn-jē-ō-kăr-dē-ŎG-ră-fē
angiogram	ĂN-jē-ō-grăm
angiospasm	ĂN-jē-ō-spăzm
aorta	ā-ŎR-tă
arrhythmia	ā-RĬTH-mē-ă
arteriolitis	ăr-tē-rē-ō-LĪ-tĭs

arteriorrhaphy	ăr-tē-rē-ŎR-ă-fē
arteriosclerosis	ăr-tē-rē-ō-sklĕ-RŌ-sĭs
atheroma	ăth-ĕr-Ō-mă
atherosclerosis	ăth-ĕr-ō-sklĕ-RŌ-sĭs
atrioventricular	ā-trē-ō-vĕn-TRĬK-ū-lăr
atrium; atria	Ā-trē-ŭm; Ā-trē-ă
bradycardia	brăd-ē-KĂR-dē-ă
bundle of His	BŬN-d'l of Hĭs
capillary	KĂP-ĭ-lār-ē
cardiac catheterization	KĂR-dē-ăk kăth-ĕ-tĕr-ĭ-ZĀ-shŭn
cardiomegaly	kăr-dē-ō-MĔG-ă-lē
cardiomyopathy	kăr-dē-ō-mī-OP-ă-thē
cardioversion	kăr-dē-ō-VĔR-zhŭn
coarctation	kō-ărk-TĀ-shŭn
coronary	KŎR-ŏ-nār-ē
cyanosis	sī-ă-NŌ-sĭs
diastole	dī-ĂS-tō-lē
digitalis	dĭj-ĭ-TĂL-ĭs
echocardiography	ĕk-ō-kăr-dē-ŎG-ră-fē
electrocardiography	ē-lĕk-trō-kăr-dē-ŎG-ră-fē
embolus; emboli	ĔM-bō-lŭs; ĔM-bō-lī
endarterectomy	ĕnd-ăr-tĕr-ĔK-tō-mē
fibrillation	fĭb-rĭ-LĀ-shŭn
hemangioma	hĕ-măn-jē-Ō-mă
hemorrhoids	HĔM-ō-roydz
hypercholesterolemia	hī-pĕr-kō-lĕs-tĕr-ŏl-Ē-mē-ă
idiopathic	ĭd-ē-ō-PĂTH-ĭk
infarction	ĭn-FĂRK-shŭn
mitral valve	MĪ-trăl vălv
myocardium	mī-ō-KĂR-dē-ŭm
nitroglycerin	nī-trō-GLĬS-ĕr-ĭn
occlusion	ŏ-KLOO̅-zhŭn

patent	PĀ-tĕnt
petechiae	pĕ-TĒ-kē-ē
pericardium	pĕr-ĭ-KĂR-dē-ŭm
phlebitis	flĕ-BĪ-tĭs
phlebotomy	flĕ-BŎT-ō-mē
pulmonary	PŬL-mō-nĕr-ē
Raynaud's phenomenon	rā-NŌZ fĕ-NŎM-ĕ-nŏn
rheumatic heart disease	rōō-MĂT-ĭk hărt dĭ-ZĒZ
septum; septa	SĔP-tŭm; SĔP-tă
sinoatrial	sī-nō-Ā-trē-ăl
sphygmomanometer	sfĭg-mō-mă-NŎM-ĕ-tĕr
stethoscope	STĔTH-ō-skōp
systole	SĬS-tō-lē
tachycardia	tăk-ē-KĂR-dē-ă
tetralogy of Fallot	tĕ-TRĂL-ō-jē of făl-Ō
tricuspid	trī-KŬS-pĭd
varicose veins	VĂR-ĭ-kōs vānz
vasoconstriction	văz-ō-kŏn-STRĬK-shŭn
vasodilation	văz-ō-dī-LĀ-shŭn
vegetations	vĕj-ĕ-TĀ-shŭnz
vena cava; venae cavae	VĒ-nă KĀ-vă; VĒ-nē KĀ-vē
venotomy	vē-NŎT-ō-mē
venous	VĒ-nŭs
ventricle	VĔN-trĭ-k'l
ventriculotomy	vĕn-trĭk-ū-LŎT-ō-mē
venulitis	vĕn-ū-LĪ-tĭs

REVIEW SHEET 11

Combining Forms

aneurysm/o ____________________

angi/o ____________________

aort/o ____________________

arteri/o ____________________

arteriol/o ____________________

ather/o ____________________

atri/o ____________________

axill/o ____________________

brachi/o ____________________

cardi/o ____________________

coron/o ____________________

isch/o ____________________

ox/o ____________________

phleb/o ____________________

pulmon/o ____________________

sphygm/o ____________________

steth/o ____________________

thromb/o ____________________

valv/o ____________________

vas/o ____________________

ven/o ____________________

ventricul/o ____________________

venul/o ____________________

Suffixes

-emia ____________________

-rrhaphy ____________________

-megaly ____________________

-meter ____________________

-sclerosis ____________________

-spasm ____________________

-stasis ____________________

-stenosis ____________________

Prefixes

brady- ____________________

de- ____________________

endo- ____________________

hyper- ____________________

hypo-	______________	tachy-	______________
inter-	______________	tetra-	______________
peri-	______________	tri-	______________

Additional Terms

aneurysm (288)

angina pectoris (283)

aorta (279)

arrhythmia (284)

arterial hypertension (287)

atrioventricular node (279)

atrium (279)

bacterial endocarditis (285)

beta blockers (289)

bundle of His (279)

calcium blockers (290)

cardiac catheterization (291)

cardiac scan (291)

cardioversion (292)

coarctation of the aorta (287)

congestive heart failure (286)

coronary arteries (279)

coronary bypass surgery (292)

diastole (279)

digitalis (290)

digital subtraction angiography (291)

echocardiography (291)

emboli (290)

endarterectomy (292)

essential hypertension (287)

fibrillation (284)

flutter (284)

heart block (284)

heart-lung machine (292)

heart murmur (285)

hemorrhoids (289)

hypertensive heart disease (286)

idiopathic (290)

infarction (290)

intracoronary thrombolytic therapy (293)

lipid tests (290)

lipoprotein electrophoresis (291)

mitral valve (279)

myocardial infarction (283)

nitroglycerin (290)

occlusion (290)

pacemaker (279)

patent (290)

patent ductus arteriosus (287)

percutaneous transluminal coronary angioplasty (293)

petechiae (290)

propranolol (290)

pulmonary artery (279)

pulmonary vein (280)

Raynaud's phenomenon (289)

rheumatic heart disease (284)

secondary hypertension (287)

septum (280)

serum enzyme tests (290)

sinoatrial node (280)

sphygmomanometer (280)

stress test (292)

systole (280)

tetralogy of Fallot (286)

tricuspid valve (280)

varicose veins (289)

vegetations (290)

venae cavae (280)

ventricle (280)

CHAPTER 12

RESPIRATORY SYSTEM

In this chapter you will:

- Name the organs of the respiratory system, and describe their location and function;
- Identify various pathological conditions which affect the system;
- Recognize medical terms which pertain to respiration; and
- Identify clinical procedures and abbreviations related to the system.

This chapter is divided into the following sections:

I. INTRODUCTION

We usually think of **respiration** as the mechanical process of breathing, that is, the repetitive and, for the most part, unconscious exchange of air between the lungs and the external environment. This exchange of air at the lungs is also called **external respiration**. In external respiration, oxygen is inhaled (air inhaled contains about 21 per cent oxygen) into the air spaces (sacs) of the lungs and immediately passes into tiny capillary blood vessels surrounding the air spaces. Simultaneously, carbon dioxide, a gas produced when oxygen and food combine in cells, passes from the capillary blood vessels into the air spaces of the lungs to be exhaled (exhaled air contains about 16 per cent oxygen).

While external respiration occurs between the outside environment and the capillary bloodstream of the lungs, another form of respiration is occurring simultaneously between the individual body cells and the tiny capillary blood vessels which surround them. This process is called **internal** (cellular) **respiration**. Internal respiration is the exchange of gases not at the lungs but at the cells within all the organs of the body. In this process, oxygen passes out of the bloodstream and into the tissue cells. At the same time, carbon dioxide passes from the tissue cells into the bloodstream and is carried by the blood back to the lungs to be exhaled.

II. ANATOMY AND PHYSIOLOGY OF RESPIRATION

Label Figure 12–1 as you read the following paragraphs.

Air enters the body through the **nose** (1) and passes through the **nasal cavity** (2) which is lined with a mucous membrane and fine hairs (**cilia**) to help filter out foreign bodies, as well as to warm and moisten the air. **Paranasal sinuses** (3) are hollow, air-containing spaces within the skull that communicate with the nasal cavity. They, too, have a mucous membrane lining and

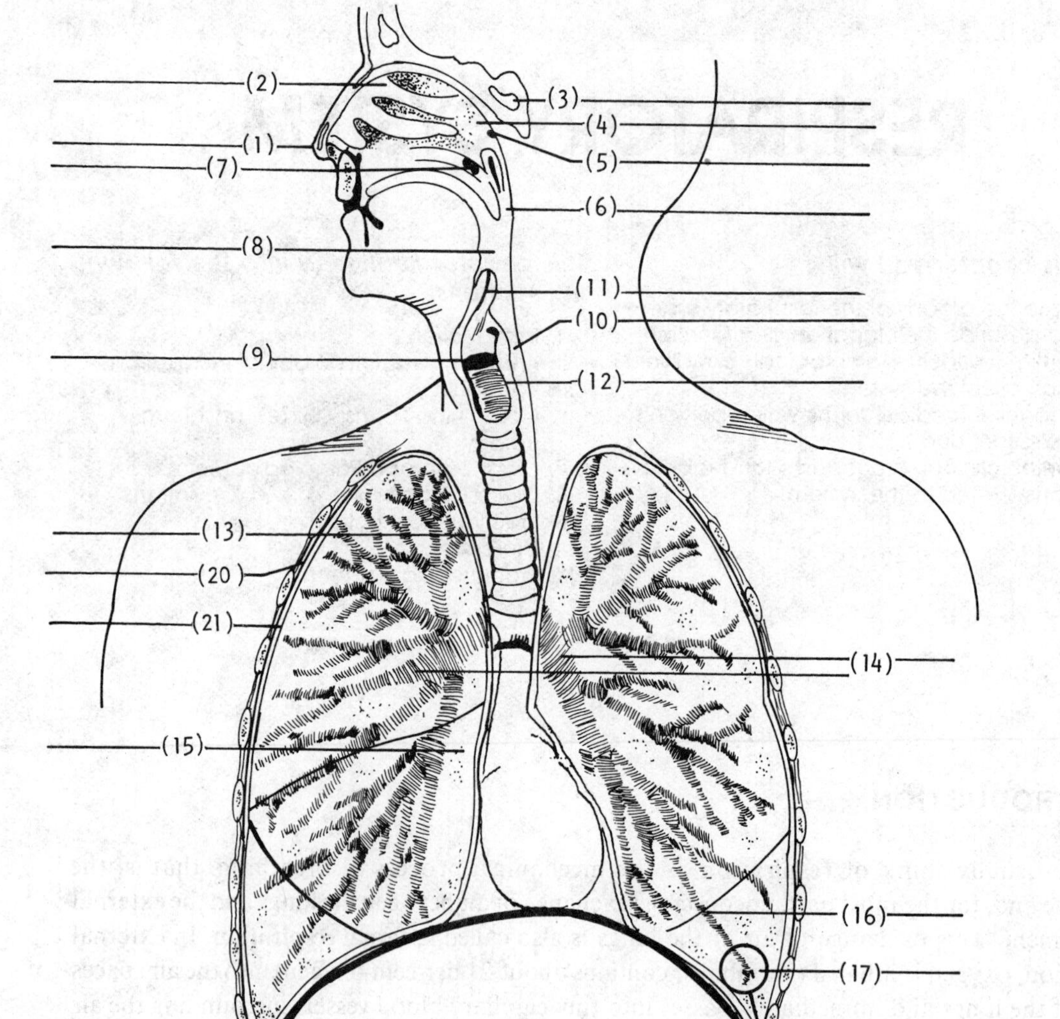

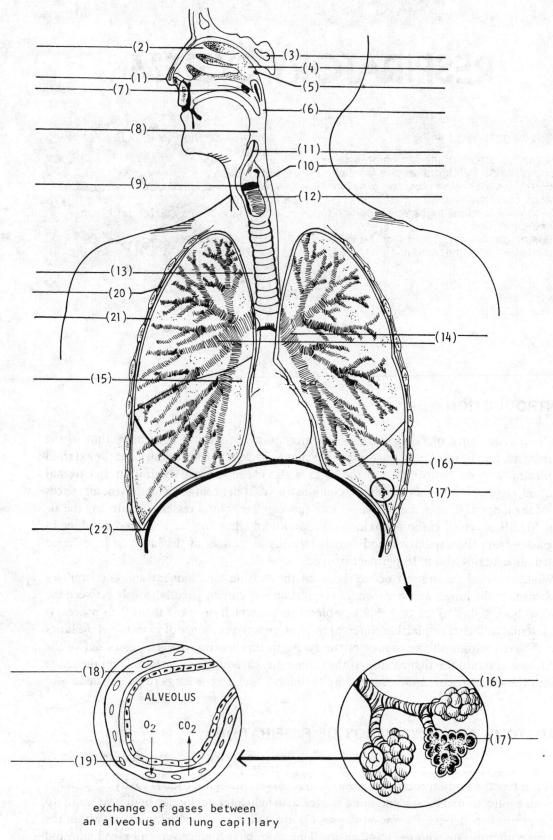

Figure 12-1 Organs of the respiratory system.

function to provide the lubricating fluid mucus, as well as to lighten the bones of the skull and help produce sound.

After passing through the nasal cavity, the air next reaches the **pharynx** (throat). There are three divisions of the pharynx. The **nasopharynx** (4) is the first division, and is nearest to the nasal cavities. It contains the **adenoids** (5), which are masses of lymphatic tissue. The adenoids (also known as the pharyngeal tonsils) are more prominent in children, and if enlarged can obstruct air passageways. Below the nasopharynx and closer to the mouth is the second division of the pharynx, the **oropharynx** (6). The **palatine tonsils** (7), two rounded masses of lymphatic tissue, are located in the oropharynx. The third division of the pharynx is the **hypopharynx** (also called the **laryngopharynx**) (8). It is in the hypopharyngeal region that the pharynx, serving as a common passageway for food from the mouth and air from the nose, divides into two branches, the **larynx** (voice box) (9), and the **esophagus** (10).

The esophagus leads into the stomach and carries food to be digested. The larynx contains the vocal cords and is surrounded by pieces of cartilage for support. Sounds are produced as air is expelled past the vocal cords and the cords vibrate. The tension of the vocal cords determines the high or low pitch of the voice.

Since food entering from the mouth and air entering from the nose mix in the pharynx, what prevents the passing of food or drink into the larynx and respiratory system after it has been swallowed? Even with a small quantity of solid or liquid matter finding its way into the air passages, breathing could be seriously blocked. A special deterrent to this event is provided for by a flap of cartilage attached to the root of the tongue which acts like a lid over the larynx. This flap of cartilage is called the **epiglottis** (11). The epiglottis lies over the entrance to the larynx. In the act of swallowing, when food and water move through the throat, the epiglottis closes off the larynx so that food cannot enter. Figure 12–2 shows the larynx from a superior view.

On its way to the lungs, air passes from the larynx to the **trachea** (windpipe) (12), a vertical tube about 4½ inches long and an inch in diameter. The trachea is kept open by 16 to 20 C-shaped rings of cartilage separated by fibrous connective tissue which stiffen the front and sides of the tube.

In the region of the **mediastinum** (13), the trachea divides into two branches called **bronchi** (14) (singular: bronchus). Each bronchus leads to a separate **lung** (15), and divides and subdivides into smaller and finer tubes, somewhat like the branches of a tree.

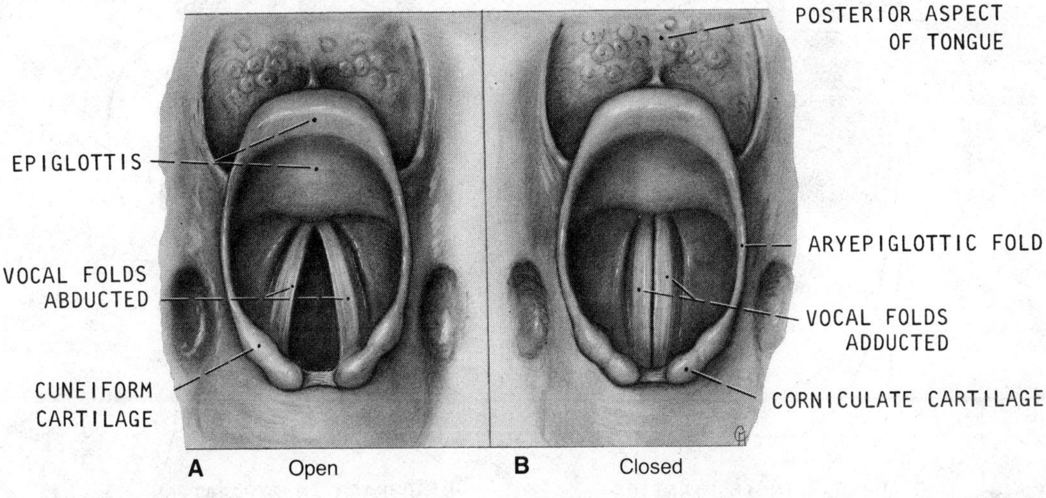

Figure 12-2 The larynx from a superior view. (From Jacob S.W., Francone, C.A., and Lossow, W.J.: Structure and Function in Man. 5th ed. Philadelphia, W.B. Saunders Co., 1982.)

The smallest of the bronchial branches are called **bronchioles** (16). At the end of the bronchioles are clusters of air sacs called **alveoli** (17) (singular: alveolus). Each alveolus is made of a one-cell layer of epithelium. The very thin wall allows for the exchange of gases between the alveolus and the **capillaries** (18) which surround and come in close contact with it. The blood that flows through the capillaries accepts the oxygen from the alveolus and deposits carbon dioxide into the alveolus to be exhaled. Oxygen is combined with a protein (hemoglobin) in **erythrocytes** (19) and carried to all parts of the body.

Each lung is enveloped in a double-folded membrane called the **pleura**. The outer layer of the pleura, nearest the ribs, is the **parietal pleura** (20), and the inner layer, closest to the lung, is the **visceral pleura** (21). The pleura is moistened with a serous (thin, watery fluid) secretion that facilitates the movements of the lungs within the chest (thorax).

The two lungs are not quite mirror images of each other. The right lung, which is the slightly larger of the two, is divided into three **lobes**, or divisions, and the left lung is divided into two lobes. It is possible for one lobe of the lung to be removed without damage to the rest, which can continue to function normally. The uppermost part of the lung is called the **apex**, and the lower area is the **base**. The **hilum** of the lung is the midline region where blood vessels, nerves, and bronchial tubes enter and exit the organ.

The lungs extend from the collarbone to the **diaphragm** (22) in the thoracic cavity. The diaphragm is a muscular partition that separates the thoracic from the abdominal cavity and aids in the process of breathing. The diaphragm contracts and descends with each **inhalation** (inspiration). The downward movement of the diaphragm enlarges the area in the thoracic cavity and reduces the internal air pressure so that air flows into the lungs to equalize the pressure. When the lungs are full, the diaphragm relaxes and elevates, making the area in the thoracic cavity smaller, and thus increasing the air pressure in the thorax. Air then is expelled out of the lungs to equalize the pressure; this is called **exhalation** (expiration). Figure 12-3 shows the position of the diaphragm in inspiration and expiration.

Figure 12–4 is a flow diagram reviewing the pathway of air from the nose, where air enters the body, to the capillaries of the lungs, where air enters the bloodstream.

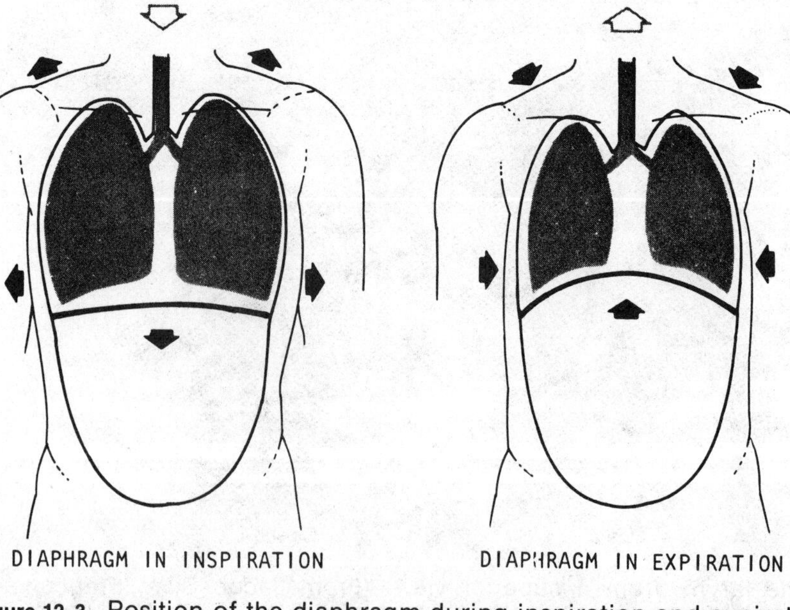

Figure 12-3 Position of the diaphragm during inspiration and expiration.

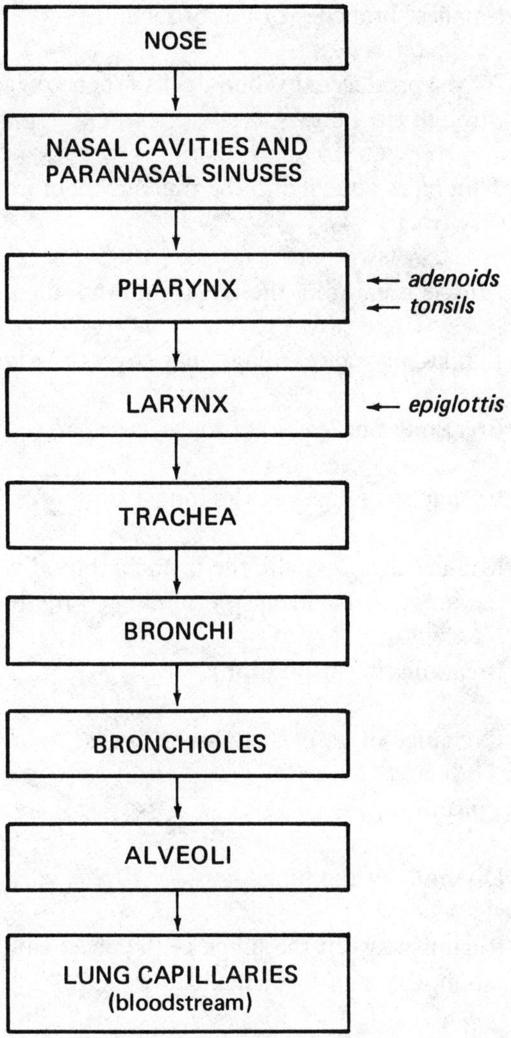

Figure 12-4 Pathway of air from the nose to the capillaries of the lungs.

III. VOCABULARY

adenoids — Collections of lymph tissue in the nasopharynx. Also called pharyngeal tonsils.

alveolus; alveoli — Air sac in the lung. (Also used to describe the sockets of the jaws in which the roots of teeth are embedded.)

apex of the lung — Uppermost portion of the lung. Apical means pertaining to the apex.

base of the lung — Lower portion of the lung.

bronchus; bronchi — Branch of the trachea (windpipe) that acts as a passageway into the air spaces of the lung.

bronchioles	Smallest branches of the bronchi.
carbon dioxide (CO_2)	A gas produced by body cells when oxygen and food combine; exhaled through the lungs.
cilia	Thin hairs attached to the mucous membrane epithelium lining the respiratory tract.
diaphragm	Muscle separating the chest and abdomen.
epiglottis	Lidlike piece of cartilage that covers the larynx.
exhalation	Breathing out (expiration).
external respiration	Exchange of gases in the lungs.
hilum (of lung)	Midline region where the bronchi, blood vessels, and nerves enter and exit the lungs. Hilar means pertaining to the hilum.
inhalation	Breathing in (inspiration).
internal respiration	Exchange of gases at the tissue cells.
larynx	Voice box.
lobes	Divisions of the lungs.
mediastinum	Region between the lungs in the chest cavity. It contains the heart, aorta, esophagus, and bronchial tubes.
oxygen (O_2)	Gas that passes into the bloodstream at the lungs, and travels to all body cells.
palatine tonsils	Rounded masses of lymph tissue in the oropharynx (palatine means roof of the mouth).
paranasal sinuses	Air-containing cavities in the bones near the nose.
parietal pleura	The outer fold of pleura lying closest to the ribs and wall of the thoracic cavity.
pharynx	Throat; composed of the nasopharynx, oropharynx, and laryngopharynx.
pleura	Double-folded membrane surrounding each lung.
pleural cavity	Space between the folds of the pleura.

pulmonary parenchyma — The essential cells of the lung, those performing its main function; the air sacs and small bronchioles.

trachea — Windpipe.

visceral pleura — The inner fold of pleura lying closest to the lung tissue.

IV. COMBINING FORMS, SUFFIXES, AND TERMINOLOGY

Combining Form	*Meaning*	*Terminology*	*Meaning*
nas/o	nose	paranasal	______________
		nasogastric tube	______________
rhin/o	nose	rhinorrhea	______________
		rhinoplasty	______________
adenoid/o	adenoids	adenoid hypertrophy	______________
		adenoidectomy	______________
tonsill/o	tonsils	tonsillectomy	______________
pharyng/o	throat	pharyngeal	______________
		nasopharyngitis	______________
laryng/o	voice box, larynx	laryngotracheobronchitis	______________
		laryngospasm	______________
		laryngeal	______________
		laryngectomy	______________
epiglott/o	epiglottis	epiglottitis	______________
trache/o	windpipe, trachea	tracheotomy	______________
		tracheoesophageal fistula	______________

		endotracheal
bronch/o bronchi/o	bronchial tube	bronchitis
		bronchiectasis
bronchiol/o	bronchiole, small bronchus	bronchiolitis
pulmon/o	lung	pulmonary
pneumon/o pneum/o	lung, air	pneumonectomy
		pneumonitis
		pneumothorax
lob/o	lobe of the lung	lobectomy
phren/o	diaphragm	phrenic nerve
thorac/o	chest	thoracoplasty
		thoracotomy
pector/o	chest	expectoration
pleur/o	pleura	pleuritis
		pleurodynia
spir/o	to breathe	expiration *Note that the "s" is omitted.*
sinus/o	sinus, cavity	sinusitis
coni/o	dust	pneumoconiosis
anthrac/o	coal dust	anthracosis
alveol/o	alveolus; air sac	alveolar
ox/o	oxygen	anoxia
		hypoxia
cyan/o	blue	cyanosis

-osmia	smell	anosmia ______________
-capnia	carbon dioxide	hypercapnia ______________
-phonia	voice, sound	dysphonia ______________ *Any voice impairment.*
-ptysis	spitting	hemoptysis ______________
-pnea	breathing	dyspnea ______________
orth/o	straight	orthopnea ______________ *Breathing is easier in an upright position.*
-sphyxia	pulse	asphyxia ______________ *Interference with respiration can ultimately lead to absence of pulse.*
-thorax	pleural cavity, chest	hemothorax ______________
em	in	empyema ______________ *-ema means quality, state or condition. Empyema can occur in any body cavity but is most common within the pleural cavity as pyothorax.*

V. DIAGNOSTIC AND PATHOLOGICAL TERMS

Diagnostic Terms

auscultation — Listening to sounds within the body.

This procedure, using a stethoscope, is used chiefly for discerning the condition of the lungs, pleura, heart, and abdomen, as well as the condition of the fetus during pregnancy.

percussion — Sharp, short blows to the surface of the body with a finger or instrument.

This technique is used to diagnose a condition by determining the density of structure from the sounds obtained.

rales — Abnormal rattling sounds heard on auscultation.

Rales may be produced by secretions within the bronchi and lungs, as well as by spasm or stenosis of the bronchial walls.

sputum — Material expelled from the chest by coughing or clearing the throat.

stridor

High-pitched, harsh sound heard during inspiration when the larynx is obstructed.

Pathological Terms

Upper Respiratory Disorders

diphtheria

An acute infectious disease of the throat and upper respiratory tract caused by the presence of diphtheria bacteria (Corynebacterium).

This disease is characterized by the appearance of inflammation and the formation of a leathery, opaque membrane in the pharynx and respiratory tract. Swelling of the larynx and pharynx leads to dyspnea, aphonia, and dysphagia. This condition can be fatal if not treated promptly with diphtheria antitoxin.

Immunity to diphtheria (production of antibodies) is induced by the administration of weakened toxins (antigens) beginning between the sixth and eighth week of life. These injections are usually given in combination with pertussis and tetanus toxins and are called DPT injections.

pertussis

Whooping cough.

This is a contagious bacterial infection of the upper respiratory tract (pharynx, larynx, and trachea). It is characterized by a **paroxysmal** (sudden) cough. Treatment is rest and antibiotics if complications such as pneumonia develop.

croup

Acute respiratory syndrome in children and infants; characterized by obstruction of the larynx, hoarseness, barking cough, and **stridor**.

Croup itself is not a disease condition but a group of symptoms which may result from infection, allergy, or foreign body in the larynx. Mist therapy (cold-steam vapor) and rest will help to relieve symptoms.

epistaxis

Nosebleed.

Bronchial Tube Disorders

asthma

Bronchial airway obstruction marked by recurrent attacks of paroxysmal dyspnea, wheezing, gasps, and cough.

Etiology may involve allergy or infection or be related to nervous tension and emotional problems. Treatment includes drugs to dilate the bronchi and relieve any underlying respiratory problem. Oxygen therapy may also be needed.

bronchogenic carcinoma

Cancerous tumor arising from a bronchus.

This malignant tumor may be either **epidermoid** (derived from the lining of the bronchus) or **oat cell** (a small cell of uncertain origin). Metastases spread readily to the brain, liver, and other organs. These types of tumors are commonly known as lung cancers.

cystic fibrosis

Inherited disease of exocrine glands (pancreas, sweat glands, and mucous membranes of the respiratory tract) leading to airway obstruction.

Chronic respiratory infections are common, as well as pancreatic insufficiency (fats are improperly digested). Therapy involves replacement of pancreatic enzymes and treatment of pulmonary obstruction and infection.

Lung Disorders

atelectasis (a/tel/ectasis)

Imperfect (atel means incomplete) expansion of the air sacs; functionless, airless lung or portion of a lung.

The bronchioles and alveoli (pulmonary parenchyma) resemble a collapsed balloon. Common causes of atelectasis include blockage of a bronchus or smaller bronchial tube after general anesthesia for surgery and a chest wound that permits air to leak into the pleural cavity. Acute atelectasis requires removal of the underlying cause (tumor, foreign body, excessive secretions) and therapy to open airways. Chronic atelectasis may necessitate lobectomy and antibiotics to combat infection of the lung.

emphysema

Distention of alveoli with swelling and inflation of lung tissue.

This degenerative disease is marked by loss of elasticity of the lungs as the walls of alveoli break down and are replaced by larger sacs. Air is trapped in the alveoli, and many bronchioles are obstructed by mucorrhea. Chronic bronchitis is a common etiological factor. As a result of dyspnea and hypoxemia, the heart must work harder to pump blood and this leads to right-sided heart failure (**cor pulmonale**).

pneumonia

Acute inflammation and infection of the alveoli; they fill with fluid, blood cells, or both.

Etiologic agents are most often pneumococci and less frequently staphylococci, fungi, or viruses. Infection damages alveolar membranes so that fluid, blood cells, and debris consolidate in the alveoli. **Lobar pneumonia** involves one or more lobes of a lung associated with consolidation. **Bronchopneumonia** begins in the terminal bronchioles. Bed rest and antibiotics are important in therapy.

Figure 12–5 illustrates the structural differences in alveoli in normal lung tissue, atelectasis, emphysema, and pneumonia.

pneumoconiosis

Abnormal condition of dust in the lungs.

Various forms of pneumoconiosis are named according to the type of dust particle inhaled:

silicosis—silica dust or glass (grinder's disease).
anthracosis—coal dust (black-lung disease).
asbestosis—asbestos particles (in shipbuilding and construction trades).
byssinosis—cotton, flax, and hemp (brown-lung disease).

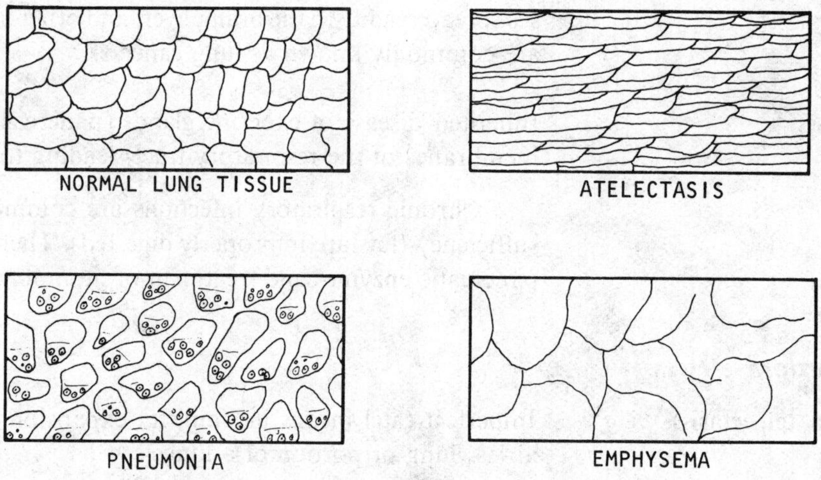

Figure 12-5 Alveoli in normal lung tissue, atelectasis, pneumonia, and emphysema.

pulmonary abscess — Localized area of pus formation in the lungs.

pulmonary edema — Swelling and fluid in the air sacs and bronchioles.

This condition is often caused by poor blood supply to the heart muscle and thus weakened ability to pump blood. Blood backs up in the pulmonary blood vessels, and fluid seeps out into alveoli and bronchioles.

pulmonary embolism — Floating clot or other material blocking the blood vessels of the lung.

A common type of embolism is one that travels from the right atrium or from the lower extremities and pelvis and blocks a branch of the pulmonary artery. This produces an area of dead (necrotic) lung tissue called a **pulmonary infarction**.

tuberculosis — An infectious disease due to Mycobacterium tuberculosis.

Rod-shaped bacteria called **bacilli** invade the lungs, producing small tubercles (nodes) of infection. These diseased tubercles (composed of bacteria, leukocytes, and fibrous connective tissue) can spread throughout the body. **INH** (isoniazid) is an effective antimicrobial agent used to treat tuberculosis.

Disorders of the Pleura

pleurisy — Inflammation of the pleura.

This condition causes pleurodynia and dyspnea and, in chronic cases, escape of fluid into the pleural cavity.

pleural effusion — Escape of fluid into the pleural cavity.

Examples of pleural effusions are **empyema** (pus in the pleural cavity) and **hemothorax** (blood in the pleural cavity). Empyema is a frequent

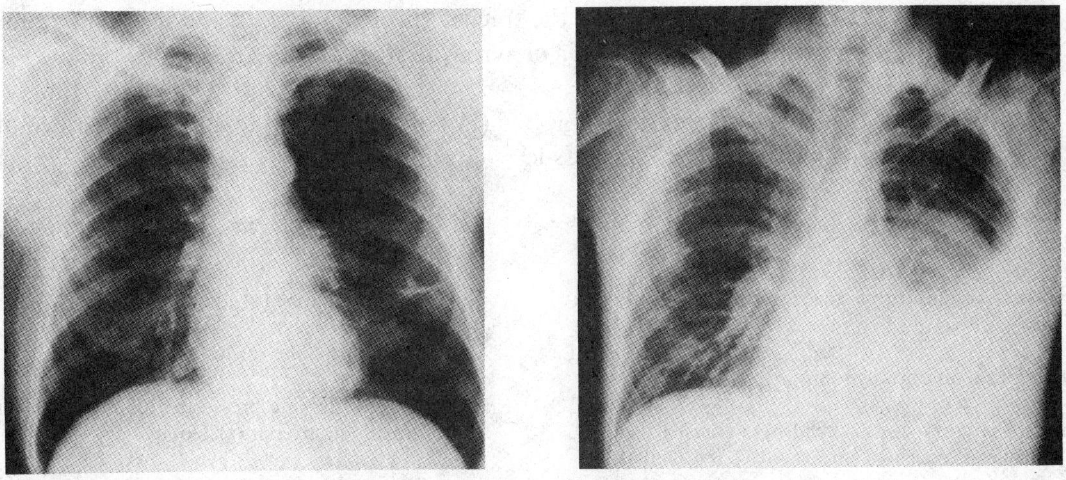

Figure 12-6 Streptococcal empyema. *Left*, Normal x-ray when admitted with high fever. *Right*, Chest x-ray 3 days after admission. (From Tunley, K.: Thoracic Wall, Pleura, Mediastinum & Lung. In: Way, L.W.: Current Surgical Diagnosis & Treatment. 6th ed. Los Altos, CA. Lange Medical Publications, 1983.)

complication of streptococcal pneumonia. Figure 12–6 shows a chest x-ray of a patient with empyema.

VI. CLINICAL PROCEDURES AND ABBREVIATIONS

Clinical Procedures

Pulmonary function tests This group of tests evaluates ventilation capabilities of the lungs. A **spirometer** measures the air taken in and out of the lungs.

Tuberculin tests Antigens such as PPD (purified protein derivative) are applied to the skin with multiple punctures (Heaf and tine tests), or intradermally (Mantoux test). A local inflammatory reaction is observed in infected persons after 48 to 96 hours.

Laryngoscopy The larynx is visualized with a laryngoscope.

Bronchoscopy Examination of the bronchi by passing a flexible fiberoptic tube into the bronchi. Specimens can be obtained for cytologic and bacterial studies by aspiration of bronchial secretions or by injecting fluid and retrieving it (**bronchial washing**). Biopsy by forceps or brush (**bronchial brushing**) can be accomplished through a catheter inserted under x-ray guidance.

Endotracheal intubation A tube is placed through the mouth, pharynx, and larynx into the trachea to establish an airway.

Thoracentesis The chest wall is punctured with a needle to obtain fluid from the pleural cavity for diagnostic studies, to drain pleural effusions, or to re-expand a collapsed lung.

Tracheostomy Cutting an opening into the trachea through the neck and inserting a tube to facilitate passage of air or removal of secretions.

Lung scan Radioactive material is injected (IV) or inhaled and images are recorded of its distribution in lung tissue.

Abbreviations

AFB	Acid-fast bacillus (type that causes tuberculosis)
A&P	Auscultation and percussion
ARDS	Adult respiratory distress syndrome (caused by injury or illness)
Broncho	Bronchoscopy
COPD	Chronic obstructive pulmonary disease (airway obstruction associated with bronchitis and emphysema)
CPR	Cardiopulmonary resuscitation (three basic steps: airway opened by tilting the head, breathing restored by mouth-to-mouth breathing, and circulation restored by external cardiac compression)
CXR	Chest x-ray
ENT	Ear, nose, and throat
INH	Isoniazid
IPPB	Intermittent positive-pressure breathing (inspiring air under pressure greater than atmospheric pressure)
LLL	Left lower lobe (of lung)
LUL	Left upper lobe (of lung)
$PaCO_2$	Carbon dioxide pressure; amount of carbon dioxide in arterial (a) blood
PaO_2	Oxygen pressure; amount of oxygen in arterial blood
PPD	Purified protein derivative
RDS	Respiratory distress syndrome (difficulty with inhalation in newborns because of lack of surfactant, a substance that lubricates alveoli; also called hyaline membrane disease)
RLL	Right lower lobe (of lung)
RUL	Right upper lobe (of lung)
SOB	Shortness of breath
TB	Tuberculosis
URI	Upper respiratory infection

VII. PRACTICAL APPLICATIONS

Case Report

A 22-year-old known heroin abuser was admitted to an emergency room comatose with shallow respirations. Routine laboratory studies and chest x-ray were done after the patient was aroused. He was then transferred to the ICU. He complained of left-sided chest pain. Examination of the chest x-ray showed three fractured ribs on the right and a large right pleural effusion. Further questioning of a friend revealed that he had fallen and struck the corner of a table after injecting heroin.

The diagnosis was traumatic hemothorax secondary to fractured ribs, and a thoracotomy tube was inserted into the right pleural space. No blood could be obtained despite maneuvering of the tube. Another chest x-ray showed that the tube was correctly placed in the right pleural space but the fractured ribs and pleural effusion were on the left. The radiologist then realized that he had reversed the first film. A second tube was inserted into the left pleural space and 1500 cc of blood was evacuated.

Necropsy Report

Adenocarcinoma, bronchogenic, left lung, with extensive mediastinal, pleural, and pericardial involvement. Metastasis to tracheobronchial lymph nodes, liver, lumbar vertebrae. Pulmonary emboli, multiple, recent, with recent infarct of left lower lobe. The tumor apparently originated at the left main bronchus and extends peripherally. Parenchyma is particularly atelectatic with a centrally located area of hemorrhage in the lower lobe.

X-ray Reports and Bronchoscopy

1. CXR: Complete opacification of left hemithorax with deviation of mediastinal structures of right side. Massive pleural effusion.
2. Chest tomograms: Mass most compatible with LUL bronchogenic carcinoma. Possible left paratracheal adenopathy or direct involvement of mediastinum.
3. Bronchoscopy: Larynx, trachea, carina [area where trachea bifurcates], and left lung all within normal limits. On the right side there was irregularity and roughening of the bronchial mucosa on the lateral aspect of the bronchial wall. This irregularity extended into the RUL, and the apical and posterior segments each contained inflamed irregular mucosa. Conclusion: suspicious for infiltrating tumor, but may be nonspecific inflammation. Bronchial washings, brushings, and bxs [biopsies] taken. Bronchial biopsy diagnosis: epidermoid carcinoma. Washings and brushings showed no malignant cells.

VIII. EXERCISES

A. *Match the following anatomical structures with their meanings below:*

mediastinum	cilia	paranasal sinuses
alveoli	bronchioles	palatine tonsils
larynx	parietal pleura	visceral pleura
pharynx	hilum	adenoids
trachea	epiglottis	bronchi

1. The outer fold of pleura lying closest to the ribs is called ________________

2. Collections of lymph tissue in the nasopharynx are the ________________

3. The windpipe is known as the ________________

4. The lidlike piece of cartilage that covers the voice box is the ______________

____

5. Branches of the windpipe that lead into the lungs are the ______________

6. The region between the lungs in the chest cavity is the ______________

7. Air-containing cavities in the bones around the nose are the ______________

8. Thin hairs attached to the mucous membrane lining the respiratory tract are called

____

9. The inner fold of pleura closest to lung tissue is called ______________

10. The throat is known as the ______________

11. Air sacs of the lung are called ______________

12. The voice box is called the ______________

13. Smallest branches of bronchi are the ______________

14. Collections of lymph tissue in the oropharynx are the ______________

15. The midline region where the bronchi, blood vessels, and nerves enter and exit the lungs is called the ______________

B. Complete the following sentences:

1. The apical part of the lung is the ______________

2. The gas that passes into the bloodstream at the lungs is ______________

3. Breathing in air is called ______________

4. Divisions of the lungs are known as ______________

5. The gas produced by cells and exhaled through the lungs is called ______________

____

6. The space between the visceral and parietal pleura is called the ______________

____

7. Breathing out air is called ______________________________

8. The essential cells of the lung performing its main function are known as the pulmonary ______________________________

9. The exchange of gases in the lung is called ______________ respiration.

10. The exchange of gases at the tissue cells is called ______________ respiration.

C. *Give meanings for the following medical terms:*

1. rhinoplasty ______________________________
2. thoracotomy ______________________________
3. bronchiectasis ______________________________
4. pleuritis ______________________________
5. pneumothorax ______________________________
6. anosmia ______________________________
7. laryngectomy ______________________________
8. nasopharyngitis ______________________________
9. phrenic ______________________________
10. alveolar ______________________________

D. *Name the following respiratory symptoms from their descriptions:*

1. Excessive amount of carbon dioxide in the blood ______________
2. Breathing is possible only in an upright position ______________
3. Difficult breathing ______________________________
4. Condition of blueness of skin ______________________________
5. Spitting blood ______________________________
6. Deficiency of oxygen ______________________________

7. Condition of pus in the pleural cavity ______________________

8. High pitched, harsh sound heard during inspiration ______________________

9. Inability to make sounds ______________________

10. Blood in the pleural cavity ______________________

E. *Match the following terms with their descriptions below:*

rales	atelectasis
pertussis	emphysema
percussion	croup
auscultation	diphtheria
epistaxis	asthma
cystic fibrosis	oat cell carcinoma

1. Nosebleed ______________________

2. Acute respiratory syndrome in children and infants marked by obstruction of the larynx and stridor ______________________

3. Alveoli become distended and overinflated ______________________

4. Sharp, short blows to the surface of the body with a finger or instrument ______________________

5. Bronchi are obstructed, along with recurrent attacks of dyspnea, wheezing, and coughs ______________________

6. Lungs or portion of lung is collapsed ______________________

7. Malignant neoplasm originating in a bronchus ______________________

8. Whooping cough ______________________

9. Inherited disease of exocrine glands that leads to airway obstruction ______________________

10. Listening to sounds with a stethoscope ______________________

11. Abnormal rattling sounds heard on auscultation ______________________

12. An acute infectious disease of the throat caused by Corynebacterium ________

____

F. Give meanings for the following medical terms:

1. pulmonary abscess ________
2. pulmonary edema ________
3. pneumoconiosis ________
4. pneumonia ________
5. pulmonary embolism ________
6. paroxysmal ________
7. tuberculosis ________
8. pleural effusion ________
9. pleurisy ________
10. anthracosis ________

G. Identify the clinical procedure or abbreviation:

1. A tube is placed through the mouth into the trachea to establish an airway

____

2. Radioactive material is injected or inhaled and images of the lung are recorded

____

3. PPD and tine tests ________

4. The chest wall is punctured with a needle to obtain fluid from the pleural cavity

____

5. Tests that measure the ventilation capacity of the lung ________

6. An opening is made into the trachea through the neck to establish an airway

____

7. Visual examination of the bronchi ______________________

8. Fluid is injected into the bronchi and then removed for examination ______________________

9. $PaCO_2$ ______________________

10. RDS ______________________

11. COPD ______________________

12. CXR ______________________

13. CPR ______________________

14. URI ______________________

15. ARDS ______________________

ANSWERS

A.

1. parietal pleura
2. adenoids
3. trachea
4. epiglottis
5. bronchi
6. mediastinum
7. paranasal sinuses
8. cilia
9. visceral pleura
10. pharynx
11. alveoli
12. larynx
13. bronchioles
14. palatine tonsils
15. hilum

B.

1. uppermost part
2. oxygen
3. inspiration; inhalation
4. lobes
5. carbon dioxide
6. pleural cavity
7. expiration; exhalation
8. parenchyma
9. external
10. internal

C.

1. surgical repair of the nose
2. incision of the chest
3. dilation, widening of bronchi
4. inflammation of pleura
5. air in the chest (pleural cavity)
6. lack of sense of smell
7. removal of the voice box
8. inflammation of the nose and throat
9. pertaining to the diaphragm
10. pertaining to an air sac

D.

1. hypercapnia
2. orthopnea
3. dyspnea
4. cyanosis
5. hemoptysis
6. hypoxia
7. pyothorax; empyema
8. stridor
9. dysphonia
10. hemothorax

E.

1. epistaxis
2. croup
3. emphysema
4. percussion
5. asthma
6. atelectasis
7. oat cell carcinoma
8. pertussis
9. cystic fibrosis
10. auscultation
11. rales
12. diphtheria

F.

1. collection of pus in the lungs
2. swelling, fluid collection in the air sacs and bronchioles
3. abnormal condition of dust in the lungs
4. acute inflammation and infection of alveoli; they become filled with fluid and blood cells
5. floating clot or other material blocking the blood vessels of the lung
6. pertaining to a sudden occurrence of symptoms
7. an infectious disease caused by rod-shaped bacilli and producing tubercles (nodes) of infection
8. collection of fluid in the pleural cavity
9. inflammation of pleura
10. abnormal condition of coal dust in the lungs (black-lung disease)

G.

1. endotracheal intubation
2. lung scan
3. tuberculin tests
4. thoracentesis
5. pulmonary function tests
6. tracheostomy
7. bronchoscopy
8. bronchial washings
9. pressure (amount) of carbon dioxide in arterial blood
10. respiratory distress syndrome; hyaline membrane disease
11. chronic obstructive pulmonary disease
12. chest x-ray
13. cardiopulmonary resuscitation
14. upper respiratory infection
15. adult respiratory distress syndrome

IX. PRONUNCIATION OF TERMS

abscess	ĂB-sĕs
adenoid	ĂD-ĕ-noyd
adenoidectomy	ăd-ĕ-noyd-ĔK-tō-mē
alveolar	ăl-VĒ-ō-lăr
alveolus	ăl-VĒ-ō-lŭs
anosmia	ăn-ŎZ-mē-ă
anoxia	ăn-ŎK-sē-ă
anthracosis	ăn-thră-KŌ-sĭs
asbestosis	ăs-bĕs-TŌ-sĭs
asphyxia	ăs-FĬK-sē-ă
asthma	ĂZ-mă
atelectasis	ă-tĕ-LĔK-tă-sĭs
auscultation	ăw-skŭl-TĀ-shŭn
bacilli	bă-SĬL-ī
bronchiectasis	brŏng-kē-ĔK-tă-sĭs
bronchiolitis	brŏng-kē-ō-LĪ-tĭs
bronchitis	brŏng-KĪ-tĭs
bronchogenic	brŏng-kō-JĔN-ĭk
bronchoscopy	brŏng-KŎS-kō-pē
bronchus	BRŎN-kŭs
cilia	SĬL-ē-ă

cyanosis	sī-ă-NŌ-sĭs
diphtheria	dĭf-THĒ-rē-ă
dysphonia	dĭs-FŌ-nē-ă
dyspnea	DĬSP-nē-ă
edema	ĕ-DĒ-mă
effusion	ĕ-FŪ-zhŭn
embolism	ĔM-bō-lĭzm
emphysema	ĕm-fĭ-ZĒ-mă; ĕm-fĭ-SĒ-mă
empyema	ĕm-pī-Ē-mă
endotracheal	ĕn-dō-TRĀ-kē-ăl
epiglottis	ĕp-ĭ-GLŎT-ĭs
epiglottitis	ĕp-ĭ-glŏ-TĪ-tĭs
expectoration	ĕk-spĕk-tō-RĀ-shŭn
hemoptysis	hē-MŎP-tĭ-sĭs
hemothorax	hē-mō-THŌ-răks
hypercapnia	hī-pĕr-KĂP-nē-ă
hypertrophy	hī-PĔR-trō-fē
hypoxia	hī-PŎK-sē-ă
laryngeal	lă-RĬN-jē-ăl; lăr-ĭn-JĒ-ăl
laryngectomy	lăr-ĭn-JĔK-tō-mē
laryngospasm	lă-RĬNG-gō-spăzm
laryngotracheobronchitis	lă-rĭng-gō-trā-kē-ō-brŏng-KĪ-tĭs
larynx	LĂR-ĭnks
lobectomy	lō-BĔK-tō-mē
mediastinum	mē-dē-ă-STĪ-nŭm
nasopharyngitis	nā-zō-făr-ĭn-JĪ-tĭs
orthopnea	ŏr-thŏp-NĒ-ă
paranasal	păr-ă-NĀ-zăl
parenchyma	pă-RĔNG-kĭ-mă
parietal	pă-RĪ-ĕ-tăl
paroxysmal	păr-ŏk-SĬZ-măl
percussion	pĕr-KŬSH-ŭn

pharyngeal	fă-RĬN-jĕ-ăl; făr-ĭn-JĒ-ăl
pharynx	FĂR-ĭnkz
phrenic	FRĔN-ĭk
pleura	PLOO͞R-ă
pleurisy	PLOO͞R-ĭ-sē
pleuritis	ploo͞-RĪ-tĭs
pleurodynia	ploo͞r-ō-DĬN-ē-ă
pneumoconiosis	nū-mō-kō-nē-Ō-sĭs
pneumonectomy	nū-mō-NĔK-tō-mē
pneumonia	nū-MŌ-nē-ă
pneumonitis	nū-mō-NĪ-tĭs
pneumothorax	nū-mō-THŎ-răks
rales	răhlz
rhinoplasty	RĪ-nō-plăs-tē
rhinorrhea	rī-nō-RĒ-ă
silicosis	sĭ-lĭ-KŌ-sĭs
sinusitis	sī-nŭ-SĪ-tĭs
sputum	SPŪ-tŭm
stridor	STRĪ-dŏr
thoracentesis	thŏ-ră-sĕn-TĒ-sĭs
thoracoplasty	thŏ-ră-kō-PLĂS-tē
thoracotomy	thŏ-ră-KŎT-ō-mē
tonsillectomy	tŏn-sĭ-LĔK-tō-mē
trachea	TRĀ-kē-ă
tracheoesophageal	trā-kē-ō-ĕ-sŏf-ă-JĒ-ăl
tracheotomy	trā-kē-ŎT-ō-mē
tuberculosis	tū-bĕr-kū-LŌ-sĭs

REVIEW SHEET 12

Combining Forms

adenoid/o	______________	ox/o	______________
alveol/o	______________	pector/o	______________
anthrac/o	______________	pharyng/o	______________
atel/o	______________	phren/o	______________
bronch/o	______________	pleur/o	______________
bronchi/o	______________	pneum/o	______________
bronchiol/o	______________	pneumon/o	______________
coni/o	______________	pulmon/o	______________
epiglott/o	______________	py/o	______________
hydr/o	______________	rhin/o	______________
laryng/o	______________	sinus/o	______________
lob/o	______________	spir/o	______________
nas/o	______________	thorac/o	______________
or/o	______________	tonsill/o	______________
orth/o	______________	trache/o	______________

Suffixes

-algia	______________	-dynia	______________
-capnia	______________	-ectasis	______________
-centesis	______________	-ectomy	______________
-lysis	______________	-rrhagia	______________
-osmia	______________	-rrhea	______________

-oxia	________	-stenosis	________
-phonia	________	-stomy	________
-plasty	________	-thorax	________
-pnea	________	-tomy	________
-ptysis	________	-trophy	________

Prefixes

brady-	________	hypo-	________
dys-	________	para-	________
em-	________	per-	________
eu-	________	re-	________
ex-	________	tachy-	________
hyper-	________		

Additional Terms

adenoids (313)

alveoli (313)

anthracosis (319)

apex of lung (313)

asbestosis (319)

asthma (318)

atelectasis (319)

auscultation (317)

bronchial brushings (321)

bronchial washings (321)

bronchiole (314)

bronchogenic carcinoma (318)

bronchus (313)

byssinosis (319)

carbon dioxide (314)

cilia (314)

croup (318)

cystic fibrosis (319)

diaphragm (314)

diphtheria (318)

emphysema (319)

empyema (320)

endotracheal intubation (321)

epiglottis (314)

epistaxis (318)

external respiration (314)

hilum of the lung (314)

internal respiration (314)

larynx (314)

lung scan (322)

mediastinum (314)

oat cell carcinoma (318)

parietal pleura (314)

palatine tonsils (314)

paroxysmal (318)

percussion (317)

pertussis (318)

pharynx (314)

pleural cavity (314)

pleural effusion (320)

pleurisy (320)

pneumoconiosis (319)

pneumonia (319)

pulmonary abscess (320)

pulmonary edema (320)

pulmonary embolism (320)

pulmonary function tests (321)

pulmonary parenchyma (315)

rales (317)

silicosis (319)

spirometer (321)

sputum (317)

stridor (318)

thoracentesis (321)

trachea (315)

tuberculin tests (321)

tuberculosis (320)

visceral pleura (315)

CHAPTER 13

BLOOD AND LYMPHATIC SYSTEMS

In this chapter you will:

- Identify terms relating to the composition, formation, and function of blood and lymph;
- Differentiate between the different types of blood groups;
- Identify terms related to blood clotting;
- Build words and recognize combining forms used in the blood and lymphatic systems;
- Describe various pathological conditions affecting blood and lymph; and
- Differentiate between various laboratory tests, clinical procedures, and abbreviations used in connection with the blood and lymph systems.

This chapter is divided into the following sections:

I. INTRODUCTION

Blood and lymph are the liquid tissues of the body; each is composed of cells suspended and carried within a watery fluid.

Blood contains **leukocytes, erythrocytes**, and **platelets (thrombocytes)** within a fluid portion called **plasma.** Plasma and cells circulate throughout the body in blood vessels called arteries, capillaries, and veins.

Lymph does not contain erythrocytes or platelets, but is rich in two types of white blood cells called **lymphocytes** and **monocytes**. The liquid medium of lymph is similar to blood plasma but contains much less protein. Lymph actually originates from the blood as fluid is squeezed out of tiny blood capillaries into the spaces between cells. This fluid is called **interstitial fluid**. The interstitial fluid passes continuously into special thin-walled vessels called lymph capillaries, which begin at the tissue spaces. The fluid, now called lymph, passes through larger lymphatic vessels and glands (nodes), finally to reach large veins in the thoracic region of the body. Lymph enters the veins and thus empties back into the bloodstream. Figure 13-1 illustrates the close relationship between the blood and lymph circulation in the body.

The blood and lymphatic systems have many functions. Blood carries vital materials such

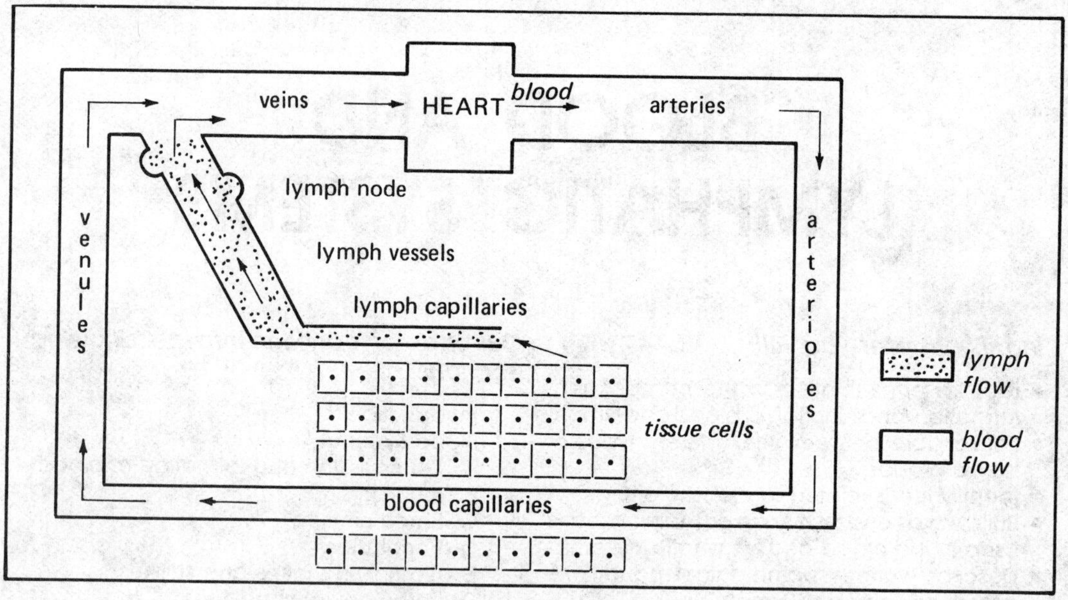

Figure 13-1 Relationship between the circulatory systems of blood and lymph.

as oxygen, nutrients, and hormones to tissue cells and transports waste materials, such as carbon dioxide and urea, away from tissue cells to be excreted from the body. Lymph transports needed proteins that have leaked out of the blood capillaries back to the bloodstream via the veins. Both blood and lymph protect the body by carrying disease-fighting cells (phagocytes) and protein substances called **antibodies** that combat infection. Also, plasma proteins and blood-clotting cells (platelets) contribute in the important **coagulation** (clotting) function of blood.

II. BLOOD SYSTEM

A. Composition and Formation of Blood

Whole blood is composed of **formed elements** (blood cells, or corpuscles) and a clear, straw-colored liquid called **plasma**.

The formed elements in the blood are the **erythrocytes** (red blood cells), **leukocytes** (white blood cells), and **platelets,** or **thrombocytes** (clotting cells). These formed elements constitute about 45 per cent of the total blood volume. The remaining 55 per cent of blood is plasma, which is composed of a solution of water and solid materials, such as proteins, sugar, salts, hormones, and vitamins.

All blood cells originate from unspecialized, immature cells called **stem cells** or **hemocytoblasts**. Hemocytoblasts mature in the red bone marrow of adults (skull, vertebrae, ribs, pelvis, breastbone, thigh, and upper arm bones) and in the liver and spleen of the fetus. The change from primitive to specialized, or **differentiated**, form involves alterations in the size and shape of the blood cell. This means that the blood cells change from large (immature cells) to small (mature forms); the size of the cell nucleus decreases (in red cells, the nucleus actually disappears); and the intensity of the stain taken up by the cytoplasm diminishes. Figure 13-2 illustrates these changes in the formation of blood cells.

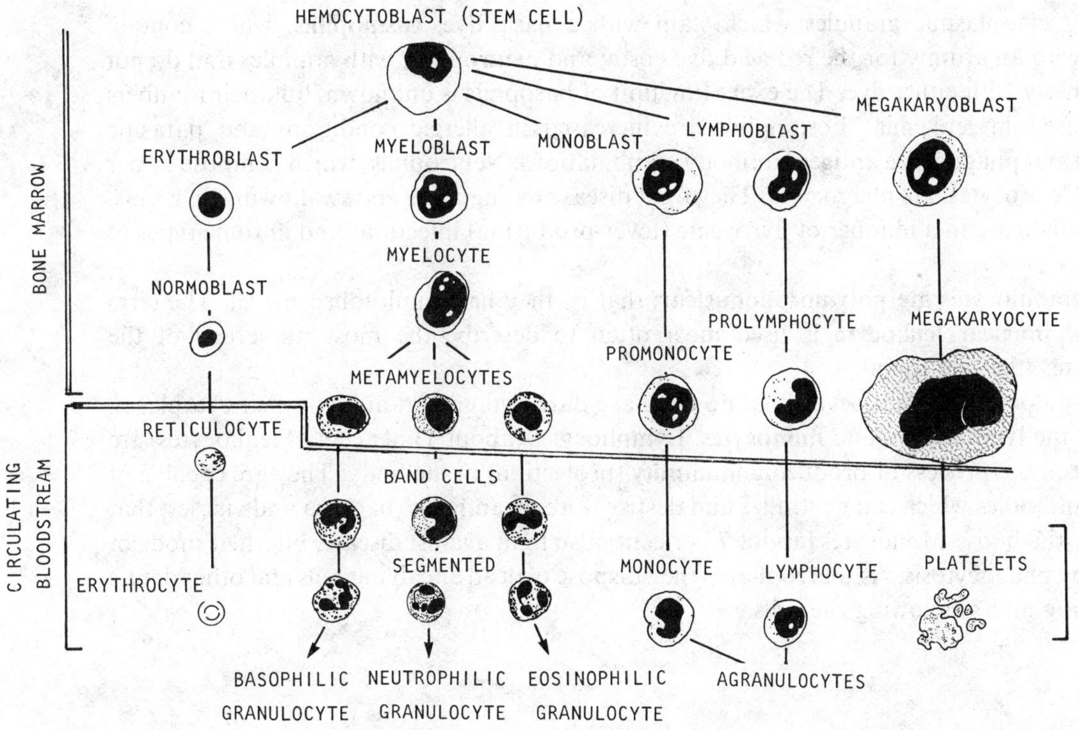

Figure 13-2 Stages in blood cell development. Band cells are identical to **segmented** granulocytes except that the nucleus is *U*-shaped and its lobes are connected by a band rather than a thin thread as in segmented cell forms.

Erythrocytes

As a red blood cell reaches maturity, its nucleus is extruded from the cell and the cell assumes the shape of a **biconcave** disk. This shape (a depressed or hollow surface on each side of the cell resembling a cough drop with a thin central portion) allows for a large surface area on the erythrocyte so that absorption and release of gases (oxygen and carbon dioxide) can take place. In addition, **hemoglobin** (a protein consisting of an iron pigment called **heme** and a protein part called **globin**) is found in mature erythrocytes. It is the hemoglobin in the erythrocytes that enables the cell to carry oxygen all through the body. The combination of oxygen and hemoglobin (oxyhemoglobin) produces the bright red color of blood.

Erythrocytes live for about 120 days in the circulating bloodstream. After this time, cells in the spleen, liver, and bone marrow destroy the worn-out erythrocytes. These cells, called **macrophages**, set the hemoglobin free from the erythrocyte and break the hemoglobin down into its heme and globin portions. The heme decomposes into **bilirubin** and **iron**. Iron is used to form new red cells or is stored in the spleen, liver, and bone marrow for later use. Bilirubin is carried to the liver and excreted through the intestines with bile.

Leukocytes

While there is only one type of mature erythrocyte, there are five types of mature leukocytes. Three of the types of leukocytes are called **granulocytes** and two are **agranulocytes**. See Figure 13-2.

Granulocytes are the most numerous leukocytes (about 60 per cent) and include **basophils,**

containing cytoplasmic granules which stain with a basic dye; **eosinophils**, which contain granules with an affinity for the red acid dye eosin; and **neutrophils**, with granules that do not stain intensely with either dye. The exact function of basophils is unknown, but their numbers are increased in leukemia. Eosinophils are increased in allergic conditions and parasitic infections and phagocytize antigen-antibody combinations. Neutrophils, which compose 57 per cent of all leukocytes, are phagocytes. They fight disease by engulfing and swallowing up germs. They also increase in a number of **pyrogenic** (fever-producing) infections and in some types of leukemia.

All granulocytes are **polymorphonuclear**; that is, they have multilobed nuclei. The term **polymorphonuclear leukocyte** is used most often to describe the most numerous of the granulocytes, the neutrophil.

Agranulocytes are leukocytes that do not have dark-staining granules in their cytoplasm. These are the **lymphocytes** and **monocytes**. Lymphocytes (about 33 per cent of leukocytes) are important in the process of producing **immunity** (protection) in the body. They are capable of making **antibodies** which can neutralize and destroy foreign **antigens** (bacteria and viruses) that may enter the body. Monocytes (about 7 per cent) also fight against disease, but their mode of action is by phagocytosis. As **macrophages** they dispose of dead and dying cells and other debris by engulfing and swallowing the cells.

Platelets

Platelets, or thrombocytes, are formed in red bone marrow from giant multinucleated cells called **megakaryocytes** (see Figure 13-2). Tiny fragments of the megakaryocyte break off from the cell to form platelets. The main function of platelets is to help in the clotting of blood. The specific terms related to blood clotting will be discussed in a later section of this chapter.

Plasma

Plasma is the liquid part of the blood. It consists of 91 per cent water and 9 per cent solid materials, which are mainly proteins, with lesser amounts of sugar, wastes, salts, hormones, and other substances. The four major plasma proteins are **albumin**, **globulin**, **fibrinogen**, and **prothrombin**. Albumin and globulin are the **serum proteins**. **Serum** is plasma from which the clotting proteins, fibrinogen and prothrombin, have been removed.

Albumin maintains the proper water content of the blood. Since albumin cannot easily pass through capillary walls, it remains in the blood and attracts water from the tissues back into the bloodstream. This opposes the water's tendency to leak out into the tissue spaces, which would cause **edema** (swelling). If albumin escapes from the capillaries as a result of injury, such as severe burn, water cannot be held in the blood and the blood volume drops. Shock can result if the loss of water is too great.

The globulin portion of plasma contains antibodies which, as part of the body's immune system, fight off foreign antigens. There are three different kinds of globulins in plasma. They are called **alpha**, **beta**, and **gamma**, and they can be distinguished by the process of **electrophoresis**. This technique involves placing the plasma in a special solution and passing an electric current through the solution. The different protein molecules in the plasma separate out as they migrate at different speeds to the source of the electricity. **Immunoglobulins** are a specific type of gamma globulin that are capable of acting as antibodies. Examples of immunoglobulin antibodies are **IgG** (present in the fetus before and at birth) and **IgA** (found in breast milk, saliva, tears, and respiratory mucus). Other immunoglobulins are **IgM**, **IgD**, and **IgE**.

Plasmapheresis (apheresis means to remove) is the process of separating plasma from the formed elements in the blood. This separation is mechanical, not electrical as is electrophoresis. The entire blood sample is spun around in a centrifuge machine, and the plasma, being lighter in weight than the blood cells, is found at the top of the sample.

Figure 13-3 reviews the composition of blood.

B. Blood Groups

Transfusions of "whole blood" (cells and plasma) are used to replace blood lost after injury, during surgery, or in severe shock. A transfusion cannot be made between any two people at random, however. Human blood falls into four main groups called A, B, AB, and O, and there are harmful effects of transfusing blood from a donor of one blood group into a recipient who is of another blood group.

Each of the blood groups has a specific combination of factors (antigens and antibodies) which are inherited. These antigen (also called agglutinogen) and antibody (also called agglutinin) factors of the various blood types are:

Type A, containing **A antigen** and **anti-B antibody**

Type B, containing **B antigen** and **anti-A antibody**

Type AB, containing **A and B antigens** and **no anti-A or anti-B antibodies**

Type O, containing **no A or B antigens** and **both anti-A and anti-B antibodies**

The problem in transfusing blood from a type A donor into a type B recipient is that A antigens (from the A donor) will react adversely with the anti-A antibodies in the recipient's type B bloodstream. The adverse reaction is called **agglutination**, or clumping, of the recipient's blood. Damage to the erythrocytes also occurs, so that hemoglobin leaks out of the cell (hemolysis). The agglutination is fatal to the recipient because it stops the flow of blood. Similar problems can occur in other transfusions if the donor's antigens are incompatible with the recipient's antibodies. People with type O blood are known as universal donors because their blood contains neither A nor B antigens. Those with type AB blood are known as universal recipients because their blood contains neither anti-A nor anti-B antibodies.

Besides A and B antigens, there are many other antigens located on the surface of red blood cells. One of these is called the **Rh factor** (named because it was first found in the blood of a rhesus monkey). The term Rh-positive refers to a person who is born with the Rh antigen on his

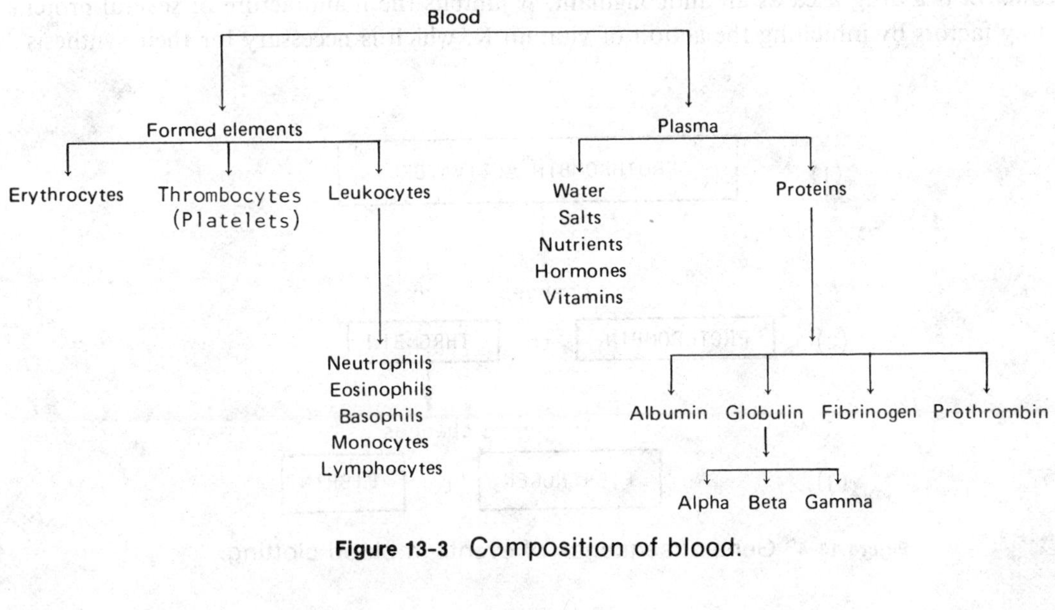

Figure 13-3 Composition of blood.

or her red blood cells. An Rh-negative person does not have the Rh antigen. There are no anti-Rh antibodies normally present in the blood of an Rh-positive or an Rh-negative person. However, if Rh-positive blood is transfused into an Rh-negative person, the recipient will begin to develop antibodies which would agglutinate any Rh-positive blood if another transfusion were to occur subsequently.

The same reactions occur during pregnancy if the fetus of an Rh-negative woman happens to be Rh-positive. This situation is described in Chapter 4, as an example of an antigen-antibody reaction.

C. Blood Clotting

Blood clotting, or **coagulation**, is a complicated process involving many different substances and chemical reactions. The final result of the process is the formation of a **fibrin clot** from the plasma protein **fibrinogen**. Platelets are important in beginning the process but 13 other factors including calcium and vitamin K are essential. Simply stated, the process involves the following steps:

1. When a blood vessel is damaged or breaks, a **prothrombin activator** is released into the blood in response to special factors from platelets and tissues. One of these factors is the protein that is missing in patients suffering from hemophilia.

2. The prothrombin activator, along with calcium and other plasma factors, helps to convert **prothrombin** (a plasma protein) into an enzyme called **thrombin**.

3. Thrombin then converts **fibrinogen** to **fibrin** threads, which trap red blood cells, platelets, and plasma to form the clot.

Figure 13-4 reviews this basic sequence of events.

After the fibrin threads of a clot form, most of the plasma leaves the clot. This plasma fluid, which lacks the clotting proteins and clotting factors, is called **serum**. The clot thus begins to contract and the edges of the broken blood vessel are pulled together, ending the coagulation process.

Normally, clots (thrombi) do not form in blood vessels unless the vessel is damaged or the flow of blood is impeded. Anticoagulant substances in the bloodstream inhibit blood clotting so thrombi or emboli (floating clots) do not form. **Heparin**, produced by specialized tissue cells, is an example of an anticoagulant. It blocks several steps in the generation of thrombin. **Dicumarol** is a drug used as an anticoagulant. It inhibits the manufacture of several protein clotting factors by inhibiting the action of vitamin K, which is necessary for their synthesis.

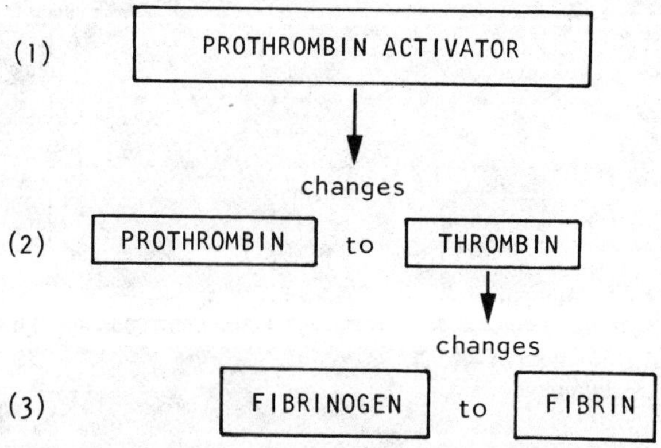

Figure 13-4 General sequence of events in blood clotting.

D. Vocabulary

agglutination — Clumping of recipient's blood cells when incompatible bloods are mixed.

albumin — Protein found in blood; maintains the proper amount of water in the blood. Also called serum albumin.

antibodies — Protein substances whose formation is stimulated by the presence of antigens in the body. An antibody then helps neutralize or inactivate the antigen that stimulated its formation.

antigens — Foreign material that causes the production of an antibody. Naturally occurring antigens are the blood type factors A and B that are present at birth in some individuals.

basophil — White blood cell with large, dark-staining granules that have an affinity for basic dyes.

bilirubin — Orange-yellowish pigment produced from hemoglobin when red blood cells are destroyed. Bilirubin is concentrated in bile by the liver and excreted in the feces.

coagulation — Blood clotting.

corpuscle — "Little body"—refers to blood cells.

dicumarol — An anticoagulant drug; used to prevent thromboembolic clotting disorders.

differentiation — Change in structure and function of a cell as it matures; specialization.

electrophoresis — Method of separating out plasma proteins by electrical charge.

eosinophil — White blood cell with dense, reddish granules having an affinity for the red acid dye eosin.

erythrocyte — A red blood cell.

fibrin — Protein threads that form the basis of a blood clot.

fibrinogen — Plasma protein that is converted to fibrin in the clotting process.

formed elements — The cellular elements in blood.

globin — The protein part of hemoglobin.

globulin — Plasma protein; separates into alpha, beta, and gamma types by electrophoresis.

granulocytes — White blood cells with granules: eosinophils, neutrophils, and basophils.

heme Iron-containing nonprotein portion of the hemoglobin molecule.

hemocytoblast Primitive stem cell found in the bone marrow from which all blood cells are thought to arise.

hemoglobin Blood protein found in red blood cells; enables the red blood cell to carry oxygen and carbon dioxide.

heparin An anticoagulant found in blood and tissues.

immune reaction Reaction between an antigen and an antibody in which the antigen is neutralized or inactivated by the antibody.

immunoglobulin Type of gamma globulin; IgG, IgM, IgA, IgE, IgD.

interstitial fluid Fluid in the extracellular spaces.

leukocyte A white blood cell.

lymphocyte White blood cell (agranulocyte) found in lymph tissue; produces antibodies.

macrophages Large phagocytes that destroy worn-out red blood cells and engulf foreign material.

megakaryocyte Platelet precursor (forerunner) formed in the bone marrow.

monocyte White blood cell (agranulocyte) formed in lymph tissue; phagocyte.

neutrophil White blood cell (granulocyte) formed in bone marrow; a phagocyte with neutral-staining granules.

plasma Liquid portion of blood; contains water, proteins, salts, nutrients, hormones, and vitamins.

plasmapheresis Process of using a centrifuge to separate the formed elements from the blood plasma. Formed elements are retransfused into the donor and fresh frozen plasma is used to replace withdrawn plasma.

platelet Smallest formed element in the blood; a thrombocyte.

prothrombin Plasma protein; converted to thrombin in the clotting process.

Rh factor An antigen normally found on red blood cells of Rh-positive individuals.

serum Plasma minus clotting proteins and cells.

stem cell A cell in bone marrow that gives rise to different types of blood cells; also called a hemocytoblast.

thrombin An enzyme that helps to convert fibrinogen to fibrin during coagulation.

thrombocyte Platelet.

E. Combining Forms and Suffixes

Combining Form	*Definition*	*Terminology*	*Meaning*
hem/o hemat/o	blood	hematocrit ______________ *See laboratory tests.*	
		hemolysis ______________	
erythr/o	red	erythropoiesis ______________	
is/o	same, equal	anisocytosis ______________ *Variation in the size of erythrocytes (-osis, with blood cell terms, indicates a slight increase in numbers).*	
chrom/o	color	hypochromia ______________ *Reduction in hemoglobin in red cells.*	
poikil/o	varied, irregular	poikilocytosis ______________ *Variation in shape of erythrocyte.*	
spher/o	globe, round	spherocytosis ______________ *One type of poikilocytosis found in hemolytic anemias. The normal shape of the erythrocyte is a biconcave disk.*	
leuk/o	white	leukopenia ______________	
eosin/o	red, dawn, rosy	eosinophilia ______________ *-philia indicates a condition of more than the normal numbers of cells.*	
bas/o	base, opposite of acid	basophil ______________	
neutr/o	neither, neutral *(neither base nor acid)*	neutropenia ______________	
granul/o	granules	granulocytosis ______________	

myel/o	bone marrow	myeloblast ____________
		-blast indicates an immature cell.
phag/o	eat, swallow	phagocyte ____________
mon/o	one, single	monocyte ____________
		monocytosis ____________
thromb/o	clot	thrombocytopenia ____________
		thrombocytosis ____________
		thrombosis ____________
nucle/o	nucleus	nucleated ____________
kary/o	nucleus	megakaryocyte ____________
morph/o	shape, form	morphology ____________
		polymorphonuclear ____________ ____________
		Granulocytes are polymorphonuclear leukocytes.
reticul/o	network	reticulocyte ____________
		This developing erythrocyte contains a network of granules in its cytoplasm.
agglutin/o	clumping, sticking together	agglutination ____________
immun/o	safe, protection	immunology ____________
sider/o	iron	sideropenia ____________
-globin	protein	hemoglobin ____________
-globulin	protein	gamma globulin ____________
-blast	embryonic, immature	monoblast ____________
-emia	blood condition	leukemia ____________
		See under pathological conditions.

-cytosis	condition of cells *(slight increase in cell numbers)*	macrocytosis ________________ *Refers to the size of erythrocytes.*
-philia	attraction for *(usually increase in numbers)*	neutrophilia ________________ ________________
-poiesis	formation	myelopoietic ________________ *-sis changes to -tic in the adjectival form.*
-stasis	stop, control	hemostasis ________________
-apheresis	removal *(use of a centrifuge to spin down blood to separate out elements)*	plasmapheresis ________________
		plateletpheresis ________________ *Platelets are removed from donor's blood and the remainder of the blood is retransfused into the donor.*
		leukapheresis ________________
-phoresis	carrying, transmission	electrophoresis ________________

F. Pathological Conditions

Any abnormal or pathological condition of the blood is generally referred to as a blood **dyscrasia** (disease). The blood dyscrasias discussed in this section are organized in the following manner: diseases of red blood cells, disorders of blood clotting, diseases of white blood cells, and bone marrow disease.

Diseases of Red Blood Cells

anemia

Deficiency in erythrocytes or hemoglobin.

Anemia implies a reduction in red blood cells. This can be exhibited by a decrease in number of red cells or decrease in the amount of hemoglobin in red cells. The most common type is **iron-deficiency anemia** caused by a lack of iron, which is required for hemoglobin production (see Figure 13-5). Other types of anemia include:

pernicious anemia

Lack of mature erythrocytes due to inability to absorb vitamin B_{12} into the body.

Vitamin B_{12} is necessary for the proper development and maturation of erythrocytes. While vitamin B_{12} is a common constituent of food matter, it cannot be absorbed into the bloodstream without the aid of a special

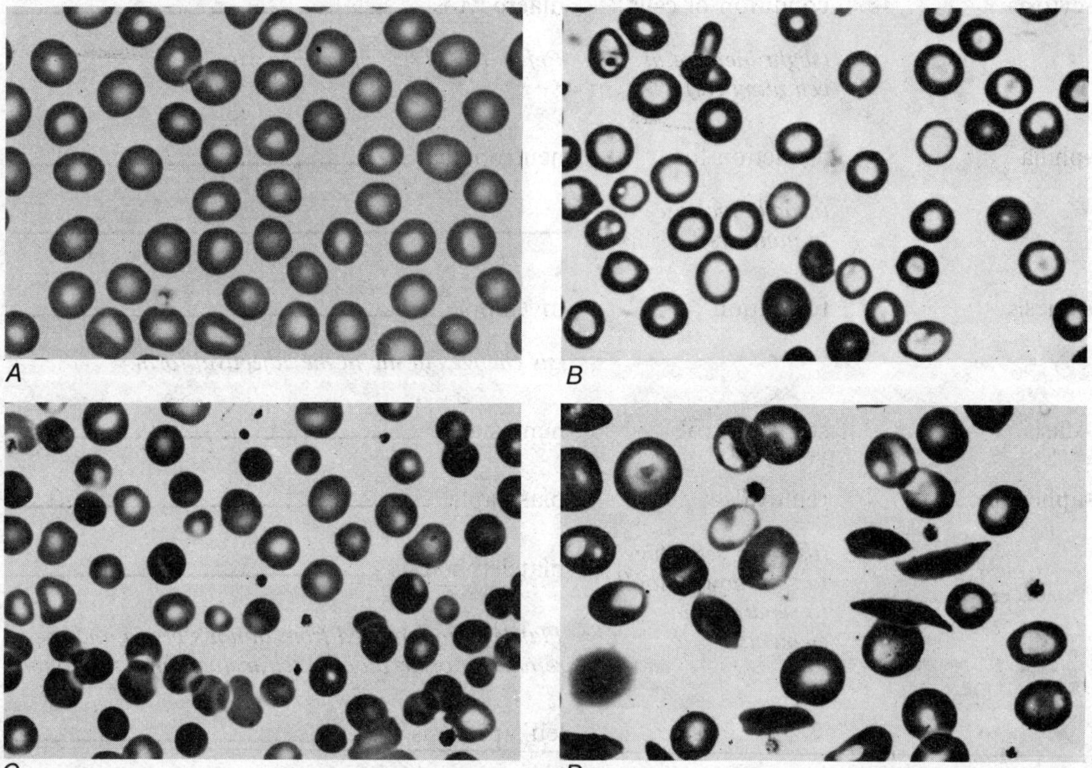

Figure 13-5 *A*, Normal blood film. *B*, Iron deficiency anemia, with hypochromic, microcytic cells. *C*, Hereditary spherocytosis, with small RBCs of spherical shape (little or no central pallor). *D*, Sickle-cell anemia with poikilocytosis. (From Nelson, D.A., in Henry, J.B.: Clinical Diagnosis and Management by Laboratory Methods. 17th ed. Philadelphia, W.B. Saunders Co., 1984.)

substance called intrinsic factor that is normally found in gastric juice. Individuals with pernicious anemia lack this factor in their gastric juice, and the result is unsuccessful maturation of red cells, with an excess of large, immature, nucleated, and poorly functioning red cells (**megaloblasts**) in the circulation. Treatment is administration of vitamin B_{12} for life.

aplastic anemia Failure of blood cell production due to aplasia (absence of development, formation) of bone marrow cells.

The cause of most cases of aplastic anemia is often unknown (idiopathic), but some cases have been linked to benzene exposure and to antibiotics such as chloramphenicol. **Pancytopenia** occurs as stem cells fail to produce leukocytes, platelets, and erythrocytes. Blood transfusions prolong life until the marrow resumes its normal functioning, and antibiotics are used to control infections. Bone marrow transplants have been successful, particularly those conducted with marrow from an identical twin.

hemolytic anemia Reduction in red cells due to excessive destruction.

One example of hemolytic anemia is **congenital spherocytic anemia**. Instead of their normal biconcave shape, erythrocytes are spheroidal (see Figure 13-5). This shape makes them very fragile and easily destroyed (hemolysis), leading to anemia. The spherocytosis causes increased numbers of reticulocytes in the circulating blood as the bone marrow attempts to compensate for the hemolysis of mature erythrocytes. The excessive hemolysis leads to jaundice because of accumulation of bilirubin in the circulating bloodstream. Since the spleen is an organ where red cells are destroyed, it may be removed with helpful results.

sickle-cell anemia

Hereditary condition characterized by abnormal shape of erythrocytes and by hemolysis.

The crescent or sickle shape of the erythrocyte is caused by an abnormal type of hemoglobin (hemoglobin S) in the red cell (see Figure 13-5). The distorted, fragile erythrocytes clump together and block blood vessels, leading to thrombosis and infarction (dead tissue). Symptoms include arthralgias, acute attacks of abdominal pain, and ulcerations of the extremities. The genetic defect (presence of the hemoglobin S gene) is found predominantly in blacks and appears with different degrees of severity depending on the presence of one or two inherited genes for the trait.

thalassemia

An inherited defect in the ability to produce hemoglobin, usually seen in persons of Mediterranean (thalass = sea) background.

This condition, consisting of various forms and degrees of severity (the most severe form is called **Cooley's anemia**), usually leads to hypochromic anemia (diminished hemoglobin content in red cells).

polycythemia vera

Malignant condition associated with an increase in red blood cells (erythremia).

Blood consistency is viscous (sticky) because of greatly increased numbers of erythrocytes. The bone marrow is hyperplastic, and leukocytosis and thrombocytosis accompany the increase in red blood cells. Treatment consists of reduction of red cell volume to normal levels by phlebotomy (removal of blood from a vein) and by suppressing production with myelotoxic drugs.

hemochromatosis

Excessive deposits of iron throughout the body.

Hepatomegaly occurs and the skin is pigmented so that it has a bronze hue; diabetes can occur, and frequently cardiac failure. The condition is usually seen in males over 40 years of age.

Disorders of Blood Clotting

hemophilia

Excessive bleeding caused by a congenital lack of a substance necessary for blood clotting.

While the platelet count of a hemophiliac is normal, there is a marked deficiency in a plasma clotting factor (Factor VIII), which results in a very prolonged coagulation time. Treatment consists of administration of the deficient factor.

purpura

Multiple pinpoint hemorrhages and accumulation of blood under the skin

Purpura means purple, and in this bleeding condition, hemorrhages into the skin and mucous membranes produce red-purple discoloration of the skin. The bleeding is caused by a fall in the number of platelets (thrombocytopenia). The etiology of the disorder may be immunologic, meaning that the body produces an antiplatelet factor that harms its own platelets. Splenectomy (spleen is the site of platelet destruction) and drug therapy to discourage antibody synthesis are methods of treatment. Purpura is also seen in any other condition associated with a low platelet count, such as leukemia and drug reactions.

Diseases of White Blood Cells

leukemia

Excessive increase in white blood cells.

This is a cancerous disease of the bone marrow with malignant leukocytes filling the marrow and bloodstream. There are several types of leukemia, depending on the particular leukocyte involved. Four forms of the disease are:

acute myelogenous leukemia (AML)—Immature granulocytes (myeloblasts) predominate. Platelets and erythrocytes are diminished because of infiltration and replacement of the bone marrow by large numbers of myeloblasts.

acute lymphocytic leukemia (ALL)—Immature lymphocytes (lymphoblasts) predominate. This form is seen most often in children and adolescents; onset is sudden.

chronic myelogenous leukemia (CML)—Both mature and immature granulocytes are present in the marrow and bloodstream. This is a slowly progressive illness in which patients may live for many years without encountering life-threatening problems.

chronic lymphocytic leukemia (CLL)—Abnormal numbers of relatively mature lymphocytes predominate in the marrow, lymph nodes, and spleen. This form of leukemia occurs later in life and follows a slowly progressive course.

All forms of leukemia are treated with chemotherapy, using drugs that prevent cell division and selectively injure rapidly dividing cells. Effective treatment can lead to a **remission** (disappearance of signs of disease). **Relapse** occurs when leukemia cells reappear in the blood and bone marrow, necessitating further treatment.

granulocytosis

Abnormal increase in granulocytes in the blood.

An increase in granulocytes in the blood may occur in response to infection or inflammation of any type. **Eosinophilia** is an increase in eosinophilic granulocytes, which is seen in certain allergic conditions, such as asthma, or in parasitic infections (tapeworm, pinworm). **Basophilia** is an increase in basophilic granulocytes seen in certain types of leukemia.

Disease of Bone Marrow

multiple myeloma Malignant tumor of bone marrow.

This is a progressive tumor of antibody-producing cells. The malignant cells invade the bone marrow and destroy bony structures. The tumors lead to overproduction of immunoglobulins and **Bence Jones protein**. Often, the condition leads to osteolytic lesions, hypercalcemia, anemia, renal damage, and increased susceptibility to infection. Treatment is with analgesics, radiotherapy, **palliative** (relieving, not curing) doses of chemotherapy, and special orthopedic supports.

III. LYMPHATIC SYSTEM

A. Composition, Anatomy, and Function

Composition

Lymph is tissue fluid found in special lymphatic vessels all over the body. Lymph is clear and colorless and contains less protein than blood plasma. Other noncellular constituents of lymph are water, salts, sugar, and wastes of metabolism, such as urea and creatinine. Lymph passing from the villi of the small intestine is called **chyle**, and it is milky in appearance from fats absorbed through the villi into the intestinal lymph vessels which are called **lacteals**. The cellular composition of lymph includes lymphocytes, monocytes, and a few platelets and erythrocytes.

Label Figure 13-6 as you read the following paragraphs.

Anatomy

Lymph capillaries (1) begin at the tissue spaces from microscopic blind ends. They, like blood capillaries, are thin-walled tubes. Lymph capillaries carry lymph from the tissue spaces to larger **lymphatic vessels** (2). Lymphatic vessels are thicker than lymph capillaries and, like veins, contain valves so that lymph fluid flows only in one direction, toward the thoracic cavity. Two ducts in the thoracic cavity receive the lymph from the lymph vessels. These ducts are the **right lymphatic duct** (3) and the **thoracic duct** (4). They empty lymph into **veins** (5) in the upper thoracic region.

Function

By serving as a channel for the flow of substances from tissue spaces to the bloodstream, lymph has an important function in the body. Valuable proteins which may have leaked out of blood capillaries at the tissue spaces can be returned to the bloodstream by flowing through the lymphatic fluid. Also, lymph vessels called lacteals are the channels for the absorption of fats from the small intestine into the bloodstream. The lymphatic system serves, as well, as a passageway for toxic or disease substances which leave tissue spaces and get trapped in **lymph nodes** (6).

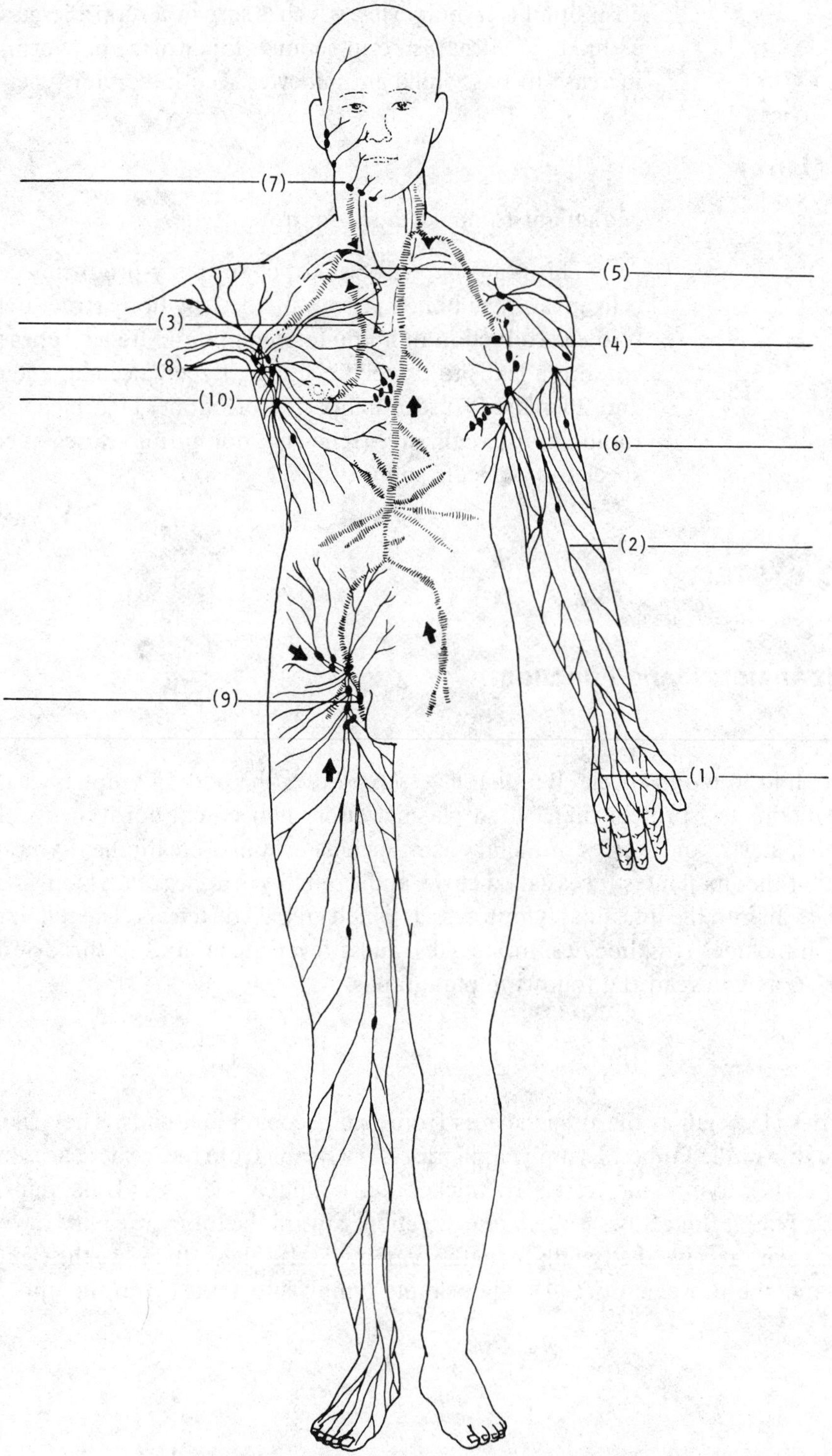

Figure 13-6 Lymphatic system.

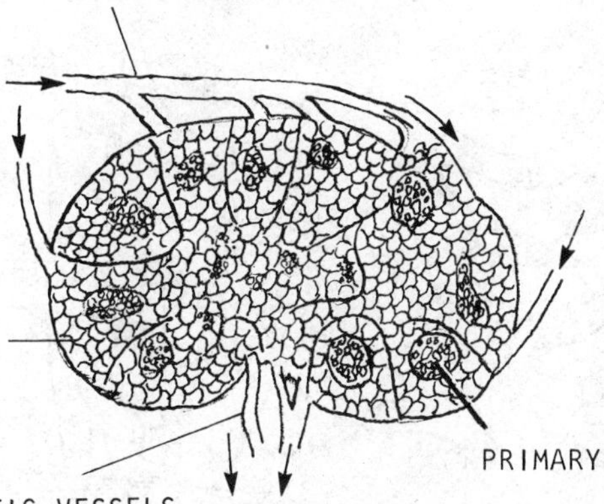

Figure 13-7 A lymph node.

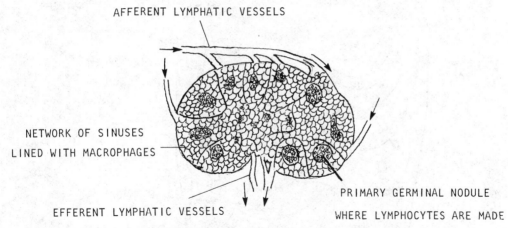

A lymph node contains lymphocytes and lymphatic channels that are held together by a fibrous connective tissue capsule. The lymph nodes have many functions. They trap and filter toxic and malignant substances from inflammatory and cancerous lesions. There are also special cells in lymph nodes that can phagocytize foreign substances and digest them. These phagocytic cells are called macrophages (or histiocytes). Macrophages are found in the liver, spleen, bone marrow, lungs, brain, and spinal cord, as well as in lymph nodes.

Lymph nodes also fight disease by antibody production from lymphocytes present in nodes. The major sites of lymph node concentration are the **cervical** (7), **axillary** (8), **inguinal** (9), and **mediastinal** (10) regions of the body. Figure 13-7 shows the contents of a lymph node.

B. Related Lymphatic Organs

The **spleen** and **thymus gland** are organs composed of lymphatic tissue.

Spleen

The spleen (pictured in Figure 13-8) is located in the left upper quadrant of the abdomen, adjacent to the stomach. While the spleen is not essential to life, it has several important functions:

1. Destruction of old erythrocytes by macrophages. Because of hemolytic activity in the spleen, bilirubin is formed there and added to the bloodstream.
2. Filtration of microorganisms and other foreign material from the blood.
3. Production of antibodies and immunity, chiefly by leukocytes.
4. Storage of blood, especially red blood cells. Blood is released by the spleen as the body needs it.
5. Production of blood cells such as lymphocytes and monocytes. Also, the spleen seems to have a stimulatory effect on the production of blood from the bone marrow.

Thymus and Immunity

The thymus gland (pictured in Figure 13-9) is located in the mediastinum, posterior to the breastbone and between the lungs. It plays an important role in the body's immunologic system, especially in fetal life and the early years of growth. It is known that thymectomy performed in

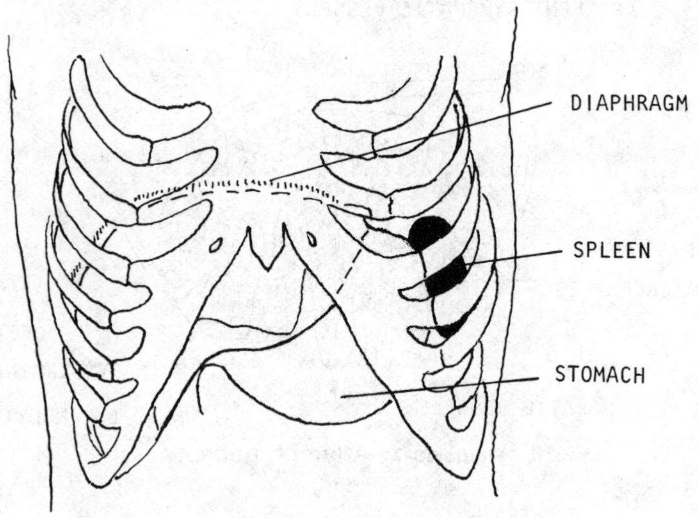

Figure 13-8 The spleen and adjacent organs.

animals during the first few weeks of life impairs the ability of the animal to make antibodies to fight against foreign antigens.

The body's immune response involves the production of two types of lymphocytes, **T-cells** and **B-cells**. T-cells (thymic cells) are found in the thymus. They migrate from the thymus into the bloodstream, and from there to the site of antigens (foreign substances such as bacteria and viruses). T-cells are able to attach to the antigen and destroy it. B-cells are produced in the bone marrow. A B-cell, when confronted with a specific type of antigen, transforms into an antibody-producing cell called a **plasma cell**. The antibodies that are made by plasma cells are called **immunoglobulins**, such as IgM, IgG, IgD, IgE, and IgA.

The type of immune response in which antibodies are produced is called **humoral immunity**. Antibodies can destroy antigens in many ways. One of these ways is to activate a complex series of proteins in the blood. These proteins are called **complement**. Complement can then aid the antibody in destroying the antigen. Complement also aids phagocytes in the destruction of antigens.

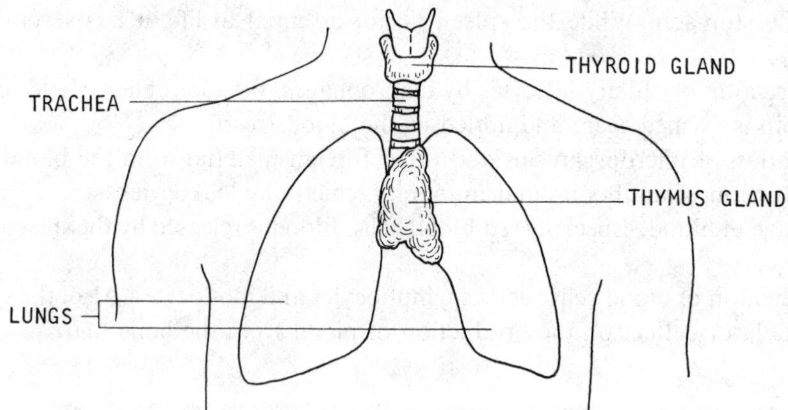

Figure 13-9 The thymus gland.

CELL-MEDIATED IMMUNITY

T-CELLS (THYMUS)

1. Attach to antigens and destroy them
2. Stimulate macrophages to recognize and ingest antigens
3. Secrete proteins (lymphokines and interferon) that help other cells to respond to antigens
4. Act as helper cells to promote antibody synthesis by B-cells
5. Act as suppressor cells to inhibit antibody synthesis

HUMORAL IMMUNITY

B-CELLS (BONE MARROW)

1. Transform into plasma cells and secrete antibodies called immunoglobulins

Figure 13-10 Functions of T-cell and B-cell lymphocytes.

Another type of immune response is called **cell-mediated immunity**. This type of immune response is dependent on T-cell lymphocytes and is seen in the fight against chronic bacterial infections (such as tuberculosis), viral and fungal diseases, malignant cell growth, and cells of transplanted organs. T-cell lymphocytes involved in cell-mediated immunity are active in destruction of foreign materials, such as bacteria, viruses, and foreign tissues such as skin grafts. The T-cells produce chemicals called **lymphokines** that help **macrophages** (large phagocytes found in lymph nodes and other body tissues) do their job. Another chemical called **interferon** is produced by T-cell lymphocytes and other cells after viral infections. Interferon inhibits the ability of viruses to infect uninfected cells.

T-cells can be subdivided according to their ability to help or retard antibody production by B-cells. Some T-cell lymphocytes are called **suppressor cells**. These cells suppress antibody production by B-cells, and in addition produce chemicals that damage the cell membranes of foreign cells. Other T-cells aid the B-cells in their response. These cells are called **helper cells**.

Figure 13-10 summarizes the functions of T-cells and B-cells.

C. Vocabulary

B-cells	Lymphocytes formed in the bone marrow; transform into plasma cells and secrete antibodies.
cell-mediated immunity	An immune response involving T-cells.
chyle	Lymph fluid filled with absorbed fats from the villi of the small intestine.

complement	Proteins that aid antibodies in destroying antigens.
histiocyte	Macrophage; a large phagocyte.
humoral immunity	Immune response in which B-cells transform into plasma cells and secrete antibodies.
immunoglobulins	Antibodies such as IgA, IgE, IgG, IgM, and IgD; secreted by plasma cells.
interferon	An antiviral protein secreted by T-cells and other cells.
lacteal	Lymph vessel found in the villi of the intestine.
lymph capillaries	Tiniest lymph vessels.
lymph nodes	Stationary lymph tissue along lymph vessels.
lymphokines	Substances produced by lymphocytes that play a role in cell-mediated immunity.
lymph vessels	Carriers of lymph throughout the body; lymph vessels empty into veins in the chest.
macrophage	Large phagocyte found in lymph nodes and other tissues of the body; histiocyte.
plasma cell	A cell that secretes antibody.
right lymphatic duct	Large lymph vessel in the chest.
spleen	Organ near the stomach that helps in blood cell storage, elimination, and production.
T-cells	Lymphocytes formed in the thymus; they are cytotoxic to antigens.
thoracic duct	Large lymph vessel in the chest.
thymus gland	Organ in the mediastinum that produces T-cell lymphocytes and aids in the immune response.

D. Combining Forms

Combining Form	*Structure or Substance*	*Terminology*	*Meaning*
lymph/o	lymph	lymphopoiesis	____________________
		lymphedema	____________________
		See elephantiasis, under pathological conditions.	

lymphaden/o	lymph gland	lymphadenopathy ____________
lymphangi/o	lymph vessels	lymphangiogram ____________
splen/o	spleen	splenomegaly ____________
		splenectomy ____________
thym/o	thymus gland	thymectomy ____________
		thymoma ____________

E. Pathological Conditions

Hodgkin's disease — Malignant tumor arising in lymphatic tissue such as lymph nodes and spleen.

This disease of unknown etiology produces lymph node enlargement, fever, and weight loss. A malignant cell, called a Reed-Sternberg cell, is characteristically found in the lymph nodes. There may be metastases to other organs in the more advanced stages of the disease. Radiation and chemotherapy are effective methods of treatment.

lymphosarcoma (lymphoma) — Malignant tumor of lymph nodes which closely resembles Hodgkin's disease.

This disease, also called **non-Hodgkin's lymphoma**, affects the lymph nodes, spleen, bone marrow, and other organs. There are several types of lymphoma, including **lymphocytic** (composed of lymphocytes) and **histiocytic** (composed of large lymphocytes that resemble histiocytes). Chemotherapy and radiation are used to stop the progress of the disease.

Burkitt's lymphoma — Malignant tumor of lymph nodes; usually affects children and is most common in Central Africa.

sarcoidosis — Inflammatory disease in which small nodules, or tubercles form in lymph nodes and other organs.

Lesions develop on the skin and in the spleen, lungs, lymph nodes, and liver. The disease process resembles the tubercles of tuberculosis but the etiology of this condition is unknown.

mycosis fungoides — Rare, chronic lymphoma which affects primarily the skin and lymph nodes. May be preceded by an intense reddening of the skin, termed Sézary syndrome.

lymphadenitis — Inflammation of lymph nodes, usually due to infection.

mononucleosis — Acute infectious disease with enlarged lymph nodes and spleen and increased numbers of lymphocytes and monocytes in bloodstream.

This disease is caused by a virus. Lymphadenopathy is present, with sore throat and enlarged, tender nodes in the cervical and sometimes axillary and inguinal regions. Splenomegaly, hepatomegaly, and marked asthenia (weakness) are also present.

lymphocytosis Increased numbers of lymphocytes in the blood and bone marrow.

elephantiasis Blockage of lymph vessels with swelling (lymphedema) of tissues due to fluid accumulation.

The condition characteristically affects the lower extremities and scrotum and is most common in tropical countries where it is caused by infestation with a worm. The disease can also be congenital.

hypersplenism A syndrome that occurs in various disorders. In these cases, splenomegaly is associated with destruction of blood cells in the spleen, resulting in anemia, leukopenia, and thrombocytopenia.

AIDS (acquired immunodeficiency syndrome) A disease marked by a decrease in the immune response.

AIDS occurs predominantly in homosexual males, intravenous drug abusers, and Haitians or Africans. Patients have severe depletion of helper T-cell lymphocytes, acquire unusual life-threatening infections, and may develop tumors such as Kaposi's sarcoma (a skin and lymphoid cancer) or lymphoma.

IV. LABORATORY TESTS, CLINICAL PROCEDURES, AND ABBREVIATIONS

Laboratory Tests

Hemoglobin test This is a measurement of the amount of hemoglobin in a blood sample.

Hematocrit This test measures the percentage of erythrocytes in a volume of blood. A sample of blood is spun around in a centrifuge so that the erythrocytes fall to the bottom of the sample.

White blood cell count This is the number of white blood cells per cubic millimeter. Automatic counting devices can record numbers within seconds. Leukocytes normally average between 5000 and 10,000 per cu mm.

White blood cell differential count This test determines the numbers of different types of leukocytes (immature and mature forms). The cells are stained and counted under a microscope by a technician. A minimum of 100 cells is counted and the percentages for neutrophils, lymphocytes, monocytes, basophils, and eosinophils are given.

The term **shift to the left** is used to describe a condition in which there is an increase in immature neutrophils and a decrease in mature forms in the blood.

Platelet count The number of platelets per cubic millimeter of blood is determined. Platelets normally average between 200,000 and 500,000 per cu mm.

Red blood cell count

This test gives the number of erythrocytes per cubic millimeter of blood. The normal number is about 5 million per cu mm.

Red blood cell morphology

A blood smear is examined to determine the shape or form of individual red cells. The presence of anisocytosis, poikilocytosis, sickle cells, "target cells" (they have a central dense area of hemoglobin), and hypochromia can be noted.

Erythrocyte sedimentation rate

This test measures the speed at which erythrocytes settle out of plasma. Venous blood is collected, anticoagulant is added, and the blood is placed in a tube in a vertical position. The distance that the erythrocytes fall in a given period of time is the sedimentation rate. The rate is altered in disease conditions, such as infections, joint inflammation, and tumor, which increase the immunoglobulin content of the blood.

Bleeding time

This is a measurement of the time it takes for a small puncture wound to stop bleeding. Normal time is 8 minutes or less. Bleeding time is prolonged in platelet disorders such as thrombocytopenia.

Coagulation time

This is the time required for venous blood to clot in a test tube. Normal time is less than 15 minutes.

Prothrombin time

This is a test of the ability of the blood to clot. It measures the time elapsed between the addition of calcium to a plasma sample and the appearance of a visible clot. The test is used to follow patients taking blood thinners, such as sodium warfarin (Coumadin).

Partial thromboplastin time

This test determines the presence of important clotting factors in the blood. There are 13 factors, 11 of which are readily measurable.

Antiglobulin test (Coombs' test)

This test demonstrates whether the patient's erythrocytes are coated with antibody and is useful in determining the presence of antibodies in infants of Rh^- women.

Clinical Procedures

Bone marrow biopsy

A needle is introduced into the bone marrow cavity and a small amount of marrow is aspirated. The marrow is then examined under a microscope. This procedure is helpful in the diagnosis of blood disorders such as anemia, cytopenias, and leukemia.

Bone marrow transplant

Bone marrow cells from a donor whose tissue and blood cells match those of the recipient are infused into a patient with leukemia or aplastic anemia. First the patient is given total-body irradiation or aggressive chemotherapy to kill all diseased cells. The donor's marrow is then intravenously infused into the patient and repopulates the marrow with normal cells. Problems encountered subsequently are serious infection, graft versus host disease (immune reaction of the donor's cells to the recipient), and relapse of the original disease (such as leukemia) despite the treatment.

Lymphangiogram Dye is injected into lymph vessels in the foot, and x-rays are taken to show the path of lymph flow as it moves into the chest region.

Abbreviations

ABO	Three main blood types
AHF	Antihemophilic factor (one of 13 clotting factors)
AIDS	Acquired immunodeficiency syndrome
ALL	Acute lymphocytic leukemia
AML	Acute myelogenous leukemia
baso	Basophils
CBC	Complete blood count
CLL	Chronic lymphocytic leukemia
CML	Chronic myelogenous leukemia
diff.	Differential count (white blood cells)
eosins	Eosinophils
ESR	Erythrocyte sedimentation rate
Hb	Hemoglobin
Hct	Hematocrit
Hgb	Hemoglobin
IgA, IgD, IgG, IgM, IgE	Immunoglobulins
lymphs	Lymphocytes
MCH	Amount of hemoglobin per cell (mean corpuscular hemoglobin)
MCHC	Average concentration of hemoglobin per red cells (mean corpuscular hemoglobin concentration)
MCV	Average volume of a red blood cell (mean corpuscular volume)
metamyl	Metamyelocyte (immature granulocyte)
mon, mono	Monocyte
myelocyt	Myelocyte (immature granulocyte)
poly	Polymorphonuclear leukocyte
PMN	Polymorphonuclear leukocyte
PT	Prothrombin
PTT	Partial thromboplastin time
RBC	Red blood cell (red blood cell count)
segs	Segmented, mature white blood cells
WBC	White blood cell (white blood cell count)

V. PRACTICAL APPLICATIONS

Laboratory Report: Hematology (normal values are in brackets)

CBC

1. WBC [5–10,000] __________ /cu mm
2. Hgb
   M [14–16] __________ gm
   F [13–15] __________ gm
3. Hct
   M [42–50] __________ %
   F [35–45] __________ %
4. RBC
   M [4.5–6.0] __________ million
   F [4.0–5.5] __________ million

5. Platelets
   [140–400,000] __________ /cu mm
6. Differential
   Bands __________
   Segs (Polys) __________
   Lymphs __________
   Eosins __________
   Baso __________
   Mono __________
   Metamyl __________
   Myelocyt __________
7. RBC morphology
   anisocyt __________
   poikilocyt __________
   hypochro __________
   polychro __________
   microcyte __________
   macrocyte __________
   sickle cells __________
8. Reticulocytes __________ %
9. ESR __________ mm/hr

Sentences Using Medical Terms

1. The patient is a 45-year-old woman with a diagnosis of Hodgkin's disease, Stage III [stage of the disease indicates the extent of spread—Stage I is more localized than Stage IV], with cervical, axillary, periaortic, and inguinal lymphadenopathy.
2. Thrombocytopenia is frequently associated with purpura.
3. Multiple myeloma is a neoplastic proliferation of plasma cells. The clinical manifestations of the disease result from the effects of the myeloma tumor cell mass in the bone marrow, as well as from the myeloma proteins produced by the malignant cells. The effects of the tumor cell mass include lytic skeletal lesions, hypercalcemia, anemia, leukopenia, and thrombocytopenia. Clinical features related to the myeloma proteins include hyperviscosity [excessive stickiness], coagulopathy, and renal insufficiency [tubules get plugged with protein material].

VI. EXERCISES

A. Match each of the following with its description below:

albumin	thrombocyte	megakaryocyte
eosinophil	serum	hemocytoblast
hemoglobin	lymphocyte	globulin
fibrinogen	monocyte	bilirubin
neutrophil	erythrocyte	heparin

1. A platelet __________
2. Plasma minus clotting proteins and cells __________
3. Leukocyte with dense, reddish granules __________
4. Orange-yellowish pigment produced when red blood cells are destroyed

   ____

5. A plasma protein that is converted to fibrin in coagulation ______________

6. A plasma protein that maintains the proper amount of water in the blood

____

7. A granulocyte with neutral staining granules ______________

8. Blood protein found in red blood cells ______________

9. An anticoagulant found in blood and tissues ______________

10. An agranulocyte that produces antibodies ______________

11. A plasma protein that separates into alpha, beta, and gamma types ______________

____

12. A phagocytic agranulocyte found in lymph nodes ______________

13. Platelet precursor formed in the bone marrow ______________

14. A red blood cell ______________

15. Primitive stem cell found in the bone marrow ______________

B. *Give meanings for the following terms:*

1. agglutination ______________
2. antigen ______________
3. antibody ______________
4. electrophoresis ______________
5. immunoglobulin ______________
6. macrophage ______________
7. plasmapheresis ______________
8. coagulation ______________
9. thrombin ______________
10. dicumarol ______________

C. *Give answers for the following:*

1. Name four plasma proteins: ______________________________

2. What is the Rh factor? ______________________________

3. A person with type B blood has ______________ antigens and ______________ antibodies in his or her blood.

4. A person with type O blood has ______________ antigens and ______________ antibodies in his or her blood.

5. A person with type AB blood has ______________ antigens and ______________ antibodies in his or her blood.

D. *Describe the following abnormal conditions in red blood cell morphology:*

1. anisocytosis ______________________________
2. hypochromia ______________________________
3. spherocytosis ______________________________
4. poikilocytosis ______________________________
5. macrocytosis ______________________________

E. *Give meanings for the following terms:*

1. neutropenia ______________________________
2. erythropoiesis ______________________________
3. eosinophilia ______________________________
4. reticulocyte ______________________________
5. hemolysis ______________________________
6. thrombocytopenia ______________________________
7. leukapheresis ______________________________
8. polymorphonuclear ______________________________

9. blood dyscrasia ________________

10. hematocrit ________________

F. *Give the combining form or suffix for the following:*

Combining Forms	*Suffixes*
1. iron ________	6. blood condition ________
2. bone marrow ________	7. embryonic, immature ________
3. nucleus (2) ________ ________	8. formation (2) ________ ________
4. irregular ________	9. stop, control ________
5. eat, swallow ________	10. removal ________

G. *Match the abnormal condition in Column I with an associated symptom in Column II:*

Column I

1. purpura ______
2. pernicious anemia ______
3. hemophilia ______
4. polycythemia vera ______
5. thalassemia ______
6. sickle-cell anemia ______
7. aplastic anemia ______
8. iron-deficiency anemia ______
9. hemolytic anemia ______
10. hemochromatosis ______

Column II

A. pancytopenia
B. erythrocytes are spheroidal and easily destroyed; reticulocytosis occurs
C. malignant condition associated with erythremia
D. iron deposits in body tissues such as the heart and liver
E. hereditary abnormality in type of hemoglobin; RBCs clump together leading to infarction
F. thrombocytopenia and multiple pinpoint hemorrhages are major symptoms
G. sideropenia
H. hypochromia occurs with hereditary hemoglobin abnormality; Cooley's anemia
I. congenital deficiency in a clotting factor leads to prolonged coagulation time
J. Vitamin B_{12} cannot be absorbed and RBCs do not develop properly

H. Give meanings for the following terms or abbreviations:

1. ALL ______
2. CML ______
3. relapse ______
4. multiple myeloma ______
5. AML ______
6. CLL ______
7. remission ______
8. granulocytosis ______
9. eosinophilia ______
10. palliative ______

I. Match the following terms with their meanings below:

macrophage	lacteal	cell-mediated immunity
spleen	chyle	interferon
thymus gland	B-cells	thoracic duct
humoral immunity	T-cells	plasma cell
lymphokines	immunoglobulins	

1. Lymphocytes formed in the bone marrow; transform into plasma cells

   ______

2. Substances produced by T-cell lymphocytes that play a role in cell-mediated immunity ______
3. Large lymphatic vessel in the chest ______
4. Immune response in which B-cells transform into plasma cells and secrete antibodies ______
5. Organ in the mediastinum that produces T-cell lymphocytes ______

6. A specialized cell that secretes antibody ____________

7. Immune response involving T-cell lymphocytes ____________

8. Anitbodies such as IgA, IgG, IgD, IgE, and IgM ____________

9. An antiviral protein secreted by T-cell lymphocytes and other cells ____________

10. Lymph vessel found in the villi of the intestine ____________

11. Organ near the stomach that helps in blood cell storage, elimination, and production ____________

12. Lymph fluid filled with absorbed fats ____________

13. Lymphocytes formed in the thymus; involved in cell-mediated immunity ____________

14. A large phagocyte found in lymph nodes and other tissues of the body; histiocyte ____________

J. Build medical terms:

1. Formation of lymph ____________

2. Removal of the thymus gland ____________

3. Enlargement of the spleen ____________

4. Record (x-ray) of lymph vessels ____________

5. Tumor (malignant) of lymph nodes ____________

6. Disease of lymph glands ____________

7. Increased numbers of lymphocytes in the bloodstream ____________

8. Study of shape or form ____________

9. Deficiency of iron ____________

10. Swelling of lymph vessels (and surrounding tissue) ____________

K. *Select from the following pathological conditions, laboratory tests, and clinical procedures to match their descriptions below:*

elephantiasis	Burkitt's lymphoma	WBC differential count
mononucleosis	Hodgkin's disease	bleeding time
mycosis fungoides	hematocrit	coagulation time
AIDS	bone marrow biopsy	
sarcoidosis	bone marrow transplant	

1. Test that measures the percentage of RBCs in a volume of blood ________________

2. Test that measures the time required for venous blood to clot in a test tube

____

3. Bone marrow is aspirated and examined under the microscope ________________

____

4. Rare, chronic lymphoma that primarily affects the skin ________________

5. Acute infectious disease of enlarged lymph nodes and spleen ________________

____

6. Malignant tumor of lymph nodes and spleen; Reed-Sternberg cell is a characteristic finding ________________

7. Test to determine the numbers of different types of leukocytes ________________

____

8. Blockage of lymph vessels with swelling of tissues ________________

9. Inflammatory disease in which small nodules form in lymph nodes, skin, spleen, and lungs ________________

10. Healthy bone marrow cells are introduced into a patient suffering from leukemia or aplastic anemia ________________

11. Test that measures the time it takes for a small puncture wound to stop bleeding

____

12. Malignant tumor of lymph nodes; usually affecting children in Africa ____________

____

13. Disease marked by failure of the immune response; predominantly in homosexual men, intravenous drug abusers, and Haitians ____________________

L. Give the meanings of the following abbreviations:

1. ESR ________________________________
2. Hgb ________________________________
3. CBC ________________________________
4. PMN ________________________________
5. Hct ________________________________

ANSWERS

A.

1. thrombocyte
2. serum
3. eosinophil
4. bilirubin
5. fibrinogen
6. albumin
7. neutrophil
8. hemoglobin
9. heparin
10. lymphocyte
11. globulin
12. monocyte
13. megakaryocyte
14. erythrocyte
15. hemocytoblast

B.

1. clumping of recipient's blood cells when incompatible bloods are mixed
2. foreign material that causes the production of antibodies
3. protein substance produced in the body in reaction to the presence of an antigen
4. method of separating proteins by use of electrical charge
5. type of gamma globulin; IgG, IgM, IgD, IgE, and IgA are examples
6. a large phagocyte which engulfs foreign material (antigens) and destroys worn-out red blood cells
7. process of removing formed elements from the blood plasma
8. blood clotting
9. an enzyme that helps convert fibrinogen to fibrin
10. an anticoagulant drug used to prevent disorders of clot formation

C.

1. albumin, globulin, fibrinogen, and prothrombin
2. an antigen found on the red blood cells of Rh-positive individuals
3. B antigens; anti-A antibodies
4. no A or B antigens; anti-A and anti-B antibodies
5. A and B antigens; no anti-A or anti-B antibodies

D.

1. Cells are unequal sizes.
2. Cells are deficient in hemoglobin; abnormally pale.
3. Cells are spheroidal instead of normal biconcave disk shape.
4. Cells are irregularly shaped.
5. Cells are abnormally large.

E.

1. deficiency in neutrophils
2. formation of red blood cells
3. increase in numbers of eosinophils
4. a young red blood cell showing a network of granules in its cytoplasm
5. destruction of red blood cells
6. deficiency of clotting cells (platelets or thrombocytes)
7. removal of white blood cells from blood and return of other blood components to the donor
8. pertaining to a cell that has a nucleus with many lobes (shapes); a granulocytic leukocyte
9. a blood disorder
10. the percentage of red blood cells in a volume of blood

F.

1. sider/o
2. myel/o
3. kary/o; nucle/o
4. poikil/o
5. phag/o
6. -emia
7. -blast
8. -poiesis; -plasia
9. -stasis
10. -apheresis

G.

1. F
2. J
3. I
4. C
5. H
6. E
7. A
8. G
9. B
10. D

H.

1. acute lymphocytic leukemia
2. chronic myelogenous leukemia
3. return of symptoms of disease
4. malignant tumor of bone marrow
5. acute myelogenous leukemia
6. chronic lymphocytic leukemia
7. disappearance of symptoms of disease
8. abnormal condition of increase in numbers of granulocytes
9. increase in numbers of eosinophils
10. relieving, not curing

I.

1. B-cells
2. lymphokines
3. thoracic duct
4. humoral immunity
5. thymus gland
6. plasma cell
7. cell-mediated immunity
8. immunoglobulins
9. interferon
10. lacteal
11. spleen
12. chyle
13. T-cell
14. macrophage

J.

1. lymphopoiesis
2. thymectomy
3. splenomegaly
4. lymphangiogram
5. lymphosarcoma (lymphoma)
6. lymphadenopathy
7. lymphocytosis
8. morphology
9. sideropenia
10. lymphedema

K.

1. hematocrit
2. coagulation time
3. bone marrow biopsy
4. mycosis fungoides
5. mononucleosis
6. Hodgkin's disease
7. WBC differential count
8. elephantiasis
9. sarcoidosis
10. bone marrow transplant
11. bleeding time
12. Burkitt's lymphoma
13. AIDS

L.

1. erythrocyte sedimentation rate
2. hemoglobin
3. complete blood count
4. polymorphonuclear leukocyte
5. hematocrit

VII. PRONUNCIATION OF TERMS

agglutination	ă-gloo-tĭ-NĀ-shŭn
albumin	ăl-BŪ-mĭn
anisocytosis	ăn-ī-sō-sī-TŌ-sĭs
antibody	ĂN-tĭ-bŏd-ē
antigen	ĂN-tĭ-jĕn
basophil	BĀ-sō-fĭl
bilirubin	bĭl-ĭ-ROO-bĭn
chyle	kīl
coagulation	kō-ăg-ū-LĀ-shŭn
corpuscle	KŎR-pŭs'l
differentiation	dĭf-ĕr-ĕn-shē-Ā-shŭn
dyscrasia	dĭs-KRĀ-zē-ă
electrophoresis	ē-lĕk-trō-fō-RĒ-sĭs
elephantiasis	ĕl-ĕ-făn-TĪ-ă-sĭs
eosinophil	ē-ō-SĬN-ō-fĭl
erythrocyte	ĕ-RĬTH-rō-sīt
erythropenia	ĕ-rĭth-rō-PĒ-nē-ă
erythropoiesis	ĕ-rĭth-rō-poy-Ē-sĭs
fibrin	FĪ-brĭn
fibrinogen	fī-BRĬN-ō-jĕn
globulin	GLŎB-ū-lĭn
granulocyte	GRĂN-ū-lō-sīt
granulocytosis	grăn-ū-lō-sī-TŌ-sĭs
hematocrit	hē-MĂT-ō-krĭt
hemochromatosis	hē-mō-krō-mă-TŌ-sĭs
hemocytoblast	hē-mō-SĪ-tō-blăst
hemoglobin	HĒ-mō-glō-bĭn
hemolysis	hē-MŎL-ĭ-sĭs
hemophilia	hē-mō-FĬL-ē-ă
hemostasis	hē-mō-STĀ-sĭs
heparin	HĔP-ă-rĭn

histiocyte	HĬS-tē-ō-sīt
hypersplenism	hī-pĕr-SPLĔN-ĭzm
hypochromia	hī-pō-KRŌ-mē-ă
immunogenic	ĭm-ū-nō-JĔN-ĭk
immunoglobulin	ĭm-ū-nō-GLŎB-ū-lĭn
immunology	ĭm-ū-NŎL-ō-jē
lacteal	LĂK-tē-ăl
leukopenia	lo͞o-kō-PĒ-nē-ă
lymphadenitis	lĭm-făd-ĕ-NĪ-tĭs
lymphadenopathy	lĭm-făd-ĕ-NŎP-ă-thē
lymphangiogram	lĭm-FAN-jē-ŏ-grăm
lymphedema	lĭm-fĕ-DĒ-mă
lymphocytosis	lĭm-fō-sī-TŌ-sĭs
lymphopoiesis	lĭm-fō-poy-Ē-sĭs
lymphosarcoma	lĭm-fō-săr-KŌ-mă
macrocytosis	măk-rō-sī-TŌ-sĭs
macrophage	MĂK-rō-fāj
megakaryocyte	mĕg-ă-KĂR-ē-ō-sīt
microcytosis	mī-krō-sī-TŌ-sĭs
monoblast	MŎN-ō-blăst
monocyte	MŎN-ō-sīt
mononucleosis	mŏn-ō-nū-klē-Ō-sĭs
morphology	mŏr-FŎL-ō-jē
mycosis fungoides	mī-KŌ-sĭs fŭng-GOY-dēz
myeloblast	MĪ-ĕ-lō-blăst
myelogenous	mī-ĕ-LŎJ-ĕ-nŭs
myeloma	mī-ĕ-LŌ-mă
myelopoietic	mī-ĕ-lō-poy-ĔT-ĭk
neutropenia	nū-trō-PĒ-nē-ă
neutrophil	NŪ-trō-fĭl
pernicious anemia	pĕr-NĬSH-ŭs ă-NĒ-mē-ă
phagocytosis	făg-ō-sī-TŌ-sĭs

plasmapheresis	plăz-mă-fĕ-RĒ-sĭs
plateletpheresis	plāt-lĕt-fĕ-RĒ-sĭs
poikilocytosis	poy-kĭ-lō-sī-TŌ-sĭs
polycythemia vera	pŏl-ē-sī-THĒ-mē-ă VĔR-ă
polymorphonuclear	pŏl-ē-mŏr-fō-NŪ-klē-ăr
prothrombin	prō-THRŎM-bĭn
purpura	PŬR-pū-ră
reticulocyte	rĕ-TĬK-ū-lō-sīt
sarcoidosis	săr-koy-DŌ-sĭs
serum	SĒ-rŭm
sideropenia	sĭd-ĕr-ō-PĒ-nē-ă
spherocytosis	sphĕr-ō-sī-TŌ-sĭs
splenectomy	splē-NĔK-tō-mē
splenomegaly	splē-nō-MĔG-ă-lē
thalassemia	thăl-ă-SĒ-mē-ă
thrombocytopenia	thrŏm-bō-sī-tō-PĒ-nē-ă
thymectomy	thī-MĔK-tō-mē
thymoma	thī-MŌ-mă
thymus	THĪ-mŭs

REVIEW SHEET 13

Combining Forms

agglutin/o	______	micr/o	______
bas/o	______	mon/o	______
chrom/o	______	morph/o	______
eosin/o	______	myel/o	______
erythr/o	______	neutr/o	______
granul/o	______	nucle/o	______
hem/o	______	phag/o	______
hemat/o	______	poikil/o	______
immun/o	______	reticul/o	______
is/o	______	sider/o	______
kary/o	______	spher/o	______
leuk/o	______	splen/o	______
lymphaden/o	______	thromb/o	______
lymphangi/o	______	thym/o	______
macr/o	______		

Suffixes

-blast	______	-emia	______
-cytosis	______	-genic	______
-globulin	______	-phoresis	______
-penia	______	-poiesis	______
-philia	______	-stasis	______

Additional Terms

agglutination (341)

AIDS (356)

albumin (341)

anemia (345)

antibodies (341)

antigens (341)

aplastic anemia (346)

basophil (341)

B-cell lymphocyte (353)

bilirubin (341)

bleeding time (357)

blood dyscrasia (345)

bone marrow biopsy (357)

bone marrow transplant (357)

Burkitt's lymphoma (355)

cell-mediated immunity (353)

chyle (353)

coagulation time (357)

corpuscle (341)

dicumarol (340)

electrophoresis (341)

elephantiasis (356)

eosinophil (341)

fibrin (341)

fibrinogen (341)

globin (341)

globulin (341)

granulocytes (341)

granulocytosis (348)

hematocrit (356)

heme (337)

hemochromatosis (347)

hemoglobin (337)

hemolytic anemia (346)

hemophilia (347)

heparin (340)

histiocyte (354)

Hodgkin's disease (355)

humoral immunity (354)

hypersplenism (356)

immunoglobulin (354)

infectious mononucleosis (355)

interferon (354)

interstitial fluid (335)

lacteals (349)

leukemia (348)

lymphokines (354)

lymphosarcoma (355)

macrophage (354)

megakaryocyte (338)

monocyte (338)

multiple myeloma (349)

mycosis fungoides (355)

neutrophil (338)

palliative (349)

pernicious anemia (345)

plasma (338)

plasma cell (354)

plasmapheresis (338)

plateletpheresis (345)

polycythemia vera (347)

prothrombin (340)

purpura (348)

relapse (348)

remission (348)

reticulocyte (344)

Rh factor (339)

right lymphatic duct (354)

sarcoidosis (355)

serum (340)

sickle-cell anemia (347)

spleen (354)

stem cell (336)

T-cell lymphocyte (354)

thalassemia (347)

thoracic duct (354)

thrombin (341)

thymus gland (354)

CHAPTER 14

MUSCULOSKELETAL SYSTEM

In this chapter you will:

- Define terms relating to the structure and function of bones, joints, and muscles;
- Describe the process of bone formation and growth;
- Locate and name the major bones of the body;
- Analyze the combining forms, prefixes, and suffixes used to describe bones, joints, and muscles;
- Explain various musculoskeletal disease conditions and terms related to bone fractures; and
- Identify important laboratory tests, clinical procedures, and abbreviations relating to the musculoskeletal system.

This chapter is divided into the following sections:

I. Introduction
II. Bones
  A. Formation and Structure
  B. Processes and Depressions in Bones
  C. Cranial Bones
  D. Facial Bones
  E. Vertebral Column and Structure of Vertebrae
  F. Bones of the Thorax, Pelvis, and Extremities
  G. Vocabulary
  H. Combining Forms and Suffixes
  I. Pathological Conditions and Fractures
III. Joints
  A. Classification of Joints
  B. Bursae
  C. Vocabulary
  D. Combining Forms
  E. Pathological Conditions
IV. Muscles
  A. Types of Muscles
  B. Actions of Skeletal Muscles
  C. Vocabulary
  D. Combining Forms
  E. Pathological Conditions
V. Laboratory Tests, Clinical Procedures, and Abbreviations
VI. Practical Applications
VII. Exercises
VIII. Pronunciation of Terms

I. INTRODUCTION

The musculoskeletal system includes the bones, muscles, and joints. Each has several important functions in the body. **Bones**, by providing the framework around which the body is constructed, protect and support our internal organs. Also, by serving as a point of attachment for muscles, bones assist in body movement. The inner core of bones is composed of hematopoietic tissue (red bone marrow manufactures blood cells), while other parts are storage areas for minerals necessary for growth, such as **calcium** and **phosphorus.**

Joints are the places where bones come together. Several different types of joints are found within the body. The type of joint found in any specific location is determined by the need for greater or lesser flexibility of movement.

Muscles, whether attached to bones or to internal organs and blood vessels, are responsible for movement. Internal movement involves the contraction and relaxation of muscles that are a part of viscera, and external movement is accomplished by the contraction and relaxation of muscles that are attached to the bones.

II. BONES

A. Formation and Structure

Formation

Bones are complete organs, chiefly composed of connective tissue called **osseous** (bony) **tissue** plus a rich supply of blood vessels and nerves. Osseous tissue is a dense connective tissue that consists of **osteocytes** (bone cells) surrounded by a hard, intercellular substance filled with calcium salts.

During fetal development, the bones of the fetus are composed of **cartilage tissue**, which resembles osseous tissue but is more flexible and less dense because of a lack of calcium salts in its intercellular spaces. As the embryo develops, the process of depositing calcium salts in the soft, cartilaginous bones occurs, and continues throughout the life of the individual after birth. The gradual replacement of cartilage and its intercellular substance by immature bone cells and calcium deposits is called **ossification** (bone formation).

Osteoblasts are the immature osteocytes that produce the bony tissue that replaces cartilage during ossification. **Osteoclasts** (-clast means to break) are large cells that function to reabsorb, or digest, bony tissue. Osteoclasts (also called bone phagocytes) digest dead bone tissue from the inner sides of bones and thus enlarge the inner bone cavity so that the bone does not become overly thick and heavy. When a bone breaks, osteoblasts lay down the mineral bone matter (calcium salts) and osteoclasts remove excess bone debris (smooth out the bone).

The formation of bone is dependent to a great extent on a proper supply of **calcium** and **phosphorus** to the bone tissue. These minerals must be taken into the body along with a sufficient amount of vitamin D. Vitamin D helps the passage of calcium through the lining of the small intestine and into the bloodstream. Once calcium and phosphorus are in the bones, osteoblastic activity produces an enzyme that causes the formation of a calcium-phosphate compound giving bone its characteristic hard quality.

Not only are calcium and phosphorus part of the hard structure of bone tissue, but calcium is also stored in bones and small quantities are present in the blood. If the proper amount of calcium is lacking in the blood, nerve fibers are unable to transmit impulses effectively to muscles; heart muscle becomes weak and muscles attached to bones undergo spasms.

The necessary level of calcium in the blood is maintained by the parathyroid gland, which secretes a hormone to release calcium from bone storage. Excess of the hormone (caused by tumor or other pathological process) will raise blood calcium at the expense of the bones, which become weakened by the loss of calcium.

Structure

Bones all over the body are of several different types. **Long bones** are found in the thigh, lower leg, and upper and lower arm. These bones are very strong, are broad at the ends where they join with other bones, and have large surface areas for muscle attachment.

Short bones are found in the wrist and ankle and have small, irregular shapes. **Flat bones** are found covering soft body parts. These are the shoulder bone, ribs, and pelvic bones. **Sesamoid bones** are small, rounded bones resembling a grain of sesame in shape. They are found near joints; the knee cap is the largest example of this type of bone.

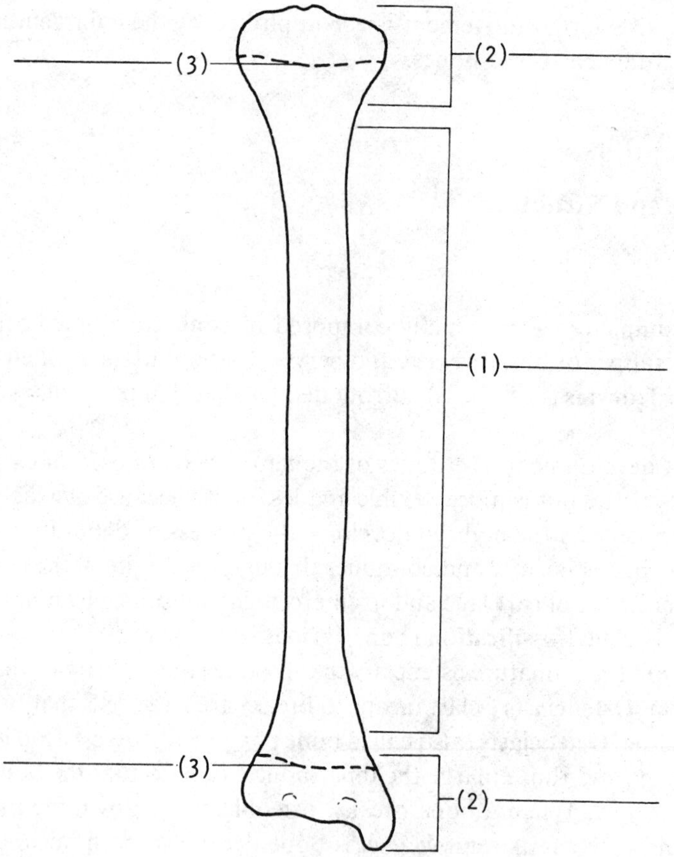

Figure 14-1 Divisions of a long bone.

Figure 14-1 shows the anatomical divisions of a long bone such as the thigh bone or upper arm bone. Label the figure as you read the following.

The shaft, or middle region, of a long bone is called the **diaphysis** (1). Each end of a long bone is called an **epiphysis** (2). The **epiphyseal line** or **plate** (3) represents an area of cartilage tissue which is constantly being replaced by new bony tissue as the bone grows. Cartilage cells at the edges of the epiphyseal plate form new bone and this is responsible for the lengthening of bones during childhood and adolescence. The plate calcifies and disappears when the bone has achieved its full growth.

Figure 14-2 shows some of the structures that are part of the composition of the epiphysis and diaphysis. The **periosteum** (1) is a strong, fibrous, vascular membrane that covers the surface of a long bone, except at the ends of the epiphyses. Bones other than long bones are completely covered by the periosteum. Beneath the periosteum is the layer of osteoblasts which deposit calcium-phosphorus compounds in the bony tissue.

The ends of long bones are covered by a thin layer of cartilage called **articular cartilage** (2). This cartilage layer cushions the bones at the place where they meet with other bones (joints).

Compact (cortical) bone (3) is a layer of hard, dense tissue that lies under the periosteum in all bones and chiefly around the diaphysis of long bones. Within the compact bone is a system of small canals containing blood vessels that bring oxygen and nutrients to the bone and remove waste produces such as carbon dioxide. The inset in Figure 14-2 shows these channels, called **haversian canals** (4), in the compact bone. Compact bone is tunneled out in the shaft of the long

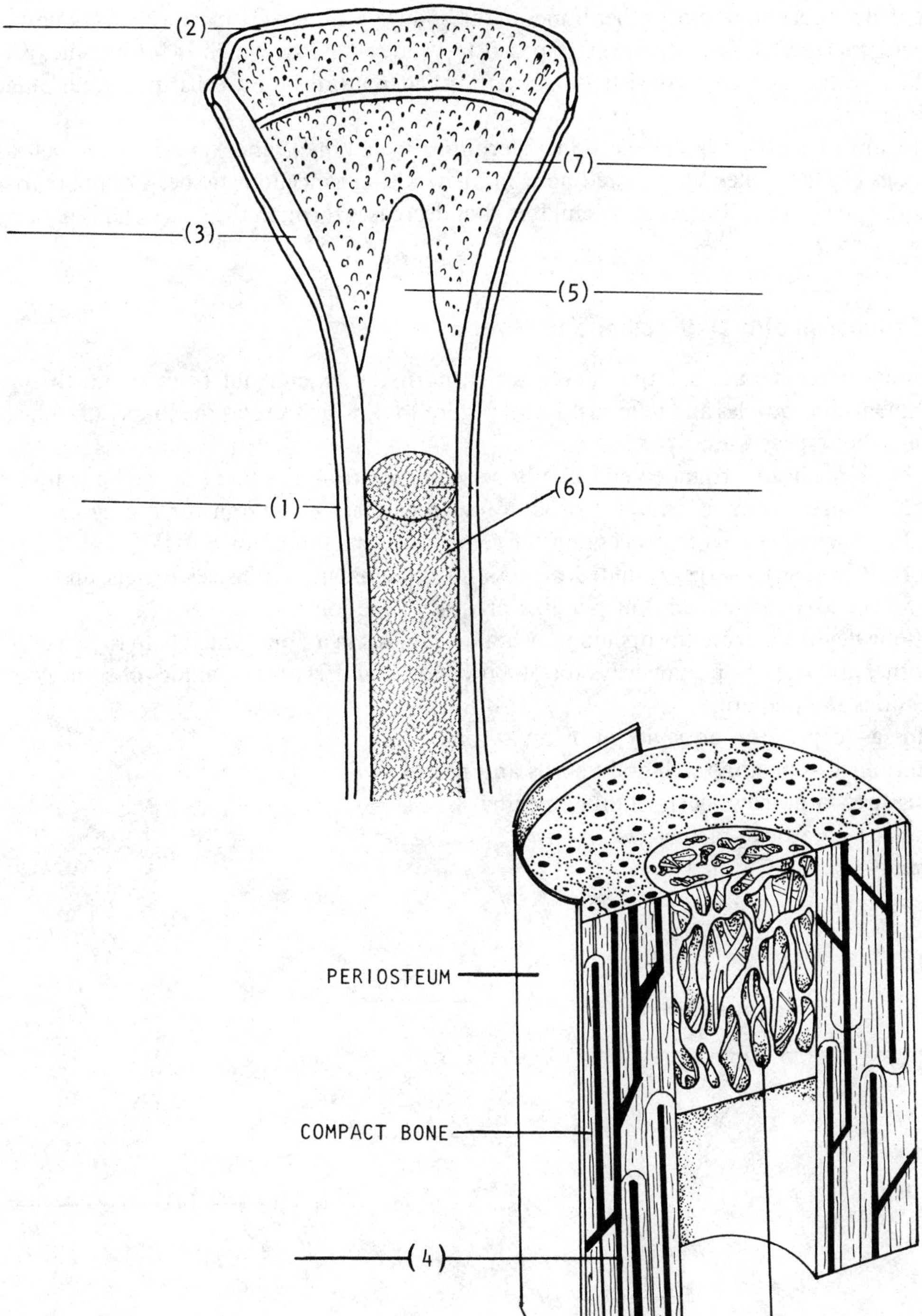

Figure 14-2 Interior bone structure.

bones by a central **medullary cavity** (5) which contains **yellow bone marrow** (6). Yellow bone marrow is chiefly composed of fat cells.

Cancellous bone (7), sometimes called spongy bone, is much more porous and less dense than compact bone. The mineral matter in it is laid down in a series of separated bony fibers called a spongy latticework or **trabeculae**. It is found largely in the epiphyses of long bones and in the middle portion of most other bones of the body as well. Spaces in cancellous bone contain **red bone marrow**. This marrow, as opposed to yellow marrow which is fatty tissue, is richly supplied with blood and consists of immature and mature blood cells in various stages of development.

In an adult, the ribs, pelvic bone, sternum (breastbone), and vertebrae, as well as the epiphyses of long bones, contain red bone marrow within cancellous tissue. The red marrow in the long bones is plentiful in young children, but decreases through the years and is replaced by yellow marrow.

B. Processes and Depressions in Bones

Bone processes are enlarged tissue which normally extend out from bones to serve as attachments for muscles and tendons. Label Figure 14-3, which shows the shapes of some of the common bony processes:

(1) **bone head**—rounded end of a bone separated from the body of the bone by a neck.
(2) **tubercle**—small, rounded process for attachment of tendons or muscles.
(3) **trochanter**—large process on the femur for attachment of muscle.
(4) **tuberosity**—large, rounded process for attachment of muscles or tendons.
(5) **condyle**—rounded, knuckle-like process at the joint.

Bone depressions are the openings or hollow regions in a bone which help to join one bone to another and serve as passageways for blood vessels and nerves. The names of some common depressions in bone are:

fossa—depression or cavity in or on a bone.
foramen—opening for blood vessels and nerves.
fissure—a narrow, deep, slitlike opening.
sulcus—a groove or furrow.
sinus—cavity within a bone.

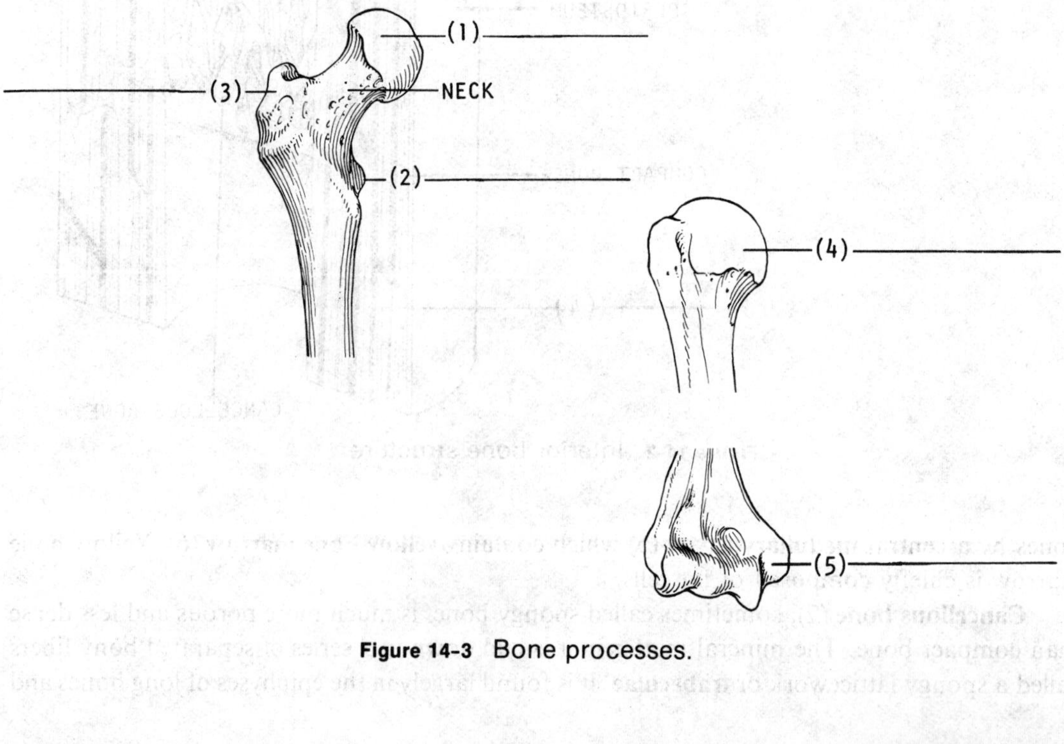

Figure 14-3 Bone processes.

C. Cranial Bones

The bones of the skull, or cranium, protect the brain and structures related to it, such as the sense organs. Muscles for controlling head movements and chewing motions are connected to the cranial bones.

The cranial bones of a newborn child are not completely joined. There are gaps of unossified tissue in the skull at birth. These are called soft spots, or **fontanelles** (little fountains). The pulse of blood vessels can be felt under the skin in those areas.

Figure 14-4 illustrates the bones of the cranium. Label them as you read the following descriptions:

(1) **frontal bone**—forms the forehead and bony sockets that contain the eyes.

(2) **parietal bone**—there are two parietal bones which form the roof and upper part of the sides of the cranium.

(3) **temporal bone**—two temporal bones form the lower sides and base of the cranium. Each bone encloses an ear and contains a fossa for joining with the mandible (lower jaw bone). The **mastoid process** is a round process of the temporal bone behind the ear.

(4) **occipital bone**—forms the back and base of the skull and joins the parietal and temporal bones, forming a **suture** (juncture line of cranial bones). The inferior portion of the occipital bone has an opening called the **foramen magnum** through which the spinal cord passes. See Figure 14-5.

(5) **sphenoid bone**—this bat-shaped bone extends behind the eyes and forms part of the base of the skull. Because it joins with the frontal, occipital, and ethmoid bones, it serves as an anchor to hold those skull bones together. (Sphen/o means wedge.)

(6) **ethmoid bone**—this thin, delicate bone is composed primarily of spongy, cancellous bone. It supports the nasal cavity and forms part of the orbits of the eyes. (Ethm/o means sieve.)

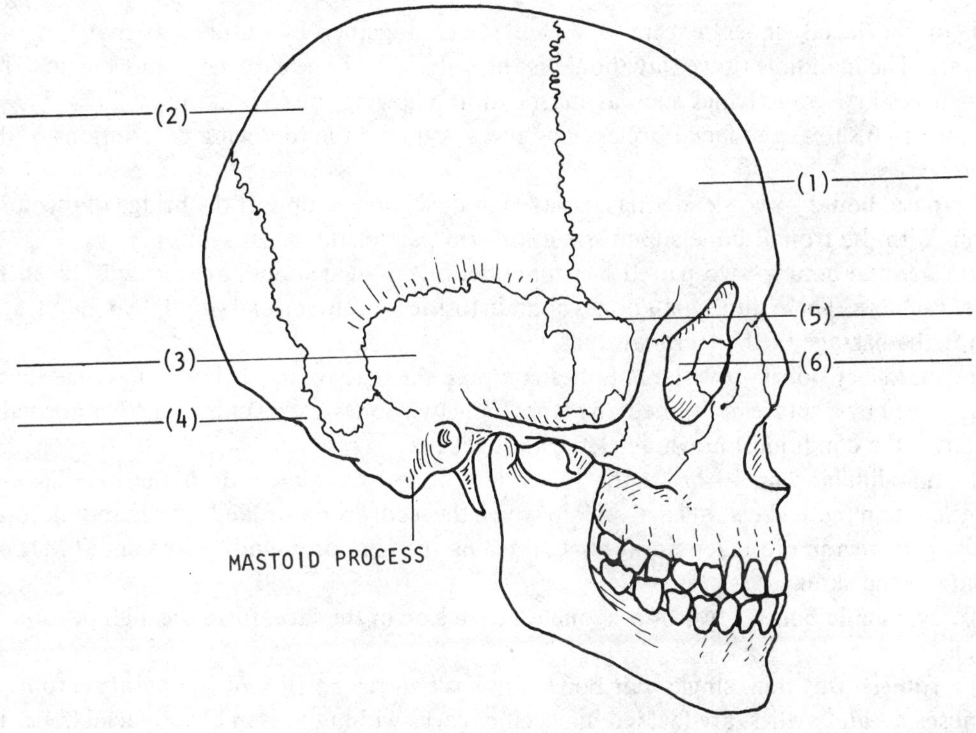

Figure 14-4 Cranial bones, lateral view.

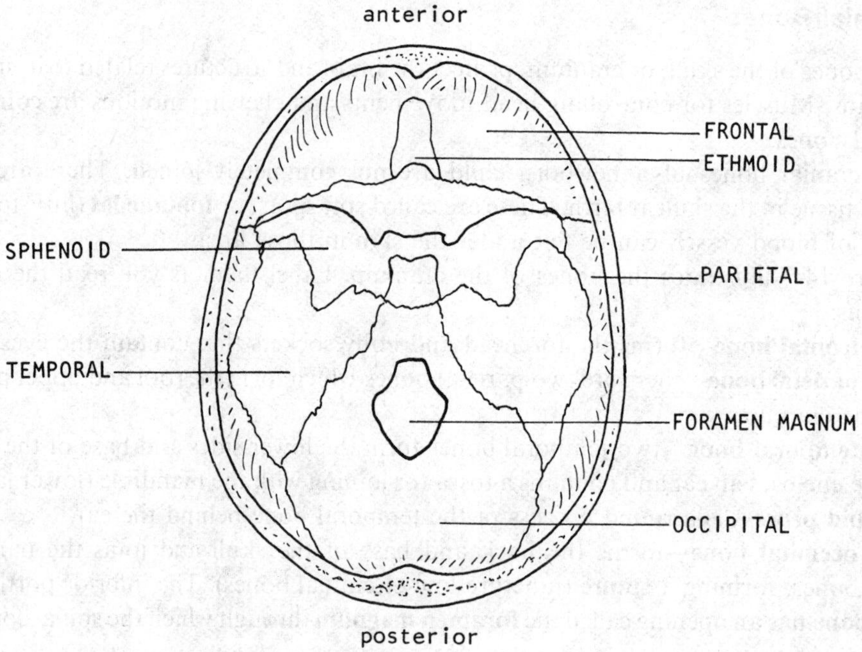

Figure 14-5 Bones of the skull viewed from the floor of the cranial cavity.

Study Figure 14-5, which shows the above-mentioned cranial bones as viewed through the floor of the cranial cavity.

D. Facial Bones

All of the facial bones, except one, are joined together by sutures so that they are immovable. The mandible (lower jaw bone) is the only facial bone capable of movement. This ability is necessary for activities such as mastication (chewing) and speaking.

Figure 14-6 shows the facial bones; label it as you read the following descriptions of the facial bones:

(1) **nasal bones**—two slender nasal (nas/o = nose) bones support the bridge of the nose. They join with the frontal bone superiorly and form part of the nasal septum.

(2) **lacrimal bones**—two paired lacrimal (lacrim/o = tear) bones are located one at the corner of each eye. These thin, small bones contain fossae for the lacrimal gland (tear gland) and canals for the passage of the lacrimal duct.

(3) **maxillary bones**—two large bones compose the massive upper jaw bones (maxillae). They are joined by a suture in the median plane. If the two bones do not come together normally before birth, the condition known as **cleft palate** results.

(4) **mandibular bone**—this is the lower jaw bone (**mandible**). Both the maxilla and mandible contain the sockets called alveoli in which the teeth are embedded. The mandible joins the skull at the region of the temporal bone, forming the **temporomandibular joint** (TMJ) on either side of the skull.

(5) **zygomatic bones**—two bones, one on each side of the face, form the high portion of the cheek.

(6) **vomer**—this thin, single, flat bone forms the lower portion of the nasal septum.

Sinuses, or air cavities, are located in specific places within the cranial and facial bones to lighten the skull and warm and moisten air as it passes through. Figure 14-7 shows the sinuses of the skull.

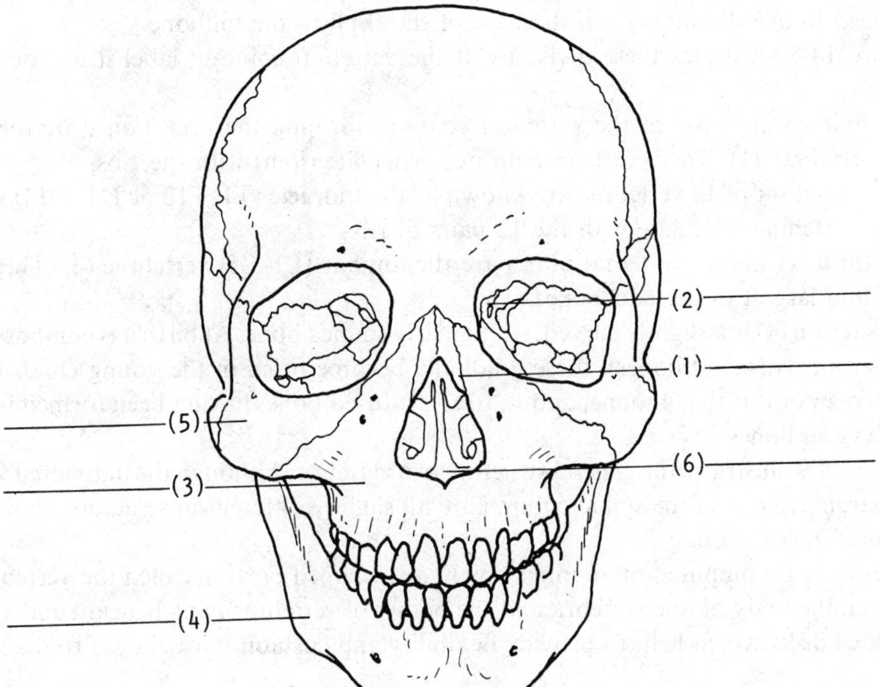

Figure 14-6 Facial bones.

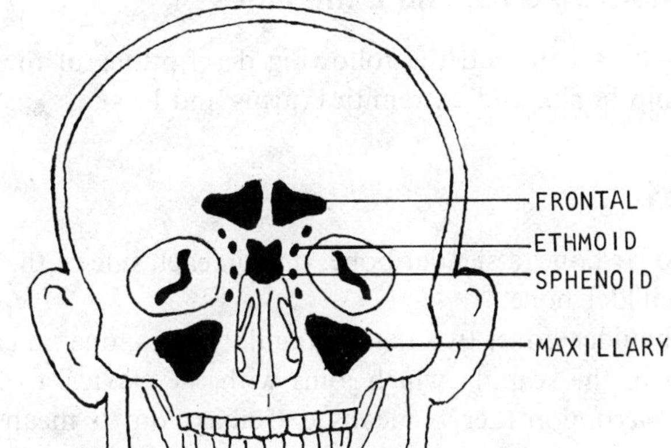

Figure 14-7 Sinuses of the skull.

E. Vertebral Column and Structure of Vertebrae

The **vertebral**, or spinal, **column** is composed of 26 bone segments, called vertebrae, which are arranged in five divisions from the base of the skull to the tailbone.

Figure 14-8 illustrates these divisions of the vertebral column; label it as you read the following:

The first seven bones of the vertebral column, forming the neck bone, are the **cervical** (C1–C7) **vertebrae** (1). These vertebrae do not articulate (join) with the ribs.

The second set of 12 vertebrae are known as the **thoracic** (T1–T12 or D1–D12) **vertebrae** (2). These vertebrae articulate with the 12 pairs of ribs.

The third set of five vertebral bones are the **lumbar** (L1–L5) **vertebrae** (3). They are the strongest and largest of the backbones.

The **sacrum** (4) is a slightly curved, triangularly shaped bone. At birth it is composed of five separate segments (sacral bones); these gradually become fused in the young child.

The **coccyx** (5) is the tailbone, and it, too, is a fused bone, having been formed from four small coccygeal bones.

Figure 14-9 illustrates the general structure of a vertebra. Although the individual vertebrae in the separate regions of the spinal column are all slightly different in structure, they do have several parts in common.

A vertebra is composed of an inner, thick, disk-shaped portion called the **vertebral body** (1). Between the body of one vertebra and the bodies of vertebrae lying beneath and above are **cartilaginous disks** which help to provide flexibility and cushion most shocks to the vertebral column.

The **vertebral arch** (2) is the posterior part of the vertebra, and consists of a **spinous process** (3), **transverse processes** (4), and **laminae** (5). The **neural canal** (6) is the space between the vertebral body and the vertebral arch through which the spinal cord passes.

F. Bones of the Thorax, Pelvis, and Extremities

Label Figure 14-10 as you read the following descriptions of the bones of the thorax (chest cavity), pelvis (hip bone), and extremities (arms and legs):

Bones of the Thorax

(1) **clavicle**—collar bone; a slender bone, one on each side of the body, connecting the breastbone to each shoulder bone.

(2) **scapula**—shoulder bone; two flat, triangular bones, one on each dorsal side of the thorax. The extension of the scapula which joins with the clavicle to form the joint of the shoulder is called the **acromion** (acr/o means extremity; om/o means shoulder). See Figure 14-11 for a posterior view of the scapula.

(3) **sternum**—breastbone; a flat bone extending down the midline of the chest. The uppermost part of the sternum articulates on the sides with the clavicle and ribs, while the lower, narrower portion is attached to the diaphragm and abdominal muscles. The lower portion of the sternum is called the **xiphoid process** (xiph/o means sword).

(4) **ribs**—there are 12 pairs of ribs. The first seven pairs join the sternum anteriorly through cartilaginous attachments called costal cartilages. Ribs 1–7 are called **true ribs**. They join with the sternum anteriorly and with the vertebral column in the back. Ribs 8–10 are called **false ribs**. They join with the vertebral column in the back but join the 7th rib anteriorly, instead of attaching to the sternum. Ribs 11 and 12 are the **floating ribs** because they are completely free at their anterior extremity. See Figure 14-11 for a posterior view of the rib cage.

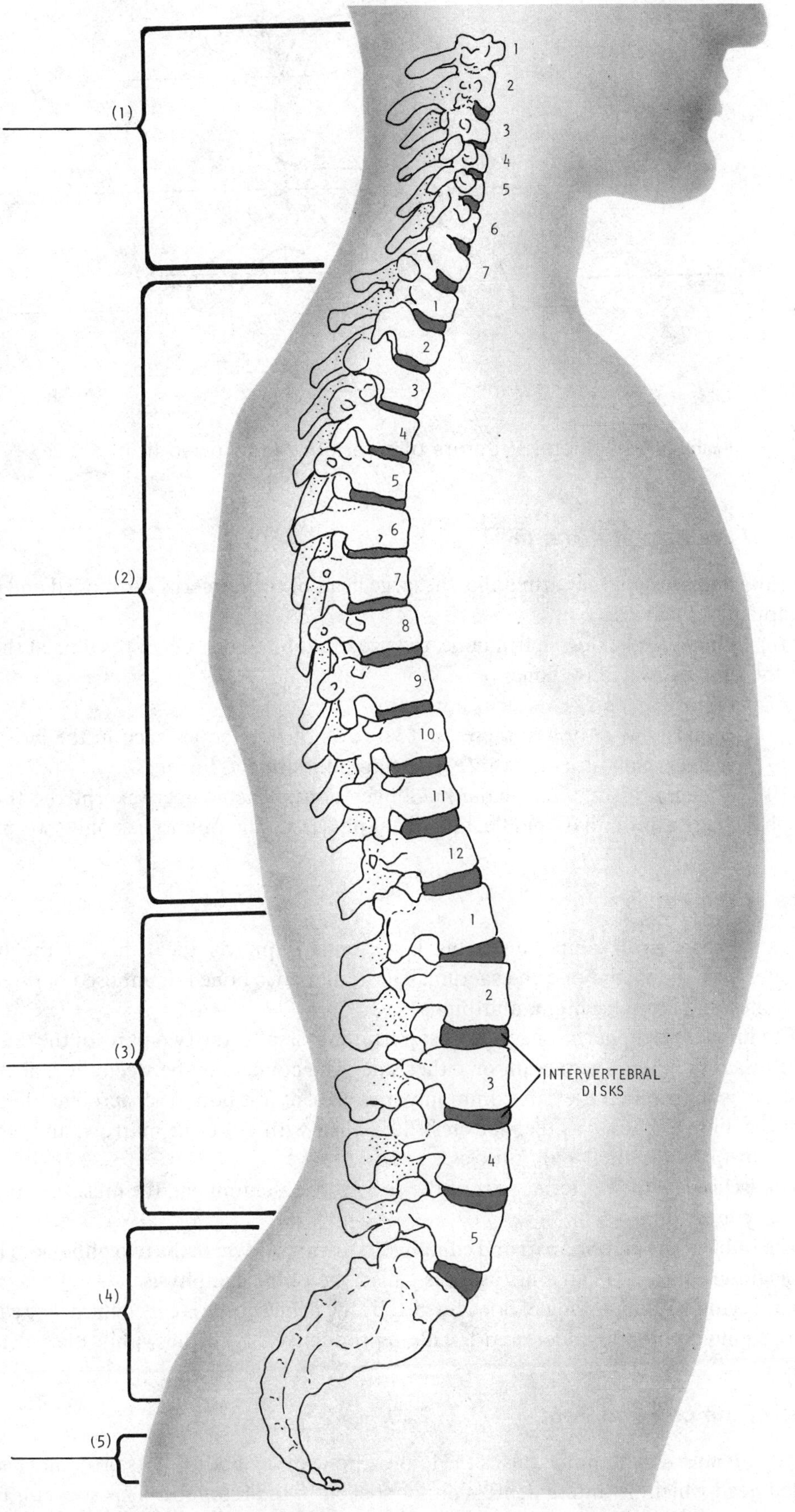

Figure 14-8 Vertebral column.

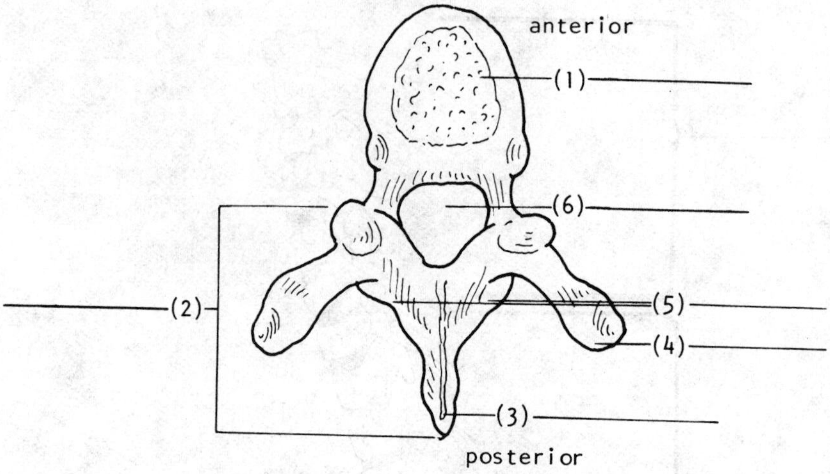

Figure 14-9 General structure of a vertebra (as viewed from above).

Bones of the Arm and Hand

(5) **humerus**—upper arm bone; the large head of the humerus is rounded and joins with the scapula and clavicle.

(6) **ulna**—medial lower arm bone; the proximal bony process of the ulna at the elbow is called the **olecranon** (elbow bone).

(7) **radius**—lateral lower arm bone.

(8) **carpals**—wrist bones; there are two rows of four bones each in the wrist.

(9) **metacarpals**—these are five radiating bones to the fingers.

(10) **phalanges** (singular: phalanx)—finger bones; each finger (except the thumb) has three phalanges: a proximal, middle, and distal phalanx. The thumb has only two phalanges.

Bones of the Pelvis

(11) **pelvic girdle**—hip bone; this large bone supports the trunk of the body and articulates with the thigh bone and sacrum. The adult pelvic bone is composed of three pairs of fused bones: the ilium, ischium, and pubis.

The **ilium** is the uppermost and largest portion. Dorsally, the two parts of the ilium do not meet. Rather, they join the sacrum on either side. The connection between the iliac bones and the sacrum is so firm that they are commonly spoken of as one bone: the sacroiliac. The superior part of the ilium is known as the iliac crest. It is filled with red bone marrow, and serves as an attachment for abdominal wall muscles.

The **ischium** is the posterior part of the pelvis. The ischium and the muscles attached to it are what you sit on.

The **pubis** is the anterior part and contains suture marks where the two pubes join by way of a cartilaginous disk. This area of fusion is called the **pubic symphysis**.

The region within the ring of bone formed by the pelvic girdle is called the pelvic cavity. The rectum, sigmoid colon, bladder, and female reproductive organs lie within the pelvic cavity.

Bones of the Leg and Foot

(12) **femur**—thigh bone; this is the longest bone in the body. At its proximal end it has a rounded head which fits into a depression, or socket, in the hip bone. This socket is called the

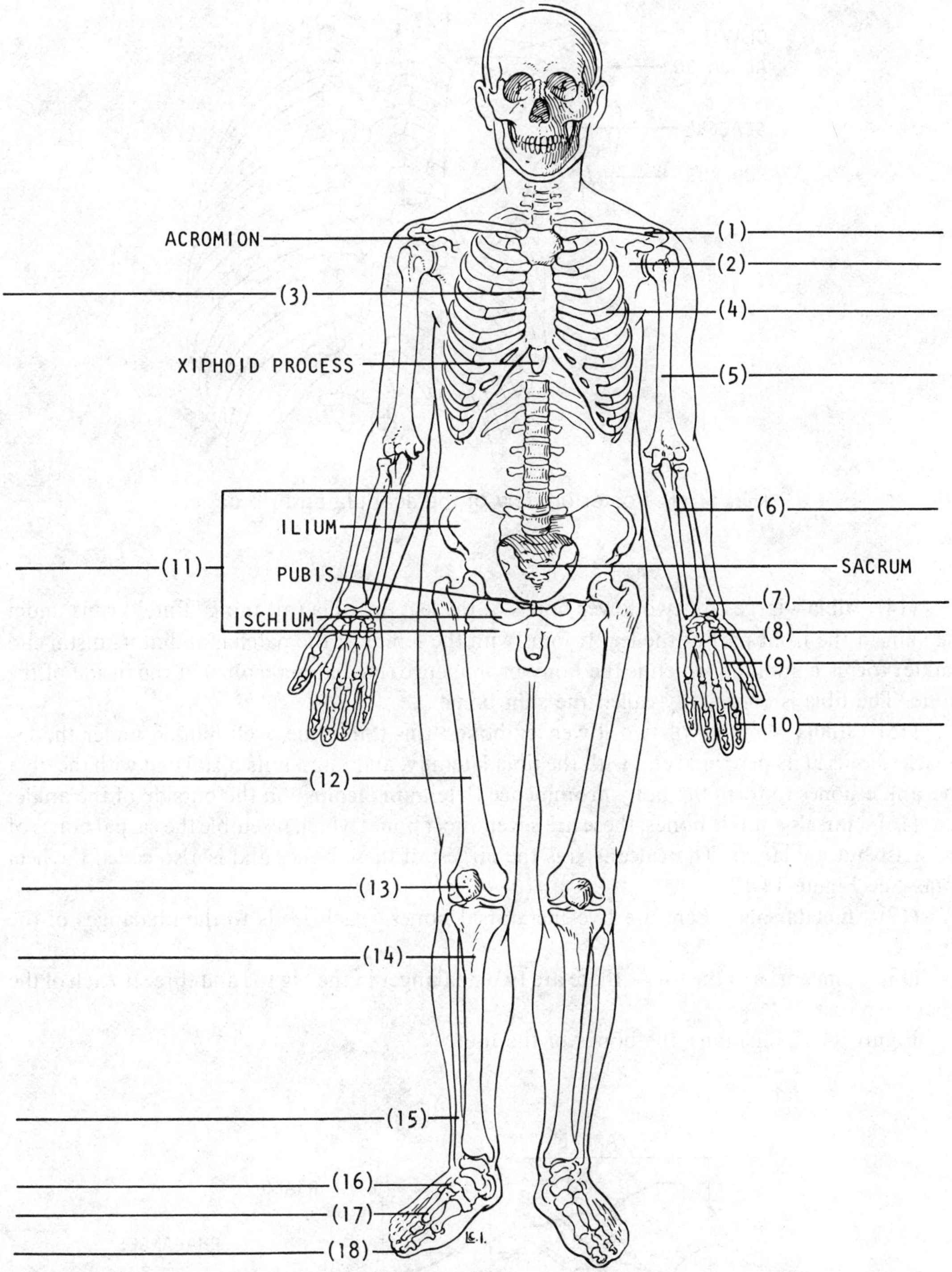

Figure 14-10 Bones of the thorax, pelvis, and extremities.

acetabulum. The acetabulum was named because of its resemblance to a rounded cup the Romans used for vinegar (acetum).

(13) **patella**—kneecap; this is a small, flat bone which lies in front of the articulation between the femur and one of the lower leg bones called the tibia. It is surrounded by protective tendons and held in place by muscle attachments.

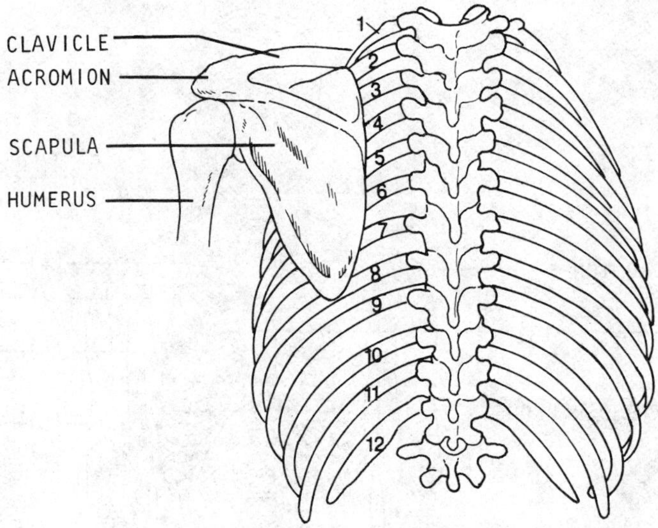

Figure 14-11 Posterior view of the scapula and rib cage.

(14) **tibia**—largest of two lower bones of the leg; the tibia (meaning "flute") runs under the skin in the front part of the leg. It joins with the femur at the patella, and at its distal end (ankle) forms a swelling which is the bony prominence (medial **malleolus**) at the inside of the ankle. The tibia is commonly called the **shin bone**.

(15) **fibula**—smaller of two lower leg bones; this thin bone, well hidden under the leg muscles, joins at its proximal end with the tibia laterally, and joins at its distal end with the tibia and ankle bones to form the bony prominence (lateral **malleolus**) on the outside of the ankle.

(16) **tarsals**—ankle bones; these are seven short bones which resemble the carpal bones of the wrist but are larger. The **calcaneus** is the largest of these bones and is also called the heel bone. See Figure 14-12.

(17) **metatarsals**—there are five metatarsal bones—each leads to the phalanges of the toes.

(18) **phalanges of the toes**—there are two phalanges in the big toe and three in each of the other four toes.

Figure 14-12 illustrates the bones of the foot.

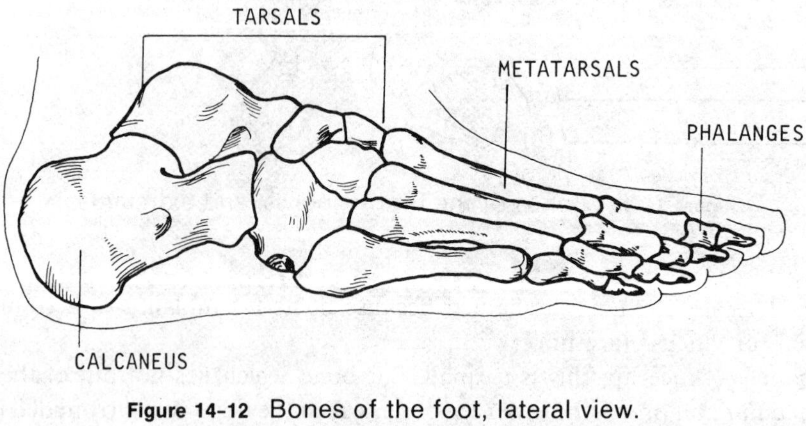

Figure 14-12 Bones of the foot, lateral view.

G. Vocabulary

acetabulum	Rounded depression, or socket, in the pelvic bone where the thigh bone joins with the pelvis.
acromion	Outward extension of the shoulder bone forming the point of the shoulder.
articular cartilage	Thin layer of cartilage at the ends of long bones.
calcium	One of the mineral constituents of bone.
cancellous bone	Spongy, porous bone tissue.
cartilage tissue	Flexible, rubbery connective tissue found on joint surfaces and in the embryonic skeleton.
compact bone	Hard, dense bone tissue.
condyle	Knuckle-like process at the end of a bone near the joint.
cranial bones	Skull bones: ethmoid, frontal, occipital, parietal, sphenoid, and temporal.
diaphysis	Shaft, or midportion, of a long bone.
disk (disc)	A flat, round, platelike structure. An intervertebral disk is a fibrocartilage substance between the vertebrae.
epiphyseal plate	Cartilaginous area at the ends of long bones where lengthwise growth takes place.
epiphysis	Each end of a long bone.
facial bones	Bones of the face: lacrimal, mandible, maxillae, nasal, vomer, and zygomatic.
false ribs	Ribs 8–10.
fissure	Narrow, slitlike opening between bones.
floating ribs	Ribs 11 and 12.
fontanelle	Soft spot (incomplete bone formation) between the skull bones of an infant.
foramen	Opening or passage in bones where blood vessels and nerves enter and leave. The foramen magnum is the opening of the occipital bone through which the spinal cord passes.
fossa	Depression or cavity in a bone.
haversian canals	Minute spaces filled with blood vessels, found in compact bone.

malleolus	Round process on both sides of the ankle joint.
mastoid process	Round projection on the temporal bone behind the ear.
medullary cavity	Central, hollowed-out area in the shaft of a long bone.
olecranon	Large process forming the elbow.
osseous tissue	Bone tissue.
ossification	Process of bone formation.
osteoblast	Bone cell that helps form bone tissue.
osteoclast	Bone cell that absorbs and removes unwanted bone tissue.
periosteum	Membrane surrounding bones.
phosphorus	Mineral substance found in bones in combination with calcium.
pubic symphysis	Area of fusion of the two pubic bones.
red bone marrow	Found in cancellous bone; site of hemopoiesis.
sinus	Cavity within a bone.
sulcus	Groovelike depression.
trabeculae	Supporting bundles of bony fibers in cancellous (spongy) bone.
trochanter	Large process below the neck of the femur.
tubercle	Small, rounded process on a bone.
tuberosity	Large, rounded process on a bone.
vertebra	Backbone, composed of: vertebral body, vertebral arch, spinous process, transverse processes, lamina, and neural canal.
xiphoid process	Lower, narrow portion of the sternum.
yellow bone marrow	Fatty tissue found in the diaphyses of long bones.

H. Combining Forms and Suffixes

These are divided into two groups: general terms and terms related to specific bones.

General Terms

Combining Form	*Definition*	*Terminology*	*Meaning*
oste/o	bone	osteitis	____________
		osteodystrophy	____________
		osteolysis	____________
		osteogenesis	____________
		Osteogenesis imperfecta is an inherited congenital anomaly marked by brittle bones and multiple fractures.	
orth/o	straight	orthopedic	____________
		Originally orthopedics was a science dealing with correcting deformities in children (ped/o means child).	
calc/o	calcium	decalcification	____________
		de- means lack of; fic/ means to make.	
		hypercalcemia	____________
vertebr/o *(used to describe the structure)*	vertebra	vertebral	____________
spondyl/o *(used to make words about conditions of the structure)*	vertebra	spondylitis	____________
		spondylolisthesis	____________
		-listhesis means a slipping or subluxation.	
rachi/o	spinal column, vertebrae	rachialgia	____________
lamin/o	lamina *(part of the vertebral arch)*	laminectomy	____________
		An operation often performed to relieve the symptoms of a ruptured intervertebral disk.	

kyph/o	humpback *(posterior curvature in the thoracic region)*	kyphosis ______
lord/o	curve, swayback *(anterior curvature in the lumbar region)*	lordosis ______ *This term is used to describe both the normal anterior curvature of the spinal column in the lumbar region and an excessive, abnormal anterior curvature, or swayback, condition.*
scoli/o	crooked, bent *(lateral curvature)*	scoliosis ______
myel/o	bone marrow	myelopoiesis ______
lumb/o	loins, lower back	lumbar ______ lumbodynia ______ *Also called lumbago.*
-blast	embryonic or immature cell	osteoblast ______
-clast -clasis	to break	osteoclast ______ osteoclasis ______ *Surgical fracture to remedy a deformity.*
-schisis	to split	rachischisis ______ *Pronounced (rā-KIS-kĭ-sĭs). Congenital condition; spina bifida.*
-physis	to grow	epiphysis ______ pubic symphysis ______
-malacia	softening	osteomalacia ______ *A condition in which vitamin D deficiency leads to decalcification of bones. Also called rickets.*
-porosis	passage	osteoporosis ______ *See pathological conditions.*

Specific Bones

crani/o	skull bones	craniotomy ____________
maxill/o	upper jaw bone	maxillary ____________
mandibul/o	lower jaw bone	mandibular ____________
clavicul/o	clavicle	clavicular ____________
scapul/o	scapula	scapular ____________
cost/o	ribs	costal ____________
		chondrocostal ____________
stern/o	sternum	sternal ____________
humer/o	humerus	humeral ____________
uln/o	ulna	ulnar ____________
olecran/o	elbow	olecranal ____________
radi/o	radius; ray	radial ____________
carp/o	wrist bones	carpal ____________
metacarp/o	metacarpals	metacarpectomy ____________
phalang/o	phalanges	phalangeal ____________
pelv/i	pelvic bone	pelvimetry ____________
ili/o	ilium	iliac ____________
ischi/o	ischium	ischial ____________
pub/o	pubis	pubic ____________
acetabul/o	acetabulum	acetabular ____________
femor/o	femur	femoral ____________
patell/o patell/a	patella	patellar ____________
		patellapexy ____________

tibi/o	tibia	tibial ________________
fibul/o	fibula	fibular ________________
perone/o	fibula	peroneal ________________
calcane/o	calcaneus	calcaneal ________________
malleol/o	malleolus	malleolar ________________

I. Pathological Conditions and Fractures

osteoporosis

Decrease in bone density; thinning and weakening of bone due to loss of calcium salts.

This condition commonly occurs in older women as one of the serious consequences of estrogen deficiency. Estrogen deficiency promotes excessive bone resorption (osteoclast activity) and less bone deposition. Weakened bones are subject to fractures (as in the hip); loss of height and kyphosis occur when vertebrae collapse. Estrogen replacement therapy and increased intake of calcium may be helpful for some patiens. Osteoporosis may also occur in men as part of the aging process or as a consequence of corticosteroid therapy.

osteitis fibrosa cystica

Inflammation of bone with fibrous changes in the bone tissue.

When the parathyroid gland produces an excess of **parathyroid hormone** (hyperparathyroidism), calcium is removed from the bones and appears in the blood. The bones become porous (osteoporosis) and decalcified, leading to curvature and cyst formation as well as fractures. Blood calcium accumulation may lead to renal and cystic calculi (stones).

rickets (rachitis)

Inflammation of the spinal column.

Rickets is an osteodystrophy characterized by **osteomalacia.** It is primarily a disease of infancy and childhood when bones are forming but fail to receive calcium and phosphorus. Vitamin D is usually deficient in the diet and this prevents calcium and phosphorus from being absorbed into the bloodstream from the intestines. The bones become soft and bend easily, leading to kyphosis as well as other bone curvatures.

osteomyelitis

Inflammation of the bone and bone marrow due to a pyogenic infection.

The etiology of osteomyelitis is bacterial. Bacteria enter the body through a wound, spread from an infection near the bone, or come from a skin or throat infection. Children, particularly boys, are most often affected and the infection usually occurs in the long bones of the legs and arms.

Bone infection can lead to **abscess** (inflammation with pus collection), and if the bone dies, a **sequestrum** (segment of dead bone) may result.

Antibiotic therapy can correct the condition so that abscess can be averted.

talipes

Clubfoot.

This term refers to a congenital deformity of the bones of the foot.

exostoses

Bony growths (benign tumors) arising from the surface of the bone.

Osteochondromas are exostoses and are usually found on the diaphysis of long bones near the epiphyseal plate.

osteogenic sarcoma

Malignant tumor arising from bone.

Osteoblasts multiply without control and form large tumors, especially at the ends of long bones (half the lesions are located just below or above the knee). Surgical resection with chemotherapy improves the survival rate.

Ewing's tumor

Malignant bone tumor (Ewing's sarcoma).

Pain and swelling are common, with the tumor sometimes involving the entire shaft of a long bone. Radiation therapy with chemotherapy represents the best chance for cure.

fracture

Sudden breaking of a bone.

Some terms describing fractures and related injuries are:

closed fracture—A bone is broken but there is no open wound in the skin (**simple fracture**).

open fracture—A broken bone with an open wound in the skin (**compound fracture**). See Figure 14-13.

comminuted fracture—Bone is splintered or crushed. See Figure 14-13.

impacted fracture—The bone is broken, and one end is wedged into the anterior of the other. See Figure 14-13.

greenstick fracture—The bone is partially bent and partially broken, as when a green stick breaks. See Figure 14-13.

compression fracture—The bone is compressed. This often occurs to the vertebrae.

crepitation—Crackling sensation felt and heard as the ends of a broken bone move together.

Treatment of fractures involves **reduction**, which is the restoration of the fracture to its normal position. A **closed reduction** is manipulative reduction without an incision; in an **open reduction** an incision is made into the fracture site. A **cast** (solid mold of the body part) is applied to fractures to immobilize the injured area.

III. JOINTS

A. Types of Joints

A joint (articulation) is a coming together of two or more bones. Some joints are immovable, such as the **suture joints** between the skull bones. Other joints, such as those between the vertebrae, are partially movable. Most joints, however, allow considerable

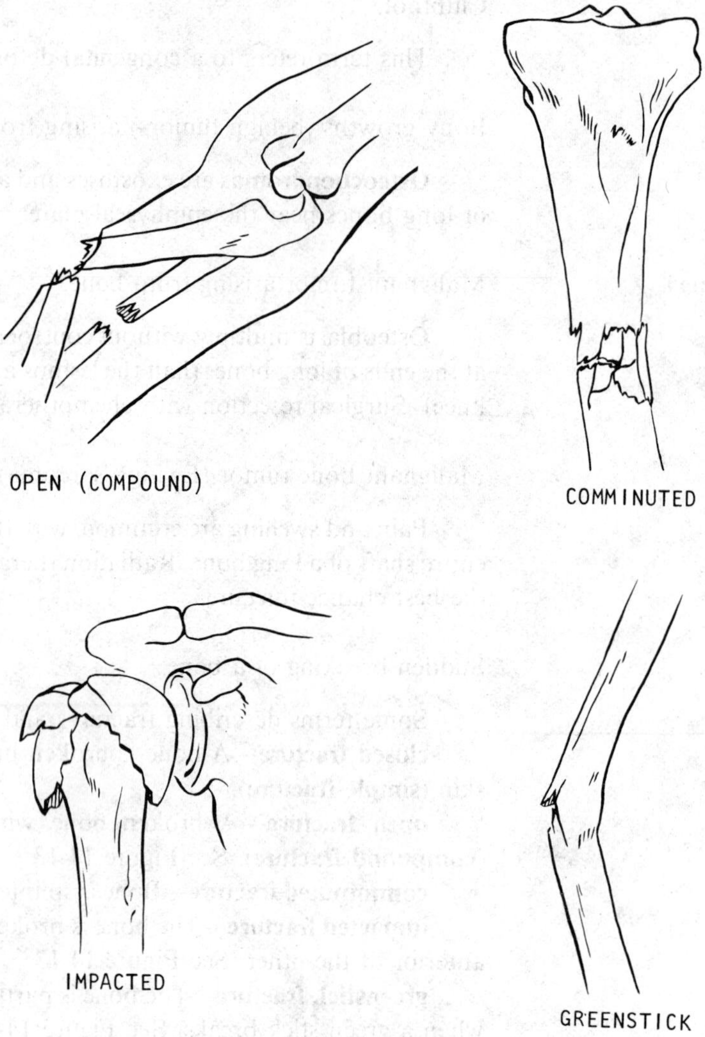

Figure 14-13 Types of fractures.

movement. These freely movable joints are called **synovial joints**. Examples of synovial joints are the ball and socket type (hip joint; the head of the femur fits into the acetabular fossa of the ilium) and hinge type (elbow, knee, and ankle joints). Label the structures in Figure 14-14 as you read the following description of a synovial joint:

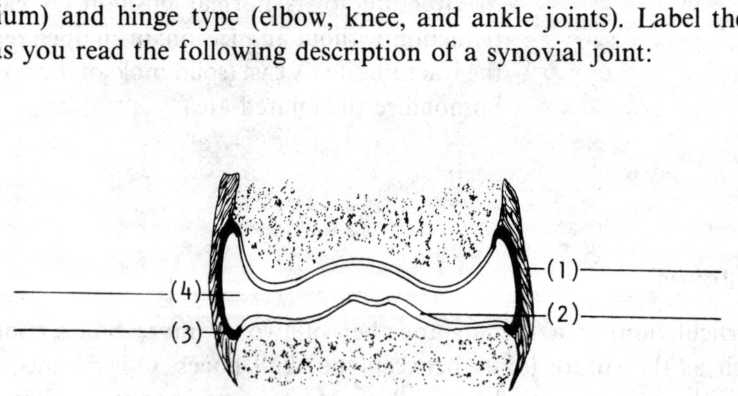

Figure 14-14 Synovial joint.

The bones in a synovial joint are separated by a **joint capsule** (1) composed of fibrous cartilage tissue. **Ligaments** (fibrous bands, or sheets, of connective tissue) often anchor the bones together around the joint capsule to strengthen it. The surface of the bones at the joint is covered with a smooth cartilage surface called the **articular cartilage** (2). The **synovial membrane** (3) lies under the joint capsule and lines the **synovial cavity** (4) between the bones. The synovial cavity is filled with a special lubricating fluid produced by the synovial membrane. This **synovial fluid** contains water and nutrients which nourish as well as lubricate the joints so that friction on the articular cartilage is minimal.

B. Bursae

Bursae are closed sacs of synovial fluid lined with a synovial membrane. They are formed in the spaces between **tendons** (connective tissue binding muscles to bones), **ligaments** (connective tissue binding bones to bones), and bones. Bursae lubricate these areas where friction would normally develop close to the joint capsule.

Some common bursae locations are at the elbow joint (olecranon bursa), knee joint (patellar bursa), and shoulder joint (subacromial bursa).

C. Vocabulary

articulation	Joint.
bursa; bursae	Sac of fluid at or around a joint.
ligament	Connective tissue binding bones to other bones.
suture joint	Type of joint in which apposed surfaces are closely united.
synovial cavity	Space between bones at a synovial joint.
synovial fluid	Viscous (sticky) fluid within the synovial cavity. Synovial fluid is similar in viscosity to egg white; this accounts for the origin of the term (syn = like; ovum = egg).
synovial joint	A freely movable joint.
synovial membrane	Membrane lining the synovial cavity.
tendon	Connective tissue which binds muscles to bones.

D. Combining Forms

Combining Form	*Definition*	*Terminology*	*Meaning*
arthr/o	joint	arthroplasty	______________________
		arthrotomy	______________________

		hemarthrosis ________
articul/o	joint	articular surface ________
synovi/o	synovial membrane, synovia *(fluid that lubricates joints)*	synovioma ________ synovectomy ________
burs/o	bursa	bursitis ________
chondr/o	cartilage	chondroma ________ chondromalacia ________ achondroplasia ________
fibros/o	fibrous connective tissue	fibrositis ________ *Also called rheumatism. Pain comes from tendons, ligaments, and muscles that are too tense, tight, and contracted for too long.*
ten/o tend/o tendin/o	tendons *(fibrous bands connecting muscles to bones)*	tendoplasty ________ tenosynovitis ________ *Synov means the sheath around the tendon.* tendinitis ________
ligament/o	ligaments	ligamentous ________
syndesm/o	ligament	syndesmoplasty ________
ankyl/o	crooked, bent, stiff	ankylosis ________ *Joint is often immobile as a result of rheumatoid arthritis.*
-desis	to bind, or tie together	arthrodesis ________ *Artificial ankylosis.*

E. Pathological Conditions

arthritis Inflammation of joints.

Some of the more common forms are:

rheumatoid arthritis

A chronic disease in which joints become inflamed and painful. It is believed to be caused by an immune reaction against joint tissues.

The small joints of the hands and feet are affected at first and larger joints later. Women are more commonly afflicted than men. Synovial membranes become inflamed and thickened, damaging the articular cartilage and preventing easy movement. Sometimes fibrous tissue forms and calcifies, creating a bony **ankylosis** (union) at the joint and preventing any movement at all. Swollen, painful joints accompanied by **pyrexia** (fever) are symptoms. Treatment consists of heat applications and drugs (aspirin, gold compounds, and corticosteroids) to reduce inflammation and pain.

ankylosing spondylitis

Chronic, progressive arthritis with stiffening of joints, primarily of the spine.

Bilateral sclerosis of the sacroiliac joints is a diagnostic sign. Joint changes are similar to those seen in rheumatoid arthritis and the condition responds to corticosteroids and anti-inflammatory drugs.

osteoarthritis

Chronic inflammation of bones and joints due to degenerative changes in cartilage.

This condition occurs mainly in the hips and legs of older individuals. Drugs reduce inflammation and pain, and physical therapy loosens impaired joints. Figure 14-15 shows the changes in a joint with osteoarthritis and rheumatoid arthritis.

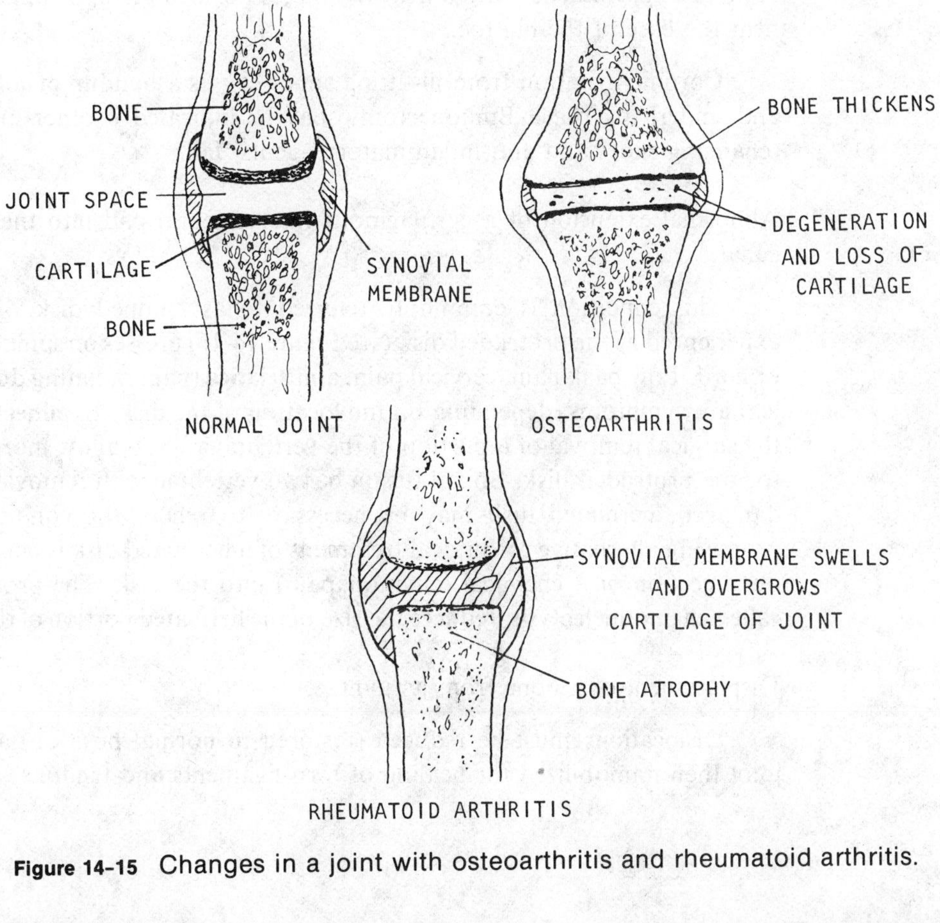

Figure 14-15 Changes in a joint with osteoarthritis and rheumatoid arthritis.

gouty arthritis (gout)

Inflammation of joints caused by excessive uric acid in the body.

An inherited defect in metabolism causes too much uric acid to accumulate in blood (hyperuricemia), joints, and soft tissues near joints. The uric acid crystals destroy the articular cartilage and damage the synovial membrane. A joint chiefly affected is the big toe; hence the condition is often known as **podagra** (pod = foot, -agra = excessive pain). Treatment consists of drugs to lower uric acid production (allopurinol) and to prevent inflammation (colchicine), and a special diet that avoids foods (red meat) rich in uric acid.

systemic lupus erythematosus (SLE)

Chronic inflammatory disease involving joints, skin, kidneys, nervous system, heart, and lungs.

Patients, usually women, experience joint pain (polyarthralgias), fever, and malaise. Etiology is unknown, but may be related to a disorder of the immune system (antigen-antibody complexes).

bursitis

Inflammation of bursae.

Etiology may be related to stress placed on the bursa or diseases such as gout or rheumatoid arthritis. Movement becomes limited and painful. Intrabursal injection of corticosteroids as well as rest and splinting of the limb are helpful in treatment.

bunion

Abnormal prominence with bursal swelling at the metatarsophalangeal joint near the base of the big toe.

Chronic irritation from ill-fitting shoes causes a buildup of soft tissue and underlying bone. Bunionectomy may be indicated if other measures (changing shoes and anti-inflammatory agents) fail.

protrusion of an intervertebral disk (disc)

Abnormal extension of a cartilaginous intervertebral pad into the neural canal.

This condition is commonly referred to as "slipped disk." Pain is experienced as the protruded disk (see Figure 14-16) presses on spinal nerves or cord. Low back pain, cervical pain, and **sciatica** (pain radiating down the leg) are symptoms, depending on the location of the disk. **Laminectomy** is the surgical removal of a portion of the vertebral arch to allow more room for the protruded disk. Spinal fusion of two vertebrae with removal of the damaged, herniated disk may be necessary to relieve the condition. A promising alternative to surgical treatment of a herniated disk is percutaneous injection of a chemical (chymopapain) into the disk. The procedure, called **chemonucleolysis**, reduces the size of the herniated portion of the disk.

dislocation

Displacement of a bone from its joint.

Dislocations must be reduced (restored to normal position) and the joint then immobilized for healing of torn ligaments and tendons.

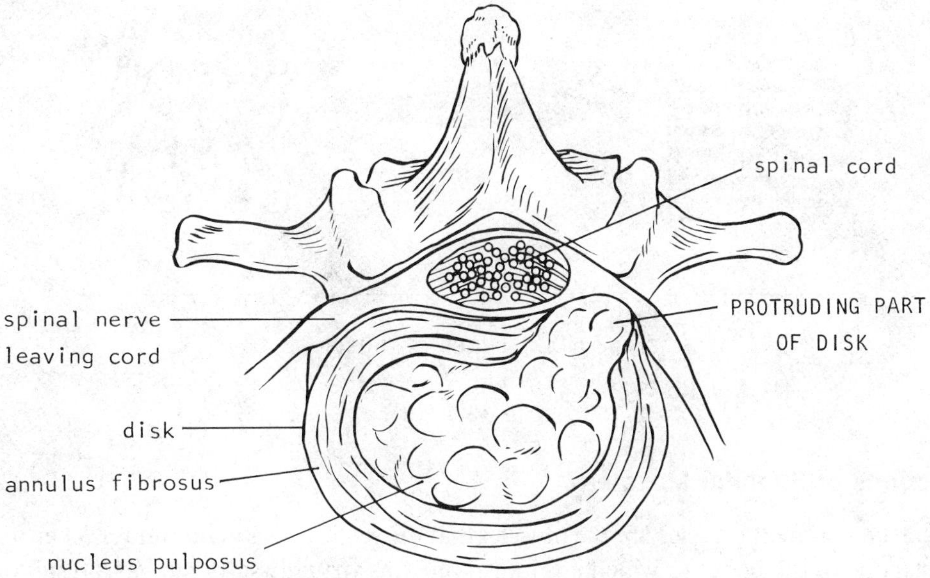

Figure 14-16 Protrusion of an intervertebral disk (looking down on a vertebra). Note how the inner portion (nucleus pulposus) of the disk herniates and presses on the spinal nerve.

sprain Trauma to a joint, with pain, swelling, and injury to ligaments.

Sprains may also involve damage to blood vessels, muscles, tendons, and nerves. A **strain** is a less serious injury with overstretching of muscle. Application of ice and elevation of the joint are immediate measures to relieve pain and prevent swelling due to sprains.

IV. MUSCLES

A. Types of Muscles

There are three types of muscles in the body. Label Figure 14-17 as you read the following descriptions of the various types of muscles:

Striated muscles (1), also called **voluntary** or **skeletal** muscles, are the muscle fibers that move all bones, as well as the face and eyes. We have conscious control over the activity of this type of muscle. Striated muscle fibers (cells) have a pattern of dark and light bands, or fibrils, in their cytoplasm. A delicate membrane called a **sarcolemma** surrounds each skeletal muscle fiber. Fibrous tissue that envelops muscles is called **fascia.**

Smooth muscles (2), also called **involuntary** or **visceral** muscles, are those muscle fibers which move our internal organs such as the digestive tract, blood vessels, and secretory ducts leading from glands. We have no conscious control over these muscles. They are called "smooth" because they have no dark and light fibrils in their cytoplasm. While skeletal muscle fibers are arranged in bundles, smooth muscle forms sheets of fibers as it wraps around tubes and vessels.

Cardiac muscle (3) is striated in appearance but like smooth muscle in its action. Its movement cannot be consciously controlled. The fibers of cardiac muscle are branching fibers and are found in the heart.

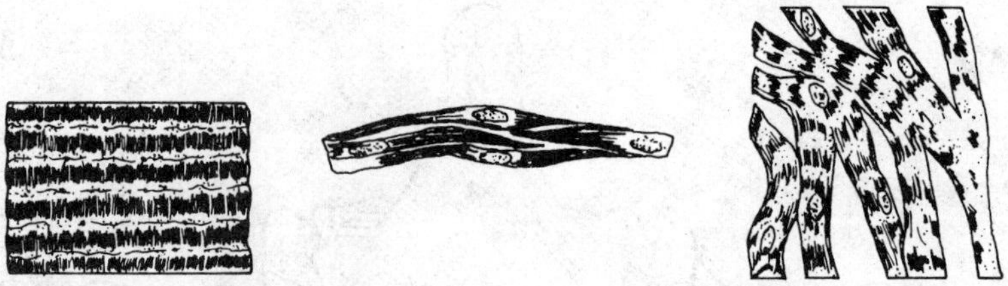

Figure 14-17 Types of muscles.

B. Actions of Skeletal Muscles

Skeletal (striated) muscles are the muscles that move the bones of our body. When a muscle contracts, one of the bones to which it is joined remains virtually stationary as a result of other muscles that hold it in place. The point of attachment of the muscle to the stationary bone is called the **origin** (beginning) of that muscle. However, when the muscle contracts, another bone to which it is attached does move. The point of junction of the muscle to the bone that moves is called the **insertion** of the muscle.

There can be more than one origin for a muscle, as is the case with the upper arm muscle (biceps brachii) where one origin is at the upper end of the humerus near the shoulder joint and a second origin is above the scapula. The insertion of the biceps brachii is at the upper end of the radius near the elbow.

Near the point of insertion, a muscle narrows and is connected to the bone by way of a **tendon**. One type of tendon that helps attach muscles to bones, as well as to their tissues, is called an **aponeurosis**.

Muscles can perform a variety of actions. Some of the terms used to describe those actions are listed below with a short description of the specific type of movement performed (see Figure 14-18):

Action	*Meaning*
Flexion	Decreasing the angle between two bones; bending a limb.
Extension	Increasing the angle between two bones; straightening out a limb.
Abduction	Movement away from the midline of the body.
Adduction	Movement toward the midline of the body.
Rotation	Circular movement around an axis.
Dorsiflexion	Decreasing the angle of the ankle joint so that the foot bends backward.
Plantar flexion	The motion that increases the angle in the ankle joint as when "pointing the toes" or extending the foot toward the ground. Plant/o means sole of the foot.

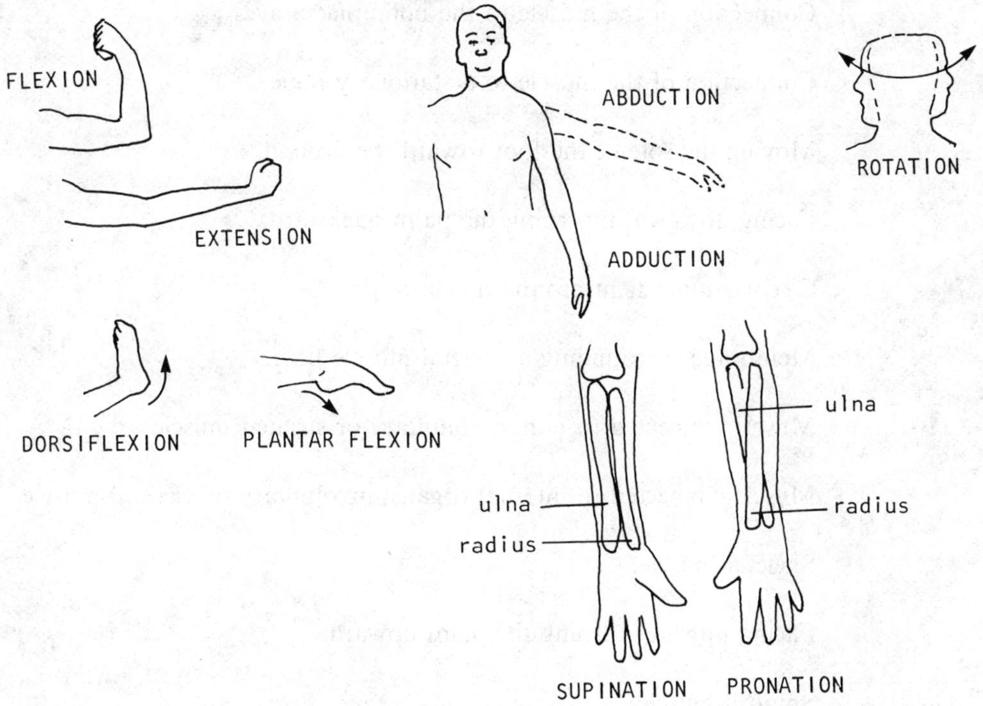

Figure 14-18 Types of muscular actions.

Supination	Facing upward; as applied to the hand, the palm moves from a posterior to an anterior position.
Pronation	Facing downward; as applied to the hand, the palm moves from an anterior to a posterior position.

Your medical dictionary will have a complete list of the muscles of the body, with a description of their origin, insertion, and various actions.

C. Vocabulary

abduction	Movement away from the midline of the body.
adduction	Movement toward the midline of the body.
aponeurosis	Broad, flat tendon connecting muscles to bones. (Neur can also mean tendon in Greek; apo means from.
dorsiflexion	Backward bending of the foot.
extension	Straightening of a flexed limb.
fascia	Fibrous membrane separating and enveloping muscles.
flexion	Bending.

insertion of a muscle	Connection of the muscle to the bone that moves.
origin of a muscle	Connection of the muscle to a stationary bone.
plantar flexion	Moving the sole of the foot toward the ground.
pronation	Facing downward; turning the palm backward.
rotation	Circular movement around a central point.
sarcolemma	Membrane surrounding a skeletal muscle fiber.
skeletal muscle	Muscle connected to bones; voluntary or striated muscle.
smooth muscle	Muscle connected to internal organs; involuntary or visceral muscle.
striated muscle	Skeletal muscle.
supination	Facing upward; turning the palm upward.
visceral muscle	Smooth muscle.

D. Combining Forms

Combining Form	*Definition*	*Terminology*	*Meaning*
my/o	muscle	myalgia	______________
		myorrhaphy	______________
myos/o	muscle	myositis	______________
leiomy/o	smooth, visceral muscle	leiomyoma	______________
rhabdomy/o	skeletal, striated muscle	rhabdomyoma	______________
sarc/o	flesh *(connective tissue)*	leiomyosarcoma	______________
myocardi/o	heart muscle	myocardial	______________
fasci/o	fascia	fasciectomy	______________
aponeur/o	aponeurosis	aponeurorrhaphy	______________
-sthenia	strength	myasthenia	______________

-trophy	development, nourishment	hypertrophy ____________________ atrophy ____________________

E. Pathological Conditions

myasthenia gravis Lack of muscle strength marked by paralysis.

This condition is characterized by extreme weakness of the muscles of the face, jaw, and eyelids and difficulty in swallowing. The etiology is unknown, but it is thought that there is some defect at the myoneural junction where the nerve enters the muscle fiber to stimulate muscle contraction. There is either a lack of **acetylcholine** to help transmit the impulse across the myoneural junction or an increase in **cholinesterase**, which is an enzyme released at the junction to destroy whatever acetylcholine remains after the impulse has passed. Treatment consists of giving a drug to interfere with cholinesterase production. Some cases are associated with benign tumors of the thymus (thymoma), and thymectomy is found to be beneficial.

muscular dystrophy A group of inherited diseases characterized by progressive weakness and degeneration of muscle fibers without involvement of the nervous system.

Pseudohypertrophic (Duchenne) muscular dystrophy is the most common form. Muscles enlarge as fat replaces functional muscle cells that have atrophied.

polymyalgia rheumatica Muscle pain, primarily of the shoulder and pelvis, with absence of arthritis and signs of muscle distress.

Treatment with low doses of corticosteroids may relieve symptoms.

amyotrophic lateral sclerosis Movement disorder (muscles atrophy) with degeneration of nerves in the spinal cord and lower region of the brain (brainstem).

Early symptoms include difficulty in swallowing and talking and weakness in the arms and legs. As the disease progresses there is increased spasticity and atrophy of muscles. Etiology and effective treatment are unknown.

V. LABORATORY TESTS, CLINICAL PROCEDURES, AND ABBREVIATIONS

Laboratory Tests

Serum calcium Measurement of the amount of calcium in the blood (serum).

Serum phosphorus Measurement of the amount of phosphorus in the blood.

Serum creatine kinase Creatine kinase (CK) is an enzyme normally present in skeletal and cardiac muscle. Serum CK levels are found elevated in muscular dystrophy, myocardial infarction, and skeletal muscle disorders.

Uric acid test
This test measures the amount of uric acid in a sample of blood. High values are associated with gouty arthritis and blood diseases such as leukemia and polycythemia.

Latex fixation test (rheumatoid factor test)
A sample of blood is tested for the presence of the rheumatoid factor (an antibody found in people suffering from rheumatoid arthritis).

Erythrocyte sedimentation rate
This test measures the rate at which erythrocytes settle out of solution when an anticoagulant is added to blood. Elevated "sed" rates are associated with several joint and muscle disorders.

Lupus erythematosus (LE) cell test
This test searches for the presence of a white blood cell containing ingested erythrocytes. This cell is found in the blood of patients with systemic lupus erythematosus.

Clinical Procedures

Bone scan
A radioactive phosphate substance is injected intravenously and uptake of the substance in bone is measured by a special scanning device. Areas that take up excessive amounts of radioactive substance may contain tumors, infection, inflammation, or other destructive changes.

Arthrocentesis
Surgical puncture of the joint space with a needle. Synovial fluid is removed for analysis.

Arthroscopy
Visual examination of the inside of a joint with an endoscope.

Arthrography
An x-ray of a joint after injection of opaque contrast medium.

Electromyography
The process or recording the strength of muscle contraction as a result of electrical stimulation.

Muscle biopsy
Removal of muscle tissue for microscopic examination.

Abbreviations

C-1, C-2, etc.	Cervical vertebrae	LE cell	Lupus erythematosus cell
Ca	Calcium	Ortho.	Orthopedics, orthopaedics
CK	Creatine kinase	P	Phosphorus
DTR	Deep tendon reflexes	RA	Rheumatoid arthritis
EMG	Electromyography	RF	Rheumatoid factor
ESR	Erythrocyte sedimentation rate	SI	Sacroiliac joint
IM	Intramuscular	SLE	Systemic lupus erythematosus
L-1, L-2, etc.	Lumbar vertebrae	T-1, T-2, etc.	Thoracic vertebrae

VI. PRACTICAL APPLICATIONS

Skeletal Memorial Hospital—Department of Radiology

PA [posterior-anterior] and lateral chest: The heart is enlarged in its transverse diameter. The lungs are fully expanded and free of active disease.

The thoracic spine shows a scoliosis of the upper thoracic spine convex to the left. There is 50 per cent wedge compression fracture of T-6 and slight wedge compression fracture of T-5. There is also anterior wedge compression fracture of T-12.

Lumbar spine shows 90 per cent compression fractures of L-1 and L-3 with 30 per cent compression fractures of L-2 and L-5. All bones are markedly osteoporotic. There is calcification within the aortic arch. There are gallstones in the right upper quadrant. The findings in the spine are most compatible with osteoporotic compression fractures. During the procedure, the patient had a sickable* episode and fell, striking her head. A skull series, done at no cost to the patient, shows no evidence of bony fracture. The pineal gland is calcified and has a midline location. The sella turcica is normal.

*This word was incorrectly transcribed. Can you guess the correct term?

Operating Schedule—Skeletal Memorial Hospital

1. Excision, osteochondroma, right calcaneus
2. Arthrodesis, right index [second digit] distal interphalangeal joint
3. Excision, bone tumor, left distal fibula, with iliac bone graft
4. Arthroscopy, left knee
5. Lumbar laminectomy
6. Open reduction, malleolar fracture
7. Left quadriceps biopsy
8. Excision, distal end right clavicle, with prob. acromioplasty

VII. EXERCISES

A. Complete the following sentences with medical terms:

1. Bones are composed of bony connective tissue called ______________________ tissue.

2. Bone cells are called ______________________________________.

3. The bones of a fetus are mainly composed of ______________________ tissue.

4. During bone development, immature bone cells called ______________________ produce bony tissue.

5. Large bone cells called ____________________________ digest bone tissue to shape the bone and smooth it out.

6. Two mineral substances necessary for proper development of bones are

_______________ and _______________.

7. A round, small bone resembling a sesame seed in shape and covering the knee joint is called a _______________ bone.

8. The shaft of a long bone is called the _______________.

9. The ends of a long bone are called the _______________.

10. The cartilaginous area at the end of long bones where growth takes place is called the _______________.

11. Red bone marrow is found in spongy or _______________ bone.

12. Yellow bone marrow is composed of _______________ tissue.

13. The strong membrane surrounding the surface of a bone is called the

_______________.

14. Hard, dense bone tissue lying under the periosteum is called _______________.

15. A series of canals containing blood vessels lie within the outer dense tissue of bone and are called the _______________ canals.

16. A thin layer of cartilage surrounding the ends of bones at the joint is called

_______________.

17. The _______________ _______________ is a central, hollowed-out area in the shaft of long bones.

B. Match the following bone processes and depressions with their proper meaning:

1. fissure _______ cavity within bone.

2. sulcus _______ opening for nerves and blood vessels.

3. tubercle _______ large process below neck of femur.

4. sinus _______ large rounded process.

5. trochanter ________ narrow slitlike opening.

6. fossa ________ groovelike depression in bone surface.

7. condyle ________ knuckle-like process at end of bone.

8. foramen ________ small rounded process.

9. tuberosity ________ furrow or cavity in bone.

C. *Match the following cranial and facial bones with their descriptions below:*

mandible	maxilla
ethmoid bone	parietal bone
zygomatic bone	sphenoid bone
nasal bone	vomer
temporal bone	lacrimal bone
occipital bone	frontal bone

1. Forms the roof and upper side parts of the skull ________________

2. Delicate bone, composed of spongy, cancellous tissue; supports the nasal cavity and orbits of the eye ________________

3. Forms the back and base of the skull ________________

4. Forms the forehead ________________

5. Bat-shaped bone that extends behind the eyes to form the base of the skull ________________

6. Bone near the ear and connecting to the lower jaw ________________

7. Cheek bone ________________

8. Bone that supports the bridge of the nose ________________

9. Thin, flat bone forming the lower portion of the nasal septum ________________

10. Lower jaw bone ________________

11. Upper jaw bone ________________

12. Two paired bones located one at the corner of each eye ________________

D. *Name the five divisions of the spinal column:*

1. ______________________ 3. ______________________

2. ______________________ 4. ______________________

5. ______________________

E. *Identify the following parts associated with a vertebra:*

1. Space through which the spinal cord passes ______________________
2. Piece of cartilage between each vertebra ______________________
3. Posterior part of a vertebra ______________________
4. Anterior part of a vertebra ______________________

F. *Give the medical names for the following bones:*

1. Shoulder bone ______________
2. Upper arm bone ______________
3. Breastbone ______________
4. Thigh bone ______________
5. Finger bones ______________
6. Hand bones ______________
7. Medial lower arm bone ______________
8. Lateral lower arm bone ______________
9. Collar bone ______________
10. Wrist bones ______________
11. Backbone ______________
12. Knee cap ______________
13. Shin bone (larger of two lower leg bones) ______________
14. Smaller of two lower leg bones ______________
15. Three parts of the hip bone are: ______________, ______________, and ______________
16. Foot bones ______________

G. *Give the meanings for the following terms associated with bones:*

1. Foramen magnum ______________________

2. Calcaneus ______________________________

3. Acromion ______________________________

4. Xiphoid process ______________________________

5. Lamina ______________________________

6. Malleolus ______________________________

7. Acetabulum ______________________________

8. Pubic symphysis ______________________________

9. Olecranon ______________________________

10. Fontanelle ______________________________

H. Give meanings for the following terms:

1. Osteogenesis ______________________________

2. Rachialgia ______________________________

3. Spondylosis ______________________________

4. Epiphyseal ______________________________

5. Decalcification ______________________________

6. Ossification ______________________________

7. Osteolysis ______________________________

8. Costoclavicular ______________________________

I. Build medical terms:

1. Pertaining to the shoulder bone ______________________________

2. Instrument to cut the skull ______________________________

3. Pertaining to the upper arm bone ______________________________

4. Fixation of the knee cap ______________________________

5. Softening of cartilage ____________________

6. Pertaining to a toe bone ____________________

7. Removal of hand bones ____________________

8. Pertaining to the shin bone ____________________

9. Pertaining to the heel bone ____________________

10. Poor bone development ____________________

11. Removal of the lamina of the vertebral arch ____________________

12. Pertaining to the sacrum and ilium ____________________

J. Give the medical term for the following:

1. Decrease in bone density due to loss of calcium salts ____________________

2. Clubfoot ____________________

3. Humpback ____________________

4. Malignant tumor of bone (two types) ____________________

   and ____________________

5. Inflammatory pyogenic infection of bone and bone marrow ____________________

   ____

6. Benign tumors arising from the bone surface ____________________

7. Condition of excessive calcium in blood ____________________

8. Lateral curvature of the spine ____________________

9. Abnormal anterior curvature of the spine ____________________

10. Inflammation of the spinal column with softening of bone due to vitamin D deficiency ____________________

11. Surgical fracture of a bone to remedy a deformity ____________________

K. *Match the term in Column I with its description in Column II:*

Column I		*Column II*
1. greenstick fracture	________	A. Trauma to a joint; injury to ligaments.
2. closed (simple) fracture	________	B. Break in bone with wound in the skin.
3. comminuted fracture	________	C. One side of the bone is fractured; the other side is bent.
4. open (compound) fracture	________	D. Bone is put in proper place without incision of skin.
5. sprain	________	E. Displacement of the bone from the joint.
6. dislocation	________	F. Bone is broken by pressure from another bone.
7. open reduction	________	G. Bone is splintered or crushed.
8. closed reduction	________	H. Bone is put in proper place after incision through the skin.
9. impacted fracture	________	I. Bone is broken and one end is wedged into the interior of the adjoining bone.
10. compression fracture	________	J. Break in the bone without an open skin wound.

L. *Give the meanings for the following terms:*

1. sequestrum ________________________________
2. osteoporosis ________________________________
3. osteitis fibrosa cystica ________________________________
4. palliative treatment ________________________________
5. crepitation ________________________________
6. trabeculae ________________________________
7. chondromalacia ________________________________

8. synovial joint ______________________

9. synovial membrane ______________________

10. bursa ______________________

11. tendons ______________________

12. ligaments ______________________

13. tenosynovitis ______________________

14. chondroplasty ______________________

15. syndesmorrhaphy ______________________

M. Name the abnormal condition described below:

1. Inflammation of joints with hyperuricemia ______________________

2. Chronic inflammation of bones and joints (degenerative changes in cartilage) ______________________

3. Arthritis of the spinal column with stiffening and hardening of tissues at the joints ______________________

4. Pain radiating down the leg as a result of a herniated disk ______________________

5. Chronic joint inflammation with stiffness and swelling of the joints (hands and feet usually first) and fever ______________________

6. Inflammation of sacs of synovial fluid near the joints ______________________

7. Inflammation of fibrous connective tissue around muscles, joints, tendons, and ligaments ______________________

8. Chronic inflammatory disease involving not only joints but skin, kidney, and lungs ______________________

9. Swelling of a metatarsophalangeal bursa ________________

10. Abnormal immobility and stiffening of a joint ________________

N. Give meanings for the following medical terms:

1. striated muscle ________________
2. sarcolemma ________________
3. smooth muscles ________________
4. aponeurosis ________________
5. rhabdomyoma ________________
6. myasthenia gravis ________________
7. tenodesis ________________
8. fasciotomy ________________
9. leiomyosarcoma ________________
10. polymyalgia rheumatica ________________
11. myocarditis ________________
12. pyrexia ________________
13. muscular dystrophy ________________
14. origin of a muscle ________________
15. insertion of a muscle ________________
16. serum calcium ________________
17. erythrocyte sedimentation rate ________________
____
18. arthrocentesis ________________
19. electromyography ________________
20. arthroscopy ________________

O. Match the term for muscle action with its meaning:

1. extension	________	movement away from the midline
2. rotation	________	facing downward; turning the palm posteriorly
3. flexion	________	facing upward; turning the palm anteriorly.
4. adduction	________	straightening out a limb.
5. supination	________	bending the sole of the foot downward.
6. abduction	________	circular movement around an axis.
7. pronation	________	bending a limb.
8. dorsiflexion	________	movement toward the midline.
9. plantar flexion	________	backward bending of the foot.

P. Match the term in Column I with its meaning in Column II:

Column I		*Column II*
1. LE cell test	________	A. Radioactive substance is injected and traced in tissue.
2. Serum creatine kinase	________	B. Chemical found in myoneural space.
3. Uric acid test	________	C. Test for presence of rheumatoid factor (antibody).
4. Latex fixation test	________	D. Substance necessary for proper bone development.
5. Bone scan	________	E. Visual examination of a joint.
6. Muscle biopsy	________	F. Test tells if patient has gouty arthritis.
7. Arthrography	________	G. Test tells if patient has systemic lupus erythematosus.
8. Acetylcholine	________	H. Removal of tissue for microscopic examination.
9. Phosphorus	________	I. Elevated levels of this enzyme are found in muscular disorders.

ANSWERS

A.

1. osseous
2. osteocytes
3. cartilage
4. osteoblasts
5. osteoclasts
6. calcium and phosphorus
7. sesamoid
8. diaphysis
9. epiphyses
10. epiphyseal plate
11. cancellous
12. fat
13. periosteum
14. compact
15. haversian
16. articular cartilage
17. medullary cavity

B.

4
8
5
9
1
2
7
3
6

C.

1. parietal bone
2. ethmoid bone
3. occipital bone
4. frontal bone
5. sphenoid bone
6. temporal bone
7. zygomatic bone
8. nasal bone
9. vomer
10. mandible
11. maxilla
12. lacrimal bones

D.

1. cervical
2. thoracic
3. lumbar
4. sacral
5. coccygeal

E.

1. neural canal
2. intervertebral disk
3. vertebral arch
4. vertebral body

F.

1. scapula
2. humerus
3. sternum
4. femur
5. phalanges
6. metacarpals
7. ulna
8. radius
9. clavicle
10. carpals
11. vertebral column
12. patella
13. tibia
14. fibula
15. ilium, ischium, pubis
16. metatarsals

G.

1. Opening of the occipital bone through which the spinal cord passes
2. Heel bone; largest of the tarsal (ankle) bones
3. Extension of the scapula
4. Lower portion of the sternum
5. Portion of the vertebral arch
6. The bulge on either side of the ankle joint; the lower end of the fibula is the lateral malleolus and the lower end of the tibia is the medial malleolus
7. Depression in the hip bone into which the femur fits
8. Area of fusion of the two pubis bones, at the midline
9. Bony process at the proximal end of the ulna; elbow joint
10. Soft spot between the bones of the skull in an infant

H.

1. Formation of bone
2. Pain in the spine
3. Abnormal condition of the vertebrae
4. Pertaining to the epiphysis
5. Removal of calcium from bones
6. Formation of bone
7. Destruction of bone
8. Pertaining to the ribs and clavicle

I.

1. scapular
2. craniotome
3. humeral
4. patellapexy
5. chondromalacia
6. phalangeal
7. metacarpectomy
8. tibial
9. calcaneal
10. osteodystrophy
11. laminectomy
12. sacroiliac

J.

1. osteoporosis
2. talipes
3. kyphosis
4. Ewing's tumor; osteogenic sarcoma
5. osteomyelitis
6. exostoses
7. hypercalcemia
8. scoliosis
9. lordosis
10. rachitis (rickets); osteomalacia
11. osteoclasis

K.

1. C
2. J
3. G
4. B
5. A
6. E
7. H
8. D
9. I
10. F

L.

1. Dead bone tissue
2. Increased porosity in bone; decrease in bone density
3. Inflammation of bone with cyst formation
4. Relieving, not curing
5. Crackling sensation as broken bones move against each other
6. Supportive bony fibers in cancellous, spongy bone
7. Softening of cartilage (usually in the knee)
8. A freely movable joint
9. The membrane that lines the synovial cavity between the bones in a joint
10. Closed sac of synovial fluid near the joints
11. Connective tissue binding muscles to bones
12. Connective tissue binding bones to bones
13. Inflammation of a tendon sheath
14. Surgical repair of cartilage
15. Suture of a ligament

M.

1. Gouty arthritis
2. Osteoarthritis
3. Ankylosing spondylitis
4. Sciatica
5. Rheumatoid arthritis
6. Bursitis
7. Fibrositis (rheumatism)
8. Systemic lupus erythematosus
9. Bunion
10. Ankylosis

N.

1. Skeletal muscle, connected to bones
2. Sheath around skeletal muscles
3. Visceral muscles, attached to internal organs
4. A broad, flat tendon
5. Tumor of skeletal muscle (benign)
6. Weakness in muscles; due to defect at the myoneural space
7. Surgical binding together of tendons
8. Incision into fascia
9. Malignant tumor of smooth muscles
10. Pain in muscles (primarily shoulder and pelvis) without signs of arthritis or atrophy of muscles
11. Inflammation of heart muscle
12. Fever
13. Inherited muscle weakness and degeneration; atrophy of muscle tissue
14. Point of attachment of a muscle to a stationary bone
15. Point of attachment of a muscle to the bone that moves
16. Measurement of calcium levels in blood (serum)
17. The time that it takes for red blood cells to settle out of blood after an anticoagulant is added. Increase frequently associated with joint inflammation
18. Surgical puncture of a joint to remove fluid
19. Process of recording the strength of a muscle to contract after electrical stimulation
20. Visual examination of a joint with an endoscope

O.

6
7
5
1
9
2
3
4
8

P.

1. G
2. I
3. F
4. C
5. A
6. H
7. E
8. B
9. D

VIII. PRONUNCIATION OF TERMS

abduction	ăb-DŬK-shŭn
acetabular	ăs-ĕ-TĂB-ū-lăr
acetabulum	ăs-ĕ-TĂB-ū-lŭm
achondroplasia	ā-kŏn-drō-PLĀ-zē-ă
acromion	ă-KRŌ-mē-ŏn
adduction	ă-DŬK-shŭn
amyotrophic lateral sclerosis	ă-mī-ō-TRŌ-fĭk LĂT-ĕr-ăl sklĕ-RŌ-sĭs
ankylosing spondylitis	ăng-kĭ-LŌ-sĭng spŏn-dĭ-LĪ-tĭs
ankylosis	ăng-kĭ-LŌ-sĭs
aponeurorrhaphy	ăp-ō-nū-RŎR-ă-fē
aponeurosis	ăp-ō-nū-RŌ-sĭs
arthrodesis	ăr-thrō-DĒ-sĭs
arthroplasty	ĂR-thrō-plăs-tē
arthrotomy	ăr-THRŎT-ō-mē
articular	ăr-TĬK-ū-lăr
articulation	ăr-tĭk-ū-LĀ-shūn
atrophy	ĂT-rō-fē
bunion	BŬN-yŭn
bursa	BŬR-să
bursitis	bŭr-SĪ-tĭs
calcaneal	kăl-KĀ-nē-ăl
calcaneus	kăl-KĀ-nē-ŭs
calcium	KĂL-sē-ŭm
cancellous	KĂN-sĕ-lŭs
carpals	KĂR-pălz
cartilage	KĂR-tĭ-lĭj
chondrocostal	kŏn-drō-KŎS-tăl
chondromalacia	kŏn-drō-mă-LĀ-shă
clavicle	KLĂV-ĭ-k'l
clavicular	klă-VĬK-ū-lăr
comminuted	KŎM-ĭ-nūt-ĕd

condyle	KŎN-dīl
costal	KŎS-tăl
craniotomy	krā-nē-ŎT-ō-mē
crepitation	krĕp-ĭ-TĀ-shŭn
decalcification	dē-kăl-sĭ-fĭ-KĀ-shŭn
diaphysis	dī-ĂF-ĭ-sĭs
dorsiflexion	dŏr-sĭ-FLĔK-shŭn
dystrophy	DĬS-trō-fē
epiphyseal	ĕp-ĭ-FĬZ-ē-ăl
epiphysis	ĕ-PĬF-ĭ-sĭs
Ewing's tumor	Ū-ĭngz TŪ-mŏr
exostosis	ĕk-sŏs-TŌ-sĭs
facial	FĀ-shăl
fascia	FĂSH-ē-ă
fasciectomy	făsh-ē-ĔK-tō-mē
femoral	FĔM-ŏr-ăl
femur	FĒ-mŭr
fibrositis	fī-brō-SĪ-tĭs
fibula	FĬB-ū-lă
fibular	FĬB-ū-lăr
fissure	FĬSH-ŭr
flexion	FLĔK-shŭn
fontanelle	fŏn-tă-NĔL
foramen	fō-RĀ-mĕn
fossa	FŎS-ă
haversian	hă-VĔR-shăn
humeral	HŪ-mĕr-ăl
humerus	HŪ-mĕr-ŭs
hypercalcemia	hī-pĕr-kăl-SĒ-mē-ă
hypertrophy	hī-PĔR-trō-fē
iliac	ĬL-ē-ăk
ilium	ĬL-ē-ŭm

ischial	ĬSH-ē-ăl or ĬS-kē-ăl
ischium	ĬSH-ē-ŭm or ĬS-kē-ŭm
kyphosis	ki-FŌ-sĭs
lamina	LĂM-ĭ-nă
laminectomy	lăm-ĭ-NĔK-tō-mē
leiomyoma	lī-ō-mī-Ō-mă
leiomyosarcoma	lī-ō-mī-ō-sar-KŌ-ma
ligament	LĬG-ă-mĕnt
lordosis	lŏr-DŌ-sĭs
lumbodynia	lŭm-bō-DĬN-ē-ă
malleolus	măl-LĒ-ō-lŭs
mandible	MĂN-dĭ-b'l
mandibular	măn-DĬB-ū-lăr
mastoid	MĂS-toyd
maxillary	MĂK-sĭ-lār-ē
medullary	MĔD-ū-lār-ē
metacarpals	mĕt-ă-KĂR-pălz
metatarsals	mĕt-ă-TĂR-sălz
myalgia	mī-ĂL-jă
myasthenia gravis	mī-ăs-THĒ-nē-ă GRĂ-vĭs
myelopoiesis	mī-ĕ-lō-poy-Ē-sĭs
myocardial	mī-ō-KĂR-dē-ăl
myocarditis	mī-ō-kăr-DĪ-tĭs
myorrhaphy	mī-ŎR-ă-fē
myositis	mī-ō-SĪ-tĭs
olecranon	ō-LĔK-ră-nŏn
orthopedic	ŏr-thō-PĒ-dĭk
osseous	ŎS-ē-ŭs
ossification	ŏs-ĭ-fĭ-KĀ-shŭn
osteitis fibrosa cystica	ŏs-tē-Ī-tĭs fī-BRŌ-să SĬS-tĭ-kă
osteoarthritis	ŏs-tē-ō-ăr-THRĪ-tĭs
osteoblast	ŎS-tē-ō-blăst

osteochondroma	ŏs-tē-ō-kŏn-DRŌ-mă
osteoclasis	ŏs-tē-ŎK-lă-sĭs
osteoclast	ŎS-tē-ō-klăst
osteodystrophy	ŏs-tē-ō-DĬS-trō-fē
osteogenic sarcoma	ŏs-tē-ō-JĔN-ĭk săr-KŌ-mă
osteolysis	ŏs-tē-ŎL-i-sĭs
osteomalacia	ŏs-tē-ō-mă-LĀ-shă
osteomyelitis	ŏs-tē-ō-mī-ĕ-LĪ-tĭs
osteoporosis	ŏs-tē-ō-pō-RŌ-sĭs
palliative	PĂL-ē-ă-tĭv
patella	pă-TĔL-ă
patellapexy	pă-TĔL-ă-pĕk-sē
pelvimetry	pĕl-VĬM-ĕ-trē
periosteum	pĕr-ē-ŎS-tē-ŭm
peroneal	pĕr-ō-NĒ-ăl
phalanges	fă-LĂN-jēz
phosphorus	FŎS-fō-rŭs
plantar	PLĂN-tăr
pronation	prō-NĀ-shŭn
pseudohypertrophic	sōō-dō-hī-pĕr-TRŌF-ĭk
pubis	PŪ-bĭs
pyrexia	pī-RĔK-sē-ă
rachialgia	rā-kē-ĂL-jă
rachischisis	rā-KĬS-kĭ-sĭs
rachitis	rā-KĪ-tĭs
radius	RĀ-dē-ŭs
rhabdomyoma	răb-dō-mī-Ō-mă
rheumatoid arthritis	RŌŌ-mă-toyd ăr-THRĪ-tĭs
sarcolemma	săr-kō-LĔM-ă
scapula	SKĂP-ū-lă
sciatica	sī-ĂT-ĭ-kă
scoliosis	skō-lē-Ō-sĭs

sequestrum	sē-KWĚS-trŭm
spondylitis	spŏn-dĭ-LĪ-tĭs
spondylolisthesis	spŏn-dĭ-lō-LĬS-thē-sĭs
sternum	STĚR-nŭm
striated	STRĪ-ā-tĕd
sulcus	SŬL-kŭs
supination	sū-pĭ-NĀ-shŭn
symphysis	SĬM-fĭ-sĭs
syndesmoplasty	sĭn-DĚZ-mō-plăs-tē
synovectomy	sĭn-ō-VĚK-tō-mē
synovial	sĭ-NŌ-vē-ăl
synovioma	sĭ-nō-vē-Ō-mă
systemic lupus erythematosus	sĭs-TĚM-ĭk LŪ-pŭs ĕ-rĭ-thē-mă-TŌ-sŭs
talipes	TĂL-ĭ-pēz
tendinitis	tĕn-dĭ-NĪ-tĭs
tendon	TĚN-dŭn
tendoplasty	TĚN-dō-plăs-tē
tenosynovitis	tĕn-ō-sĭn-ō-VĪ-tĭs
tibia	TĬB-ē-ă
trabeculae	tră-BĚK-ū-lē
trochanter	trō-KĂN-tĕr
tubercle	TŪ-bĕr-k'l
tuberosity	tū-bĕ-RŎS-ĭ-tē
ulna	ŬL-nă
vertebral	VĚR-tĕ-brăl or vĕr-TĒ-brăl
visceral	VĬS-ĕr-ăl
xiphoid	ZĬF-oyd

REVIEW SHEET

Combining Forms

acetabul/o	______	fibul/o	______
acromi/o	______	humer/o	______
ankyl/o	______	ili/o	______
aponeur/o	______	ischi/o	______
arthr/o	______	kyph/o	______
articul/o	______	lamin/o	______
burs/o	______	leiomy/o	______
calcane/o	______	ligament/o	______
calci/o	______	lord/o	______
carp/o	______	lumb/o	______
cervic/o	______	malleol/o	______
chondr/o	______	mandibul/o	______
clavicul/o	______	maxill/o	______
coccyg/o	______	metacarp/o	______
cost/o	______	my/o	______
crani/o	______	myel/o	______
fasci/o	______	myocardi/o	______
femor/o	______	myos/o	______
fibr/o	______	olecran/o	______
fibros/o	______	oste/o	______

patell/o ______________________

pelv/o ______________________

perone/o ______________________

phalang/o ______________________

pub/o ______________________

pubi/o ______________________

pyr/o ______________________

rachi/o ______________________

radi/o ______________________

rhabdomy/o ______________________

sacr/o ______________________

sarc/o ______________________

scapul/o ______________________

scoli/o ______________________

spondyl/o ______________________

stern/o ______________________

syndesm/o ______________________

synovi/o ______________________

ten/o ______________________

tend/o ______________________

tenon/o ______________________

thorac/o ______________________

tibi/o ______________________

uln/o ______________________

vertebr/o ______________________

Suffixes

-blast ______________________

-clast ______________________

-desis ______________________

-lemma ______________________

-malacia ______________________

-physis ______________________

-porosis ______________________

-schisis ______________________

-sthenia ______________________

-trophy ______________________

Prefixes

de- ______________________

peri- ______________________

sym- ______________________

Additional Terms

Specific Bones and Processes

acetabulum (387)

acromion (387)

calcaneus (386)

carpals (384)

cervical vertebrae (382)

clavicle (382)

coccyx (382)

ethmoid bone (379)

femur (384)

fibula (386)

frontal bone (379)

humerus (384)

ilium (384)

ischium (384)

lacrimal bones (380)

lumbar vertebrae (382)

malleolus (388)

mandible (380)

mastoid process (388)

maxillary bones (380)

metacarpals (384)

metatarsals (386)

nasal bones (380)

occipital bone (379)

parietal bones (379)

patella (385)

pelvic bone (384)

pubis (384)

radius (384)

sacral vertebrae (382)

scapula (382)

sphenoid bone (379)

spinous process (382)

sternum (382)

tarsals (386)

temporal bones (379)

thoracic vertebrae (382)

tibia (386)

transverse process (382)

ulna (384)

vomer (380)

xiphoid process (388)

zygomatic bones (380)

Terms Related to Bones

cancellous (387)

compact bone (387)

condyle (387)

diaphysis (387)

epiphysis (387)

Ewing's sarcoma (393)

exostoses (393)

false ribs (387)

fissure (387)

floating ribs (387)

fontanelle (387)

foramen (387)

fossa (387)

fractures (393)

haversian canals (387)

lamina (382)

medullary cavity (388)

osseous tissue (388)

osteitis fibrosa cystica (392)

osteodystrophy (389)

osteogenic sarcoma (393)

osteomyelitis (392)

osteoporosis (392)

red bone marrow (388)

reduction of fractures (393)

rickets (rachitis) (392)

sequestrum (392)

sinus (388)

sulcus (388)

trabeculae (388)

trochanter (388)

true ribs (382)

tubercle (388)

tuberosity (388)

vertebral arch (382)

yellow bone marrow (388)

Terms Related to Joints and Muscles

abduction (401)

adduction (401)

amyotrophic lateral sclerosis (403)

ankylosing spondylitis (397)

aponeurosis (401)

articular cartilage (395)

articulation (395)

bunion (398)

bursa (395)

dislocation (395)

dorsiflexion (401)

extension (401)

fascia (401)

fibrositis (396)

flexion (401)

gouty arthritis (398)

insertion of muscle (402)

intervertebral disk (398)

latex fixation test (404)

LE cell test (404)

ligaments (395)

muscular dystrophy (403)

myasthenia gravis (403)

origin of a muscle (402)

osteoarthritis (397)

plantar flexion (402)

polymyalgia rheumatica (403)

pronation (402)

rheumatoid arthritis (397)

rotation (402)

sarcolemma (402)

sciatica (398)

serum creatine kinase (403)

skeletal muscle (402)

sprain (399)

supination (402)

suture (395)

synovial joint (395)

synovial membrane (395)

systemic lupus erythematosus (398)

tendons (395)

uric acid test (404)

CHAPTER 15

SKIN

In this chapter you will:

- Identify the layers of the skin and the accessory structures associated with the skin;
- Build medical words using the combining forms that are related to the specialty of dermatology;
- Describe lesions, symptoms, and pathological conditions that relate to the skin; and
- Identify laboratory tests, clinical procedures, and abbreviations that pertain to the skin.

The chapter is divided into the following sections:

I. INTRODUCTION

The skin and its accessory organs (hair, nails, and glands) are known as the **integumentary system** of the body. Integument means covering, and the skin is the outer covering for the body. It is, however, more than a simple body covering. The skin, as a complex system of specialized tissues, contains glands which secrete several types of fluids, nerves which carry impulses, and blood vessels which aid in the regulation of the body temperature. The following paragraphs review the many important functions of the skin.

First, as a protective membrane over the entire body, the skin guards the deeper tissues of the body against excessive loss of water, salts, and heat and against invasion by pathogens and their toxins. Secretions from the skin are slightly acid in nature and this contributes to the skin's ability to prevent bacterial invasion.

Second, the skin contains two types of glands which produce important secretions. These glands under the skin are the **sebaceous** and **sweat glands**. The sebaceous glands produce an oily secretion called **sebum**, while the sweat glands produce a watery secretion called **sweat**. Sebum and sweat are carried to the outer edges of the skin by ducts, and excreted from the skin through openings, or pores. Sebum helps to lubricate the surface of the skin, and sweat helps to cool the body as it evaporates from the skin surface.

Third, nerve fibers located under the skin act as receptors for sensations such as pain, temperature, pressure, and touch. The adjustment of an individual to his or her environment is thus dependent on the sensory messages relayed to the brain and spinal cord by the sensitive nerve endings in the skin.

Fourth, several different tissues in the skin aid in maintaining the body temperature (thermoregulation). Nerve fibers coordinate thermoregulation by carrying messages to the skin from heat centers in the brain which are sensitive to increases and decreases in body temperature. Impulses from these fibers cause blood vessels to dilate to bring blood to the surface and cause sweat glands to produce the watery secretion which carries heat away.

II. STRUCTURE OF THE SKIN

Figure 15-1 shows the three layers of the skin. Label these layers from the outer surface inward:

(1) **Epidermis**—a thin, cellular membrane layer.
(2) **Corium** or **dermis**—dense, fibrous, connective tissue layer.
(3) **Subcutaneous tissue**—thick, fat-containing tissue.

Epidermis

The epidermis is the outermost, totally cellular layer of the skin. It is composed of **squamous epithelium**. Epithelium is the covering of both the internal and external surfaces of the body. Squamous epithelial cells are flat and scalelike. In the outer layer of the skin, these cells

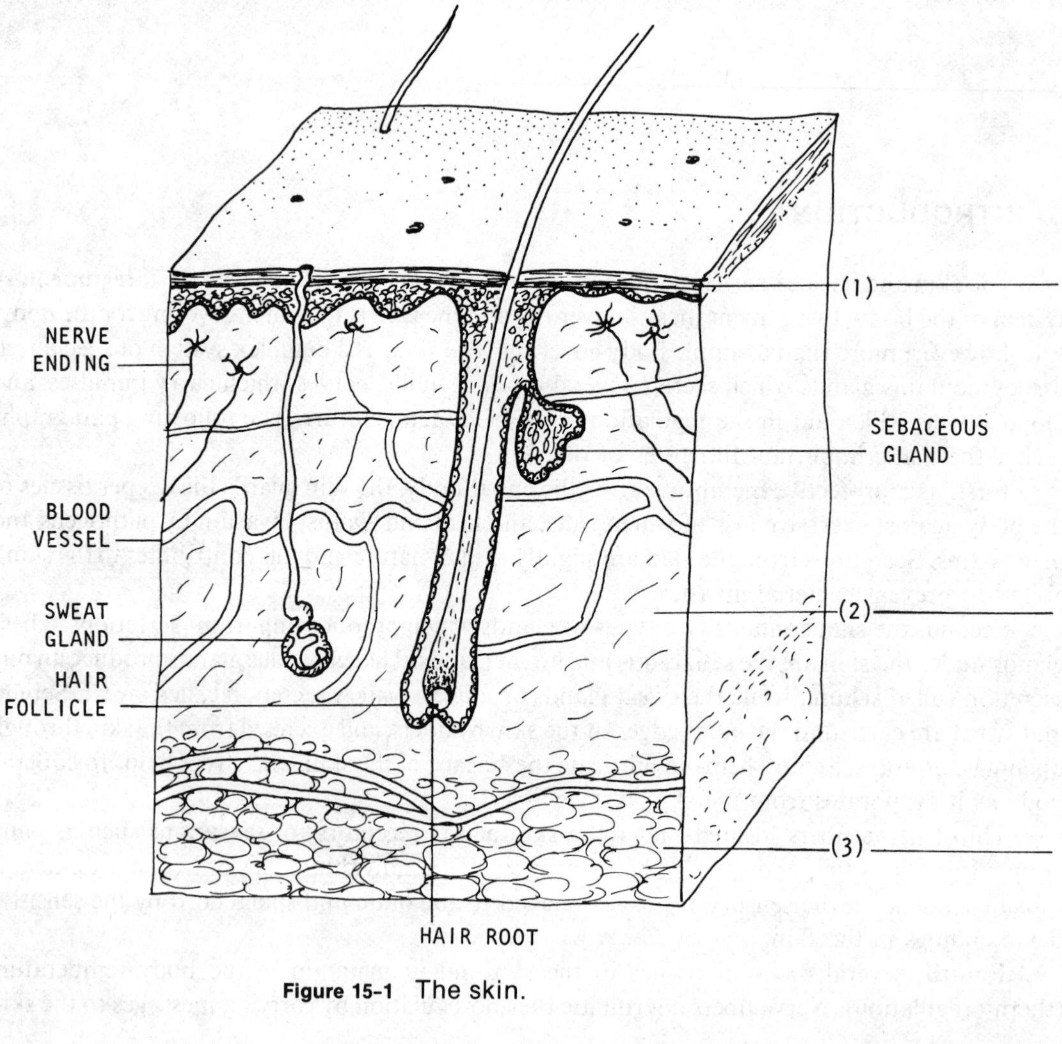

Figure 15-1 The skin.

are arranged in several layers (**strata**) and are, therefore, called **stratified squamous epithelium**.

The epidermis lacks blood vessels, lymphatic vessels, and connective tissue (elastic fibers, cartilage, fat) and is, therefore, dependent on the deeper corium layer and its rich network of capillaries for nourishment. In fact, oxygen and nutrients seep out of the capillaries in the corium, pass through tissue fluid, and supply nourishment to the deeper layers of the epidermis.

Figure 15-2 illustrates the multilayered cells of the epidermis. The deepest layer is called the **basal layer** (1). The cells in the basal layer are constantly growing and multiplying and give rise to all the other cells in the epidermis. As the basal layer cells divide, they are pushed upward and away from the blood supply of the corium layer by a steady stream of younger cells. In their movement toward the most superficial layer of the epidermis, called the **stratum corneum** (2), the cells flatten, shrink, lose their nuclei, and die, becoming filled with a protein called **keratin**. The cells are then called **horny cells**, reflecting their composition of keratin, which is a hard, protein material. Finally, within 3 to 4 weeks after beginning as a basal cell in the deepest part of the epidermis, the horny, keratinized cell is sloughed off from the surface of the skin. The epidermis is thus constantly renewing itself, cells dying at the same rate at which they are born.

The basal layer of the epidermis contains special cells called **melanocytes** (3). Melanocytes form and contain a black pigment called **melanin**. The amount of black pigment accounts for the color differences among the races. Individuals with darker skin possess more active melanocytes, not a greater number of melanocytes. Also, the presence of melanin in the epidermis is vital for protection against the harmful effects of ultraviolet radiation which can manifest themselves as skin cancer. Individuals who, through a flaw in their chemical makeup,

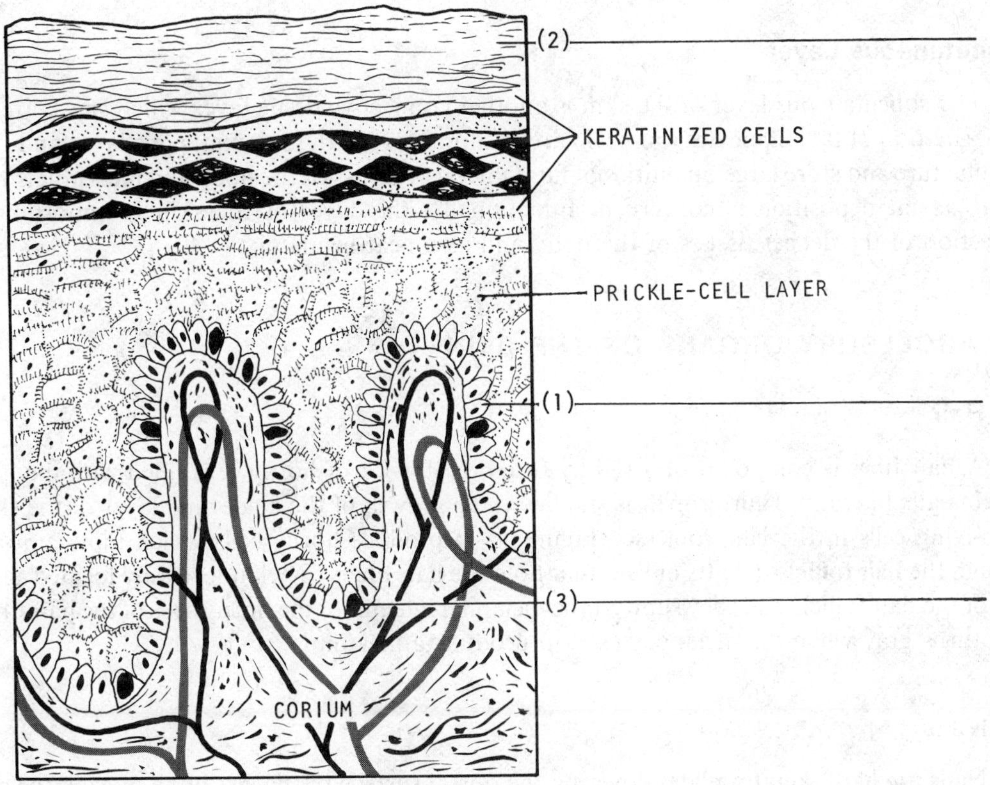

Figure 15-2 The epidermis.

are incapable of forming melanin at all are called **albino** (meaning "white"). Skin and hair are white, and the eyes are red because in the absence of pigment the tiny blood vessels are visible in the iris (normally pigmented portion) of the eye.

Corium (Dermis)

The corium layer, directly below the epidermis, is also called the **dermis**. In contrast to the epidermis, it is living tissue composed of blood and lymph vessels and nerve fibers, as well as the accessory organs of the skin, which are the hair follicles, sweat glands, and sebaceous glands. To support the elaborate system of nerves, vessels, and glands, the corium contains connective tissue cells and fibers.

There are several types of connective tissue cells in the corium: **fibroblasts**, **histiocytes** (macrophages), and **mast cells**. Fibroblasts are fiber-producing cells that are active in repair of injury. These cells are found in connective tissue all over the body. **Histiocytes** (macrophages) are phagocytic cells that protect the body by engulfing foreign materials. **Mast cells** are specialized cells that contain quantities of **histamine** (a substance released in allergies which produces itching) and **heparin** (an anticoagulant substance).

The fibers in the dermis, or corium, are mainly composed of **collagen**. Collagen (colla means glue) is a fibrous protein material found in bone, cartilage, tendons, and ligaments, as well as in the skin. It is tough and resistant but also flexible. In the infant, collagen is loose and delicate, and it becomes harder as the body ages. Collagen fibers support and protect the blood and nerve networks that pass through the corium. Collagen diseases affect connective tissues of the body. Examples of these connective tissue collagen disorders are systemic lupus erythematosus (see Pathological Conditions section), scleroderma, and rheumatoid arthritis.

Subcutaneous Layer

The subcutaneous layer of the skin is another connective tissue layer which specializes in the formation of fat. **Lipocytes** (fat cells) are predominant in the subcutaneous layer and they manufacture and store large quantities of fat. Obviously, areas of the body and individuals vary as far as fat deposition is concerned. Functionally, this layer of the skin is important in protection of the deeper tissues of the body and as a heat insulator.

III. ACCESSORY ORGANS OF THE SKIN

A. Hair

A hair fiber is composed of a tightly fused meshwork of horny cells filled with the hard protein called keratin. Hair growth is similar to the growth of the epidermal layer of the skin. Deep-lying cells in the hair root (see Figure 15-1) produce horny cells which move upward through the **hair follicles** (shafts or sacs that hold the hair fibers). Melanocytes are located at the root of the hair follicle and they support the melanin pigment for the horny cells of the hair fiber. Hair turns gray when the melanocytes stop producing melanin.

B. Nails

Nails are hard, keratin plates covering the dorsal surface of the last bone of each toe and finger. They are composed of horny cells that are cemented together tightly and can extend

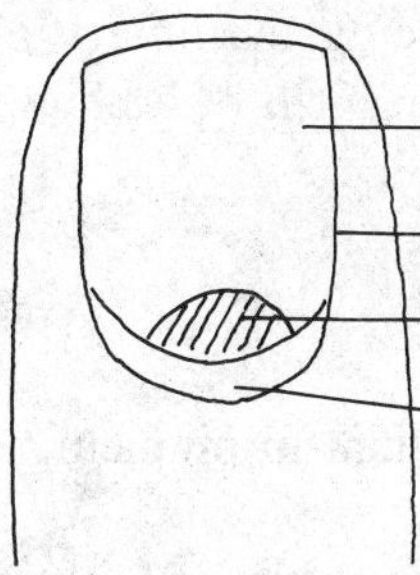

Figure 15-3 Parts of the nail.

indefinitely unless cut or broken. A nail grows in thickness and length as a result of division of cells in the region of the nail root which is at the base (proximal portion) of the nail plate.

Most nails grow about 1 mm a week, which means that fingernails may regrow in 3 to 5 months. Toenails grow more slowly than fingernails.

The **lunula** is a semilunar (half-moon) white region at the base of the nail plate, and is generally found in the thumbnail of most people and in varying degrees in other fingers. Air mixed in with keratin and cells rich in nuclei give the lunula its whitish color. The narrow band of epidermis that extends from the nail wall onto the surface is called the **cuticle** or **eponychium** (onych means nail). Figure 15-3 illustates the parts of a nail.

C. Glands

Sebaceous Glands

Sebaceous glands are located in the corium layer of the skin, and secrete an oily substance called **sebum**. Sebaceous glands are closely associated with hair follicles, and their ducts open into the hair follicle through which the sebum is released. Figure 15-1 shows the relationship of the sebaceous gland to the hair follicle. The sebaceous glands are influenced by sex hormones, which cause them to hypertrophy at puberty and atrophy in old age.

Sweat Glands

Sweat glands are tiny, coiled glands found on almost all body surfaces (about 2 million in the body). They are most numerous in the palm of the hand (3000 glands per square inch) and on the sole of the foot. Figure 15-1 illustrates how the coiled sweat gland originates deep in the corium and straightens out to extend up through the epidermis. The tiny opening on the surface is called a **pore**.

Sweat, or perspiration, is almost pure water, with dissolved materials such as salt making up less than 1 per cent of the total composition. It is colorless and odorless. The odor produced when sweat accumulates on the skin is due to the action of bacteria on the sweat.

Sweat cools the body as it evaporates into the air. Perspiration is controlled by the sympathetic nervous system whose nerve fibers are activated by the heart regulatory center in the hypothalamic region of the brain which stimulates sweating.

A special variety of sweat gland, active only from puberty onward and larger than the ordinary kind, is concentrated in a few areas of the body near the reproductive organs and in the armpits. These glands secrete an odorless sweat, but it contains certain substances that are easily broken down by bacteria on the skin. The breakdown products are responsible for the characteristic human body odor. The milk-producing mammary gland is another type of modified sweat gland; it secretes milk only after the birth of a child.

IV. VOCABULARY

albino	A person with skin deficient in pigment.
basal layer	The deepest region of the epidermis; it gives rise to all the epidermal cells.
collagen	Structural protein found in the skin and connective tissue.
corium	The middle layer of the skin; dermis.
cuticle	Band of epidermis extending from the nail wall onto the nail surface; eponychium.
dermis	The corium.
epidermis	The outermost layer of the skin.
epithelium	The layer of skin cells forming the outer and inner surfaces of the body.
eponychium	Cuticle.
fibroblast	A fiber-producing cell from which connective tissue cells develop.
hair follicle	The sac or tube within which each hair grows.
heparin	An anticoagulant substance released by special cells (mast cells) in the corium.
histamine	A substance released by mast cells in the corium during an allergic reaction.
histiocyte	A large phagocyte present in connective tissue of the skin; macrophage.
horny cell	A keratin-filled cell in the epidermis.
integumentary system	The skin and its accessory structures such as hair and nails.
keratin	A hard, protein material found in the epidermis, hair, and nails. Keratin means "horn" and is commonly found in the horns of animals.
lipocyte	A fat cell.
lunula	The half-moon–shaped white area at the base of a nail.
macrophage	Histiocyte.

mast cell A cell found in connective tissue and in the corium layer of the skin. It secretes histamine and heparin.

melanin A black pigment formed by melanocytes in the epidermis.

sebaceous gland An oil-secreting gland in the corium which is associated with hair follicles.

sebum An oil substance secreted by sebaceous glands.

squamous epithelium Flat, scalelike cells composing the epidermis.

strata Layers (of cells).

stratified Arranged in layers.

stratum corneum The outermost layer of the epidermis which consists of flattened, keratinized (horny) cells.

subcutaneous tissue Innermost layer of the skin, containing fat tissue.

V. COMBINING FORMS

Combining Form	*Definition*	*Terminology*	*Meaning*
derm/o dermat/o	skin	hypodermic	________________
		dermatitis	________________
		dermatoplasty	________________
		erythroderma	________________
		epidermolysis	________________
		Loosening of the epidermis.	
cutane/o	skin	subcutaneous	________________
xer/o	dry	xeroderma	________________
ichthy/o	dry, scaly *(fishlike)*	ichthyosis	________________
pachy/o	thick, heavy	pachyderma	________________
xanth/o	yellow	xanthoderma	________________

		xanthoma ________________
		Nodules develop under the skin owing to excess lipid deposits.
melan/o	black	melanocyte ________________
leuk/o	white	leukoderma ________________
alb/o albin/o	white	albinism ________________
erythem/o	flushed, redness	erythema ________________
kerat/o	horny, hard	keratosis ________________
	(also used to describe the cornea of the eye)	*Condition of the skin marked by horny keratinized growths (a callus, for example).*
acanth/o	thorny, spiny	acanthosis ________________
	(refers to an epidermal layer called the prickle-cell layer)	*Thickening of the epidermis.*
onych/o	nail	eponychium ________________
	(used to describe nail conditions)	onychophagia ________________
		paronychia ________________
		Inflammation of soft tissue around the nail.
ungu/o	nail	subungual ________________
myc/o	fungus, a type of plant	onychomycosis ________________
		dermatomycosis ________________
seb/o	sebum	seborrhea ________________
	(secretion from sebaceous glands)	*Seborrheic dermatitis is commonly known as dandruff.*
diaphor/o	profuse sweating	diaphoresis ________________
hidr/o	sweat	anhidrosis ________________
		hidradenitis ________________
squam/o	scale	squamous ________________

histi/o	tissue	histiocyte ________________
adip/o	fat	adipose ________________
steat/o	fat, sebum	steatoma ________________ *Sebaceous cyst; fatty mass within a sebaceous gland.*
lip/o	fat	lipoma ________________
trich/o	hair	trichomycosis ________________
pil/o	hair	pilosebaceous ________________
caus/o	burn	causalgia ________________ *Sensations are commonly felt in skin and muscles.*
-phyte	plant	dermatophytosis ________________ *Examples are fungal infections of the hands and feet.*
de-	lack of	depigmentation ________________

VI. LESIONS, SYMPTOMS, AND PATHOLOGICAL CONDITIONS OF THE SKIN

Cutaneous Lesions

A **lesion** is a pathological or traumatic discontinuity in tissue. The following terms describe common skin lesions, which are illustrated in Figure 15-4:

macule Discolored (especially reddened) flat lesion.

Freckles, tattoo marks, and flat moles are examples.

papule Solid elevation of the skin.

Warts (verrucae), which are caused by a virus infection, are an example. Papules differ in size and location within the corium and subcutaneous tissue.

wheal Smooth, slightly elevated, edematous area that is redder or paler than the surrounding skin.

A wheal is a type of papule which may be circumscribed, as in a mosquito bite, or involve a wide area, as in allergic reactions. Wheals are commonly known as **hives**, and are often accompanied by itching.

vesicle Circumscribed collection of clear fluid (blister).

Vesicles are found in burns, allergy, and dermatitis. **Bullae** (singular: bulla) are large blisters.

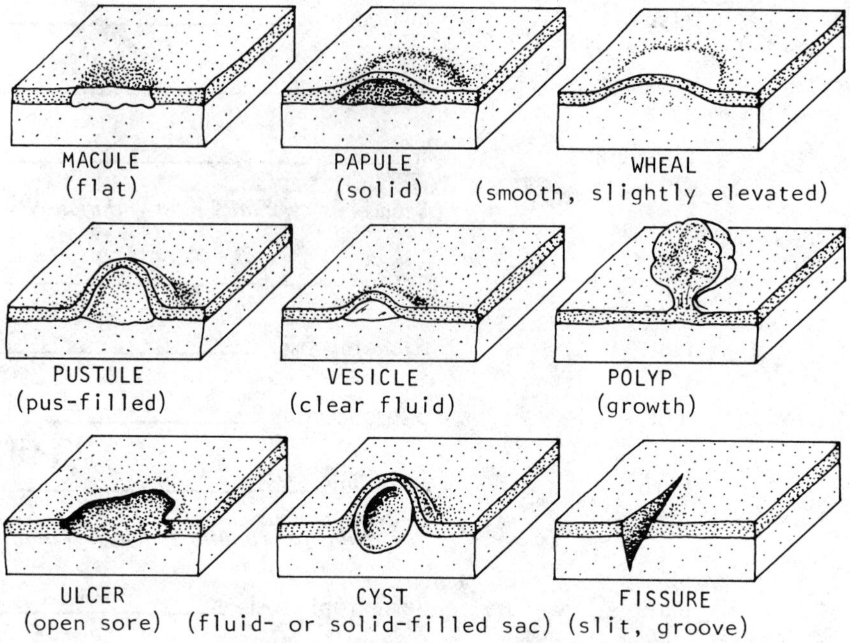

Figure 15-4 Cutaneous lesions.

pustule Circumscribed collection of pus (abscess of the skin).

Since vesicles commonly coexist with pustules, the term vesicopustular is common.

polyp A mushroom-like growth extending on a stalk from the surface of a mucous membrane.

Polyps are most commonly found in the uterus, nose, mouth, urinary bladder, and tubes of the digestive tract.

ulcer An open sore or erosion of the skin or mucous membrane.

Ulcers usually involve loss of tissue substance and formation of pus (abscess).

cyst A closed sac or pouch containing fluid or semisolid material.

Examples of cysts are: **pilonidal cyst**, which is found over the sacral area of the back in the midline and contains hairs (pil- means hair; nid- means nest); and **follicular cyst**, which arises from glandular sacs in the ovary.

fissure A groove or cracklike sore.

Naturally occurring fissures are found in the brain, spinal cord, and liver; pathological fissures, which resemble ulcer-like sores, can occur in the anal region.

Symptoms

alopecia

Baldness.

This condition can result normally from the aging process, or be induced by drugs, illness, or forms of dermatitis. It occurs when replacement of hair fibers fails to keep up with normal hair loss.

urticaria

Hives.

This condition is basically a localized edema (swelling) in association with itching. Etiology may be allergy to foods or drugs or psychological stimuli.

pruritus

Itching.

Pruritus is associated with most forms of dermatitis, and other conditions as well. It arises as a result of stimulation of the nerve network in the skin by enzymes released in allergic reactions and by irritations caused by substances from the blood or foreign bodies.

ecchymosis

Purplish, macular patch.

Ecchymoses (ec- means out; chym- means to pour) are caused by hemorrhages into the skin. They are commonly known as black and blue marks or bruises.

petechiae

Small, pinpoint hemorrhages.

Petechiae are smaller versions of ecchymoses.

purpura

Merging ecchymoses and petechiae over any part of the body.

cicatrix

Scar left by a healed wound.

Keloids are abnormally raised, thickened scars that form in the skin after trauma or surgical incision.

vitiligo

Loss of pigment in areas of the skin (milk-white patches).

The condition is often found in the tropics and the etiology is unknown.

Pathological Conditions

acne

Inflammatory papular and pustular eruption of the skin.

Acne vulgaris (ordinary) is the common variety of acne. It is caused by the build-up of sebum and keratin in pores of the skin. This material forms **comedones** (singular: **comedo**) or blackheads. Bacteria in the skin break down the sebum, producing inflammation in the surrounding tissue. Papules, pustules, abscesses, and cysts can thus form. Treatment consists of long-term antibiotic use (a solution can be applied directly to the skin) and medications to dry the skin. Retinoic acid is an effective new treatment for severe cystic acne.

burns

Lesion caused by heat contact.

Burn lesions are usually classified into three types: **first degree burns** (no blisters; superficial lesions mainly in the epidermis; hyperesthesia; and erythema); **second degree burns** (damage to the epidermis and corium; blisters; erythema; and hyperesthesia); and **third degree burns** (both the epidermis and corium are destroyed and subcutaneous layer is damaged, leaving charred, white tissue).

Burns may be due to caustic chemicals, radiation, heat, or the rubbing of objects against the skin.

tinea

Infection of the skin caused by a fungus (a type of plant).

There are many different forms of this fungus skin disease. Examples are ringworm and athlete's foot. Scaling, pruritus, and red patches on the skin are symptoms. Fungistatic preparations for application on the skin can be helpful.

decubitus ulcer

Bedsore.

Decubitus means "lying down." Ulcers occur over bony areas that have been subjected to pressure against a hard external object such as a bed.

gangrene

Death of tissue associated with loss of blood supply.

In this condition, ischemia resulting from injury, inflammation, frostbite, diseases such as diabetes, or arteriosclerosis can lead to necrosis of tissue, followed by bacterial invasion and putrefaction.

eczema

Inflammatory skin disease with erythematous, papulovesicular lesions.

This chronic or acute dermatitis is often accompanied by pruritus and is often of unknown cause. Eczema is a common allergic reaction in children, but can also occur in adults. Allergy is often to foods, or to dust and pollens.

psoriasis

Chronic, recurrent dermatosis marked by silvery gray scales covering red patches on the skin.

Psoriasis commonly occurs at the knee, elbow, or scalp. It is neither contagious nor infectious, but is due to an increased rate of growth of the basal layer of the epidermis. Its etiology is unknown. Topical lubricants, keratolytics, and steroids are treatments, but none is a cure. Phototherapy with ultraviolet light and the administration of drugs to enhance the ultraviolet light are under investigation.

impetigo

Bacterial inflammatory skin disease characterized by vesicles, pustules, and crusted-over lesions.

This is a contagious pyoderma and is usually caused by staphylococci or streptococci. Systemic use of antibiotics and proper cleansing of lesions are effective treatment.

pemphigus

Blistering (bullous) eruptions affecting the skin and mucous membranes. Pemphix is the Greek word for blister.

An adult condition in which bullous lesions appear asymptomatically and absorb into the skin, leaving pigmented spots. In severe cases, the disorder may require treatment by anti-inflammatory drugs such as a corticosteroid (hormone from the adrenal gland). Etiology is unknown.

systemic lupus erythematosus (SLE)

Inflammatory disease of the joints and collagen of the skin, as well as any organ of the body.

Lupus (meaning "wolflike"; physicians thought the shape and color of the skin lesions resembled the bite of a wolf) produces a characteristic "butterfly" pattern of redness over the cheeks and nose. In more severe cases, the extent of erythema increases and all exposed areas of the skin may be involved. The condition can affect the kidneys, joints, nervous system, and mucous membranes. Primarily a disease of females, lupus is an autoimmune condition. High levels of antibodies (ANA—antinuclear antibodies) and LE cells (leukocytes composed of nuclei that have been ejected from other antibody-damaged white blood cells) are found in the patient's blood. Ultraviolet light should be avoided; corticosteroids and immunosuppressive drugs (azathioprine; Imuran) are used to control symptoms.

SLE should be differentiated from chronic **discoid lupus erythematosus**, which is a milder scaling, plaquelike, superficial eruption of the skin confined to the face, scalp, ears, chest, arms, and back. The reddish patches heal and leave scars.

scleroderma

A chronic disease of the skin, caused by infiltration of fibrous or scar tissue into the skin.

Scleroderma leads to hardening, pigmentation, and atrophy of the skin and internal organs, such as the kidneys, lungs, and esophagus. Treatment consists of physiotherapy and palliative administration of drugs (steroids).

scabies

A contagious, parasitic infection of the skin with intense pruritus (scabere means to scratch).

Scabies is often acquired through sexual contact. Treatment with topical (on the skin) medication is effective in eliminating the scabies mite.

exanthematous viral diseases

Eruption (exanthem) of the skin due to a viral infection.

Examples of exanthematous viral illness are: **rubeola**—measles; **rubella**—German measles; and **varicella**—chickenpox.

Skin Neoplasia

Benign Neoplasms

nevus; nevi

Congenital proliferation of blood vessels or pigmented cells on the skin surface.

Moles and hemangiomas are examples.

keratoses

Thickened areas of the epidermis.

Some keratoses are pigmented and due to excessive exposure to sunlight (actinic keratosis). Seborrheic keratoses are called senile warts and occur in older patients.

leukoplakia

White, thickened patches on mucous membrane tissue of the tongue or cheek.

This may be a precancerous lesion. It is common in smokers, and may be caused by chronic inflammation.

Cancerous Lesions

basal cell carcinoma

Malignant tumor of the basal cell layer of the epidermis.

This is the most frequent type of skin cancer. It is a slow-growing tumor of the basal layer of the epidermis. It usually occurs on the upper half of the face, near the nose, and is nonmetastasizing.

squamous cell carcinoma

Malignant tumor of the squamous epithelial cells of the epidermis.

The tumor may grow in places other than the skin, wherever squamous epithelium is found (mouth, larynx, bladder, esophagus, and so forth). It may arise from **actinic** (sun-related) **keratoses** and metastasize to lymph nodes. Treatment for both basal and squamous cell carcinomas is surgical excision or radiation therapy.

malignant melanoma

Cancerous tumor composed of melanocytes.

Tumors often metastasize to the lung, liver, and brain after arising in areas of the body where pigmented cells occur. Treatment includes excision of the tumor, regional lymphadenectomy, and chemotherapy to prevent metastases.

mycosis fungoides

Rare, chronic skin disease caused by the infiltration of malignant lymphocytes.

Mycosis fungoides is characterized by generalized erythroderma and large reddish raised areas (tumors) that spread and ulcerate. In some cases, the malignant cells may involve lymph nodes and other organs. Treatment with topical nitrogen mustard and radiation can be effective in controlling the disease.

VII. LABORATORY TESTS, CLINICAL PROCEDURES, AND ABBREVIATIONS

Laboratory Tests

Bacterial analyses

Samples of **purulent** (pus-filled) material or **exudate** (fluid that accumulates in a space or passes out of tissues) are sent to the laboratory for examination to determine what type of bacteria are present.

Fungal tests

Scrapings from skin lesions are placed on a growth medium for several weeks and then examined microscopically for evidence of fungal growth.

Clinical Procedures

Skin biopsy

Skin lesions, such as pigmented nevi, chronic dermatoses, or any lesion in which there is the possibility of present or future malignant change, are removed and sent to the pathology laboratory for examination. A **punch biopsy** (used to obtain tissue in cases in which complete excision is not feasible) involves use of a surgical instrument that removes a core of tissue by rotation of its sharp, circular edge.

Skin testing for allergy or disease

The **patch test** is performed by applying to the skin a small piece of gauze or filter paper on which has been placed a suspected allergy-causing substance. If the area becomes reddened or swollen, the result is considered positive. The **scratch test** involves making several scratches in the skin and inserting a very minute amount of test material in the scratches. The test is considered negative if no reaction occurs. **Intradermal tests** are performed by injection of a reactive substance between layers of the skin and observing the skin for a subsequent reaction. This test is used for the detection of sensitivity to infectious agents such as tuberculosis (**Mantoux tests, PPD test**) or diphtheria (**Schick test**). Strong reactions indicate ongoing infection.

Abbreviations

bx	Biopsy	SLE	Systemic lupus erythematosus
Derm.	Dermatology	Subcu.	Subcutaneous
DLE	Discoid lupus erythematosus	ung.	Ointment

VIII. PRACTICAL APPLICATIONS

Pathology Report

Gross: A triangular segment of skin measuring 4 cm at its longest diameter and 2.3 cm in its lateral diameter. Skin surface presenting an irregular pigmented lesion which measures 1.4 by 1.3 cm in size. The margins of the pigmented lesion are irregular.

Micro: Sections show numerous nests of often bizarre and pleomorphic [variations in shape] malignant cells in the epidermis. Malignant cells are invading the papillary dermis, but not into the reticular dermis. Present in one section is an intradermal nevus. The melanoma is found to invade to 0.37 mm (Breslow's microstaging method).*

Final diagnosis: Malignant melanoma, superficial spreading type, Level II (Clark's staging method).*

*Breslow's and Clark's staging systems are classifications showing extent of invasion of malignant melanoma.

Disease Descriptions

1. **Candidiasis** [Candida is a yeastlike fungus]: This fungus is normally found on mucous membranes, skin, and vaginal mucosa. Under certain circumstances (excessive warmth, administration of birth control pills, antibiotics and corticosteroids, debilitated states, infancy) it can change to a pathogen and cause localized or generalized mucocutaneous disease. Examples are paronychial lesions, lesions in areas of the body where rubbing opposed surfaces is common (groin, perianal, axillary, inframammary, and interdigital), thrush (white plaques attached to oral or vaginal mucous membranes), and vulvovaginitis.
2. **Cellulitis:** This is a common nonsuppurative infection of connective tissue with severe inflammation of the dermal and subcutaneous layers of the skin. Cellulitis appears on an extremity as a reddish brown area of edematous skin. A surgical wound, puncture, skin ulcer, or patch of dermatitis is the usual means of entry for bacteria (most cases are caused by streptococci). Therapy entails rest, elevation, hot wet packs, and penicillin. Any cellulitis on the face should be given special attention because the infection may extend directly to the brain.

IX. EXERCISES

A. Complete the following sentences using the terms listed below:

corium	heparin	lunula
melanin	histamine	histiocyte
keratin	sebum	stratum corneum
collagen	basal layer	lipocyte

1. An anticoagulant substance released by mast cells is called ________________.
2. A fat cell is known as a ________________.
3. The half-moon-shaped white area at the base of a nail is called the ________________.
4. A structural protein found in the skin and in connective tissue is called ________________.

5. A black pigment found in the epidermis is called ________________.

6. A substance released by mast cells during an allergic reaction is known as ________________.

7. The deepest region of the epidermis is called the ________________.

8. The outermost layer of the epidermis which consists of flattened, keratinized cells is called the ________________.

9. An oily substance secreted by sebaceous glands is called ________________.

10. The middle layer of the skin is called the dermis or the ________________.

11. A large phagocyte present in the connective tissue of the skin is called a ________________.

12. A hard, protein material found in the epidermis, hair, and nails is called ________________.

B. Give meanings for the following terms:

1. fibroblast ________________________________
2. epidermis ________________________________
3. stratified ________________________________
4. albino ________________________________
5. diaphoresis ________________________________
6. erythema ________________________________
7. seborrhea ________________________________
8. paronychia ________________________________
9. dermatophytosis ________________________________
10. causalgia ________________________________

11. integumentary system ______________________

12. hair follicle ______________________

C. *Match the term in Column I with a related term in Column II:*

Column I	*Column II*
1. squamous epithelium ______	A. keratin
2. eponychium ______	B. dermis
3. macrophage ______	C. scalelike cells
4. horny cell ______	D. heparin
5. subcutaneous tissue ______	E. histiocyte
6. mast cell ______	F. melanin
7. corium ______	G. cuticle
8. melanocyte ______	H. lipocyte

D. *Build medical terms:*

1. Surgical repair of the skin ______________________
2. Thick, heavy skin ______________________
3. Inflammation of sweat glands ______________________
4. Abnormal condition of proliferation of horny, keratinized cells ______________________
5. Abnormal condition of dry, scaly skin ______________________
6. Loosening of the epidermis ______________________
7. Yellow tumor (nodule under the skin) ______________________
8. Under the nail ______________________
9. Abnormal condition of fungus in the hair ______________________
10. Abnormal condition of lack of sweat ______________________

E. *Give meanings for the following combining forms:*

1. pachy/o ______________
2. adip/o ______________
3. acanth/o ______________
4. xanth/o ______________
5. myc/o ______________
6. onych/o ______________
7. pil/o ______________
8. xer/o ______________
9. steat/o ______________
10. trich/o ______________

F. *Match the cutaneous lesion with its description below:*

polyp
papule
vesicle
pustule
wheal
ulcer
fissure
macule
cyst

1. Circumscribed collection of clear fluid (blister) ______________
2. Smooth, slightly elevated edematous area (hive) ______________
3. Discolored, flat lesion (freckle) ______________
4. A groove or cracklike sore ______________
5. A mushroom-like growth extending from the surface of a mucous membrane

   ____
6. Circumscribed collection of pus (abscess) ______________
7. A closed sac containing fluid or semisolid material ______________
8. Open sore or erosion of the skin ______________
9. Solid elevation of the skin (wart) ______________

G. *Give medical terms for the following:*

1. baldness ______________
2. purplish, macular patch caused by hemorrhages into the skin ______________
3. itching ______________

4. scar left by a healed wound ______________________

5. loss of pigment in areas of the skin ______________________

6. merging ecchymoses over the body ______________________

7. blackhead ______________________

8. small pinpoint hemorrhages ______________________

H. *Match the pathological skin condition with its description:*

impetigo	malignant melanoma
psoriasis	basal cell carcinoma
gangrene	squamous cell carcinoma
eczema	pemphigus
tinea	decubitus ulcer
scleroderma	systemic lupus erythematosus

1. Malignant neoplasm originating in scalelike cells of the epidermis ______________________

2. Bullous eruptions on the skin ______________________

3. Fungal skin infection ______________________

4. Hard, fibrous, scar tissue infiltrates the skin ______________________

5. Bedsore ______________________

6. Necrosis of skin tissue resulting from ischemia ______________________

7. Chronic inflammatory skin disease with erythematous, pustular, or papular lesions ______________________

8. Widespread inflammatory disease of the joints and collagen of the skin with "butterfly" rash on the face ______________________

9. Cancerous tumor composed of melanocytes ______________________

10. Chronic, recurrent dermatosis marked by silvery gray scales covering red patches on the skin ______________________

11. Malignant neoplasm originating from the basal layer of the epidermis ______________

____

12. Contagious, infectious pyoderma ______________

I. Give meanings for the following terms:

1. scabies ______________
2. rubeola ______________
3. varicella ______________
4. rubella ______________
5. mycosis fungoides ______________
6. leukoplakia ______________
7. discoid lupus erythematosus ______________
8. exanthematous ______________
9. actinic keratosis ______________
10. keloid ______________
11. bullae ______________
12. nevus ______________
13. pilonidal cyst ______________
14. urticaria ______________
15. comedo ______________

J. Describe the following types of burns:

1. Second degree burn ______________
2. First degree burn ______________
3. Third degree burn ______________

K. Give short answers:

1. Two skin tests for allergy are ________________ and ________________.

2. The ________________ test is an intradermal test for diphtheria.

3. The ________________ test or ________________ test is a test for tuberculosis.

4. Purulent means ________________.

5. A surgical procedure to core out a disk of skin tissue for microscopic examination is called a ________________.

ANSWERS

A.

1. heparin
2. lipocyte
3. lunula
4. collagen
5. melanin
6. histamine
7. basal layer
8. stratum corneum
9. sebum
10. corium
11. histiocyte
12. keratin

B.

1. a fiber-producing cell present in skin and connective tissues
2. the outermost layer of the skin
3. arranged in layers
4. one who has skin deficient in pigment
5. profuse sweating
6. redness of the skin
7. excessive discharge from sebaceous glands
8. inflammation involving the tissue surrounding the fingernail
9. fungal infection of the skin; athlete's foot is a dermatophytosis
10. a burning pain
11. the skin and its accessory structures such as hair and nails
12. the sac within which each hair grows

C.

1. C
2. G
3. E
4. A
5. H
6. D
7. B
8. F

D.

1. dermatoplasty
2. pachyderma
3. hidradenitis
4. keratosis
5. ichthyosis
6. epidermolysis
7. xanthoma
8. subungual
9. trichomycosis
10. anhidrosis

E.

1. thick
2. fat
3. thorny, spiny
4. yellow
5. fungus
6. nail
7. hair
8. dry
9. fat, sebum
10. hair

F.

1. vesicle
2. wheal
3. macule
4. fissure
5. polyp
6. pustule
7. cyst
8. ulcer
9. papule

G.

1. alopecia
2. ecchymosis
3. pruritus
4. cicatrix
5. vitiligo
6. purpura
7. comedo
8. petechiae

H.

1. squamous cell carcinoma
2. pemphigus
3. tinea
4. scleroderma
5. decubitus ulcer
6. gangrene
7. eczema
8. systemic lupus erythematosus
9. malignant melanoma
10. psoriasis
11. basal cell carcinoma
12. impetigo

I.

1. contagious parasitic infection of the skin with intense pruritus
2. measles
3. chickenpox
4. German measles
5. chronic skin disease caused by infiltration of the skin by malignant lymphocytes
6. white patches on mucous membranes of the tongue or cheek
7. scaling, plaquelike superficial eruption of the skin; mild form of systemic lupus erythematosus
8. characterized by an eruption or rash
9. thickening of the epidermis related to excessive exposure to sunlight
10. abnormally raised, thickened scars which form after surgery or trauma to the skin
11. large blisters (vesicles)
12. mole
13. sac of fluid and hair over the sacral region of the back
14. hives
15. blackhead

J.

1. damage to the epidermis and corium with blisters, erythema, and hyperesthesia
2. damage to the epidermis with erythema and hyperesthesia; no blisters
3. destruction of both epidermis and corium and damage to subcutaneous layer

K.

1. scratch; patch
2. Schick
3. Mantoux; PPD
4. pus-filled
5. punch biopsy

X. PRONUNCIATION OF TERMS

acanthosis	ăk-ăn-THŌ-sĭs
acne	ĂK-nē
adipose	ĂD-ĭ-pōs
albinism	ĂL-bĭ-nĭzm

albino	ăl-BĪ-nō
anhidrosis	ăn-hĭ-DRŌ-sĭs
basal	BĀ-săl
bulla	BŬL-ă
causalgia	kăw-ZĂL-jă
cicatrix	SĬK-ă-trĭks; sĭ-KĀ-trĭks
collagen	KŎL-ă-jĕn
comedo	KŎM-ĕ-dō
corium	KŌ-rē-ŭm
cuticle	KŪ-tĭ-k'l
decubitus	dē-KŪ-bĭ-tŭs
depigmentation	dē-pĭg-mĕn-TĀ-shŭn
dermatomycosis	dĕr-mă-tō-mī-KŌ-sĭs
dermatophytosis	dĕr-mă-tō-fī-TŌ-sĭs
dermatoplasty	DĔR-mă-tō-plăs-tē
dermis	DĔR-mĭs
diaphoresis	dī-ă-fō-RĒ-sĭs
ecchymosis	ĕk-ĭ-MŌ-sĭs
eczema	ĔK-zĕ-mă
epidermolysis	ĕp-ĭ-dĕr-MŎL-ĭ-sĭs
eponychium	ĕp-ō-NĬK-ē-ŭm
erythema	ĕr-ĭ-THĒ-mă
erythroderma	ĕ-rĭth-rō-DĔR-mă
exanthematous	ĕks-ăn-THĔM-ă-tŭs
fibroblast	FĪ-brō-blăst
fissure	FĬSH-ŭr
follicle	FŎL-ĭ-k'l
gangrene	GĂNG-grēn
hidradenitis	hī-drăd-ĕ-NĪ-tĭs
histamine	HĬS-tă-mēn
histiocyte	HĬS-tē-ō-sīt
impetigo	ĭm-pĕ-TĪ-gō

integumentary	ĭn-tĕg-ū-MĔN-tăr-ē
keloid	KĒ-loyd
keratin	KĔR-ă-tĭn
keratosis	kĕr-ă-TŌ-sĭs
leukoplakia	lū-kō-PLĀ-kē-ă
lipocyte	LĬP-ō-sīt
lipoma	lī-PŌ-mă or lĭ-PŌ-mă
lunula	LŪ-nū-lă
lupus erythematosus	LŪ-pŭs ĕr-ĭ-thē-mă-TŌ-sŭs
macule	MĂK-ūl
melanin	MĔL-ă-nĭn
melanocyte	mĕ-LĂN-ō-sīt; MĔL-ă-nō-sīt
melanoma	mĕl-ă-NŌ-mă
mycosis fungoides	mī-KŌ-sĭs fŭng-GOY-dēz
nevus	NĒ-vŭs
onychophagia	ŏn-ĭ-kō-FĀ-jē-ă
papule	PĂP-ūl
paronychia	păr-ō-NĬK-ē-ă
pemphigus	PĔM-fĭ-gŭs
petechiae	pĕ-TĒ-kē-ē
pilonidal	pī-lō-NĪ-dăl
pilosebaceous	pī-lō-sĕ-BĀ-shŭs
polyp	PŎL-ĭp
pruritus	proo-RĪ-tŭs
psoriasis	sō-RĪ-ă-sĭs
purulent	PŪ-roo-lĕnt
pustule	PŬS-tūl
sebaceous	sĕ-BĀ-shŭs
seborrheic	sĕb-ō-RĒ-ĭk
sebum	SĒ-bŭm
squamous	SKWĀ-mŭs
steatoma	stē-ă-TŌ-mă

stratified	STRĂT-ĭ-fīd
stratum	STRĂ-tŭm; STRĀ-tŭm
subcutaneous	sŭb-kū-TĀ-nē-ŭs
tinea	TĬN-ē-ă
trichomycosis	trĭk-ō-mī-KŌ-sĭs
urticaria	ŭr-tĭ-KĀ-rē-ă
verruca	vĕ-RO͞O-kă
vesicle	VĔS-ĭ-k'l
vitiligo	vĭt-ĭ-LĪ-gō
wheal	hwēl; wēl
xanthoderma	zăn-thō-DĔR-mă
xanthoma	zăn-THŌ-mă
xeroderma	zē-rō-DĔR-mă

REVIEW SHEET 15

Combining Forms

acanth/o	______________	lip/o	______________
adip/o	______________	melan/o	______________
alb/o	______________	myc/o	______________
albin/o	______________	onych/o	______________
caus/o	______________	pachy/o	______________
cutane/o	______________	pil/o	______________
derm/o	______________	py/o	______________
dermat/o	______________	seb/o	______________
diaphor/o	______________	squam/o	______________
erythem/o	______________	steat/o	______________
hidr/o	______________	trich/o	______________
histi/o	______________	ungu/o	______________
ichthy/o	______________	xanth/o	______________
kerat/o	______________	xer/o	______________
leuk/o	______________		

Additional Terms

acne (437)

actinic keratosis (440)

alopecia (437)

basal cell carcinoma (440)

basal layer (432)

bullae (435)

burns (438)

cicatrix (437)

collagen (432)

comedo (437)

corium (432)

cuticle (432)

cyst (436)

decubitus ulcer (438)

dermis (432)

discoid lupus erythematosus (439)

ecchymosis (437)

eczema (438)

epidermis (432)

epithelium (432)

eponychium (432)

exanthematous viral diseases (439)

exudate (441)

fibroblast (432)

fissure (436)

follicular cyst (436)

gangrene (438)

hair follicle (432)

heparin (432)

histamine (432)

histiocyte (432)

hives (435)

horny cell (432)

impetigo (438)

integumentary system (432)

intradermal tests (441)

keloid (437)

keratin (432)

keratosis (440)

leukoplakia (440)

lunula (432)

macrophage (432)

macule (435)

malignant melanoma (440)

Mantoux test (441)

mast cell (433)

melanin (433)

mycosis fungoides (440)

nevus (440)

papule (435)

paronychia (434)

patch test (441)

pemphigus (439)

petechiae (437)

pilonidal cyst (436)

polyp (436)

PPD test (441)

pruritus (437)

psoriasis (438)

punch biopsy (441)

purpura (437)

purulent (441)

pustule (436)

rubella (439)

rubeola (439)

scabies (439)

Schick test (441)

scleroderma (439)

scratch test (441)

sebaceous cyst (435)

sebaceous gland (433)

seborrheic dermatitis (434)

sebum (433)

squamous cell carcinoma (440)

strata (433)

stratum corneum (433)

systemic lupus erythematosus (439)

tinea (438)

ulcer (436)

urticaria (437)

varicella (439)

verrucae (435)

vesicle (435)

vitiligo (435)

warts (435)

wheal (435)

CHAPTER 16

SENSE ORGANS: THE EYE AND THE EAR

In this chapter you will:

- Identify the location and function of the major parts of the eye and the ear;
- Name the combining forms, prefixes, and suffixes most commonly used to describe these organs and their parts;
- Describe the pathological conditions which may affect the eye and ear; and
- Identify clinical procedures which pertain to ophthalmology and otology.

This chapter is divided into the following sections:

I. INTRODUCTION

In the previous chapter, we learned that the sensitive nerve endings in the corium layer of the skin receive impulses from various stimuli applied to the external surfaces of the body. These nerve endings transmit electrical messages, initiated by the stimuli, to regions of the brain (cerebrum and thalamus) so that we can recognize sensations such as temperature, touch, pain, and pressure. In Chapter 10 (Nervous System), we learned that nerve cells which carry impulses from a sense organ or sensory receptor area, such as the skin, taste buds, and **olfactory** regions (centers of smell in the nose) to the brain are called **afferent sensory neurons**.

The **eye** and the **ear** are sense organs, like the skin, taste buds, and olfactory regions. As such, they are receptors whose sensitive cells may be activated by a particular form of energy or stimulus in the external or internal environment. The sensitive cells in the eye and ear respond to the stimulus by initiating a series of nerve impulses along afferent sensory neurons which lead to the brain.

No matter what kind of stimulus is applied to a particular receptor, the sensation felt is determined by the regions in the brain which are connected to that receptor. Thus, mechanical injury which might stimulate receptor cells in the eye and the ear would produce sensations of vision (flashes of light) and sound (ringing in the ears). Similarly, if one could make a nerve connection between the sensitive receptor cells of the ear and the area in the brain associated with sight, it would be possible to perceive, or "see," sounds.

STIMULUS —applied to→ RECEPTOR CELLS IN EAR AND EYE —which excite→ AFFERENT NERVE FIBERS —which carry impulse to→ BRAIN } where nerve impulses are translated into sound sensations and visual images

Figure 16-1 Pattern of events in stimulation of a sense organ.

Figure 16–1 is a flow diagram recapitulating the general pattern of events when such stimuli as light and sound are applied to sense organs such as the eye and ear.

II. THE EYE

A. Anatomy and Physiology

Label Figure 16–2 as you read the following:

Light rays enter the dark center of the eye, the **pupil** (1). The **conjunctiva** (2) is a mucous membrane that lines the eyelids and coats the anterior portion of the eyeball over the white of the eye. The **cornea** (3) is a fibrous, transparent tissue that extends over the pupil and colored portion of the eye. The function of the cornea is to bend, or **refract**, the rays of light so that they are focused properly on the sensitive receptor cells in the posterior region of the eye. The **sclera**

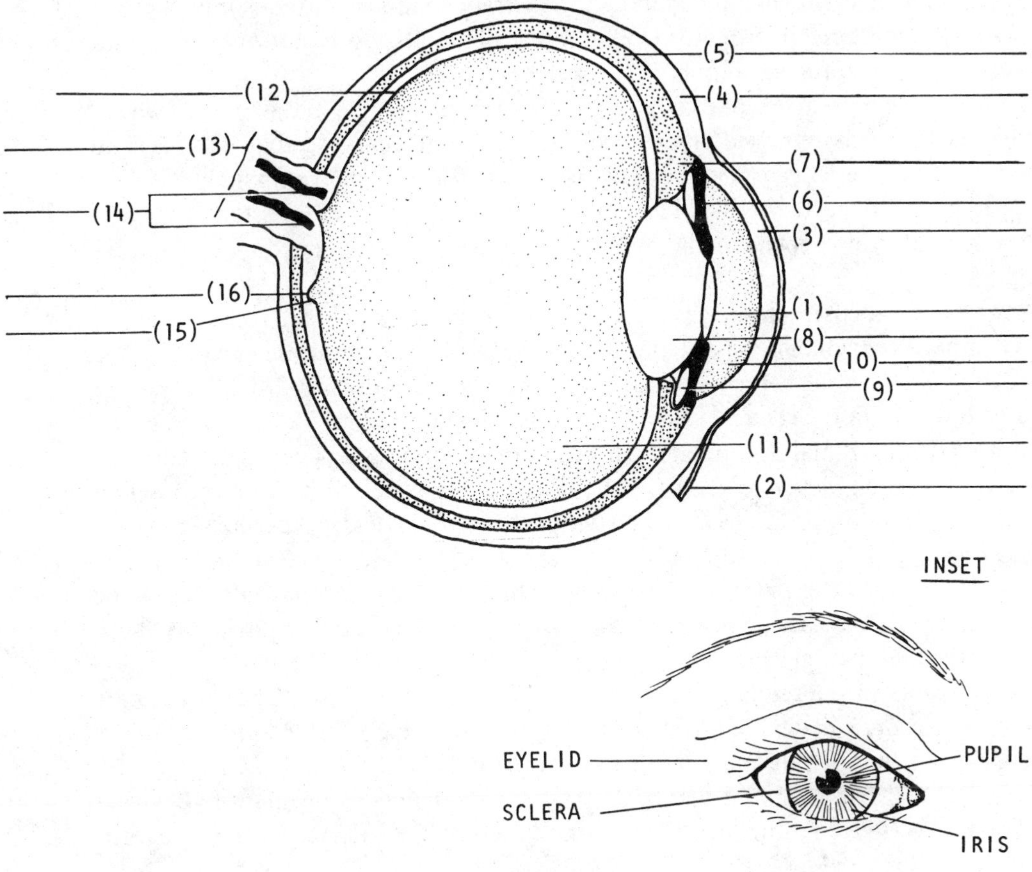

Figure 16-2 The eye.

(4), or white of the eye, is a tough, fibrous supportive tissue that extends from the optic nerve in the back of the eye to the cornea on the anterior surface of the eyeball.

The **choroid** (5) is a membranous lining inside the sclera and contains many blood vessels which supply nutrients to the eye. This vascular layer is continuous with the **iris** (6) and the **ciliary body** (7) on the anterior surface of the eye.

The iris is the colored portion of the eye which surrounds the pupil. Two sets of iris muscles (circular and radial) respond to bright and dim light by contracting. The circular muscles constrict the pupil in bright light, and the radial muscles dilate the pupil in dim light, thereby regulating the amount of light admitted to the interior of the eyeball. The inset in Figure 16–2 shows the iris and its relationship to the pupil.

The ciliary body, on each side of the **crystalline lens** (8), contains ciliary muscles which can adjust the shape and thickness of the lens. These changes in the shape of the lens (which lies posterior to the iris) aid in the **refraction** (bending) of light rays. When objects are less than 20 feet away, the rays of light coming from them would tend to be focused improperly if only the cornea were to bend the light rays. The cornea's refractive powers are not adequate to properly focus the image directly on the sensitive receptor cells at the back of the eye. Therefore, the lens is constricted and thickened by the ciliary body and further refracts the rays of light so that the image is properly focused. This refractive power of the lens is called **accommodation**.

Besides regulating the shape of the lens, the ciliary body also secretes a fluid called **aqueous humor**, which flows through the **posterior chamber** (9) and **anterior chamber** (10) of the eye. The fluid is constantly produced and leaves the eye through veins which carry it into the bloodstream. Another cavity of the eye is called the **vitreous chamber** (11), which is a large region behind the lens filled with a soft jelly-like material, the **vitreous humor**. Vitreous humor is not constantly reformed and its escape from the eye can cause blindness. Both the aqueous and the vitreous humors function to further refract light rays.

The **retina** (12) is the sensitive nerve layer of the eye. As light energy, in the form of waves, travels through the eye, it is refracted (by the cornea, lens, and fluids) so that it focuses on sensitive receptor cells of the retina called the **rods** and **cones**. There are approximately 6 million cones and 120 million rods in the retina. The cones are more sensitive in light than the rods. Color and sharpness of vision depend on the cone cells. Rods function better in dim light and are helpful in night vision.

Light energy, when focused on the retina, causes a chemical change in the rods and cones, initiating nerve impulses which then travel from the eye to the brain via the **optic nerve** (13). The region in the eye where the optic nerve meets the retina is called the **optic disk** (14). The **macula lutea** (15) is a yellow spot in the center of the retina which contains a pit, or depression, called the **fovea centralis** (16). This small section of the retina, largely composed of cones, functions as the area of sharpest vision. Figure 16–3 shows the retina of a normal eye as seen through an ophthalmoscope. The **fundus** of the eye is this posterior, inner part which is visualized through the ophthalmoscope.

Figure 16–4 illustrates the pathway of the light-stimulated nervous impulse from the sensitive cells of the retina to the visual region of the cerebral cortex in the brain. Label this figure as you read the following paragraph:

The rods and cones in the **retina** (A) synapse (meet) with neurons that lead to the **optic nerve fibers** (B). As the optic nerve fibers travel into the brain, the fibers located more medially cross in an area called the **optic chiasma** (C). Nerve fibers from the right half of each retina now form an **optic tract** (D), synapsing in the **thalamus** (E) of the brain and ending in the right visual region of the **cerebral cortex** (F). Similarly, fibers from the left half of each retina merge to form

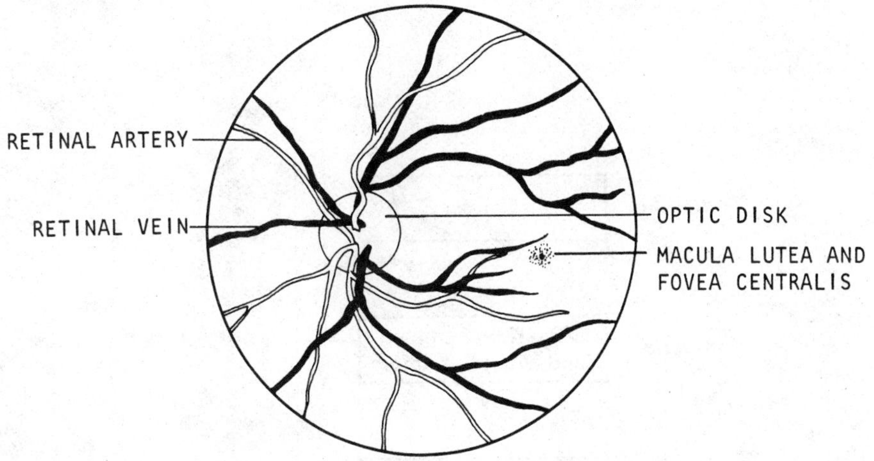

Figure 16-3 The posterior, inner part (fundus) of the eye, showing the retina as seen through an ophthalmoscope.

the optic tract and pass from the thalamus to the left region of the **cerebral cortex** (G). In the visual area of the cerebral cortex, the images are fused and a single visual sensation with a three-dimensional effect is experienced. This is called **binocular vision**.

Study Figure 16–5, which summarizes the pathway of light rays from the conjunctival membrane to the inner visual region in the cerebral cortex of the brain.

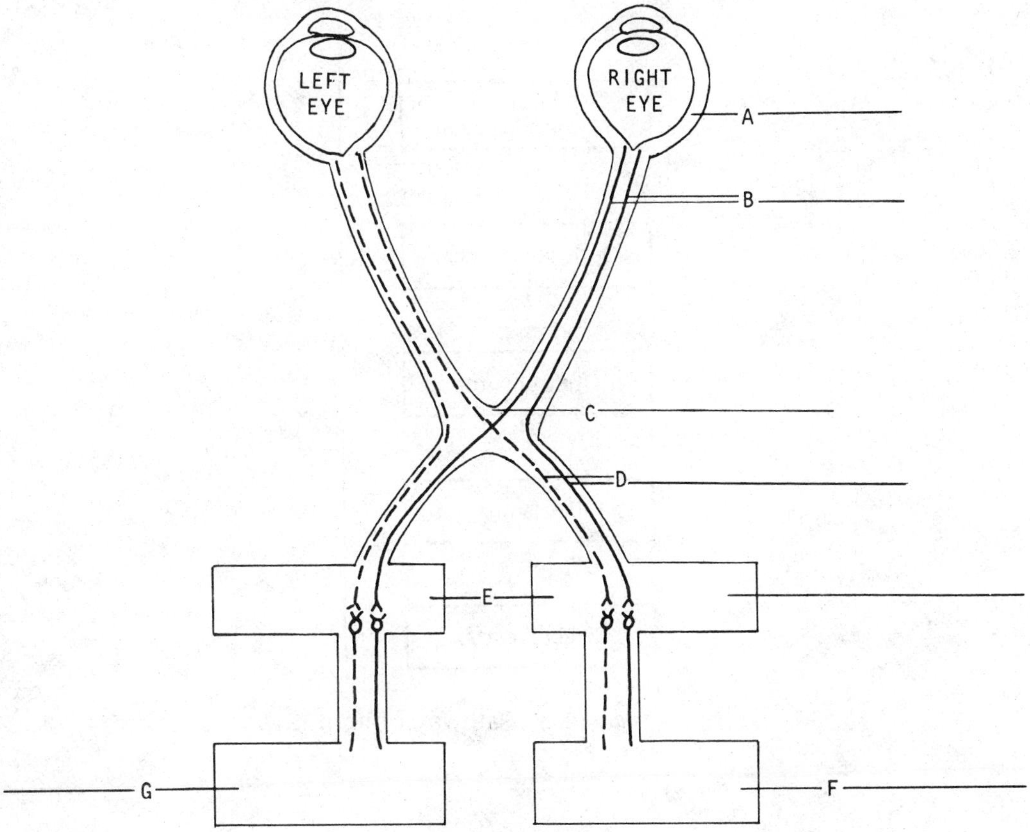

Figure 16-4 Visual pathway.

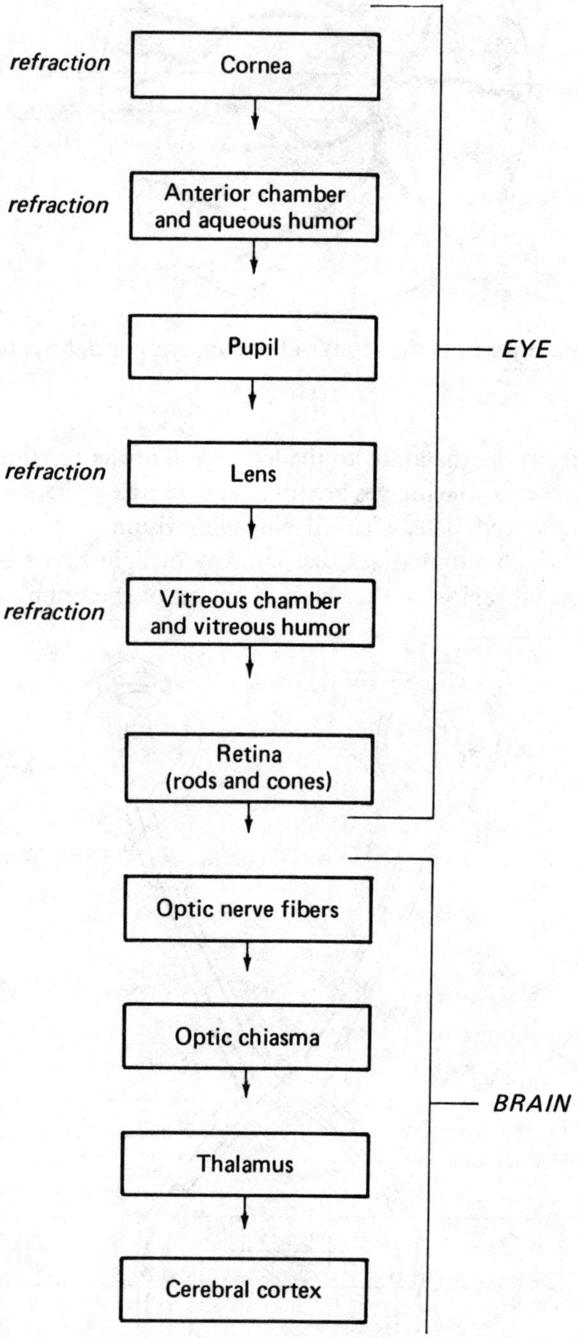

Figure 16-5 Pathway of light rays.

B. Vocabulary

accommodation	The normal adjustment of the crystalline lens by the ciliary muscle, which makes the lens fatter or thinner to bring an object into focus on the retina.
anterior chamber	The area behind the cornea and in front of the crystalline lens and iris. It contains aqueous humor.
aqueous humor	Fluid produced by the ciliary body and found in the anterior and posterior chambers.
biconvex	Having two sides which are rounded, elevated, and curved evenly, like part of a sphere.
binocular vision	Normal vision with two (bi-) eyes.
choroid layer	The middle, vascular layer of the eye, between the retina and the sclera.
ciliary body	A structure on each side of the crystalline lens which connects the choroid and the iris. It contains the ciliary muscles, which control the shape of the lens, and secretes aqueous humor.
cones	Photosensitive receptor cells in the retina that change light energy into a nerve impulse. Cones make the perception of color possible.
conjunctiva	A delicate membrane lining the eyelids and covering the exposed surfaces of the sclera.
cornea	A fibrous layer of clear tissue that extends over the anterior portion of the eyeball.
crystalline lens	A transparent, biconvex body behind the pupil of the eye. It can bend light rays to bring them in focus on the retina.
fovea centralis	The tiny pit or depression in the retina that is the region of clearest vision.
fundus of the eye	The posterior, inner part of the eye.
iris	The colored portion of the eye.
macula lutea	A yellowish region on the retina; contains the fovea centralis.
olfactory	Pertaining to the sense of smell.
optic chiasma	The point at which the fibers of the optic nerve cross in the brain (chiasma means crossing).
optic disk	The region at the back of the eye where the optic nerve meets the retina.

optic nerve	The cranial nerve that carries impulses from the retina to the brain (cerebral cortex).
posterior chamber	The area behind the iris; contains aqueous humor.
pupil	The dark opening of the eye, surrounded by the iris, through which light rays pass.
refraction	Bending of light rays by the cornea, lens, and fluids of the eye to bring the rays into focus on the retina. Refract means to break (fract) back (re-).
retina	The sensitive nerve cell layer of the eye which contains receptor cells called rods and cones.
rods	Photosensitive receptor cells of the retina that transmit light waves into a nerve impulse. Rods contain rhodopsin (a pigment), which is essential for vision in dim light.
sclera	The tough, white, outer coat of the eyeball.
vitreous chamber	Area behind the lens of the eye. It contains vitreous humor.
vitreous humor	Soft, jelly-like material that fills the large, inner, vitreous chamber of the eye.

C. Combining Forms and Suffixes

Combining Form	*Definition*	*Terminology*	*Meaning*
ophthalm/o	eye	ophthalmologist	______
		A physician who specializes in disorders of the eye.	
		ophthalmoplegia	______
		ophthalmic	______
ocul/o	eye	intraocular	______
opt/o	eye, vision	optic	______
		optician	______
		A person who grinds lenses and fits glasses.	
		optometrist	______
		Can examine eyes to determine vision problems and prescribe lenses.	

core/o cor/o	pupil	corectopia ________________
		corectasis ________________
pupill/o	pupil	pupillary ________________
kerat/o	cornea, horny substance	keratitis ________________
		keratopathy ________________
		keratomalacia ________________
corne/o	cornea	corneal ulcer ________________
scler/o	sclera	scleritis ________________
	(white of the eye)	corneoscleral ________________
ir/o irid/o	iris	iritis ________________
	(colored portion of the eye on either side of the pupil)	iridotomy ________________
		iridectomy ________________
choroid/o	choroid layer	choroiditis ________________
retin/o	retina	diabetic retinopathy ________________ *See under pathological conditions.*
		retinitis ________________
cycl/o	ciliary body of the eye	cycloplegia ________________ *Cycl/o refers to the ciliary muscle in this term.*
		iridocyclitis ________________
phac/o phak/o	crystalline lens	phacoemulsification ________________
		aphakia ________________ *This may be congenital, but most often is a result of extraction of a cataract.*
uve/o	the iris, ciliary body, and choroid	uveitis ________________
lacrim/o	tear, tear duct, lacrimal duct	lacrimal ________________

dacry/o	tear, lacrimal duct	dacryostenosis ______
dacryocyst/o	lacrimal sac, tear sac	dacryocystitis ______
	(See Fig. 16-6 for illustration of the lacrimal sac, nasolacrimal duct, and lacrimal ducts)	______ dacryocystorhinostomy ______ ______
conjunctiv/o	conjunctiva	conjunctivitis ______ *Commonly called "pinkeye."*
blephar/o	eyelid	blepharoptosis ______ *Commonly called simply "ptosis."*
palpebr/o	eyelid	palpebral ______
aque/o	water	aqueous humor ______
vitre/o	glassy	vitreous humor ______
xer/o	dry	xerophthalmia ______
phot/o	light	photophobia ______ *Sensitivity to light.*

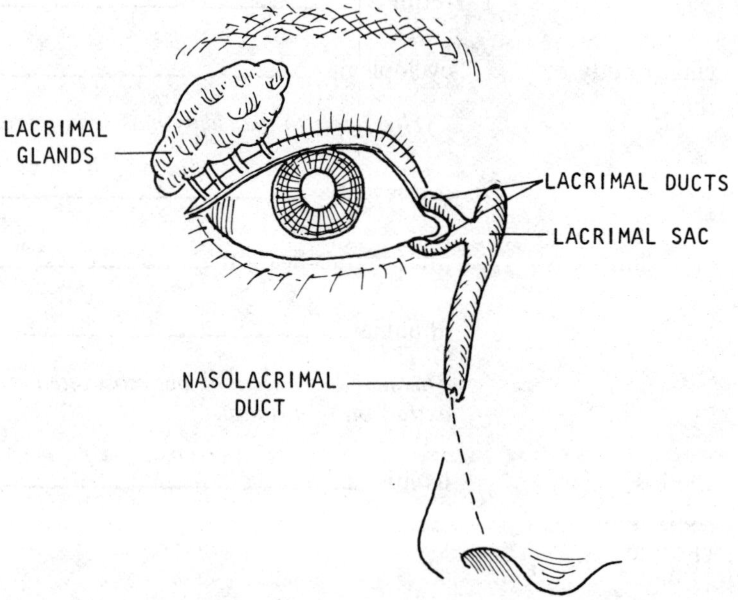

Figure 16-6 Lacrimal sac, nasolacrimal duct, and lacrimal ducts.

is/o	equal	anisocoria ______
mi/o	smaller, less	miotic ______
		Miosis means contraction of the pupil. Pilocarpine is a miotic.
mydri/o	wide	mydriatic ______
		Atropine and cocaine cause dilation of pupils.
myc/o	fungus *(immature plant)*	keratomycosis ______
glauc/o	gray	glaucoma ______
		From the dull gray-green gleam of the affected eye. See pathological conditions.
ambly/o	dull, dim	amblyopia ______
		Can be caused by alcohol, tobacco, or disease.
presby/o	old age	presbyopia ______
emmetr/o	in due measure	emmetropia ______
		Figure 16–7 shows how light rays focus on the retina in the emmetropic eye.
-opia	vision	diplopia ______
-tropia	to turn	esotropia ______
		"Crossed eyes."
-chalasis	relaxation	blepharochalasis ______
		The upper eyelid hypertrophies and loses elasticity.

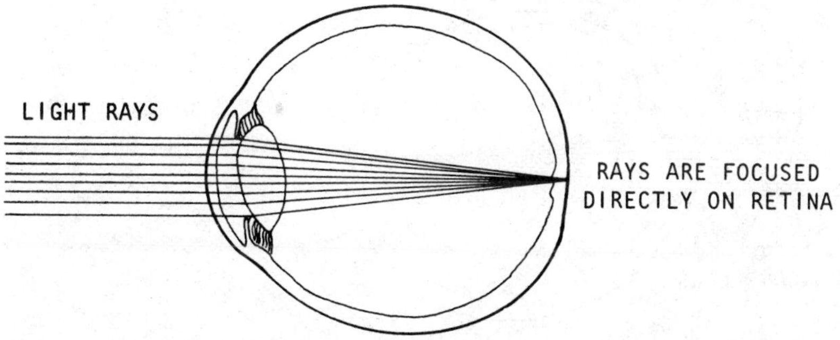

Figure 16–7 Emmetropia (ideal, normal vision).

D. Errors of Refraction

myopia

Nearsightedness.

In myopia (my- comes from "myein" meaning "to shut," referring to the observation that myopic persons usually peer through half closed eyelids) the eyeball is too long or the refractive power of the lens so strong that light rays do not properly focus on the retina. The image perceived is blurred because the light rays are focused in front of the retina. Concave glasses (thicker at the periphery than in the middle) correct this condition because the lenses spread the rays out before they reach the cornea and thus they can be properly focused directly on the retina. See Figure 16–8.

hyperopia (hypermetropia)

Farsightedness.

As Figure 16–9 illustrates, the eyeball in this condition is too short or the refractive power of the lens is too weak. Parallel rays of light tend to focus

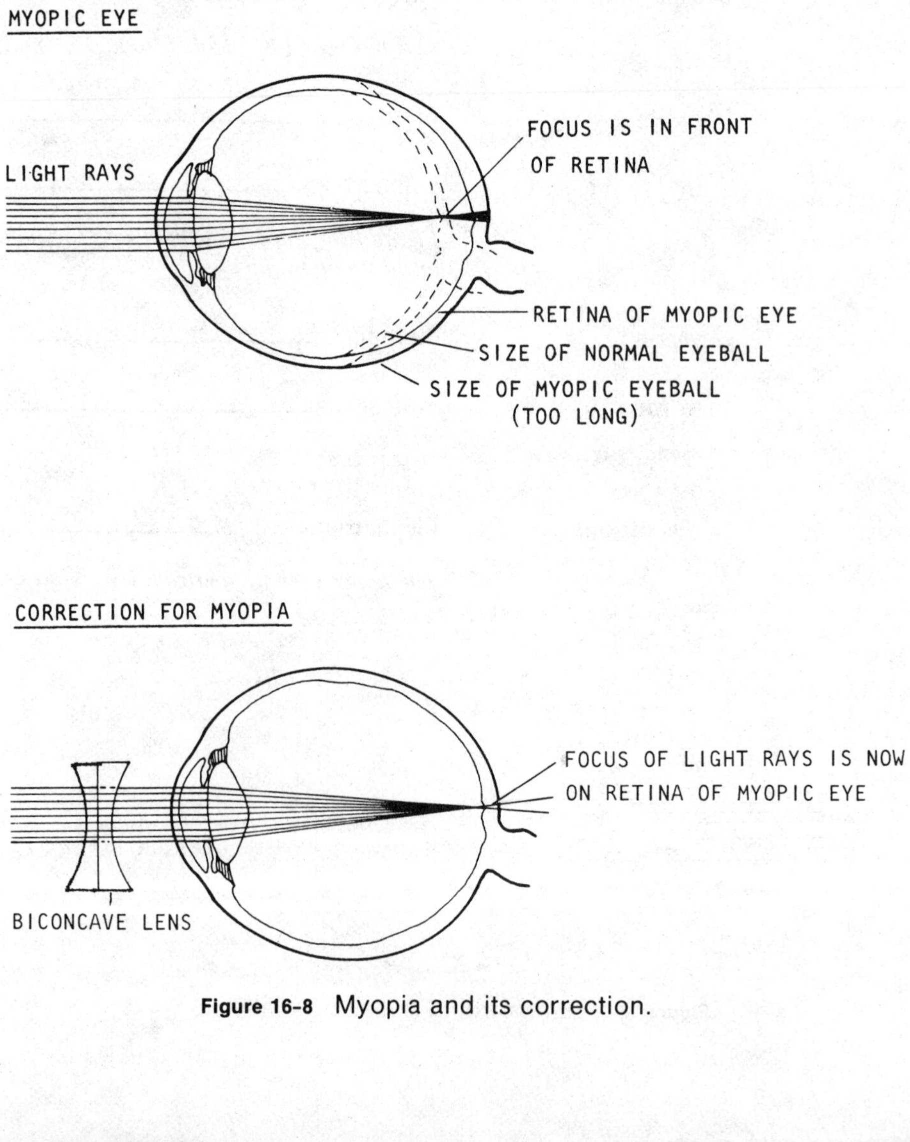

Figure 16-8 Myopia and its correction.

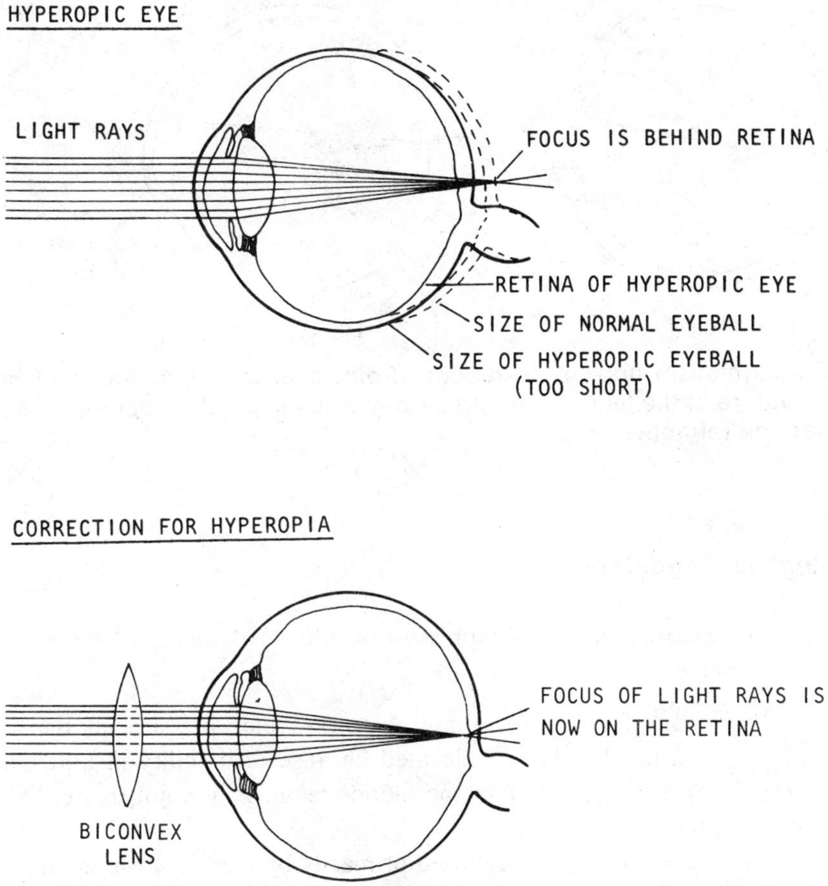

Figure 16-9 Hyperopia and its correction.

behind the retina, and this results in a blurred image. A convex lens (thicker in the middle than at the sides) bends the rays inward before they reach the cornea, and thus the rays can be focused properly on the retina.

presbyopia

Impairment of vision due to old age.

With increasing age, loss of elasticity of the ciliary body impairs its ability to adjust the lens for accommodation to near vision. The lens of the eye cannot become fat to bend the rays coming from near objects (less than 20 feet). The light rays focus behind the retina, as in hyperopia. Therefore, a convex lens is needed to refract the rays coming from objects closer than 20 feet.

astigmatism

Defective curvature of the cornea of the eye.

This problem results from one or more abnormal curvatures of the cornea. This causes light rays to be unevenly and not sharply focused on the retina so that the image is distorted. A cylindrical lens placed in the proper position in front of the eye can correct this problem. See Figure 16–10.

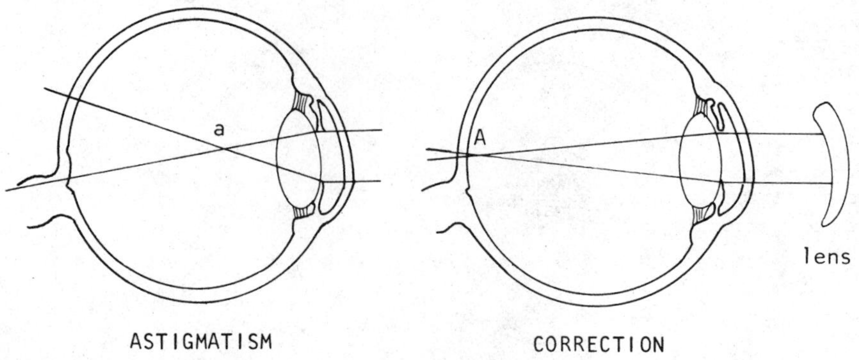

Figure 16-10 Astigmatism and its correction. Point a is improper focus of light due to abnormal curvature of the lens and cornea. Point A is the point of focus after a proper lens has corrected the refractive error.

E. Abnormal and Pathological Conditions

glaucoma

Increased intraocular pressure results in damage to the retina and optic nerve.

In this disease condition, intraocular pressure in the anterior and posterior chambers is elevated because of inability of aqueous humor to leave the eye and enter the bloodstream. If it is not treated, blindness can result.

Glaucoma is diagnosed primarily by means of **tonometry** (see Clinical Procedures), with an instrument applied externally to the eye after local anesthesia.

Administration of drugs to reduce the rate of formation of aqueous humor or to constrict the pupil (miotics) may prove effective in controlling the condition. Sometimes an operation (iridectomy) is necessary to open the anterior chamber allowing fluid to leak out slowly and continuously.

cataract

Clouding of the lens, causing decreased vision.

Cataracts are thought to be linked to the process of aging (senile cataract) and heredity. Causes of secondary cataracts include diabetes mellitus, uveitis, and prolonged high-dose corticosteroid administration. Vision appears blurred as the lens clouds over and becomes opaque. Lens cloudiness can be seen with an ophthalmoscope or the naked eye. Surgical removal of the lens, intact or by **phacoemulsification** (see Clinical Procedures), and eyeglasses to help in refraction constitute effective treatment for cataracts. Lens implants are used with success on some patients.

nystagmus

Involuntary, rapid, rhythmic movement of the eyeball.

There are various forms of this condition, and many causes, including neurologic diseases, inner ear disorders, occupational hazards (working in darkness for long periods or constantly watching moving objects), and congenital disorders.

strabismus

Abnormal deviations of the eye.

This condition is also called **squint**. It is a failure of the eyes to "look" in the same direction because of weakness of a muscle controlling the position of one eye. Different forms of strabismus include **esotropia** (cross-eyed; one eye turns inward) and **exotropia** (wall-eyed; one eye turns outward). Treatment includes corrective lenses, eye exercises and patching the normal eye (orthoptic training), or surgery to restore the muscle balance.

diabetic retinopathy

Retinal effects of diabetes mellitus include microaneurysms, dilation of retinal veins, and new blood vessels forming near the optic disk.

Edema (swelling) occurs as fluid leaks from the blood into the retina. Fatty exudates (fluid leaking from the blood) also appear in the retina as yellow-white spots. Laser photocoagulation and vitrectomy (see Clinical Procedures) are helpful to patients in whom hemorrhaging has been severe.

retinal detachment

The retina, or part of it, becomes separated from the choroid layer.

Trauma to the eyeball, head injuries, inflammation, and ocular surgery can produce holes or tears in the retina. Patients often see flashes of light and then later notice cloudy vision or loss of central vision. Photocoagulation and cryosurgery are used to seal retinal tears.

macular degeneration

Deterioration of the macula lutea of the retina.

This condition may be inherited or drug-induced, and it leads to a severe loss of central vision. Peripheral vision (using the part of the retina outside the macular region) may be retained.

retinitis pigmentosa

Progressive retinal sclerosis, pigmentation, and atrophy.

The major characteristic of this condition is the deposition of pigmented scar on the retina. This is an inherited disease associated with decreased vision, especially night blindness (**nyctalopia**).

scotoma

Area of depressed vision surrounded by an area of normal vision.

A restricted area of loss of vision caused by damage to the retina or optic nerve; a "blind spot." Scot/o means darkness.

hemianopia (hemianopsia)

Loss of one-half of the visual field (the space of vision of each eye)

This symptom is usually due to a stroke or damage to a portion of the optic nerve or its connecting fibers.

hordeolum (stye)

A localized, purulent, inflammatory staphylococcal infection of a sebaceous gland in the eyelid.

chalazion

Small, hard mass on the eyelid; formed from a sebaceous gland enlargement.

F. Clinical Procedures and Abbreviations

Clinical Procedures (Diagnostic)

Visual acuity (clearness) A test of clarity of vision. The patient reads a chart that contains black letters in gradually decreasing size. The chart is placed at a distance of 20 feet; 20/20 indicates that a person can clearly see the letters on the chart at the distance. However, a reading of 20/50 indicates that a person is able to see at 20 feet what he is supposed to be able to see at 50 feet.

Visual field test (Goldmann) This test measures the area within which objects may be seen when the eye is fixed, looking straight ahead.

Ophthalmoscopy This is a visual examination of the interior of the eye. The pupil is dilated so that the physician can see the inner chamber and retina of the eye.

Fluorescein angiography Fluorescein (a dye) is injected intravenously. The movement of blood is then observed by ophthalmoscopy to detect lesions in the macular area of the retina.

Slit lamp biomicroscopy This test uses a combination of a slit lamp (intense light is emitted through a slit) and a biomicroscope so that a microscopic study can be made of the cornea, conjunctiva, iris, lens, and vitreous humor.

Gonioscopy This procedure involves examination of the angle (gonia means angle) of the anterior chamber of the eye. Obstruction of the angle may occur in glaucoma.

Tonometry This is measurement of the tension or pressure within the eye and is useful in detecting glaucoma.

Retinoscopy A beam of light is directed into the eye, and errors of refraction (myopia and hyperopia) are observed by the movement of the reflected light.

Clinical Procedures (Treatment)

Orthoptic training These are eye muscle exercises for the purpose of correcting squint (strabismus) and restoring normal coordination of the eyes.

Diathermy This procedure involves the use of high-frequency electric current to generate heat and coagulate blood vessels within the eye.

Laser photocoagulation In this procedure argon laser (high-energy light) beams are used to stimulate coagulation of tissue (blood vessels) in the interior of the eye. The technique is useful to treat diabetic retinopathy and senile macular degeneration, as well as other ophthalmic vascular disorders.

Cataract surgery Several different procedures can be used to remove the lens when a cataract has formed. The **cryoextraction method** uses a cold probe on the anterior surface of the lens to lift the lens out as it adheres to the probe. The **aspiration-irrigation method** employs a hollow needle to suck out the lens material and wash out the anterior chamber of the eye. **Phacoemulsification** is a more recent microsurgical technique in which ultrasonic vibration is used to break up portions of the lens. The lens is then aspirated through the ultrasonic probe.

Vitrectomy — Diseased vitreous humor is removed and replaced with a clear solution. In time, the solution is naturally replaced by healthy vitreous fluid.

Keratoplasty — This procedure, also called **corneal transplant**, involves replacement of a section of an opaque cornea with normal, transparent cornea in an effort to restore vision.

Abbreviations

Accom.	Accommodation	Ophth.	Ophthalmology
Astigm.	Astigmatism	OS	Left eye (oculus sinister)
c. gl.	Correction with glasses	OU	Each eye (oculus uterque)
cyl.	Cylindrical lens	s. gl.	Without correction (without glasses)
Em.	Emmetropia (normal vision)	VA	Visual acuity
Myop.	Myopia	VF	Visual field
OD	Right eye (oculus dexter)		

III. THE EAR

A. Anatomy and Physiology

Sound waves are received by the outer ear, conducted to special receptor cells within the ear, and transmitted by those cells to nerve fibers that lead to the auditory region of the brain in the cerebral cortex. It is within the nerve fibers of the cerebral cortex that the sensations of sound are perceived.

Label Figure 16–11 as you read the following paragraphs describing the anatomy and physiology of the ear.

The ear can be divided into three separate regions—outer ear, middle ear, and inner ear. The outer and middle ears function in the conduction of sound waves through the ear, while the inner ear contains structures that receive the auditory waves and relay them to the brain.

Outer Ear

Sound waves enter the ear through the **pinna**, also called the **auricle** (1), which is the projecting part, or flap, of the ear. The **external auditory meatus (auditory canal)** (2) leads from the pinna and is lined with numerous glands that secrete a yellowish brown, waxy substance called **cerumen**. Cerumen lubricates and protects the ear.

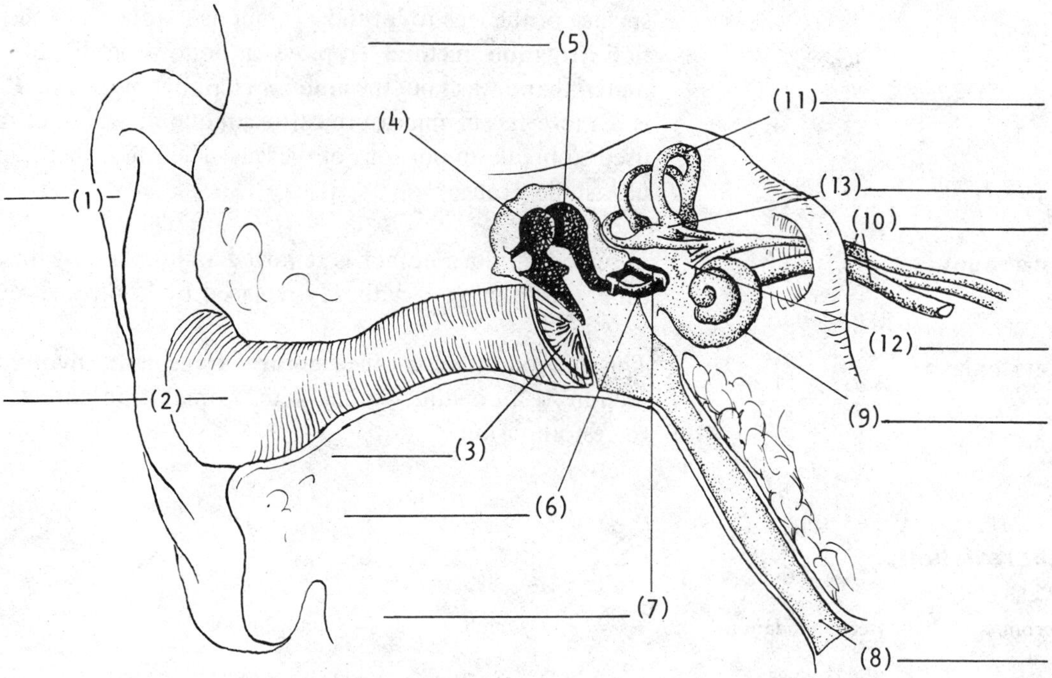

Figure 16-11 The ear.

Middle Ear

Sound waves travel through the auditory canal and strike a membrane between the outer and middle ear. This is the **tympanic membrane**, or **eardrum** (3). As the eardrum vibrates, it moves three small bones, or **ossicles**, which conduct the sound waves through the middle ear. These bones, in the order of their vibration, are the **malleus** (4), the **incus** (5), and the **stapes** (6). As the stapes moves, it touches a membrane called the **oval window** (7) which separates the middle from the inner ear.

Before proceeding with the pathway of sound conduction and reception into the inner ear, an additional structure which affects the middle ear should be mentioned. The **auditory** or **eustachian tube** (8) is a canal leading from the middle ear to the pharynx. It is normally closed but opens upon swallowing. In an efficient way, this tube can prevent damage to the eardrum and shock to the middle and inner ears. Normally the pressure of air in the middle ear is equal to the pressure of air in the external environment. However, if you ascend in the atmosphere, as in flying an airplane, climbing a high mountain, or riding a fast elevator, the atmospheric pressure, and that in the outer ear, will drop, while the pressure in the middle ear remains the same—greater than that in the outer ear. This inequality of air pressure on the inside and outside of the eardrum forces the eardrum to bulge outward and eventually to burst. Swallowing will open the eustachian tube so that air can leave the middle ear and enter the throat until the atmospheric and middle ear pressures are balanced. The eardrum then relaxes and the danger of its bursting is averted.

Inner Ear

Sound vibrations, having been transmitted by the movement of the eardrum to the bones of the middle ear, reach the inner ear via the fluctuations of the oval window which separates the middle and inner ears. The inner ear is also called the **labyrinth** because of its circular, mazelike structure. The part of the labyrinth that leads from the oval window is a bony, snail-shaped structure called the **cochlea** (9). The cochlea contains special auditory liquids called **perilymph** and **endolymph** through which the vibrations travel. Also present in the cochlea is a sensitive auditory receptor called the **organ of Corti**. In the organ of Corti, tiny hair cells called **cilia** receive vibrations from the auditory liquids and relay the sound waves to **auditory nerve fibers** (10) which end in the auditory center of the cerebral cortex, where these impulses are interpreted and "heard."

Study Figure 16–12, which is a schematic representation of the pathway of sound vibrations from the outer ear to the brain.

The ear is an important organ of equilibrium (balance), as well as an organ for hearing. Within the inner ear are three organs responsible for equilibrium. Refer back to Figure 16–11 and label these three organs: **semicircular canals** (11), **saccule** (12), and **utricle** (13). These organs contain the fluid called endolymph, as well as sensitive hair cells. In an intricate manner, the fluid and hair cells fluctuate in response to the movement of the head. This sets up impulses in nerve fibers which lead to the brain. Messages are then sent to muscles in all parts of the body to assure that equilibrium is maintained.

B. Vocabulary

auditory canal — The channel that leads from the flap of the ear to the eardrum.

auditory meatus — Auditory canal.

auditory nerve fibers — These nerves carry nerve impulses from the inner ear to the brain (cerebral cortex).

auditory tube — Channel between the middle ear and the nasopharynx; eustachian tube.

auricle — The flap of the ear; protruding part of the external ear.

cerumen — A waxy substance secreted by the external ear; also called ear wax.

cochlea — A snail-shaped, spirally wound tube in the inner ear; contains sensitive hearing receptor cells.

cilia — Hairlike processes on cells; found, in the inner ear, in the organ of Corti.

endolymph — Fluid contained in the inner ear.

eustachian tube — Auditory tube.

incus — The second ossicle (bone) of the middle ear; also called the anvil.

labyrinth — The mazelike series of canals in the inner ear. This includes the cochlea, semicircular canals, saccule, and utricle.

malleus — The first ossicle of the middle ear; also called the hammer.

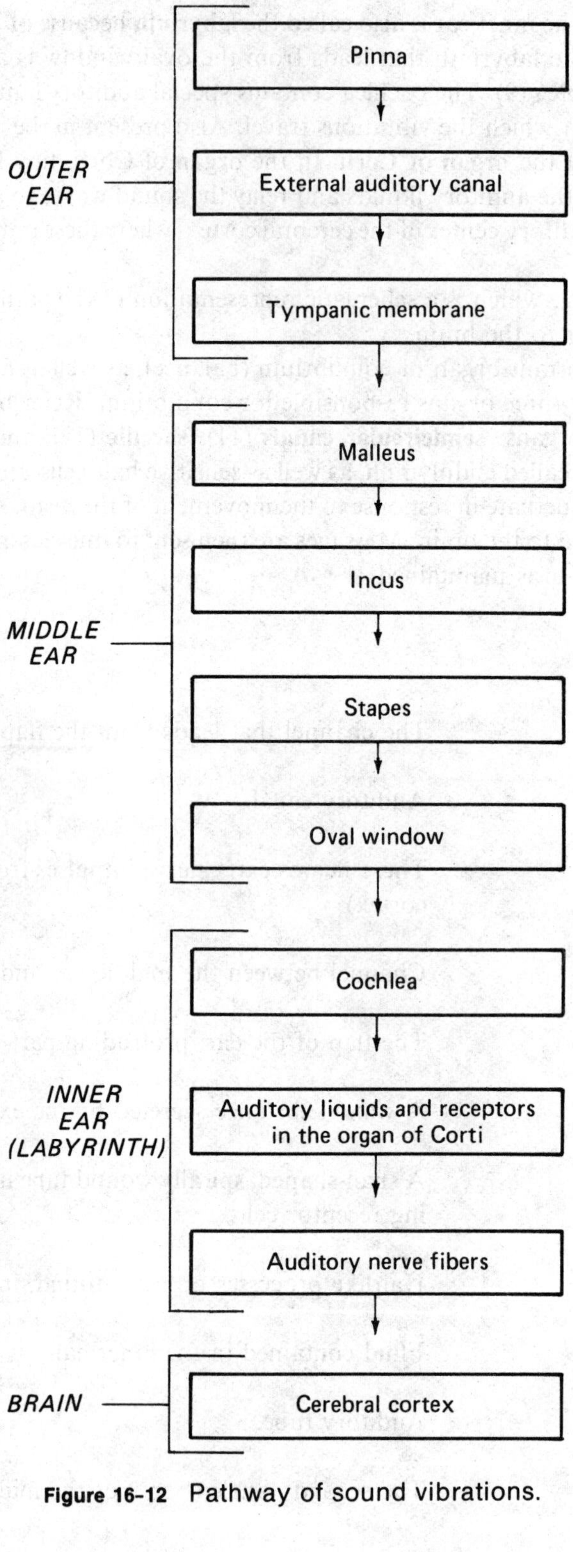

Figure 16-12 Pathway of sound vibrations.

organ of Corti A sensitive auditory receptor found in the cochlea of the inner ear.

ossicle Small bone.

oval window	A membrane between the middle and inner ears.
perilymph	Auditory fluid contained in the labyrinth of the inner ear.
pinna	The auricle; flap of the ear.
saccule	An organ in the inner ear that is associated with maintaining equilibrium; saccule means "little bag."
semicircular canals	Passages in the inner ear that are associated with maintaining equilibrium.
stapes	The third ossicle of the middle ear. Stapes means "stirrup."
tympanic membrane	A membrane between the outer and middle ear; also called the eardrum.
utricle	A tiny, saclike structure in the inner ear which, along with the saccule and semicircular canals, is associated with maintaining equilibrium.

C. Combining Forms and Suffixes

Combining Form	*Definition*	*Terminology*	*Meaning*
audi/o	hearing	audiometer	______
acous/o acou/o	hearing	acoustic	______
ot/o	ear	otoscope	______
aur/o aur/i	ear	aural discharge	______
bar/o	pressure, weight	barotitis *Changes in atmospheric pressure cause inflammation of the ear.*	______
cerumin/o	cerumen	ceruminal	______
staped/o	stapes *(3rd ossicle of the middle ear)*	stapedectomy *Prosthesis (artificial part) is used to connect incus and oval window.*	______
myring/o	eardrum, tympanic membrane	myringoplasty myringotomy	______ ______

tympan/o	eardrum, middle ear	tympanic ______________
		tympanoplasty ______________
salping/o	auditory tube, eustachian tube	salpingopharyngeal ______________
		______________
mastoid/o	referring to the mastoid process *(posterior portion of the temporal bone which extends downward behind the external auditory meatus)*	mastoidectomy ______________
		mastoiditis ______________ *Usually the result of an infection of the middle ear.*
-cusis	hearing	presbycusis ______________
-phonia	sound	dysphonia ______________

D. Abnormal and Pathological Conditions

macrotia Abnormal enlargement of the pinnae.

microtia Abnormally small pinnae.

Surgery can be performed to correct both of these congenital anomalies.

suppurative otitis media Bacterial infection of the middle ear.

Staphylococcus, streptococcus, or pneumococcus can be the infecting organism. Antibiotics are an excellent treatment. Surgical evacuation of the purulent material through the tympanic membrane will prevent hearing loss and mastoiditis. This procedure is called a myringotomy.

serous otitis media Inflammation (noninfectious) of the middle ear with accumulation of serum.

Treatment may include myringotomy to aspirate fluid and tympanostomy tubes placed in the eardrum to allow ventilation of the middle ear.

otosclerosis Hardening of the bony tissue of the labyrinth.

Bone forms around the oval window and may lead to the fixation or **ankylosis** (stiffening) of the stapes bone. This causes hearing loss and progressive deafness. Treatment is surgical. Stapedectomy with replacement by a tissue **graft** (substitute for the damaged part) using fatty tissue from the ear lobe and a **prosthesis** (an artificial part) of stainless steel wire is effective in overcoming deafness. In order to do this operation, the oval window must be **fenestrated** (opened) so that the otosclerotic areas of the stapes can be removed.

presbycusis

Hearing loss occurring with old age.

This is the most common form of nerve deafness. It occurs as a result of the physiological process of aging.

Sudden deafness may occur as a result of an infectious illness such as mumps or measles.

vertigo

Sensation of irregular or whirling motion either of oneself or of external objects.

Vertigo is dizziness often associated with nausea, and is due to a severe disturbance of the equilibrium organs in the labyrinth. The etiology is varied. It is most commonly caused by a viral illness. Cerebral concussion (brain injury), toxicity due to use of certain drugs, and syphilis (a sexually transmitted disease) are other conditions leading to vertigo, and in some cases deafness.

tinnitus

Ringing sound in the ears.

The cause and mechanism of this auditory symptom are unknown. It may be associated with chronic otitis, myringitis, or labyrinthitis, as well as other disorders. Tinnitus, a Latin-derived term, means tinkling.

Meniere's syndrome

Vertigo, hearing loss, nausea, and tinnitus, leading to progressive deafness.

This syndrome is caused by rapid, violent firing of the fibers of the auditory nerves. Increased endolymph pressure brings on attacks of vertigo. If degeneration of the organ of Corti occurs, progressive deafness is the result. Treatment is bed rest, sedation, and drugs to combat nausea and vertigo.

acoustic neuroma

Benign tumor arising from the acoustic nerve in the brain.

This tumor causes tinnitus, vertigo, and decreased hearing as its initial symptoms. Small tumors may be resected by microsurgical techniques.

cholesteatoma

Collection of skin cells and cholesterol in a sac within the middle ear.

E. Clinical Procedures and Abbreviations

Clinical Procedures

Tuning fork tests

A vibration source (tuning fork) is placed near the ear (to test hearing by air conduction) or in contact with the skull (to test hearing by bone conduction).

Audiometry — An instrument (audiometer) delivers acoustic stimuli of specific frequencies to determine the patient's hearing for each frequency. Test results are plotted on a graph called an audiogram.

Otoscopy — Visual examination of the ear with an otoscope.

Pneumatic otoscopy — Visual examination of the external ear and tympanic membrane using air to change pressure in the external auditory canal.

Tympanometry — Evaluation of middle ear function by measurement of the movement of the tympanic membrane and pressure in the middle ear. A low-frequency tone is emitted from the tip of a tympanometer probe and directed toward the tympanic membrane. Sound energy reflected off the membrane is directed back down the auditory canal and a small microphone in the probe reads the amount of reflected energy.

Abbreviations

AC	Air conduction
AD	Right ear (auris dextra)
AS	Left ear (auris sinistra)
BC	Bone conduction
HD	Hearing distance
ENT	Ear, nose, and throat
ETF	Eustachian tube function
Oto	Otology
PE tube	Polyethylene ventilating tube placed in the eardrum

IV. PRACTICAL APPLICATIONS

Audie Earring, M.D., Otolaryngologist
Selected Services and Diagnoses

Ear, Nose and Throat Services

1. Drainage, abscess, auricle
2. Drainage, hematoma, auricle
3. Myringotomy, unilat.
4. Myringotomy, bilat.
5. Removal tube
6. Removal foreign body
7. Drainage intranasal abscess
8. Excision polyps, unilat/bilat
9. Reduction, nasal fracture
10. Uvulectomy
11. I&D [incision and drainage] peritonsillar abscess

Diagnoses

1. External otitis
2. Otitis media, acute
3. Otitis media, chronic
4. Serous otitis media
5. Impacted cerumen
6. Vertigo
7. Labyrinthitis
8. Eustach. salpingitis
9. Tinnitus
10. Otalgia
11. Perforated tymp. memb.
12. Rhinitis

13. Sinusitis, acute/chronic
14. Epistaxis
15. Nasal polyps
16. Deviated nasal septum
17. Pharyngitis
18. Meniere's syndrome

Seymour I. Vision, M.D., Ophthalmologist
Selected Services and Diagnoses

Services

1. Gonioscopy
2. Retinal exam
3. Cataract evalu.
4. Glaucoma consul.
5. Strabismus evalu.
6. Refraction
7. Exc. multiple chalazia
8. Exc. & biop. lid tumor
9. Exc. corn. foreign body
10. Probing nasolac. duct
11. Retina photocoagulation
12. Fluorescein angiography
13. Fundus photos
14. Exophthalmometry
15. Mydriasis test
16. Field—Goldmann

Diagnoses

1. Ocular trauma
2. Corneal abrasion
3. Keratitis
4. Conjunctival hemorrhage
5. Scleritis
6. Uveitis
7. Aphakia
8. Dacryostenosis
9. Ptosis
10. Amblyopia
11. Epiphora (excess tears)
12. Glaucoma suspect
13. Cataract
14. Retinal vascular disease
15. Choroidal nevus
16. Myopia

Autopsy Report: Eyes

Gross examination: These are firm eyes each measuring 24 × 24 × 24 mm with 5 mm of optic nerve attached. The clear cornea measures 12 × 11 mm. The eye is opened in the horizontal plane. The anterior chamber is normal and its angle is open; the lens is in place. The iris is unremarkable; the ciliary body is unremarkable; the retina is in place. The vitreous cavity is unremarkable; the vitreous is liquid; the choroid is in place; the optic disk is flat; the sclera is unremarkable.

Microscopic examination: Exam reveals essentially normal ocular structures.

Diagnosis: Normal autopsy eyes.

V. EXERCISES

A. Match the structure in the eye with its description:

1.	pupil	______	Contains sensitive cells called rods and cones which transmit light energy to nerve fibers.
2.	conjunctiva	______	Controls the shape of the lens.
3.	cornea	______	Transparent body that lies behind the iris and in front of the vitreous humor; it refracts light rays onto the retina.
4.	sclera	______	Jelly-like material behind the lens which helps to maintain the shape of the eyeball.
5.	choroid	______	Dark center of the eye through which light rays enter the eye.
6.	iris	______	Vascular layer of the eyeball which is continuous with the iris.
7.	ciliary muscle	______	Mucous membrane over the outside of the eye and under the eyelid.
8.	lens	______	Transparent fibrous membrane which refracts light.
9.	retina	______	Colored portion of the eye; surrounds the pupil.
10.	vitreous humor	______	White of the eye; fibrous supportive tissue.

B. Build medical terms:

1. Incision of a muscle of the eye ______________________________
2. Paralysis of the eye (muscles) ______________________________
3. Unequal (size of) pupils ______________________________
4. Abnormal fungus condition of the eye ______________________________
5. Softening of the cornea ______________________________
6. Inflammation of the ciliary body ______________________________
7. Incision into a tear duct ______________________________

8. Instrument to visually examine the eye ____________________

9. Condition of disease of the retina ____________________

10. Prolapse of the eyelid ____________________

11. Relaxation of the eyelid ____________________

C. *Give the meaning of the following medical terms:*

1. macula lutea ____________________
2. refraction ____________________
3. accommodation ____________________
4. rods and cones ____________________
5. optic chiasma ____________________
6. intraocular ____________________
7. scleral icterus ____________________
8. uveitis ____________________
9. xerophthalmia ____________________
10. iridokeratitis ____________________
11. diplopia ____________________
12. olfactory ____________________
13. coreometer ____________________
14. fundus of the eye ____________________
15. corneal dystrophy ____________________
16. conjunctivitis ____________________
17. photophobia ____________________
18. emmetropia ____________________
19. biconvex ____________________
20. binocular vision ____________________

D. Match the medical term for the eye disorder with its proper definition:

1. nystagmus	______	Any abnormal deviation of the eye; squint.
2. amblyopia	______	Nearsightedness.
3. cataract	______	Turning inward of eye.
4. hyperopia	______	Defective vision or blindness in half of the visual field.
5. esotropia	______	Abnormal curvature of the cornea, leading to blurred vision.
6. myopia		
	______	Lens clouds over with opaque film and vision is impaired.
7. presbyopia		
8. exotropia	______	Blockage of circulation of aqueous humor leads to increased intraocular pressure.
9. astigmatism		
	______	Quick, jerky movement of the eye from side to side.
10. glaucoma		
	______	Farsightedness.
11. macular degeneration	______	Dull, dim vision.
12. retinitis pigmentosa	______	Tendency of the eye to turn outward.
	______	Defect of vision of old age due to loss of elasticity of the lens.
13. strabismus		
14. scotoma	______	Blind spot; area of depressed vision surrounded by an area of less depressed or normal vision.
15. hemianopia		
	______	Progressive sclerosis; pigmentation and atrophy of the inner lining of the eye.
	______	Deterioration of the macula lutea of the retina.

E. Complete the following sentences:

1. In the myopic eye, light rays do not focus properly on the ____________________.

   Either the eyeball is too ____________________ or the refractive power of the lens is

   too ____________________ so that the image is blurred and comes to a focus in

_______________ of the retina. The type of lens used to correct this refractive error is called a _______________ lens.

2. In the hyperopic eye, the eyeball is too _______________ or the refractive power of the lens too _______________ so that the image is blurred and focused in _______________ of the retina. The type of lens used to correct this refractive error is called a _______________ lens.

3. A miotic is a drug that _______________ the pupil of the eye. It is used to treat a condition called _______________.

4. A mydriatic is a drug that _______________ the pupil of the eye.

F. *Give the meanings for the following combining forms related to the eye:*

1. uve/o	_______________	7. chori/o	_______________
2. cycl/o	_______________	8. dacry/o	_______________
3. kerat/o	_______________	9. vitr/o	_______________
4. phac/o	_______________	10. palpebr/o	_______________
5. lacrim/o	_______________	11. core/o	_______________
6. irid/o	_______________	12. opt/o	_______________

G. *Name the abnormal eye condition or clinical procedure related to the eye:*

1. Acute pyogenic infection of sebaceous glands around the eye; a stye _______________

____

2. Chronic granulomatous enlargement of sebaceous glands on the eyelid _______________

____

3. Examination of the angle of the eye to detect the presence of glaucoma

____

4. High-energy light beams are used to stop retinal hemorrhaging ______________________________

5. Visual examination of the retina ______________________________

6. Corneal transplant (surgical repair) ______________________________

7. Intravenous injection of dye followed by examination of the eye and its blood vessels ______________________________

8. Ultrasonic vibrations break up the lens, and it is aspirated out of the eye ______________________________

9. Test of clearness of vision ______________________________

10. Measurement of the tension or pressure within the eye ______________________________

11. Eye muscle exercises ______________________________

12. Removal of vitreous humor ______________________________

13. The retina, or part of it, becomes detached from the choroid ______________________________

14. Test to measure the area within which objects may be seen when the eye is fixed ______________________________

15. The secondary effects (microaneurysms and neovascularization) on the eye produced by diabetes mellitus ______________________________

H. *Give the meaning of the following abbreviations:*

1. OU ______________________________
2. s. gl. ______________________________
3. VA ______________________________
4. OD ______________________________
5. OS ______________________________

6. c. gl. ____________________

7. VF ____________________

8. Myop. ____________________

9. Em. ____________________

10. Accom. ____________________

I. *Arrange the following terms in the correct order to indicate their sequence in the transmission of sound waves to the brain from the outer ear:*

incus, tympanic membrane, pinna, cochlea, malleus, oval window,

external auditory canal, auditory liquids and receptors, stapes,

auditory nerve fibers, cerebral cortex

1. ____________________
2. ____________________
3. ____________________
4. ____________________
5. ____________________
6. ____________________
7. ____________________
8. ____________________
9. ____________________
10. ____________________
11. ____________________

J. *Give the meaning of the following medical terms:*

1. labyrinth ____________________

2. semicircular canals ____________________

3. auditory (eustachian) tube ____________________

4. stapes ____________________

5. organ of Corti ____________________

6. perilymph and endolymph ____________________

7. cerumen ____________________

8. utricle ______________________________

9. oval window ______________________________

10. tympanic membrane ______________________________

K. Build medical terms:

1. Instrument to examine the ear ______________________________
2. Removal of the third bone of middle ear ______________________________
3. Pertaining to the auditory tube and throat ______________________________
4. Flow of pus from the ear ______________________________
5. Instrument to measure hearing ______________________________
6. Incision of the eardrum ______________________________
7. Surgical repair of the eardrum ______________________________
8. Deafness due to old age ______________________________
9. Small ear ______________________________
10. Inflammation of the middle ear ______________________________

L. Give the meaning of the following medical terms:

1. vertigo ______________________________
2. Meniere's syndrome ______________________________
3. otosclerosis ______________________________
4. tinnitus ______________________________
5. labyrinthitis ______________________________
6. cholesteatoma ______________________________
7. barotitis ______________________________
8. acoustic neuroma ______________________________

M. Give the meanings for the following abbreviations relating to otology:

1. oto ______________________________
2. BC ______________________________
3. AS ______________________________
4. AD ______________________________
5. AC ______________________________
6. ENT ______________________________
7. ETF ______________________________
8. HD ______________________________
9. PE tube ______________________________

ANSWERS

A.

9
7
8
10
1
5
2
3
6
4

B.

1. ophthalmomyotomy
2. ophthalmoplegia
3. anisocoria
4. ophthalmomycosis
5. keratomalacia
6. cyclitis
7. lacrimotomy
8. ophthalmoscope
9. retinopathy
10. blepharoptosis
11. blepharochalasis

C.

1. Yellow spot in the retina that contains the fovea centralis (area of clearest vision).
2. The bending of light rays by the cornea, lens, and fluids of the eye.
3. The adjustment the lens of the eye normally makes to bring an object into focus on the retina.
4. Photosensitive cells of the retina.
5. The crossing point of the fibers of the optic nerve in the brain.
6. Within the eye.
7. Abnormal yellow coloration of the white of the eye.
8. Inflammation of the vascular layer of the eyeball (the choroid and iris).
9. Condition of dryness of the eye.
10. Inflammation of the iris and the cornea.
11. Double vision.
12. Pertaining to the sense of smell.
13. Instrument to measure the pupil.
14. Posterior, inner portion of the eye.
15. Poor development of the cornea.
16. Inflammation of the conjunctiva.
17. Fear of light.
18. Condition of normal vision ("in proper measure").
19. Having two convex (rounded, elevated) surfaces.
20. Normal vision with two eyes.

D.

13
6
5
15
9
3
10
1
4
2
8
7
14
12
11

E.

1. retina; long; strong; front; concave.
2. short; weak; back; convex.
3. constricts; glaucoma.
4. dilates.

F.

1. vascular layer of the eye
2. ciliary body
3. cornea
4. crystalline lens
5. tears
6. iris
7. choroid layer
8. tear, tear duct, nasolacrimal duct
9. glassy
10. eyelid
11. pupil
12. eye

G.

1. hordeolum
2. chalazion
3. gonioscopy
4. laser photocoagulation
5. retinoscopy
6. keratoplasty
7. fluorescein angiography
8. phacoemulsification
9. visual acuity
10. tonometry
11. orthoptic training
12. vitrectomy
13. retinal detachment
14. visual field test (Goldmann)
15. diabetic retinopathy

H.

1. each eye
2. correction without glasses
3. visual acuity
4. right eye
5. left eye
6. correction with glasses
7. visual field
8. myopia
9. emmetropia (normal vision)
10. accommodation

I.

1. pinna
2. external auditory canal
3. tympanic membrane
4. malleus
5. incus
6. stapes
7. oval window
8. cochlea
9. auditory liquids and receptors
10. auditory nerve fibers
11. cerebral cortex

J.

1. Cochlea and organs of equilibrium (semicircular canals, saccule, and utricle).
2. Organ of equilibrium in the inner ear.
3. Passageway between the middle ear and the throat.
4. Third ossicle (little bone) of the middle ear.
5. Region in the cochlea which contains auditory receptors.
6. Auditory fluids circulating within the inner ear.
7. Wax in the external auditory meatus.
8. Tiny sac in the inner ear associated with the semicircular canals and important in maintaining equilibrium and balance.
9. Delicate membrane between the middle and inner ears.
10. Eardrum.

K.

1. otoscope
2. stapedectomy
3. salpingopharyngeal
4. otopyorrhea
5. audiometer
6. myringotomy (tympanotomy)
7. tympanoplasty (myringoplasty)
8. presbycusis
9. microtia
10. otitis media

L.

1. Sensation of irregular or whirling motion either of oneself or of external objects.
2. Syndrome consisting of vertigo, hearing loss, nausea, and ringing in the ears, leading to progressive deafness.
3. Abnormal condition of hardening of the bony structure of the inner ear.
4. Ringing sensation in the ears.
5. Inflammation of the labyrinth of the inner ear.
6. Collection of skin cells and cholesterol in a sac within the middle ear.
7. Inflammation of the ear produced by changes in atmospheric pressure.
8. Benign tumor arising from the acoustic nerve in the brain.

M.

1. otology
2. bone conduction
3. left ear
4. right ear
5. air conduction
6. ear, nose, and throat
7. eustachian tube function
8. hearing distance
9. ventilating tube placed in the eardrum.

VI. PRONUNCIATION OF TERMS

accommodation	ă-kŏm-ō-DĀ-shŭn
acoustic	ă-KO͞OS-tĭk
acuity	ă-KŪ-ĭ-tē
amblyopia	ăm-blē-Ō-pē-ă
anisocoria	ăn-ī-sō-KŌ-rē-ă
aphakia	ă-FĀ-kē-ă
aqueous	ĂK-wē-ŭs; Ā-kwē-ŭs
astigmatism	ă-STĬG-mă-tĭsm
audiometer	ăw-dē-ŎM-ĕ-tĕr
audiometry	ăw-dē-ŎM-ĕ-trē
auditory	ăw-dĭ-TŌ-rē
aural	ĂW-răl
auricle	ĂW-rĭ-k'l
barotitis	băr-ō-TĪ-tĭs
biconvex	bī-KŎN-vĕks
binocular	bī-NŎK-ū-lăr; bĭn-ŎK-ū-lăr
blepharochalasis	blĕf-ă-rō-kă-LĀ-sĭs
blepharoptosis	blĕf-ă-rŏp-TŌ-sĭs
cataract	KĂT-ă-răkt
cerumen	sĕ-RO͞O-mĕn
ceruminal	sĕ-RO͞O-mĭ-năl
chalazion	kă-LĀ-zē-ŏn
chiasma	kī-ĂS-mă
cholesteatoma	kō-lē-stē-ă-TŌ-mă
choroid	KŌR-oyd
cilia	SĬL-ē-ă

ciliary	SĬL-ē-ăr-ē
cochlea	KŎK-lē-ă
conjunctiva	kŏn-jŭnk-TĪ-vă
conjunctivitis	kŏn-jŭnk-tĭ-VĪ-tĭs
corectasis	kōr-ĔK-tă-sĭs
corectopia	kōr-ĕk-TŌ-pē-ă
cornea	KŌR-nē-ă
corneal	KŌR-nē-ăl
corneoscleral	kōr-nē-ō-SKLĒ-răl
cryoextraction	krī-ō-ĕks-TRĂK-shŭn
crystalline lens	KRĬS-tă-lĭn lĕnz
cycloplegia	sī-klō-PLĒ-jē-ă
dacryocystitis	dăk-rē-ō-sĭs-TĪ-tĭs
dacryocystorhinostomy	dăk-rē-ō-sĭs-tō-rī-NŎS-tō-mē
dacryostenosis	dăk-rē-ō-stĕ-NŌ-sĭs
diathermy	DĪ-ă-thĕr-mē
diplopia	dĭp-LŌ-pē-ă
dysphonia	dĭs-FŌ-nē-ă
emmetropia	ĕm-ĕ-TRŌ-pē-ă
endolymph	ĔN-dō-lĭmf
esotropia	ĕs-ō-TRŌ-pē-ă
eustachian	ū-STĀ-shŭn; ū-STĀ-kē-ăn
exotropia	ĕk-sō-TRŌ-pē-ă
fenestrated	FĔN-ĕs-trāt-ĕd
fluorescein angiography	flo͞o-ō-RĔS-ē-ĭn ăn-jē-ŎG-ră-fē
fovea centralis	FŌ-vē-ă sĕn-TRĂ-lĭs
fundus	FŬN-dŭs
glaucoma	glăw-KŌ-mă
gonioscopy	gō-nē-ŎS-kō-pē
hemianopia	hĕ-mē-ă-NŌ-pē-ă
hordeolum	hōr-DĒ-ō-lŭm
hyperopia	hī-pĕr-Ō-pē-ă

incus	ĬNG-kŭs
intraocular	ĭn-tră-ŎK-ū-lăr
iridectomy	ĭr-ĭ-DĔK-tō-mē
iridocyclitis	ĭr-ĭ-dō-sī-KLĪ-tĭs
iridotomy	ĭr-ĭ-DŎT-ō-mē
iritis	ī-RĪ-tĭs
keratitis	kĕr-ă-TĪ-tĭs
keratomalacia	kĕr-ă-tō-mă-LĀ-shă
keratomycosis	kĕr-ă-tō-mī-KŌ-sĭs
keratopathy	kĕr-ă-TŎP-ă-thē
labyrinth	LĂB-ĭ-rĭnth
lacrimal	LĂK-rĭ-măl
laser photocoagulation	LĀ-zĕr fō-tō-kō-ăg-ū-LĀ-shŭn
macrotia	măk-RŌ-shē-ă
macula lutea	MĂK-ū-lă LŪ-tē-ă
malleus	MĂL-ē-ŭs
mastoidectomy	măs-toy-DĔK-tō-mē
mastoiditis	măs-toy-DĪ-tĭs
meatus	mē-Ā-tŭs
Meniere's	mĕn-ē-ĀRZ
microtia	mī-KRŌ-shē-ă
miotic	mī-ŎT-ĭk
mydriatic	mĭd-rē-ĂT-ĭk
myopia	mī-Ō-pē-ă
myringoplasty	mī-RĬNG-gō-plăs-tē
myringotomy	mĭr-ĭn-GŎT-ō-mē
nyctalopia	nĭk-tă-LŌ-pē-ă
nystagmus	nĭ-STĂG-mŭs
olfactory	ŏl-FĂK-tō-rē
ophthalmic	ŏf-THĂL-mĭk
ophthalmologist	ŏf-thăl-MŎL-ō-jĭst
ophthalmoplegia	ŏf-thăl-mō-PLĒ-jă

ophthalmoscopy	ŏf-thăl-MŎS-kō-pē
optic	ŎP-tĭk
optician	ŏp-TĬSH-ăn
optometrist	ŏp-TŎM-ĕ-trĭst
orthoptic	ŏr-THŎP-tĭk
ossicle	ŎS-ĭ-k'l
otosclerosis	ō-tō-sklĕ-RŌ-sĭs
otoscope	Ō-tō-skōp
otoscopy	ō-TŎS-kō-pē
palpebral	PĂL-pĕ-brăl
perilymph	PĔR-ĭ-lĭmf
phacoemulsification	făk-ō-ē-mŭl-sĭ-fĭ-KĀ-shŭn
phacolysis	fă-KŎL-ĭ-sĭs
photophobia	fō-tō-FŌ-bē-ă
pinna	PĬN-ă
presbycusis	prĕz-bē-KŪ-sĭs
presbyopia	prĕz-bē-Ō-pē-ă
prosthesis	prŏs-THĒ-sĭs
pupillary	PŪ-pĭ-lăr-ē
refraction	rē-FRĂK-shŭn
retina	RĔT-ĭ-nă
retinitis pigmentosa	rĕt-ĭ-NĪ-tĭs pĭg-mĕn-TŌ-să
retinopathy	rĕt-ĭ-NŎP-ă-thē
retinoscopy	rĕt-ĭ-NŎS-kō-pē
saccule	SĂK-ūl
salpingopharyngeal	săl-pĭng-gō-fă-RĬN-gē-ăl
sclera	SKLĒ-ră
scleritis	sklē-RĪ-tĭs
scotoma	skō-TŌ-mă
stapedectomy	stā-pĕ-DĔK-tō-mē
stapes	STĀ-pēz
strabismus	stră-BĬZ-mŭs

subconjunctival	sŭb-kŏn-jŭnk-TĪ-văl
suppuration	sŭp-ū-RĀ-shŭn
tinnitus	tĭ-NĪ-tĭs
tonometry	tō-NŎM-ĕ-trē
tympanic	tĭm-PĂN-ĭk
tympanometry	tĭm-pă-NŎM-ĕ-trē
tympanoplasty	tĭm-păn-ō-PLĂS-tē
utricle	Ū-trĭ-k'l
uveitis	ū-vē-Ī-tĭs
vertigo	VĔR-tĭ-gō
vitrectomy	vĭ-TRĔK-tō-mē
vitreous	VĬT-rē-ŭs
xerophthalmia	zĕr-ŏf-THĂL-mē-ă

REVIEW SHEET 16

Combining Forms

acou/o	______	ir/o	______
acous/o	______	irid/o	______
ambly/o	______	is/o	______
aque/o	______	kerat/o	______
audi/o	______	lacrim/o	______
aur/o	______	mastoid/o	______
auri/o	______	mi/o	______
bar/o	______	myc/o	______
blephar/o	______	mydri/o	______
cerumin/o	______	myring/o	______
choroid/o	______	ocul/o	______
conjunctiv/o	______	ophthalm/o	______
cor/o	______	opt/o	______
core/o	______	ot/o	______
corne/o	______	palpebr/o	______
cycl/o	______	phac/o	______
dacry/o	______	phak/o	______
dacryocyst/o	______	phot/o	______
emmetr/o	______	presby/o	______
glauc/o	______	pupill/o	______

retin/o ______________________ tympan/o ______________________

salping/o ______________________ uve/o ______________________

scler/o ______________________ vitre/o ______________________

staped/o ______________________ xer/o ______________________

Suffixes

-chalasis ______________________ -phonia ______________________

-cusis ______________________ -tropia ______________________

-opia ______________________

Additional Terms Relating to the Eye

accommodation (461)

anterior chamber (461)

aqueous humor (461)

astigmatism (467)

biconcave lens (466)

biconvex lens (461)

binocular vision (461)

cataract (468)

chalazion (469)

choroid layer (461)

ciliary body (461)

cones (461)

conjunctiva (461)

cornea (461)

cryoextraction (470)

crystalline lens (461)

diabetic retinopathy (468)

diathermy (470)

esotropia (469)

exotropia (469)

fluorescein angiography (470)

fovea centralis (461)

fundus (461)

glaucoma (468)

gonioscopy (470)

hemianopia (469)

hordeolum (469)

hyperopia (466)

iris (461)

keratoplasty (471)

laser photocoagulation (470)

macula lutea (461)

macular degeneration (469)

miotic (465)

mydriatic (465)

myopia (466)

nystagmus (468)

optic chiasma (461)

optic disk (461)

optic nerve (462)

orthoptic training (470)

phacoemulsification (471)

posterior chamber (462)

presbyopia (467)

pupil (462)

refraction (462)

retina (462)

retinal detachment (469)

retinitis pigmentosa (469)

retinoscopy (470)

rods (462)

sclera (462)

scotoma (469)

slit lamp biomicroscopy (470)

strabismus (469)

tonometry (470)

visual field test (470)

vitrectomy (471)

vitreous chamber (462)

vitreous humor (462)

Additional Terms Relating to the Ear

acoustic neuroma (477)

audiometry (478)

auditory meatus (473)

auditory tube (473)

auricle (473)

cerumen (473)

cholesteatoma (477)

cochlea (473)

cilia (473)

endolymph (473)

eustachian tube (473)

fenestration (477)

graft (476)

incus (473)

labyrinth (473)

macrotia (476)

malleus (473)

Meniere's syndrome (477)

microtia (476)

organ of Corti (474)

ossicle (474)

otosclerosis (476)

otoscopy (478)

oval window (475)

perilymph (475)

pinna (475)

presbycusis (477)

prosthesis (476)

saccule (475)

semicircular canals (475)

serous otitis media (476)

stapes (475)

suppurative otitis media (476)

tinnitus (477)

tympanic membrane (475)

tympanometry (478)

utricle (475)

vertigo (477)

CHAPTER 17

ENDOCRINE SYSTEM

In this chapter you will:

- Identify the endocrine glands and their hormones;
- Gain an understanding of the functions of these hormones in the body;
- Analyze medical terms related to the endocrine glands and their hormones;
- Describe the pathological conditions resulting from excessive and deficient secretions of the endocrine glands; and
- Identify laboratory tests, clinical procedures, and abbreviations related to endocrinology.

This chapter is divided into the following sections:

I. INTRODUCTION

The endocrine system is composed of **glands** located in many different regions of the body, all of which release specific chemical substances directly into the bloodstream. These chemical substances, called **hormones** (from the Greek word *hormōn*, meaning urging on), can regulate the many and varied functions of an organism. For example, one hormone stimulates the growth of bones, another causes the maturation of sex organs and reproductive cells, and another controls the metabolic rate (metabolism) within all the individual cells of the body. In addition, one powerful endocrine gland near the brain secretes a wide variety of different hormones that travel through the bloodstream and regulate the activities of other endocrine glands.

Hormones produce their effects by binding to **receptors**, which are recognition sites in the various **target** tissues upon which the hormones act. The receptors initiate specific biological effects when the hormones bind to them. Each hormone has its own receptor, and binding of receptor by hormone is much like the interaction of a key and a lock.

All the **endocrine** glands, no matter which hormones they produce, secrete their hormones directly into the bloodstream rather than into ducts leading to the exterior of the body. Those glands which send their chemical substances into ducts and out of the body are called **exocrine glands**. Examples of exocrine glands are sweat, mammary, mucous, salivary, and lacrimal (tear) glands.

The ductless, internally secreting **endocrine glands** are listed below. Locate these glands on Figure 17–1.

(1) thyroid gland
(2) parathyroid glands (four glands)
(3) adrenal glands (one pair)
(4) pancreas
(5) pituitary gland
(6) ovaries in female (one pair)
(7) testes in male (one pair)
(8) pineal gland
(9) thymus gland

The last two glands on this list, the pineal and thymus glands, are included as endocrine glands because they are ductless, although little is known about their endocrine function in the human body. The pineal gland, located in the central portion of the brain, is believed to secrete a substance called **melatonin**. Melatonin contributes to the process of skin pigmentation in lower animals, such as frogs and fishes. In mammals, melatonin is believed to affect the brain and influence the rate of gonad (ovary and testis) maturation. Calcification of the pineal gland can occur and can be an important radiological landmark when x-rays of the brain are examined.

The thymus gland, located behind the sternum in the mediastinum, resembles a lymph

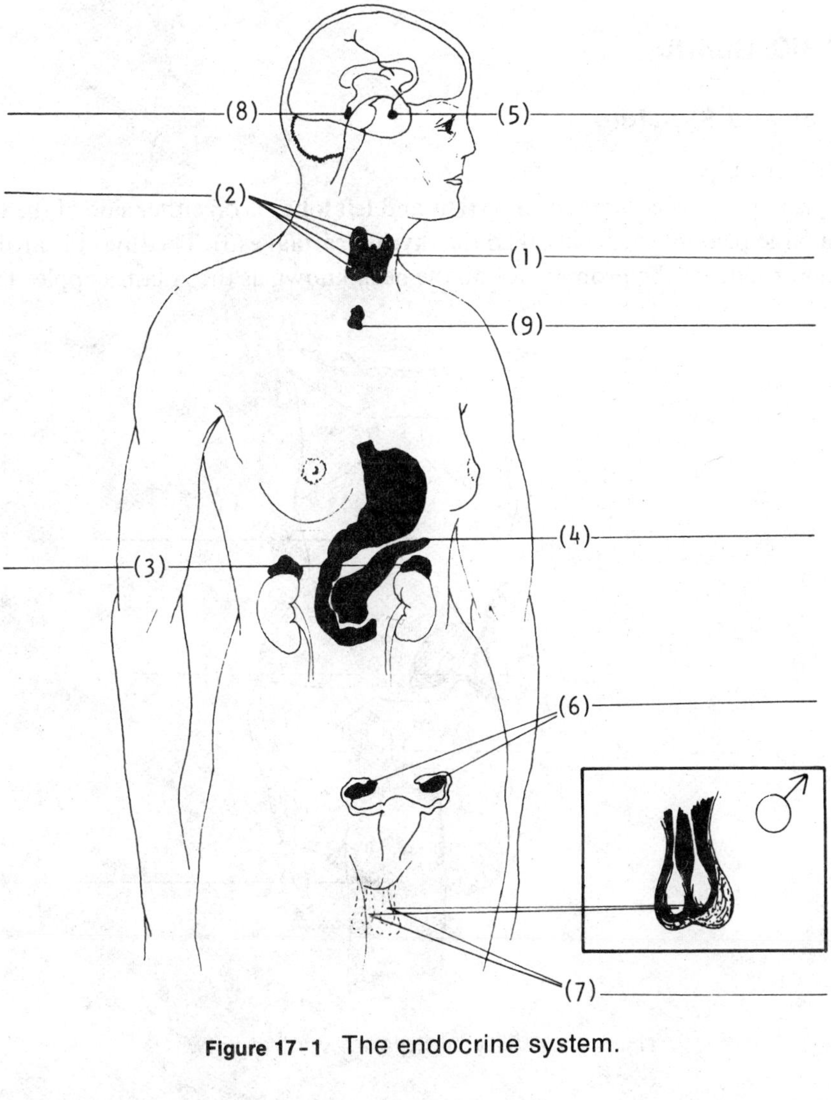

Figure 17-1 The endocrine system.

gland in structure. It contains lymphatic tissue and antibody-producing lymphocytes. The gland is important in the development of immune responses in newborns (it is large in children but shrinks in adults), but its endocrine function is not well understood. Removal of the thymus gland is helpful in treating a muscular-neurological disorder called myasthenia gravis.

Some hormones are produced by organs other than the endocrine glands already mentioned. For example, the kidney secretes two hormones, **renin** and **erythropoietin**. Renin participates in the control of blood pressure, and erythropoietin stimulates the production of red blood cells by the bone marrow. The gastrointestinal tract secretes three hormones, **gastrin**, **secretin**, and **cholecystokinin**. These hormones stimulate the secretion of gastric acid and enzymes (gastrin), the secretion of pancreatic enzymes (secretin), and contraction of the gallbladder (cholecystokinin). The skin produces **vitamin D**, which is also considered a hormone. Vitamin D stimulates the absorption of calcium from the gastrointestinal tract and is necessary for the maintenance of proper amounts of calcium in the bones and in the bloodstream.

Prostaglandins are hormone-like substances that affect the body in many ways. First found in semen but now recognized in cells throughout the body, prostaglandins stimulate the contraction of the uterus, regulate body temperature, platelet aggregation, and acid secretion in the stomach, and have the ability to lower blood pressure.

II. THYROID GLAND

A. Location and Structure

Label Figure 17-2:

The thyroid gland is composed of a **right** and **left lobe** (1) on either side of the **trachea** (2), just below a large piece of cartilage called the **thyroid cartilage** (3). The thyroid cartilage covers the larynx and produces the prominence on the neck known as the Adam's apple. The **isthmus**

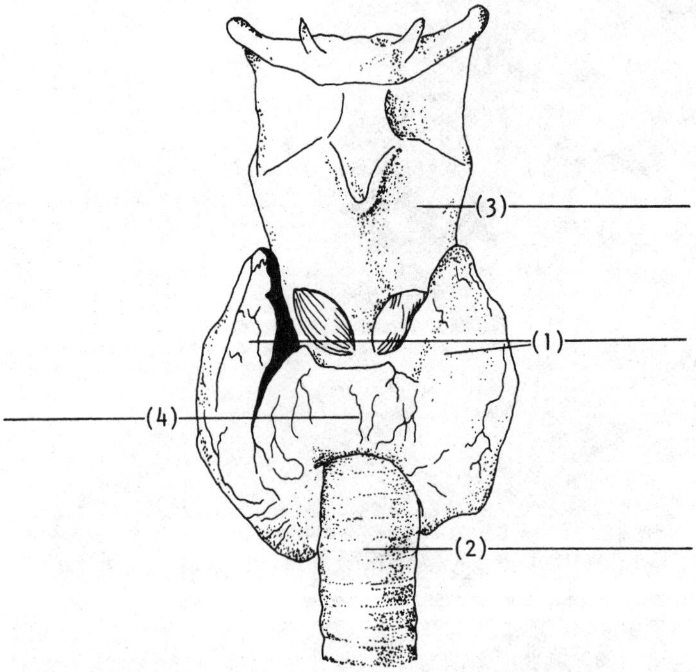

Figure 17-2 Thyroid gland, ventral view.

(4) of the thyroid gland is a narrow strip of glandular tissue that connects the two lobes on the ventral surface of the trachea.

B. Function

The two hormones secreted by the thyroid gland are called **thyroxine (T_4)** and **triiodothyronine (T_3)**. These hormones are synthesized in the thyroid gland from **iodine**, which is picked up from the blood circulating through the gland, and from an amino acid called tyrosine. T_4 (containing four atoms of iodine) is much more concentrated in the blood, while T_3 (containing three atoms of iodine) is far more potent in affecting the metabolism of cells. Most thyroid hormone is bound to protein molecules as it travels in the bloodstream.

T_4 and T_3 are necessary in the body to maintain a normal level of metabolism in all body cells. Cells need oxygen to carry on metabolic processes, one aspect of which is the burning of food to release the energy stored within the food. Thyroid hormone aids cells in their uptake of oxygen and thus supports the metabolic rate in the body. Injections of thyroid hormone will raise the metabolic rate, while removal of the thyroid gland, diminishing thyroid hormone content in the body, will result in a lower metabolic rate, heat loss, and poor physical and mental development.

A more recently discovered hormone produced by the thyroid gland is called **calcitonin (thyrocalcitonin)**. Calcitonin is secreted when calcium levels in the blood are high. It stimulates the passage of calcium into bones from the blood.

III. PARATHYROID GLANDS

A. Location and Structure

Label Figure 17-3:

The **parathyroid glands** are four small oval bodies (1) located on the dorsal aspect of the **thyroid gland** (2).

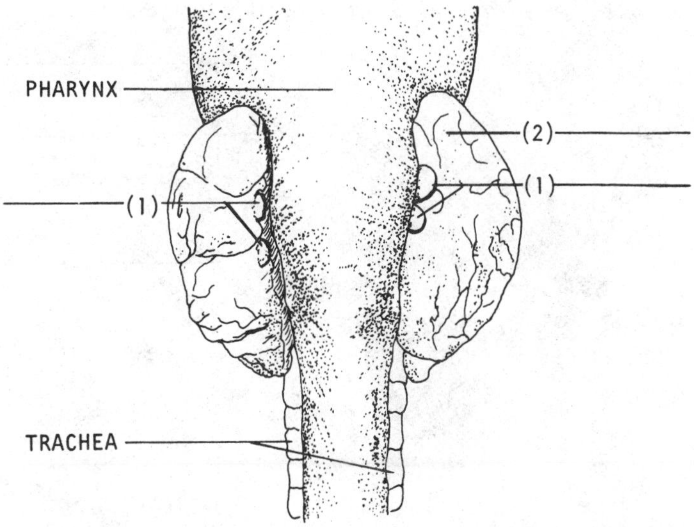

Figure 17-3 Parathyroid glands, dorsal view.

B. Function

Parathyroid hormone (PTH) is secreted by the parathyroid glands. This hormone (also known as **parathormone**) mobilizes **calcium** (a mineral substance) from bones into the bloodstream, where the calcium is necessary for the proper functioning of body tissues, especially muscles. Normally, calcium in the food we eat is absorbed from the intestine and carried, by the blood, to the bones, where it is stored. The adjustment of the level of calcium in the blood is a good example of the way hormones in general control the **homeostasis** (equilibrium or constancy in the internal environment) of the body. If there is a decrease in blood calcium (as in pregnancy or rickets, a vitamin D deficiency disease), parathyroid hormone is secreted in larger amounts to cause calcium to leave the bones and enter the bloodstream. Thus, blood calcium levels are brought back to normal. Conversely, any situation of increase in calcium in the bloodstream, such as excess quantity of calcium or vitamin D in the diet, will lead to decreased parathyroid hormone secretion, decreasing blood calcium so that homeostasis is again achieved.

IV. ADRENAL GLANDS

A. Location and Structure

Label Figure 17-4:

The adrenal glands, also called the **suprarenal glands**, are two small glands situated one on top of each **kidney** (1). Each gland consists of two parts, an outer portion called the **adrenal cortex** (2) and an inner portion called the **adrenal medulla** (3). The cortex and medulla are two glands in one, each secreting its own different endocrine hormones. The cortex secretes hormones called **steroids** (complex chemicals derived from cholesterol), and the medulla secretes hormones called **catecholamines** (chemicals derived from an amino acid).

B. Function

The adrenal cortex secretes three types of steroid hormones:

1. **Mineralocorticoids**—These hormones are essential to life because they regulate the

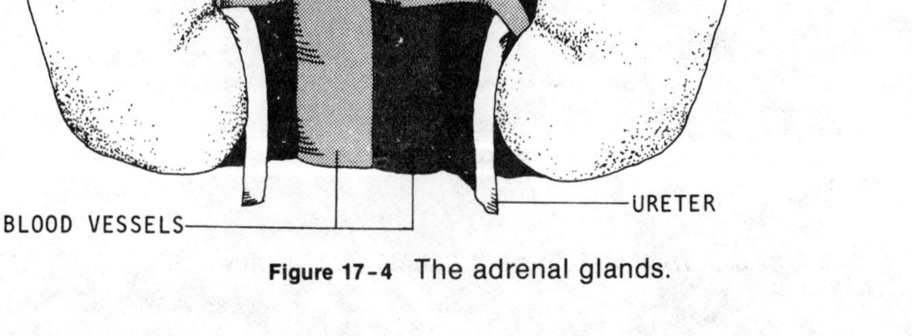

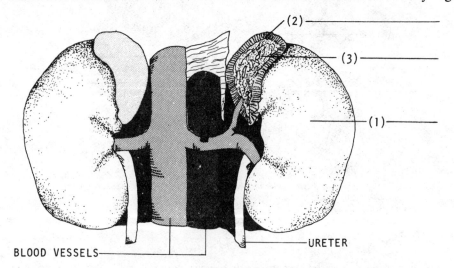

Figure 17-4 The adrenal glands.

amounts of mineral salts (also called **electrolytes**) that are retained in the body. A proper balance of water and salts in the blood and tissues is essential to the normal functioning of the body.

The most important mineralocorticoid hormone is called **aldosterone**. The secretion of aldosterone by the adrenal cortex increases the reabsorption of **sodium** (a mineral electrolyte commonly found in salts) by the kidney tubules. At the same time, aldosterone stimulates the excretion of another electrolyte called **potassium**.

The secretion of aldosterone increases manyfold in the face of a severe sodium-restricted diet, thereby enabling the body to hold needed salt in the bloodstream.

2. **Glucocorticoids**—These hormones have an important influence on the metabolism of sugars, fats, and proteins within all body cells.

Cortisol (also called **hydrocortisone**) is the most important glucocorticoid hormone. Cortisol increases the ability of cells to make new sugars out of fats and proteins (gluconeogenesis) and regulates the quantity of sugars, fats, and proteins in the blood and cells.

Cortisone is a hormone very similar to cortisol and can be prepared synthetically. Cortisone is useful in treating inflammatory ailments such as rheumatoid arthritis.

3. **Androgens, Estrogens, and Progestins**—These are male and female hormones that maintain the secondary sex characteristics, such as beard and breast development, and are necessary for reproduction. Most of these hormones are also produced in the ovaries and testes. Excess adrenal androgen secretion in females leads to **virilism** (development of male characteristics), and excess adrenal estrogen and progestin secretion in males produces abnormal feminine characteristics.

The adrenal medulla secretes two types of **catecholamine** hormones:

1. **Epinephrine (adrenaline)**—This hormone increases cardiac activity, dilates bronchial tubes, and stimulates the production of glucose from a storage substance called glycogen when glucose is needed by the body.

2. **Norepinephrine (noradrenaline)**—This hormone constricts vessels and raises blood pressure.

Both epinephrine and norepinephrine are called **sympathomimetic** agents because they mimic, or copy, the actions of the sympathetic nervous system. During times of stress, these hormones are secreted by the adrenal medulla in response to nervous stimulation. They help the body respond to crisis situations by raising blood pressure, increasing heartbeat and respiration, and bringing sugar out of storage in the cells.

V. PANCREAS

A. Location and Structure

Label Figure 17-5:

The **pancreas** (1) is located behind the **stomach** (2) in the region of the 1st and 2nd lumbar **vertebrae** (3). The specialized cells in the pancreas that produce hormones are called the **islets of Langerhans**.

B. Function

The islets of Langerhans produce two hormones called **insulin** and **glucagon**. Both of these hormones play a role in the proper metabolism of sugars and starches in the body. Insulin is necessary in the bloodstream so that sugars can pass from the blood into the cells

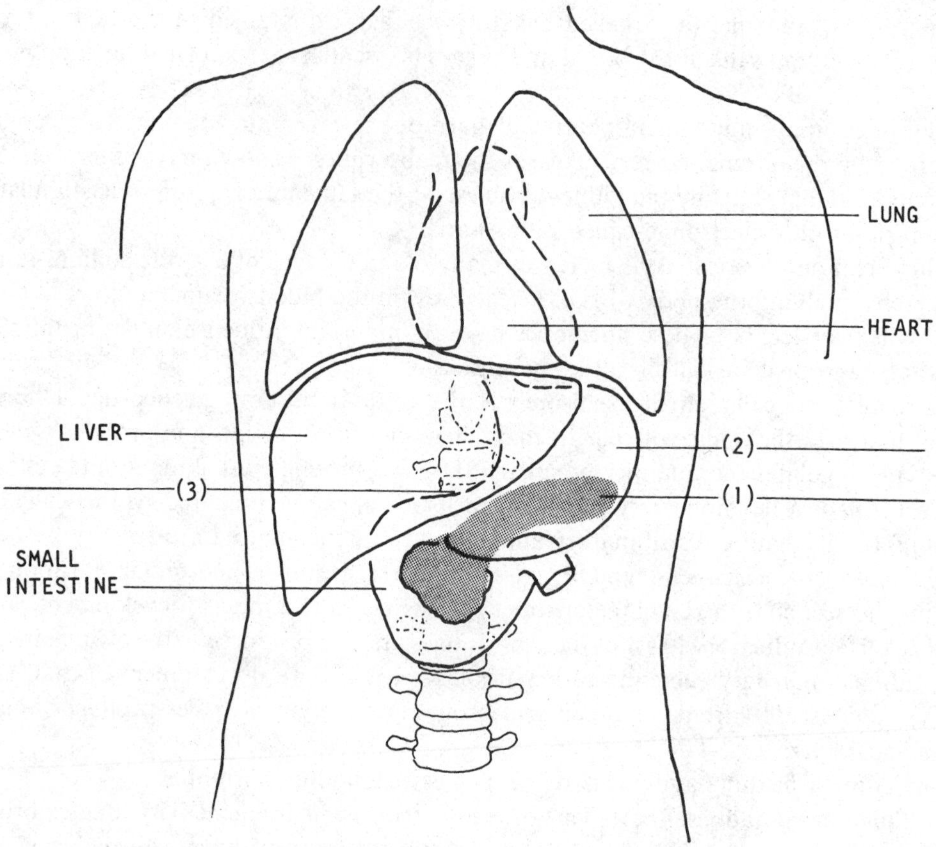

Figure 17-5 The pancreas.

of the body where they are burned to release energy. When blood sugar (glucose) is above normal, insulin is released by the islet cells of the pancreas. The insulin causes sugar to enter body cells to be burned and stimulates the conversion of glucose to **glycogen** (a starch-storage form of sugar) in the liver. Thus, sugar can leave the blood to be stored (as glycogen) or used to release energy. Glucagon, the opposite "twin" of insulin, is released into the blood when sugar levels are below normal. It causes the breakdown of liver glycogen to sugar (glucose), so that there is a rise in the sugar content of blood leaving the liver.

The islet cells of Langerhans include two major types, containing granules that stain differently. The **alpha cells** (10 to 30 per cent of the cells) stain red and produce glucagon. The **beta cells** (60 to 90 per cent) stain blue and produce insulin.

While the islets of Langerhans carry on the endocrine functions of the pancreas, other cells within the organ carry on its exocrine functions. These cells secrete digestive enzymes and juices into the gastrointestinal tract (see Chapter 5).

VI. PITUITARY GLAND

A. Location and Structure

Label Figure 17-6:

The pituitary gland, also called the **hypophysis**, is a small, pea-sized gland located at the base of the brain in a small pocket-like depression of the skull called the **sella turcica**. It is a

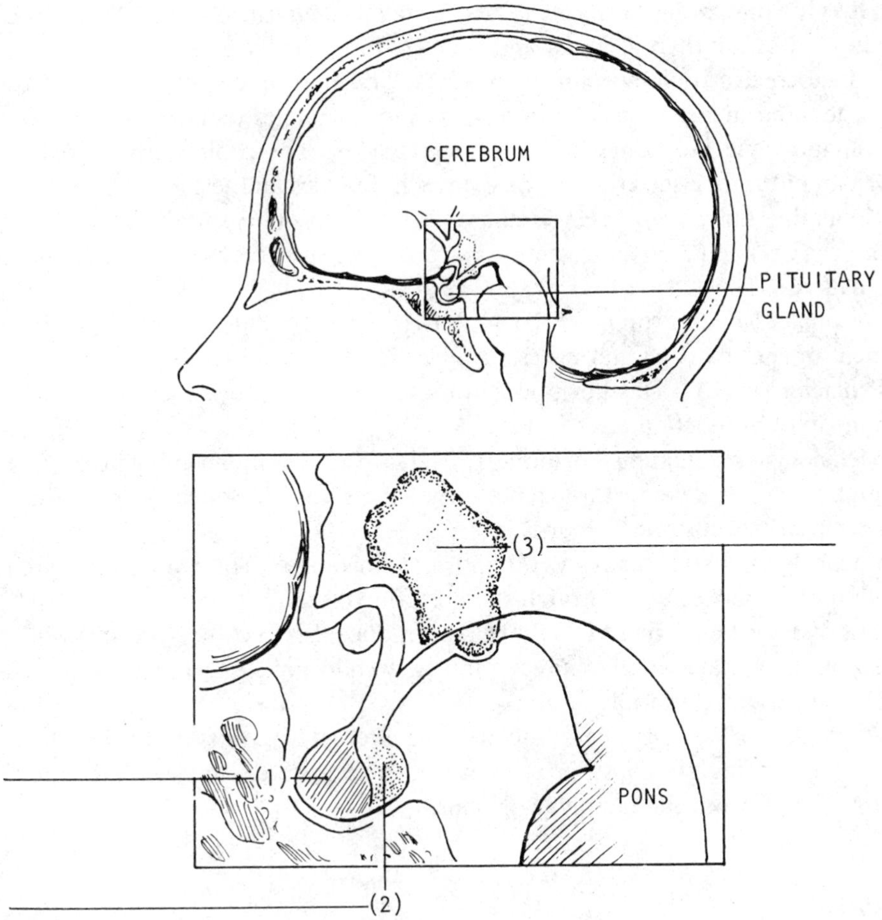

Figure 17-6 Pituitary gland.

well protected gland with the entire mass of the brain above it and the nasal cavity below. The ancient Greeks imagined that its function was to produce "pituita" or nasal secretion.

The pituitary consists of two distinct parts: an anterior lobe called the **adenohypophysis** (1), which is formed by an upgrowth from the pharynx and is glandular in nature; and a posterior lobe called the **neurohypophysis** (2), which is derived from a downgrowth from the base of the brain, and is composed of nervous tissue. The **hypothalamus** (3) is a region of the brain that is in close proximity to the pituitary gland. Signals transmitted from the hypothalamus control almost all the secretions by the pituitary gland. Secretion from the neurohypophysis is controlled by nerve fibers originating in the hypothalamus and ending in the neurohypophysis. Secretion by the adenohypophysis is controlled by special hormones called **releasing** and **inhibiting factors**. These hormones are secreted by the hypothalamus and pass to the adenohypophysis by way of special capillaries.

B. Function

The hormones of the **adenohypophysis** are:

1. **Growth hormone (GH** or **hGH** in humans; also called **somatotropin)**—This hormone acts on bone tissue to accelerate its growth in the body.

2. **Thyroid-stimulating hormone (TSH**; also called **thyrotropin)**—This hormone stimulates the growth of the thyroid gland and its secretion of thyroxine.

3. **Adrenocorticotropic hormone (ACTH)**—This hormone stimulates the growth of the adrenal cortex and increases its secretion of steroid hormones (primarily cortisol).

4. **Gonadotropic hormones**—There are several gonadotropic hormones that influence the growth and hormone secretion of the ovaries in females and testes in males. In the female, **follicle-stimulating hormone (FSH)** stimulates the growth of eggs in the ovaries, and **luteinizing hormone (LH)** induces the secretion of progesterone (pregnancy-sustaining hormone) from the ovaries.

In the male, gonadotropins (FSH and LH) from the adenohypophysis influence the development of spermatozoa and testes.

5. **Prolactin (PRL)**—This hormone promotes the growth of breast tissue and stimulates and sustains milk production after birth.

6. **Melanocyte-stimulating hormone (MSH)**—This hormone influences the formation of melanin and causes increased pigmentation of the skin. This effect is observed only when hypersecretion of the hormone occurs.

The **neurohypophysis** secretes two important hormones. These hormones are formed in the hypothalamus but secreted through the posterior pituitary gland:

1. **Antidiuretic hormone (ADH)**—This hormone, also known as **vasopressin**, stimulates the reabsorption of water by the kidney tubules. In addition, ADH can also increase blood pressure by constricting arterioles.

2. **Oxytocin**—This hormone stimulates the uterus to contract during childbirth and maintains labor during childbirth. Oxytocin is also secreted during suckling, and causes the production of milk from the mammary glands.

VII. OVARIES

A. Location and Structure

The ovaries are two small glands located in the lower abdominal region of the female. The ovaries produce the female sex cell, the ovum, as well as hormones that are responsible for female sex characteristics and regulation of the menstrual cycle.

B. Function

The ovarian hormones are **estradiol** (an estrogen) and **progesterone**. Estradiol is responsible for the development and maintenance of secondary sex characteristics, such as hair and breast development. Progesterone is responsible for the preparation and maintenance of the uterus in pregnancy.

VIII. TESTES

A. Location and Structure

The testes are two small, ovoid glands suspended from the inguinal region of the male by the spermatic cord and surrounded by the scrotal sac. The testes produce the male sex cells, spermatozoa, as well as the male hormone called **testosterone**.

B. Function

Testosterone is an **androgen** (male steroid hormone) that stimulates and promotes the growth of secondary sex characteristics in the male (development of beard and pubic hair, deepening of voice, and distribution of fat).

Table 17-1 reviews the major endocrine glands and the hormones they produce.

Table 17-1 MAJOR ENDOCRINE GLANDS AND THE HORMONES THEY PRODUCE

Endocrine Gland	Hormone	Action
Thyroid	Thyroxine, triiodothyronine	Regulate metabolism in body cells
	Calcitonin	Stimulates passage of calcium into bones from blood
Parathyroids	Parathyroid hormone	Regulates calcium in the blood
Adrenals:		
Cortex	Aldosterone (mineralocorticoid)	Regulates the amount of salts in the body
	Cortisol (glucocorticoid)	Regulates the quantities of sugars, fats, and proteins in cells
	Androgens, estrogens, and progestins	Maintain secondary sex characteristics
Medulla	Epinephrine (adrenaline)	Sympathomimetic
	Norepinephrine (noradrenaline)	Sympathomimetic
Pancreas:		
Islets of Langerhans	Insulin	Regulates the transport of glucose to the body cells
	Glucagon	Increases blood sugar by causing conversion of glycogen to glucose
Pituitary (hypophysis):		
Anterior lobe (adenohypophysis)	Pituitary growth hormone (GH; somatotropin)	Increases bone growth
	Thyroid-stimulating hormone (TSH)	Stimulates production of thyroxine and growth of the thyroid gland
	Adrenocorticotropin (ACTH)	Stimulates secretion of hormones from the adrenal cortex, especially cortisol
	Gonadotropins:	
	Follicle-stimulating hormone (FSH)	Stimulates growth of eggs in the ovaries
	Luteinizing hormone (LH)	Important in sustaining pregnancy
	Prolactin (PRL)	Promotes growth of breast tissue and milk secretion
	Melanocyte-stimulating hormone (MSH)	Increases pigmentation of the skin
Posterior lobe (neurohypophysis)	Antidiuretic hormone (ADH; vasopressin)	Stimulates reabsorption of water by kidney tubules
	Oxytocin	Stimulates contraction of the uterus during labor and childbirth
Ovaries	Estradiol	Development and maintenance of secondary sex characteristics in the female
	Progesterone	Preparation and maintenance of the uterus in pregnancy
Testes	Testosterone	Growth and maintenance of secondary sex characteristics in the male

IX. VOCABULARY

adenohypophysis	Anterior lobe of the pituitary gland.
adrenal cortex	The outer section of the adrenal gland.
adrenal medulla	The inner section of the adrenal gland.
adrenaline	Epinephrine (adrenaline is the name used in England; Adrenalin is a trademark for preparations of epinephrine in the United States).
adrenocorticotropic hormone (ACTH)	A hormone secreted by the adenohypophysis. ACTH stimulates the adrenal cortex to produce hormones.
aldosterone	A hormone secreted by the adrenal cortex; stimulates kidney tubules to retain salt in the body.
androgens	Male hormones secreted primarily by the testes, and to a lesser extent by the adrenal cortex.
antidiuretic hormone (ADH)	A hormone secreted by the neurohypophysis; stimulates reabsorption of water by the kidney tubules. Also called vasopressin.
calcitonin	A hormone produced by the thyroid gland; causes calcium to leave the bloodstream and pass into bones. Also called thyrocalcitonin.
calcium	A mineral substance necessary for the proper functioning of body tissues and bones.
catecholamines	Complex substances derived from an amino acid; epinephrine and norepinephrine are examples.
cholecystokinin	A hormone secreted by the gastrointestinal tract, stimulates contraction of the gallbladder.
cortisol	A hormone secreted by the adrenal cortex; regulates the metabolism of sugars, fats, and proteins in cells.
cortisone	A synthetic substance derived from cortisol that has identical action and is useful in treating inflammatory conditions.
electrolyte	A mineral salt found in the blood and tissues and necessary for proper functioning of body cells. Potassium, sodium, and calcium are examples.
endocrine glands	Ductless glands that secrete hormones directly into the bloodstream.
epinephrine	A catecholamine hormone produced by the adrenal medulla; it is a sympathomimetic.

erythropoietin	A hormone secreted by the kidney; stimulates the bone marrow to produce red blood cells.
estradiol	The primary estrogen secreted by the ovaries.
estrogens	Female sex hormones secreted by the ovaries and adrenal cortex.
follicle-stimulating hormone (FSH)	A hormone secreted by the adenohypophysis; stimulates the maturation of ova and secretion of estrogen.
gastrin	Hormone secreted by the gastrointestinal tract to stimulate acid and enzyme secretion by the stomach.
glucagon	A hormone produced by the pancreas (islets of Langerhans); stimulates the release of sugar from glycogen.
glucocorticoids	A group of hormones secreted by the adrenal cortex; cortisol is a major example.
glucose	A simple sugar.
glycogen	Starch; a storage form of sugar.
gonadotropic hormones	Hormones secreted by the adenohypophysis to stimulate the development and functioning of the ovaries and testes.
growth hormone (GH, hGH)	A hormone secreted by the adenohypophysis; stimulates the growth of long bones. Also called somatotropin.
homeostasis	The tendency in an organism to return to equilibrium or constant, stable state.
hormone	A chemical substance produced by cells and transported by the blood to target organs on which it has a regulatory effect.
hydrocortisone	Cortisol.
hypophysis	The pituitary gland.
hypothalamus	A region of the brain that lies near the hypophysis. It stimulates the hypophysis to release hormones.
insulin	A hormone secreted by the islets of Langerhans and essential for the proper uptake and metabolism of sugar in cells. Its name comes from "insula," meaning island (islet).
iodine	A chemical element that composes a large part of thyroxine and triiodothyronine.

islets of Langerhans	Endocrine cells of the pancreas.
isthmus	A narrow strip of tissue connecting two parts (as in the two lobes of the thyroid gland on either side of the trachea).
luteinizing hormone (LH)	A gonadotropic hormone produced by the adenohypophysis; important in sustaining pregnancy.
melanocyte-stimulating hormone	An adenohypophyseal hormone that increases pigmentation of the skin.
melatonin	A hormone secreted by the pineal gland.
mineralocorticoids	Hormones secreted by the adrenal cortex; regulate the retention of salts in the body. Aldosterone is an example.
neurohypophysis	The posterior lobe of the pituitary gland.
norepinephrine	A hormone secreted by the adrenal medulla; a sympathomimetic.
oxytocin	A hormone secreted by the neurohypophysis; it stimulates the uterus to contract during labor.
parathyroid hormone (PTH)	A hormone secreted by the parathyroid gland; it regulates the amount of calcium in the blood and bones. Also called parathormone.
pineal gland	An endocrine gland located in the middle of the brain; it secretes melatonin. Named for its pine cone shape, from the French "pomme de pin" (pine cone).
progesterone	A hormone secreted by the ovaries and important in sustaining the uterine lining during pregnancy.
prolactin (PRL)	A hormone secreted by the adenohypophysis; it stimulates the secretion of milk from mammary glands of the breast.
prostaglandins	Hormone-like lipid substances found in many body cells; they lower blood pressure, stimulate contraction of the uterus, and regulate body temperature, aggregation of platelets in clotting, and acid secretion in the stomach.
receptors	Recognition sites for hormones in target tissues.
renin	Hormone secreted by the kidney to raise blood pressure.
secretin	Hormone secreted by the gastrointestinal tract to stimulate the secretion of pancreatic enzymes.
sella turcica	The cavity in the skull where the pituitary gland is located.

somatotropin Growth hormone.

steroids Complex substances (derived from cholesterol) of which many hormones are made. Examples are estrogens, androgens, and cortisol.

sympathomimetic Producing effects (tachycardia, bronchodilation, and hypertension) similar to those produced by the sympathetic nervous system.

target tissue Cells toward which the effects of a hormone are directed.

testosterone A major male hormone produced by the testes.

triiodothyronine (T_3) A hormone produced by the thyroid gland; it stimulates cellular metabolism.

thyroid-stimulating hormone (TSH) A hormone secreted by the adenohypophysis; it stimulates the thyroid gland to produce thyroxine and triiodothyronine. Also called thyrotropin.

thyroxine (T_4) A hormone secreted by the thyroid gland; it stimulates cellular metabolism.

vasopressin Antidiuretic hormone (ADH).

vitamin D A hormone produced by the skin and necessary for absorption of calcium into the body.

X. COMBINING FORMS

Combining Form	*Definition*	*Terminology*	*Meaning*
thyroid/o thyr/o	thyroid gland	thyroidectomy	______________________
		euthyroid	______________________
		thyroiditis	______________________
toxic/o	poison	thyrotoxicosis *Caused by excessive thyroid secretion; symptoms are sweating, weight loss, tachycardia, nervousness.*	______________________
home/o	sameness, unchanging, constant	homeostasis	______________________
calc/o	calcium	hypocalcemia	______________________
		hypercalcemia	______________________

		decalcification ________________
parathyroid/o	parathyroid glands	parathyroidectomy ________________
ster/o	solid structure	steroid ________________ *Complex, solid, ring-shaped molecule.*
adren/o	adrenal glands	adrenomegaly ________________
adrenal/o	adrenal glands	adrenalectomy ________________
cortic/o	cortex, outer region of an organ	corticosteroid ________________ *Glucocorticoids, mineralocorticoids, and androgens and estrogens.*
kal/i	potassium	hypokalemia ________________
natr/o	sodium	hypernatremia ________________
gluc/o	sugar	gluconeogenesis ________________ *An effect of glucagon secretion.*
glyc/o	sugar	hyperglycemia ________________
		glycogen ________________
pineal/o	pineal gland	pinealectomy ________________
thym/o	thymus gland	thymectomy ________________
somat/o	body	somatotropin ________________ *-tropin, like -trophy, means nourishment or development.*
gonad/o	sex glands *(ovaries in the female, and testes in the male)*	hypogonadism ________________ *Deficiency of gonadotropin secretion by the adenohypophysis produces this condition.*
		gonadotropin ________________
lact/o	milk	prolactin ________________
galact/o	milk	galactorrhea ________________ *Inappropriate secretion of milk from the breasts.*

gynec/o	female	gynecomastia ____________ *Excessive development of mammary tissue in the male; can be caused by excessive estrogens or deficient androgens.*
andr/o	male	androgen ____________
pancreat/o	pancreas	pancreatectomy ____________
estr/o	female	estrogen ____________
test/o	testes	testosterone ____________
dips/o	thirst	polydipsia ____________ *Symptom associated with many disease conditions, for example, diabetes insipidus and diabetes mellitus.*
ur/o	urine	antidiuretic ____________ polyuria ____________
-physis	growth	adenohypophysis ____________ *Derived from glandular tissue in the embryo.* neurohypophysis ____________ *Derived from nervous tissue in the embryo.* cryohypophysectomy ____________ ____________ hypophyseal ____________
-tocin	labor, delivery	oxytocin ____________

XI. PATHOLOGICAL CONDITIONS

Thyroid

goiter

Enlargement of the thyroid gland.

Thyroid gland enlargement may be a symptom of many different conditions. Examples of two types of goiter are:

Endemic goiter—This condition, prevalent in certain regions and peoples ("demos" means people) and marked by accumulation of colloid (gluelike or gelatinous) material in the thyroid gland, causes hypertrophy of the thyroid. The etiology is deficiency of iodine in the diet, which causes the thyroid to work harder to make hormone and thus enlarge as compensation for the scarcity of iodine. Treatment is to increase the supply of iodine in the diet.

Nodular or **adenomatous goiter**—This form of goiter is marked not only by enlargement (hyperplasia) of the thyroid, but by the formation of nodules or adenomas. Some patients develop hyperthyroidism with toxic symptoms such as rapid pulse, tremors, nervousness, and excessive sweating. Treatment consists of use of thyroid hormone to suppress the normal thyroid gland functioning.

hyperthyroidism

Overactivity of the thyroid gland.

The most common form of this condition is known as **exophthalmic goiter** (**thyrotoxicosis** or **Graves' disease**). Hyperplasia of the thyroid parenchyma occurs so that excessive hormone is produced. Metabolic rate in cells is increased, leading to thyrotoxic symptoms as in nodular goiter. In addition, **exophthalmos** (protrusion of the eyeballs) occurs as a result of swelling of tissue behind the eyeball. The etiology is unclear, although it is currently thought to be an immunologic disorder. Treatment may include thyroidectomy, management with antithyroid drugs that reduce the amount of thyroid hormone liberated from the gland, or administration of radioactive iodine, which destroys the overactive glandular tissue. Figure 17-7 shows a patient with exophthalmos.

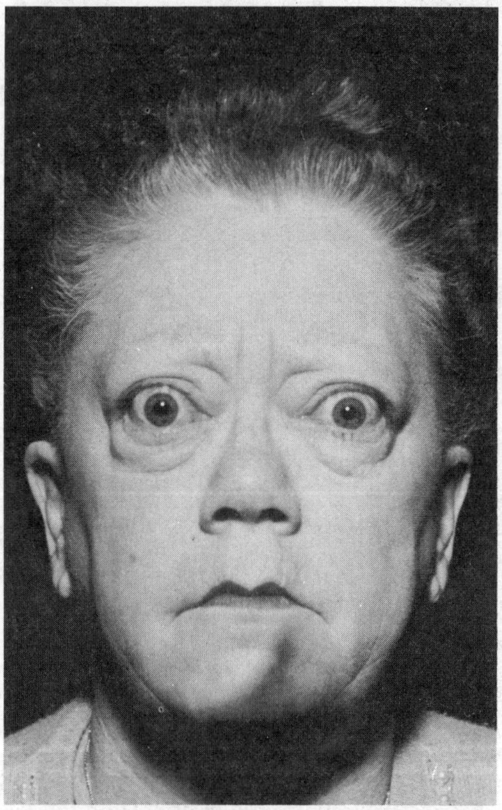

Figure 17-7 Exophthalmos in Graves' disease. (From Jacob, S.W., Francone, C.A., and Lossow, W.J.: Structure and Function in Man. 5th ed. Philadelphia, W. B. Saunders Co., 1982.)

hypothyroidism

Underactivity of the thyroid gland.

Any one of several conditions can produce hypothyroidism (thyroidectomy, endemic goiter, destruction of the gland by irradiation), but all have similar physiological effects. These include fatigue, muscular and mental sluggishness, and constipation. Two examples of hypothyroidism are:

Myxedema—This is advanced hypothyroidism in adulthood. The thyroid gland atrophies and practically no hormone is produced. The skin becomes dry and puffy (edema) because of collection of a mucus-like (myx/o means mucus) material under the skin. Many patients also develop atherosclerosis because lack of thyroid hormone increases the quantity of blood lipids (fats). Recovery may be complete if hormone is administered soon after the symptoms appear. Figure 17-8 shows a patient with myxedema.

Cretinism—Extreme hypothyroidism during infancy and childhood leads to a lack of normal physical and mental growth. Skeletal growth is more inhibited than soft tissue growth so the cretin has the appearance of an obese, short, and stocky child. Treatment consists of administration of thyroid hormone, which may be able to reverse some of the hypothyroid effects.

thyroid carcinoma

Cancer of the thyroid gland.

Some tumors are very slow growing and others may metastasize widely. Adenomas (noncancerous growths) are distinguished from carcinomas in

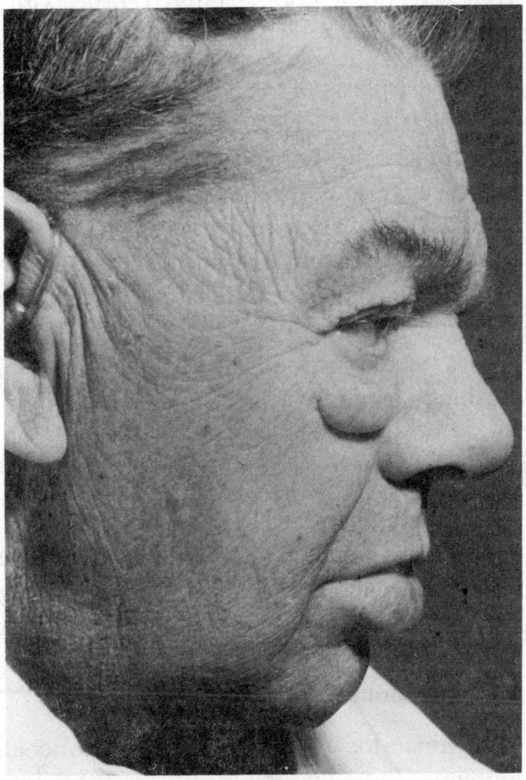

Figure 17-8 Myxedema. (From Jacob, S.W., Francone, C.A., and Lossow, W.J.: Structure and Function in Man. 5th ed. Philadelphia, W. B. Saunders Co., 1982.)

radioactive tracer studies. Hot tumor areas (those collecting more radioactivity than surrounding tissues) usually indicate benign growths; cold nodules can be either benign or malignant.

Parathyroid

hyperparathyroidism

Excessive production of parathyroid hormone.

Excessive quantities of parathyroid hormone cause calcium to leave the bones and enter the bloodstream (hypercalcemia). This leaves the bones decalcified and susceptible to fractures and cysts, as in **osteitis fibrosa cystica**. Patients also have a tendency to develop kidney stones from hypercalcemia. The cause of hyperparathyroidism is usually a tumor of one of the parathyroid glands. Treatment is surgical removal of the tumor.

hypoparathyroidism

Deficient production of parathyroid hormone.

Without sufficient parathyroid hormone, calcium is unable to enter the bloodstream from bones. This leads to muscle and nerve weakness with spasms of muscles, a condition known as **tetany**. Administration of calcium plus large quantities of vitamin D can control the calcium level in the bloodstream.

Adrenal Cortex

Cushing's disease

Hyperfunctioning of the adrenal cortex with increased glucocorticoid secretion.

Hyperplasia of the adrenal cortex results from excessive stimulation of the gland by ACTH. Obesity, moonlike fullness of the face, excess deposition of fat in the thoracic region of the back (so-called "buffalo hump"), high blood sugar, and hypertension are produced by excess secretion of adrenal steroids. Decreasing secretion of ACTH by hypophysectomy or pituitary irradiation is the usual treatment.

Occasionally, a tumor of the adrenal may be associated with excessive secretion of cortisol and the same clinical features (**Cushing's syndrome**). This is treated surgically by adrenalectomy. Figure 17-9 shows a person with Cushing's syndrome.

adrenal virilism

Excessive output of adrenal androgens.

Adrenal hyperplasia or tumor can cause this condition in adult women. Symptoms include amenorrhea, **hirsutism** (excessive hair on the face and body), acne, and deepening of the voice. Drug therapy to suppress androgen production and adrenalectomy are possible treatments.

Addison's disease

Hypofunctioning of the adrenal cortex.

Mineralocorticoids and glucocorticoids are produced in deficient amounts. Hypoglycemia (from deficient glucocorticoids), excretion of large amounts of water and salts (from deficient mineralocorticoids), weakness,

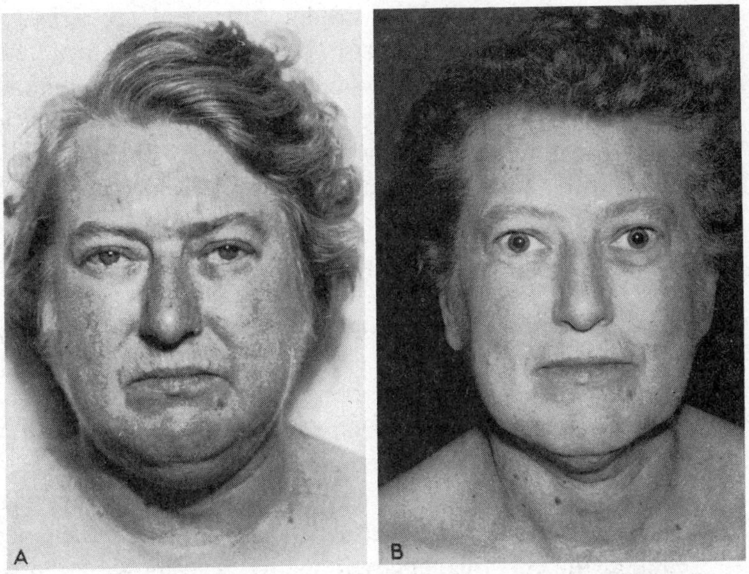

Figure 17-9 *A*, A patient with Cushing's syndrome. *B*, Signs and symptoms disappeared after adrenalectomy and therapy. (From Williams, R.H.: Textbook of Endocrinology. 4th ed. Philadelphia, W. B. Saunders Co., 1968.)

weight loss, and melanin pigmentation of the skin are symptoms of the condition. Treatment consists of daily cortisone administration and intake of salts.

Adrenal Medulla

pheochromocytoma

Tumor occurring in the adrenal medulla.

The tumor cells (which stain dark or dusky color – phe/o = dusky; chrom/o = color) produce excess secretion of the catecholamines epinephrine and norepinephrine. The excess catecholamines produce hypertension, palpitations, severe headaches, sweating, flushing of face, and muscle spasms. Surgery to remove the tumor and administration of antihypertensive drugs are possible courses of treatment.

Pancreas

diabetes mellitus

Lack of insulin secretion from the pancreas or resistance of insulin to promote carbohydrate (sugar, starch, and fat) metabolism in cells.

In diabetes mellitus sugar is prevented from leaving the blood (hyperglycemia) and cannot enter the body cells, where it is normally used to produce energy. There are two major types of diabetes mellitus:

Type I diabetes, "insulin dependent" (IDDM or juvenile-onset diabetes), seen mostly in children and adolescents, involves destruction of the beta cells of the islets of Langerhans with complete deficiency of insulin in the body. Patients are usually thin and require frequent injections of insulin to maintain a normal level of glucose in the blood.

Type II diabetes "non-insulin dependent" (NIDDM or adult-onset diabetes), is a separate disease from Type I, with a different inheritance pattern. Patients are usually older, and obesity is very common. The islets of Langerhans are not destroyed, and there is a relative deficiency of insulin secretion with a resistance by target tissues to the action of insulin. Treatment is with diet, weight reduction, exercise, and, if necessary, insulin or oral hypoglycemic agents. The oral hypoglycemic agents can stimulate the release of insulin from the pancreas and improve the body's sensitivity to insulin.

Diabetes is associated with both primary and secondary complications: **Primary complications** include **ketoacidosis** (fats are improperly burned leading to an accumulation of ketones in the body) and **hyperosmolar coma** when blood sugar concentration (osmolarity) gets too high or the patient receives insufficient amounts of insulin. **Hypoglycemia** can occur when too much insulin is taken by the patient.

Secondary (long-term) **complications** occur many years after the patient develops diabetes. These include destruction of the blood vessels of the retina of the eyes (**diabetic retinopathy**), causing visual loss and blindness; destruction of the kidneys (**diabetic nephropathy**), causing renal insufficiency and often requiring hemodialysis or renal transplantation; destruction of blood vessels, with atherosclerosis; and destruction of nerves (**diabetic neuropathy**) involving pain or loss of sensation, most commonly in the extremities.

hyperinsulinism — Excess of insulin.

This condition may be caused by a tumor of the pancreas (benign adenoma or carcinoma) or overdose of insulin. Excess insulin draws sugar out of the bloodstream, resulting in hypoglycemia. Fainting spells, convulsions, and loss of consciousness are common because a minimum level of blood sugar is necessary for proper mental functioning. If a tumor is the cause, it may be surgically resected, and drugs may be administered to prevent hyperinsulin attacks.

reactive hypoglycemia — Hypoglycemia occurring after ingestion of glucose or a meal.

This is due to an abnormality in the timing of insulin secretion in response to a meal, and is distinct from the type of hypoglycemia seen with hyperinsulinism.

Pituitary (Adenohypophysis)

gigantism — Hyperfunctioning of the pituitary gland before puberty, leading to abnormal overgrowth of the body.

Benign adenomas of the pituitary gland that occur before a child reaches puberty produce an excessive amount of growth hormone. Gigantism can be corrected by early diagnosis in childhood, followed by resection of the tumor or x-ray treatment.

acromegaly — Enlargement of the extremities caused by hyperfunctioning of the pituitary gland after puberty.

Adenomas of the pituitary gland which occur during adulthood produce acromegaly. Hypersecretion of pituitary growth hormone causes the bones in the hands, feet, face, and jaw to grow abnormally large in size, producing a characteristic Frankenstein-type facial appearance. Figure 17-10 shows a woman with acromegaly.

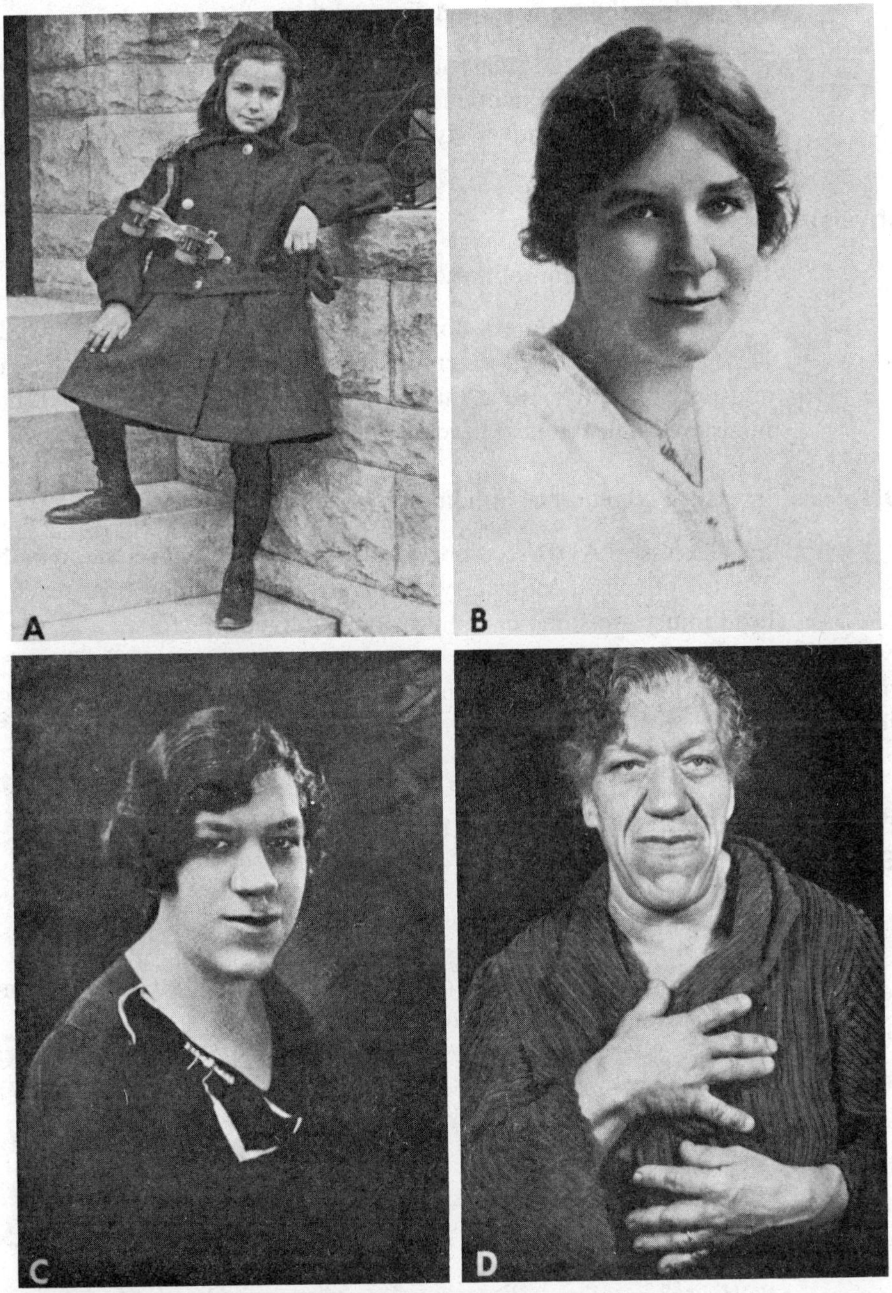

Figure 17-10 Progression of acromegaly: *A,* patient at age 9; *B,* age 16, with possible early features of acromegaly; *C,* age 33, well established acromegaly; *D,* age 52, end-stage acromegaly. (From Clinical Pathological Conference. American Journal of Medicine, *20*:133, 1956.)

dwarfism — Congenital hyposecretion of growth hormone.

The children affected are normal mentally but their bones remain small and underdeveloped. Treatment consists of administration of growth hormone. Achondroplastic dwarfs differ from hypopituitary dwarfs in that they suffer from a genetic defect in cartilage formation which adversely affects the growth of bones.

panhypopituitarism — All pituitary hormones are deficient.

Tumors of the sella turcica as well as arterial aneurysms may be etiological factors. Functions of target glands (adrenals, thyroid, ovaries, and testes) are also adversely affected.

Pituitary (Neurohypophysis)

diabetes insipidus — Insufficient secretion of antidiuretic hormone (vasopressin).

Deficient antidiuretic hormone causes the kidney tubules to fail to hold back (reabsorb) needed water and salts. Clinical symptoms include polyuria and polydipsia (excessive thirst). Synthetic preparations of ADH are administered into the nose several times a day as treatment.

inappropriate ADH (IADH) — Excessive secretion of antidiuretic hormone.

Excessive ADH secretion produces excess water retention in the body. Treatment consists of dietary water restriction. Tumor, drug reactions, and head injury are some of the possible etiological factors.

Figure 17-11 is a chart reviewing the various pathological conditions associated with hyposecretion and hypersecretion of the endocrine glands.

XII. LABORATORY TESTS, CLINICAL PROCEDURES, AND ABBREVIATIONS

Laboratory Tests

serum tests — The measurement of the following substances in serum (blood) is important in diagnosing endocrine disorders:

Substance	*Endocrine Gland Function*
calcium	parathyroid gland
cortisol	adrenal cortex
electrolytes	adrenal cortex
estradiol (estrogen)	ovaries
FSH	adenohypophysis
hGH	adenohypophysis
glucose	pancreas
insulin	pancreas

LH	adenohypophysis
parathyroid hormone	parathyroid gland
prolactin	adenohypophysis
T_3	thyroid gland
T_4	thyroid gland
free thyroxine (not bound to protein)	thyroid gland
testosterone	testes
TSH	adenohypophysis

urine tests

The following substances are measured in the urine as indicators of endocrine function:

Substance	*Endocrine Gland Function*
calcium	parathyroid gland
catecholamines	adrenal medulla
free cortisol	adrenal cortex
electrolytes	adrenal cortex
17-hydroxycorticosteroids	adrenal cortex
17-ketosteroids	adrenal cortex
ketones	pancreas
glucose	pancreas

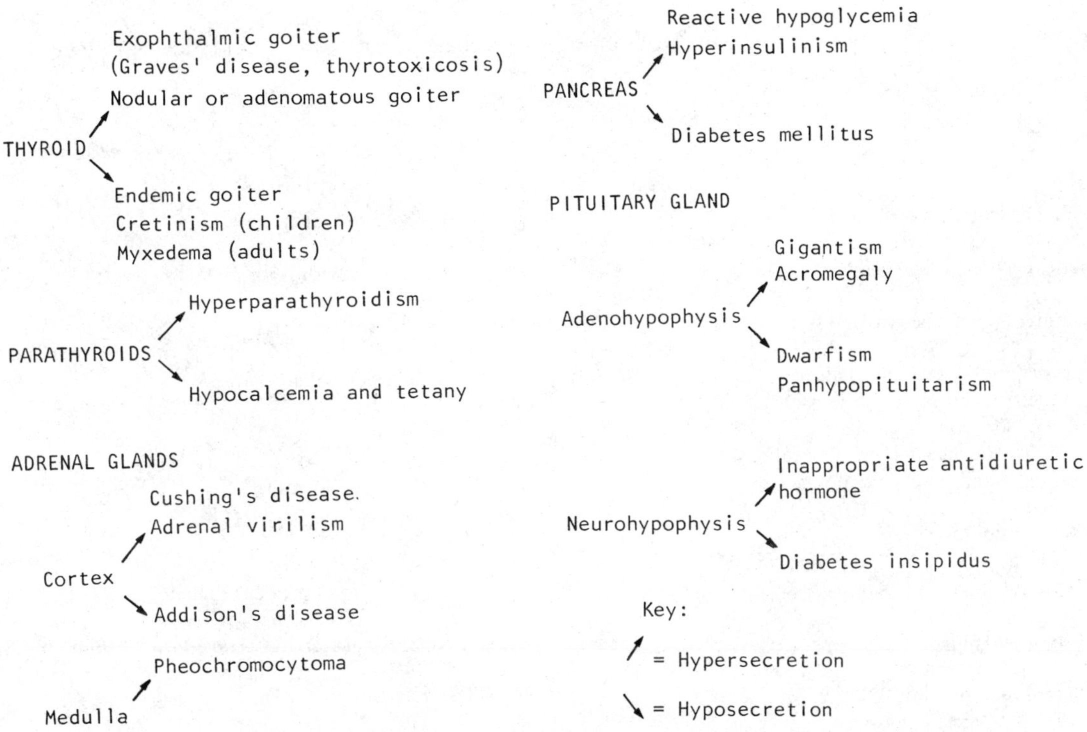

Figure 17-11 Review of pathological conditions related to endocrine organs.

glucose tolerance test — This test measures the glucose levels in a blood sample from a fasting patient (**fasting blood sugar**) and in specimens taken 30 minutes, 1 hour, 2 hours, and 3 hours after ingestion of 100 gm of glucose. Delayed return of blood glucose to normal level indicates diabetes mellitus.

radioimmunoassay (RIA) — This test measures hormone levels in plasma. The test is based on the ability of antibodies to bind specifically to radioactively labeled hormone molecules and to nonradioactively labeled molecules.

Clinical Procedures

thyroid scan — A radioactive compound is administered and localizes in the thyroid gland. The gland is then visualized with a scanner device to detect tumors or nodules.

radioactive iodine uptake — Radioactive iodine is administered orally and its uptake into the thyroid gland is measured as evidence of thyroid function.

CT scans (computerized tomography) — These transverse views of the pituitary gland and other endocrine organs are useful in diagnosis of pathological conditions.

ultrasonography — Pictures obtained from ultrasound waves as they bounce off body organs can identify pancreatic, adrenal, and thyroid masses.

skull x-ray and tomography of the sella turcica — The fossa in the base of the cranium that houses the pituitary gland is x-rayed and pictures are taken in sections to show the area in depth.

exophthalmometry — This test measures the extent of eyeball protrusion as evidenced in Graves' disease.

Abbreviations

ACTH	Adrenocorticotropic hormone
ADA	American Diabetes Association
ADH	Antidiuretic hormone (vasopressin)
BMR	Basal metabolic rate (an indicator of thyroid function, but not in current use)
CZI	Crystalline zinc insulin (regular insulin, short-acting and rapid onset of action)
DI	Diabetes insipidus
DM	Diabetes mellitus
FBS	Fasting blood sugar
FSH	Follicle-stimulating hormone
GTT	Glucose tolerance test
hGH	Human growth hormone
IADH	Inappropriate ADH
IDDM	Insulin dependent diabetes mellitus
K	Potassium
LH	Luteinizing hormone
Na	Sodium
NIDDM	Non-insulin dependent diabetes mellitus
NPH	Neutral protamine Hagedorn insulin (intermediate in duration and onset of action)

17-OH	17-Hydroxycorticosteroids
PBI	Protein-bound iodine (test of thyroid function, but not in current use)
PRL	Prolactin
PTH	Parathyroid hormone (parathormone)
PZI	Protamine zinc insulin (long duration and slow onset of action)
RAIU	Radioactive iodine uptake
RIA	Radioimmunoassay
T_3	Triiodothyronine
T_4	Thyroxine

XIII. PRACTICAL APPLICATIONS

Case Report 1

A 24-year-old college student, known diabetic, was admitted for treatment of ketoacidosis. He had a several year history of diabetes and had been taking insulin in the morning and in the evening. After the history was pieced together from the patient and his friends, it appeared that he had been getting progressively ill over several days following a flu-like episode and may well not have taken his insulin on the day of admission. He was found slightly drowsy and confused by classmates. His respirations were rapid, his pulse was 126, and he offered no sensible answers to questions. Blood sugar level was elevated at 728 mg/dl [100 mg/dl is normal] and blood ketones were positive. The patient was treated with insulin intravenously, and over the course of the next 24 hours the ketoacidosis cleared.

Case Report 2

A 42-year-old woman presented with a 6-month history of progressive weakness. She had facial and central obesity with muscle wasting in the extremities. As an initial screening test, a 24-hour urine collection for cortisol determination revealed high levels. Her ACTH level was low. On CT scan a 3-cm mass was found in the left adrenal. When the mass was resected, it proved to be a 3-cm, smooth, yellow adrenocortical adenoma that secreted cortisol. The patient's condition (Cushing's syndrome) normalized after surgery.

Case Report 3

Graves' disease, as characterized by exophthalmos and stare, was diagnosed in a 51-year-old man. Examination revealed a history of nervousness, palpitation, weight loss, diarrhea, dyspnea on exertion, insomnia, heat intolerance, and fatigue. An ECG showed atrial fibrillation with a ventricular rate of about 180 beats per minute, which was treated with digoxin and propranolol. A chest x-ray film disclosed cardiomegaly. Thyroid function tests showed T_4 and T_3 levels to be elevated, and a thyroid scan showed diffuse enlargement of the gland. The patient was treated with radioactive iodine and is now euthyroid. The exophthalmos has not resolved, however.

XIV. EXERCISES

A. Give the endocrine organs (including appropriate lobe or region) that produce the following hormones:

1. follicle-stimulating hormone ______________________
2. vasopressin ______________________
3. aldosterone ______________________
4. insulin ______________________
5. thyroxine ______________________
6. cortisol ______________________
7. gonadotropic hormones ______________________
8. epinephrine ______________________
9. oxytocin ______________________
10. prolactin ______________________
11. growth hormone ______________________
12. glucagon ______________________
13. melatonin ______________________
14. estradiol ______________________
15. progesterone ______________________
16. testosterone ______________________
17. melanocyte-stimulating hormone ______________________

B. Give the meaning of the following abbreviations:

1. ADH ______________________
2. ACTH ______________________
3. GTT ______________________
4. LH ______________________

5. FSH ______________________________

6. TSH ______________________________

7. FBS ______________________________

8. PTH ______________________________

9. hGH ______________________________

10. PRL ______________________________

11. T_4 ______________________________

12. T_3 ______________________________

C. *Indicate whether the following conditions are caused by hypersecretion or hyposecretion. Also, select from the list below the endocrine gland involved in each disease:*

thyroid	testes	adenohypophysis
adrenal cortex	adrenal medulla	parathyroid gland
pancreas	neurohypophysis	ovaries

Disease	*Hypo or Hyper*	*Gland*
1. Cushing's disease	________	______________
2. tetany	________	______________
3. Graves' disease	________	______________
4. diabetes insipidus	________	______________
5. acromegaly	________	______________
6. myxedema	________	______________
7. osteitis fibrosa cystica	________	______________
8. diabetes mellitus	________	______________
9. Addison's disease	________	______________
10. gigantism	________	______________
11. endemic goiter	________	______________

12. cretinism ________ ________________

13. panhypopituitarism ________ ________________

14. pheochromocytoma ________ ________________

15. hypocalcemia ________ ________________

16. hyperinsulinism ________ ________________

17. dwarfism ________ ________________

18. inappropriate anti-diuretic hormone ________ ________________

D. Build medical terms:

1. Abnormal condition (poison) of the thyroid gland ________________

2. Removal of the thymus gland ________________

3. Condition of deficiency or underdevelopment of the sex organs ________________

4. Excessive thirst ________________

5. Removal of the pituitary gland using cold temperatures ________________

6. Sugar in the urine ________________

7. Excessive calcium in the blood ________________

8. Inflammation of the thyroid gland ________________

9. Excessive development of mammary tissue in a male ________________

10. Enlargement of the adrenal gland ________________

E. Give the meaning of the following medical terms:

1. steroids ________________

2. catecholamines ________________

3. adenohypophysis ________________

4. tetany ______________________________

5. exophthalmic goiter ______________________________

6. mineralocorticoids ______________________________

7. homeostasis ______________________________

8. isthmus ______________________________

9. glucocorticoids ______________________________

10. epinephrine ______________________________

11. hypernatremia ______________________________

12. hypokalemia ______________________________

13. glycogenolysis ______________________________

14. galactorrhea ______________________________

15. euthyroid ______________________________

16. adrenal virilism ______________________________

F. Match the terms listed below with their meanings:

secretin
gastrin
erythropoietin
target tissue
renin
cholecystokinin
prostaglandins
hormone receptors
vitamin D

1. A hormone produced in the kidney and necessary for the formation of red blood cells

____

2. A hormone secreted by the gastrointestinal tract that stimulates the gallbladder to contract ______________________________

3. Hormone secreted by the kidney to raise blood pressure ______________________________

4. Hormone-like lipid substances that stimulate uterine contractions, lower blood pressure, and regulate body temperature and platelet aggregation in clotting

____

5. Hormone secreted by the gastrointestinal tract to stimulate the secretion of pancreatic juices (enzymes) _______________

6. Recognition sites for hormones in body tissues _______________

7. Hormone produced by the skin and necessary for absorption of calcium into the body _______________

8. Cells toward which the effects of a hormone are directed _______________

9. Hormone produced by the gastrointestinal tract to stimulate the secretion of acid and enzymes by the stomach _______________

G. *Give meanings for the following terms or abbreviations related to diabetes mellitus:*

1. IDDM _______________
2. diabetic neuropathy _______________
3. ketoacidosis _______________
4. hypoglycemia _______________
5. NIDDM _______________
6. diabetic retinopathy _______________
7. hyperosmolar coma _______________
8. diabetic nephropathy _______________

H. *Explain the following laboratory tests or clinical procedures related to the endocrine system:*

1. Thyroid scan _______________
2. Serum and urine electrolytes _______________

3. RAIU ____________________

4. Glucose tolerance test ____________________

5. 17-hydroxycorticosteroid test ____________________

6. RIA ____________________

7. Exophthalmometry ____________________

8. Skull x-ray and tomography of the sella turcica ____________________

____

9. Serum calcium ____________________

10. Serum estradiol ____________________

ANSWERS

A.

1. Anterior lobe of the pituitary gland (adenohypophysis).
2. Posterior lobe of the pituitary gland (neurohypophysis).
3. Adrenal cortex.
4. Islets of Langerhans in the pancreas.
5. Thyroid gland.
6. Adrenal cortex.
7. Anterior lobe of the pituitary (adenohypophysis).
8. Adrenal medulla.
9. Posterior lobe of the pituitary (neurohypophysis).
10. Anterior lobe of the pituitary (adenohypophysis).
11. Anterior lobe of the pituitary (adenohypophysis).
12. Islets of Langerhans in the pancreas.
13. Pineal gland.
14. Ovaries.
15. Ovaries.
16. Testes.
17. Anterior lobe of the pituitary (adenohypophysis).

B.

1. Antidiuretic hormone.
2. Adrenocorticotropin.
3. Glucose tolerance test.
4. Luteinizing hormone.
5. Follicle-stimulating hormone.
6. Thyroid-stimulating hormone.
7. Fasting blood sugar.
8. Parathyroid hormone.
9. Human growth hormone.
10. Prolactin.
11. Thyroxine.
12. Triiodothyronine.

C.

1. Hypersecretion; adrenal cortex; also hypersecretion adenohypophysis.
2. Hyposecretion; parathyroid gland.
3. Hypersecretion; thyroid gland.
4. Hyposecretion; neurohypophysis.
5. Hypersecretion; adenohypophysis.
6. Hyposecretion; thyroid gland.
7. Hypersecretion; parathyroid gland.
8. Hyposecretion; pancreas.
9. Hyposecretion; adrenal cortex.
10. Hypersecretion; adenohypophysis.
11. Hyposecretion; thyroid gland.
12. Hyposecretion; thyroid gland. A congenital condition.
13. Hyposecretion; adenohypophysis.
14. Hypersecretion; adrenal medulla.
15. Hyposecretion; parathyroid gland.
16. Hypersecretion; pancreas.
17. Hyposecretion; adenohypophysis.
18. Hypersecretion; neurohypophysis.

D.

1. Thyrotoxicosis.
2. Thymectomy.
3. Hypogonadism.
4. Polydipsia.
5. Cryohypophysectomy.
6. Glycosuria.
7. Hypercalcemia.
8. Thyroiditis.
9. Gynecomastia.
10. Adrenomegaly.

E.

1. Complex substances derived from cholesterol; hormones from the adrenal cortex (corticoids) and sex hormones are steroids.
2. Complex substances derived from an amino acid; epinephrine (adrenaline) and norepinephrine (noradrenaline) are examples.
3. Anterior lobe of the pituitary gland.
4. Continuous contractions of muscles associated with low levels of parathyroid hormone.
5. Enlargement of the thyroid gland with eyeballs that bulge outward.
6. Steroid hormones from the adrenal cortex (outer region of the adrenal gland) that influence salt (minerals such as sodium and potassium) metabolism.
7. A state of equilibrium in the body with respect to functions, fluids, and times.
8. A narrow strip of tissue connecting two parts.
9. Steroid hormones from the adrenal cortex that influence sugar metabolism in the body.
10. Catecholamine hormone from the adrenal medulla.
11. Excessive sodium in the blood.
12. Deficient potassium in the blood.
13. Breakdown of glycogen to produce sugar.
14. Inappropriate secretion of milk from the breasts.
15. Normal thyroid function.
16. Abnormal secretion of androgens from the adrenal cortex produces masculine characteristics in a female.

F.

1. erythropoietin
2. cholecystokinin
3. renin
4. prostaglandins
5. secretin
6. hormone receptors
7. vitamin D
8. target tissue
9. gastrin

G.

1. Insulin dependent diabetes mellitus; juvenile-onset type characterized by destruction of the islets of Langerhans.
2. Destruction of nerves as a secondary complication of diabetes mellitus.
3. Abnormal condition of high levels of ketones (acids) in the blood as a result of improper burning of fats. Fats are burned because the cells do not have sugar available because of lack of insulin or inability of insulin to act.
4. Too little sugar in the blood. This can occur if too much insulin is taken by a diabetic patient.
5. Non-insulin dependent diabetes mellitus; adult-onset type characterized by insulin deficiency and resistance by target tissue to the action of insulin.
6. Destruction of blood vessels in the retina as a secondary complication of diabetes mellitus.
7. Unconsciousness due to high levels of sugar in the blood; water leaves cells to balance the large amounts of sugar in the blood, leading to cellular dehydration.
8. Destruction of the kidneys as a secondary complication of diabetes mellitus.

H.

1. A radioactive compound is given and the thyroid gland is pictured with a scanner device.
2. Salts and minerals such as sodium, potassium, and chloride are measured in blood and urine samples.
3. Radioactive iodine uptake test—measures the amount of radioactive iodine that concentrates in the thyroid gland after oral administration.
4. Measurement of blood sugar levels in a fasting patient, and after intervals of 30 minutes, 1, 2, and 3 hours following ingestion of glucose.
5. Test of adrenocorticosteroids in the urine.
6. Radioimmunoassay; hormone concentrations are measured by using antibodies, nonradioactively labeled hormone, and radioactively labeled hormone.
7. Measurement of eyeball protrusion (symptom of Graves' disease).
8. X-ray of the cranium and cavity in the skull that houses the pituitary gland; serial x-rays show the gland in depth.
9. Measurement of the amount of calcium in the blood.
10. Measurement of the amount of estradiol (estrogen) in the blood.

XV. PRONUNCIATION OF TERMS

acromegaly	ăk-rō-MĔG-ă-lē
adenohypophysis	ăd-ĕ-nō-hī-PŎF-ĭ-sĭs
adenomatous goiter	ăd-ĕ-NOM-ă-tŭs GOY-tĕr
adrenal	ă-DRĒ-năl
adrenalectomy	ă-drē-năl-ĔK-tō-mē
adrenocorticotropic	ă-drē-nō-kōr-tĭ-kō-TRŎP-ĭk

adrenomegaly	ăd-rĕn-ō-MĔG-ă-lē
aldosterone	ăl-DŎS-tĕ-rōn; ăl-dō-STĔR-ōn
antidiuretic	ăn-tĭ-dī-ū-RĔT-ĭk
calcitonin	kăl-sĭ-TŌ-nĭn
calcium	KĂL-sē-ŭm
catecholamine	kăt-ĕ-KŌL-ă-mēn
cholecystokinin	kō-lē-sĭs-tō-KĪ-nĭn
corticosteroid	kōr-tĭ-kō-STĔ-royd
cortisol	KŌR-tĭ-sōl
cortisone	KŌR-tĭ-sōn
cretinism	KRĒ-tĭn-ĭzm
cryohypophysectomy	krī-ō-hī-pō-fĭ-SĔK-tō-mē
decalcification	dē-kăl-sĭ-fĭ-KĀ-shŭn
diabetes insipidus	dī-ă-BĒ-tēz ĭn-SĬP-ĭ-dŭs
diabetes mellitus	dī-ă-BĒ-tēz MĔL-ĭ-tŭs or mĕ-LĪ-tŭs
dwarfism	DWĂRF-ĭzm
electrolyte	ē-LĔK-trō-līt
endemic colloid goiter	ĕn-DĔM-ĭk KŎL-oyd GOY-tĕr
epinephrine	ĕp-ĭ-NĔF-rĭn
erythropoietin	ĕ-rĭth-rō-POY-ĕ-tĭn
estradiol	ĕs-tră-DĪ-ŏl
estrogen	ĔS-trō-jĕn
euthyroid	ū-THĪ-royd
exophthalmometry	ĕk-sŏf-thăl-MŎM-ĕ-trē
exophthalmos	ĕk-sŏf-THĂL-mŏs
galactorrhea	gă-lăk-tō-RĒ-ă
gastrin	GĂS-trĭn
gigantism	JĪ-găn-tĭzm
glucagon	GLOO-kă-gŏn
glucocorticoid	gloo-kō-KŌR-tĭ-koyd
gluconeogenesis	gloo-kō-nē-ō-JĔN-ĭ-sĭs
glycogen	GLĪ-kō-jĕn

goiter	GOY-tĕr
gonadotropic	gŏn-ăd-ō-TRŎP-ĭk
homeostasis	hō-mē-ō-STĀ-sĭs
hydrocortisone	hī-drō-KŌR-tĭ-sōn
hypercalcemia	hī-pĕr-kăl-SĒ-mē-ă
hyperglycemia	hī-pĕr-glī-SĒ-mē-ă
hyperinsulinism	hī-pĕr-ĬN-sū-lĭn-ĭzm
hypernatremia	hī-pĕr-nă-TRĒ-mē-ă
hyperparathyroidism	hī-pĕr-păr-ă-THĪ-royd-ĭzm
hyperthyroidism	hī-pĕr-THĪ-royd-ĭzm
hypocalcemia	hī-pō-kăl-SĒ-mē-ă
hypogonadism	hī-pō-GŌ-năd-ĭzm
hypokalemia	hī-pō-kā-LĒ-mē-ă
hypoparathyroidism	hī-pō-păr-ă-THĪ-royd-ĭzm
hypophyseal	hī-pō-FĬZ-ē-ăl
hypophysis	hī-PŎF-ĭ-sĭs
hypothalamus	hī-pō-THĂL-ă-mŭs
hypothyroidism	hī-pō-THĪ-royd-ĭzm
insulin	ĬN-sū-lĭn
iodine	Ī-ō-dīn
islets of Langerhans	Ī-lĕts ŏf LĂHNG-ĕr-hănz
isthmus	ĬS-mŭs
luteinizing hormone	LŪ-tē-ĭn-ī-zĭng HŌR-mōn
melatonin	mĕl-ă-TŌ-nĭn
mineralocorticoid	mĭn-ĕr-ăl-ō-KŌR-tĭ-koyd
myxedema	mĭk-sĕ-DĒ-mă
neurohypophysis	nū-rō-hī-PŎF-ĭ-sĭs
norepinephrine	nŏr-ĕp-ĭ-NĔF-rĭn
oxytocin	ŏk-sē-TŌ-sĭn
pancreatectomy	păn-krē-ă-TĔK-tō-mē
panhypopituitarism	păn-hī-pō-pĭ-TŪ-ĭ-tăr-ĭzm
parathormone	păr-ă-THŌR-mōn

parathyroid	păr-ă-THĪ-royd
parathyroidectomy	păr-ă-thī-roy-DĔK-tō-mē
pheochromocytoma	fē-ō-krō-mō-sī-TŌ-mă
pineal	PĬN-ē-ăl or pī-NĒ-ăl
polydipsia	pŏl-ē-DĬP-sē-ă
polyuria	pŏl-ē-Ū-rē-ă
progesterone	prō-JĔS-tĕ-rōn
prolactin	prō-LĂK-tĭn
prostaglandin	prŏs-tă-GLĂN-dĭn
radioimmunoassay	rā-dē-ō-ĭm-ū-nō-ĂS-ā
renin	RĒ-nĭn
secretin	sē-KRĒ-tĭn
sella turcica	SĔL-ă TŬR-sĭ-kă
somatotropin	sō-mă-tō-TRŌ-pĭn
steroid	STĔR-oyd
sympathomimetic	sĭm-pă-thō-mī-MĔT-ĭk
testosterone	tĕs-TŎS-tĕ-rōn
tetany	TĔT-ă-nē
thymectomy	thī-MĔK-tō-mē
thyroidectomy	thī-roy-DĔK-tō-mē
thyroiditis	thī-roy-DĪ-tĭs
thyrotoxicosis	thī-rō-tŏk-sĭ-KŌ-sĭs
thyroxine	thī-RŎK-sĭn
triiodothyronine	trī-ī-ō-dō-THĪ-rō-nēn
vasopressin	văz-ō-PRĔS-ĭn
virilism	VĬR-ĭ-lĭzm

REVIEW SHEET 17

Combining Forms

adren/o	______________	lact/o	______________
adrenal/o	______________	natr/o	______________
andr/o	______________	pancreat/o	______________
calc/o	______________	parathyroid/o	______________
cortic/o	______________	pineal/o	______________
dips/o	______________	somat/o	______________
estr/o	______________	ster/o	______________
galact/o	______________	test/o	______________
gluc/o	______________	thym/o	______________
glyc/o	______________	thyr/o	______________
gonad/o	______________	thyroid/o	______________
home/o	______________	toxic/o	______________
kal/i	______________	ur/o	______________

Suffixes

-ectomy	______________	-oid	______________
-emia	______________	-osis	______________
-genic	______________	-physis	______________
-lysis	______________	-stasis	______________
-megaly	______________	-tocin	______________

Additional Terms

Endocrine Glands

Know the location and function of each:

adenohypophysis (508)

adrenal cortex (508)

adrenal medulla (508)

hypophysis (509)

islets of Langerhans (510)

neurohypophysis (510)

ovaries (506)

parathyroid glands (501)

pineal gland (510)

testes (506)

thymus gland (499)

thyroid gland (500)

Hormones and Other Substances

Identify the gland or tissue that produces each:

adrenaline (508)

adrenocorticotropic hormone (508)

aldosterone (508)

androgens (508)

antidiuretic hormone (508)

calcitonin (508)

catecholamines (508)

cholecystokinin (508)

cortisol (508)

cortisone (508)

epinephrine (508)

erythropoietin (509)

estradiol (509)

estrogens (509)

follicle-stimulating hormone (509)

gastrin (509)

glucagon (509)

glucocorticoids (509)

gonadotropic hormones (509)

growth hormone (509)

hydrocortisone (509)

insulin (509)

luteinizing hormone (510)

melanocyte-stimulating hormone (510)

melatonin (510)

mineralocorticoids (510)

norepinephrine (510)

oxytocin (510)

parathyroid hormone (510)

progesterone (510)

prostaglandins (510)

prolactin (510)

renin (510)

secretin (510)

somatotropin (511)

testosterone (511)

thyroid-stimulating hormone (511)

thyroxine (511)

triiodothyronine (511)

vasopressin (511)

vitamin D (511)

Abnormal Conditions, Other Terms, Tests and Procedures

acromegaly (518)

Addison's disease (516)

adenomatous goiter (514)

adrenal virilism (516)

cretinism (515)

CT scan (522)

Cushing's disease and syndrome (516)

diabetes insipidus (520)

diabetes mellitus (517)

dwarfism (520)

electrolyte (508)

endemic goiter (513)

exophthalmic goiter (514)

exophthalmometry (522)

fasting blood sugar (522)

galactorrhea (512)

gigantism (518)

glucose tolerance test (522)

Graves' disease (514)

hirsutism (516)

homeostasis (509)

hyperinsulinism (518)

hyperparathyroidism (516)

hypogonadism (512)

hypoparathyroidism (516)

hypothalamus (509)

inappropriate ADH (520)

isthmus (510)

ketoacidosis (518)

myxedema (515)

osteitis fibrosa cystica (516)

panhypopituitarism (520)

pheochromocytoma (517)

radioactive iodine uptake (522)

radioimmunoassay (522)

reactive hypoglycemia (518)

receptors (510)

sella turcica (510)

serum tests (520)

steroids (512)

sympathomimetic (503)

tetany (516)

thyroid scan (522)

urine tests (521)

CHAPTER 18

CANCER MEDICINE (ONCOLOGY)

In this chapter you will:

- Describe medical terms related to the pathological appearance and the growth and spread of tumors;
- Recognize how tumors are classified and named;
- Understand the methods used by physicians for determining the extent of tumor spread (staging);
- Become familiar with terms related to the causes, diagnosis, and treatment of cancer; and
- Recognize combining forms, procedures, tests, and abbreviations that pertain to cancer medicine.

This chapter is divided into the following sections:

I. Introduction
II. Characteristics of Tumors
III. Classification of Cancerous Tumors
IV. Pathological Descriptions
V. Grading and Staging Systems
VI. Carcinogenesis
VII. Cancer Treatment
VIII. Vocabulary
IX. Combining Forms, Suffixes, and Prefixes
X. Laboratory Tests, Clinical Procedures, and Abbreviations
XI. Practical Applications
XII. Exercises
XIII. Pronunciation of Terms

I. INTRODUCTION

Cancer is a disease characterized by unrestrained and excessive multiplication of body cells and may occur in any body tissue at any age. Cancerous cells accumulate as growths called **malignant tumors**, which penetrate, compress, and ultimately destroy the surrounding normal tissue. In addition to local growth, cancerous cells also have the ability to invade adjacent tissues and to spread throughout the body by way of the bloodstream or lymphatic vessels. In most patients, the spread of cancers from their site of origin to distant organs is responsible for the lethality of malignant tumors.

Although half of all patients who develop cancer will be cured of their disease, it is currently the cause of almost one-fifth of all deaths in the United States. This chapter will explore the terminology related to this common, and often fatal, disease process.

II. CHARACTERISTICS OF TUMORS

Tumors (also called **neoplasms**) are masses, or growths, that arise from normal tissue. They may be either **malignant** (progressive and life-threatening) or **benign** (nonprogressive and not life-threatening). There are several differences between benign and malignant tumors. Some of these differences are:

1. Benign tumors grow slowly, while malignant tumor cells multiply rapidly.

2. Benign tumors are often **encapsulated** so that the tumor cells do not invade the surrounding tissue. Malignant tumor growth is characteristically **invasive** and **infiltrative**, extending beyond the tissue of origin into adjacent organs.

3. Benign tumors are composed of highly organized and specialized (**differentiated**) cells, which closely resemble normal, mature tissue. Malignant tumors are composed of cancerous cells that resemble primitive, or embryonic, cells that do not have the capacity for mature cellular functions. This characteristic of malignant tumors is called **anaplasia.** Anaplasia means that the cancerous cells are **dedifferentiated** (reverting to a less developed state) in contrast to the normal, differentiated tissue of their origin. Anaplastic cells lack an orderly arrangement. Instead, the tumor cells are found piled one on top of the other in a disorganized fashion. Figure 18-1 compares cells from a benign thyroid adenoma with those from a poorly differentiated thyroid carcinoma.

4. Benign tumors do not spread to form secondary tumor masses in other places in the body. Malignant tumors, however, can detach themselves from the tumor site, travel through the bloodstream and lymphatic system, and establish a new tumor site at a distant region within the body. This secondary growth is called a **metastasis.**

III. CLASSIFICATION OF CANCEROUS TUMORS

Although about half of all cancer deaths are caused by malignancies of only three organs (lung, breast, and colon), more than 100 distinct varieties of cancer are recognized, each

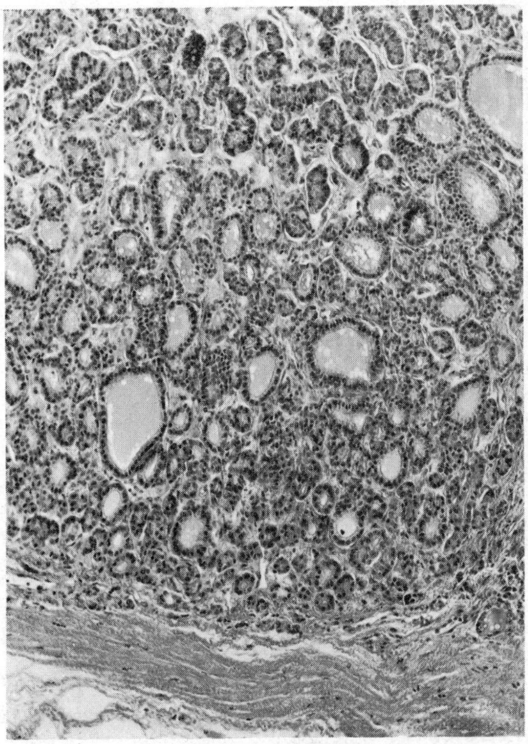

A

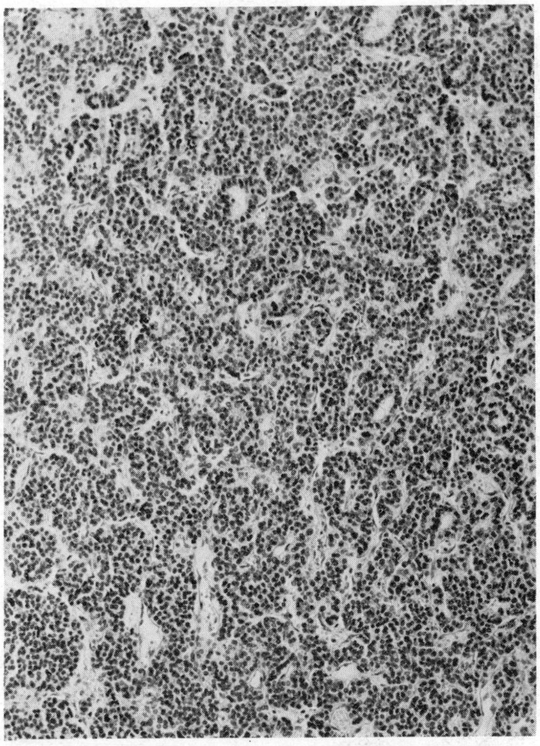

B

Figure 18-1 *A*, A well differentiated benign thyroid adenoma. *B*, A moderately poorly differentiated thyroid carcinoma. (From Robbins, S.L., and Cotran, R.S.: Pathologic Basis of Disease. 2nd ed. Philadelphia, W. B. Saunders Co., 1979.)

having a unique set of symptoms and requiring a specific type of therapy. It is possible to divide these 100 specific types of cancer into three broad groups on the basis of histogenesis—that is, by identifying the particular tissue (hist/o) from which the tumor cells have arisen (-genesis). These major groups are called **carcinomas**, **sarcomas**, and **mixed-tissue tumors**.

Carcinomas

Carcinomas, the largest group, are **solid tumors** that are derived from epithelial tissue. Epithelial tissue is found on external and internal body surfaces, including skin, glands, and digestive, urinary, and reproductive organs. Approximately 85 per cent of all maligant neoplasms are carcinomas.

Figure 18-2 gives examples of specific carcinomas and the epithelial tissue from which

Type of Epithelial Tissue	*Malignant Tumor*
Gastrointestinal tract:	
stomach	gastric adenocarcinoma
esophagus	esophageal adenocarcinoma
colon	carcinoma of the colon
Glandular tissue:	
thyroid	carcinoma of the thyroid
adrenal glands	carcinoma of the adrenals
pancreas	carcinoma of the pancreas (pancreatic adenocarcinoma)
breast	carcinoma of the breast
prostate	carcinoma of the prostate
Skin:	
squamous cell layer	squamous cell carcinoma
basal cell layer	basal cell carcinoma
melanocyte	malignant melanoma
Lung	adenocarcinoma of the lung; oat cell (small cell) carcinoma; epidermoid carcinoma
Kidney	hypernephroma (renal cell carcinoma)
Reproductive organs	cystadenocarcinoma of the ovaries; adenocarcinoma of the uterus; squamous cell (epidermoid) carcinoma of the vagina and cervix; carcinoma of the penis; seminoma (carcinoma of the testes); choriocarcinoma of the uterus or testes

Figure 18-2 Carcinomas and epithelial tissue from which they are derived.

they are derived. Benign tumors of epithelial origin are usually named by using the suffix **-oma** added to the type of tissue in which the tumor occurs. For example, a **gastric adenoma** is a benign tumor of the glandular (aden/o) epithelial cells lining the stomach. Malignant tumors of epithelial origin are named by using the term **-carcinoma** added to the type of tissue in which the tumor occurs. Thus, a **gastric adenocarcinoma** is a cancerous tumor of glandular cells lining the stomach.

Sarcomas

Sarcomas, a rarer type of cancer than carcinomas, are derived from supportive and connective tissue, such as bone, fat, muscle, cartilage, bone marrow, and lymphatic tissue, or from blood cells. Sarcomas account for approximately 10 per cent of all malignant neoplasms.

Figure 18-3 gives examples of specific types of sarcomas and the connective tissue from which they are derived. Benign tumors of connective tissue origin are named by using the suffix **-oma** added to the type of tissue in which the tumor occurs. For example, a benign tumor of bone is called an **osteoma**. Malignant tumors of connective tissue origin are often named by using the term **-sarcoma** (sarc/o = flesh) added to the type of tissue in which the tumor occurs. For example, an **osteosarcoma** is a malignant tumor of bone.

Type of Connective Tissue	*Malignant Tumor*
Bone	osteosarcoma (osteogenic sarcoma) Ewing's sarcoma
Muscle:	
smooth (visceral) muscle	leiomyosarcoma
striated (skeletal) muscle	rhabdomyosarcoma
Cartilage	chondrosarcoma
Fat	liposarcoma
Fibrous tissue	fibrosarcoma
Blood vessel tissue	hemangiosarcoma
Hematopoietic tissue:	
leukocytes	leukemia
bone marrow cells	multiple myeloma
lymphocytes	lymphosarcoma or lymphoma; reticulum cell sarcoma; Hodgkin's disease
Nerve tissue:	
embryonic nerve tissue	neuroblastoma
neuroglial tissue	astrocytoma (tumor of neuroglial cells called astrocytes)
meningeal tissue	meningeal sarcoma

Figure 18-3 Sarcomas and the connective tissue from which they are derived.

Type of Tissue	*Malignant Tumor*
Kidney	Wilms' tumor (embryonal adenosarcoma)
Ovaries and testes	teratoma (tumor composed of bone, muscle, skin, gland cells, cartilage, etc.)

Figure 18-4 Mixed-tissue tumors and where they are found.

Mixed-Tissue Tumors

Mixed-tissue tumors are derived from tissue that is capable of differentiating into epithelial as well as connective tissue. The tumors are thus composed of several different types of cells. Examples of mixed-tissue tumors (see Figure 18-4) can be found in the kidney, ovaries, and testes.

IV. PATHOLOGICAL DESCRIPTIONS

The following terms are used to describe the appearance of a malignant tumor, either on gross (visual) or on microscopic examination.

Gross Descriptions

cystic — Forming large open spaces filled with fluid. **Mucinous** tumors are filled with mucus (thick, sticky fluid), while **serous** tumors are filled with a thin, watery fluid resembling serum. Cystic tumors are commonly found in ovaries.

fungating — Mushrooming pattern of growth in which tumor cells pile one on top of another and project from a tissue surface. Fungating tumors are often found in the colon.

inflammatory — Characterized by inflammation, that is, redness, swelling, and heat. These tumors are commonly found in the breast.

medullary — Large, soft, fleshy tumors. Thyroid and breast tumors are often medullary.

necrotic — Containing dead tissue. Any type of tumor can display necrotic characteristics.

polypoid — Growths that are like projections extending outward from a membrane base. **Sessile** polypoid tumors extend from a broad base, while **pedunculated** polypoid tumors extend from a stem or stalk. These tumors are often found in the colon.

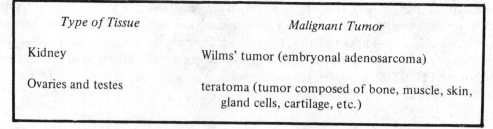

ulcerating — Characterized by an open, exposed surface resulting from death of overlying tissue. Ulcerating tumors are often found in the stomach, breast, and skin.

verrucous Resembling a wartlike growth and commonly occurring in the gingiva (cheek).

Microscopic Descriptions

alveolar Tumor cells form small, microscopic sacs; commonly found in tumors of muscle, bone, fat, and cartilage.

carcinoma *in situ* Referring to localized tumor cells that have not invaded adjacent structures. Cancer of the cervix may begin as carcinoma *in situ*.

diffuse Spreading evenly throughout the affected tissue. Malignant lymphomas may display diffuse involvement of lymph nodes.

dysplastic Displaying a highly abnormal, but not clearly cancerous appearance. Dysplastic nevi are an example.

epidermoid Resembling squamous epithelial cells (thin, platelike), often occurring in the respiratory tract.

follicular Forming small, microscopic, glandular-type sacs. Thyroid gland cancer is an example.

nodular Consisting of tightly packed clusters of cells. Malignant lymphomas may display a nodular pattern of lymph node involvement.

papillary Forming small, finger-like or nipple-like projections of cells. Bladder cancer may be described as papillary.

pleomorphic Composed of a variety of types of cells. Mixed-cell tumors are examples.

scirrhous Hard, densely packed tumors, overgrown with fibrous tissue; commonly found in the breast.

V. GRADING AND STAGING SYSTEMS

Two methods of categorizing malignant tumors are called **grading** and **staging**. They are based on different aspects of tumor growth and appearance.

When grading a tumor, the pathologist is concerned with the microscopic appearance of the tumor cells, specifically with their degree of anaplasia. In most cases, four grades are used. **Grade I** tumors are very well differentiated so that they closely resemble the normal parent tissue of their origin. **Grade IV** tumors are so anaplastic that recognition of the tumor's tissue of origin may even be difficult. **Grades II** and **III** are intermediate in appearance, moderately or poorly differentiated, as opposed to well differentiated (Grade I) and dedifferentiated (Grade IV).

Grading is of value in the prognosis of certain types of cancers, such as cancer of the urinary bladder and ovary and brain tumors (astrocytomas). Patients with Grade I tumors have a high survival rate, while patients with Grades II, III, and IV tumors have a poorer survival rate. Grading is also used in evaluating cells obtained from body fluids in preventive screening tests, such as **Pap smears** of the uterine cervix, tracheal secretions, or stomach secretions.

The staging of cancerous tumors is based on the extent of spread of the tumor rather than on its microscopic appearance. An example of a staging system is the TNM staging system. It has been applied to malignancies such as breast cancer and lung cancer, as well as many other tumors. **T** refers to the size and degree of local extension of the **tumor**; **N** refers to the number of regional lymph **nodes** that have been invaded by tumor; and **M** refers to the presence or absence of **metastases** of the tumor cells. Subscripts are used to denote size and degree of involvement: For example, 0 indicates undetectable, and 1, 2, 3, and 4 a progressive increase in size or involvement. A tumor may be described as T_1 N_2 M_0 (a tumor with palpable regional nodes, but no distant metastases). Table 18-1 is an example of the notations in the TNM staging system.

Other staging systems use letters such as A, B, C, and D or I, II, III, and IV to indicate the extent of spread of tumor in the body.

VI. CARCINOGENESIS

The transformation of a normal cell to a cancerous one is only partially understood at the present time. The key to understanding the process of malignant transformation seems to lie in the operations of the genetic material, or **DNA** (deoxyribonucleic acid), of the cell.

DNA, located in the nucleus of a cell, controls not only the production of new cells but also the cell's ability to grow, by directing the making of new proteins (protein synthesis). When a cell reproduces itself, the DNA material (located within the chromosomes) replicates (copies) itself so that exactly the same DNA is passed to new cells that are formed. This process is called **mitosis** or **self-replication**. In addition, the DNA can also send a molecular coded message to the cytoplasm of the cell so that proteins (such as hormones and enzymes) can be made for cellular growth. In the nucleus, this coded message is copied from DNA onto another molecule called **RNA** (ribonucleic acid). RNA travels from nucleus to cytoplasm carrying the molecular coded message that directs the proper formation of proteins in the cell. Figure 18-5 illustrates these two important functions of DNA.

When a cell becomes malignant, however, the process of mitosis is disturbed (cancer cells

Table 18-1 A TNM STAGING SYSTEM

Tumor	
T_0	No evidence of primary tumor.
T_{IS}	Carcinoma *in situ.*
T_1 T_2 T_3 T_4	Progressive increase in tumor size and involvement.
T_x	Tumor cannot be assessed.
Nodes	
N_o	Regional lymph nodes not demonstrably abnormal.
N_1 N_2 N_3 N_4	Increasing degrees of demonstrable abnormality of regional lymph nodes.
N_x	Regional lymph nodes cannot be assessed clinically.
Metastasis	
M_o	No evidence of distant metastasis.
M_1 M_2 M_3	Ascending degrees of distant metastasis, including metastasis to distant lymph nodes.

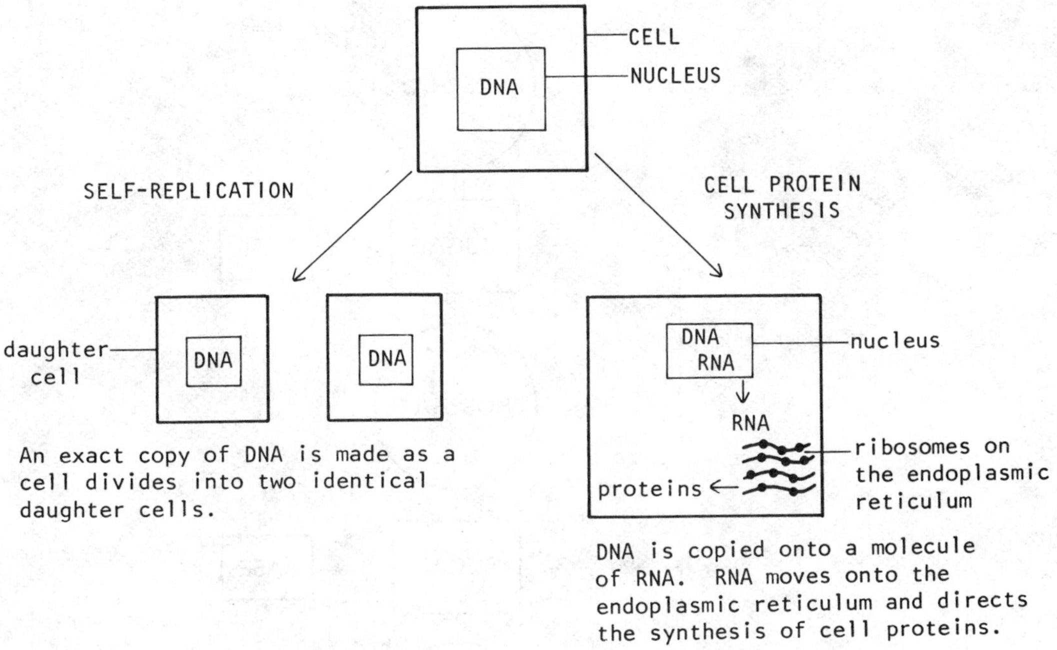

Figure 18-5 The two functions of DNA.

reproduce in an uncontrolled manner and also become anaplastic; they lose their ability to differentiate into mature cells that carry on normal functions, including synthesis of some proteins). If DNA controls mitosis and synthesis of proteins, then changes in the chemical nature of DNA can lead to permanent transformations in cell reproduction, function, and structure. Such an inheritable change in a cell is called a **mutation**, and cellular mutations can lead to malignant growths.

DNA

Understanding the chemical nature of DNA and how changes, or mutations, in its structure might occur is thus very important. DNA is a large, complex molecule composed of units called **nucleotides**. Each nucleotide unit (there are thousands in each DNA molecule) is composed of three parts: (1) a sugar called **deoxyribose**; (2) a **phosphate** group attached to the sugar; and (3) a chemical compound called a **base**. Figure 18-6 is a diagrammatic representation of three nucleotide units within a DNA molecule.

The nucleotide (sugar, phosphate, and base) units in the DNA molecule are connected by bonds between the sugar and phosphate groups, and thus form a long chain of nucleotides. Each chromosome contains two such chains, which are wound around each other in something like a twisted ladder or spiral **helix**. There are four different kinds of bases in the DNA nucleotide units. Two of the bases are called **purines**; the names of the purines are **adenine** and **guanine**. The other two bases are called **pyrimidines**; they are known as **cytosine** and **thymine**. Figure 18-7 shows the general pattern of nucleotide arrangement in DNA.

The precise order of arrangement of bases on the DNA strands is called the **molecular code (genetic code)**. This code dictates the normal way that a cell divides and how the cell makes its new proteins. (The code is transported into the cytoplasm within an RNA molecule.) Changes in the arrangement of bases in DNA or RNA can thus disrupt the cell's normal repro-

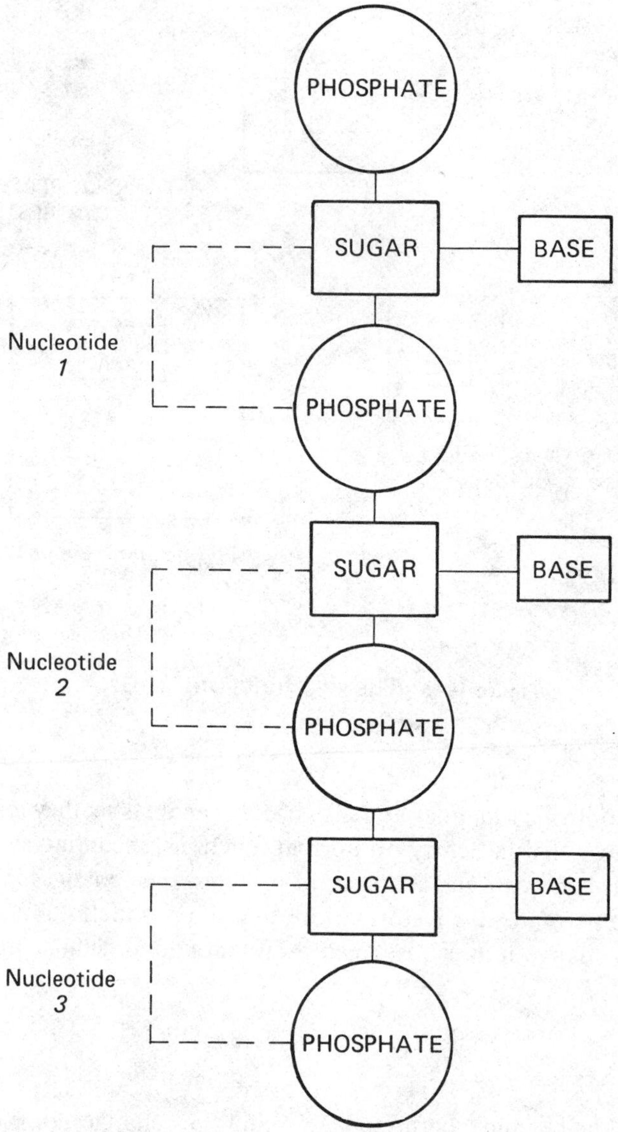

Figure 18-6 Three nucleotide units within a DNA molecule.

duction and lead to faulty protein synthesis in the cytoplasm. These changes set the stage for malignant mutations and cancerous transformations.

Environmental Agents

Agents from the environment—such as chemicals and drugs, radiation, and viruses—can cause changes in DNA and thus produce cancer. Chemical **carcinogens** include **aromatic hydrocarbons** such as **benzpyrene** (which is found in cigarette, cigar, and pipe smoke and automobile exhaust); **alkylating agents** such as mustard gas and melphalan (which produce leukemia in laboratory animals and in humans); **vinyl chloride** and **asbestos**, which are found in sprays, insulation, and industrial chemicals; and hormones such as **diethylstilbestrol (DES)**, which causes vaginal carcinomas in female offspring of women who have taken this drug during pregnancy.

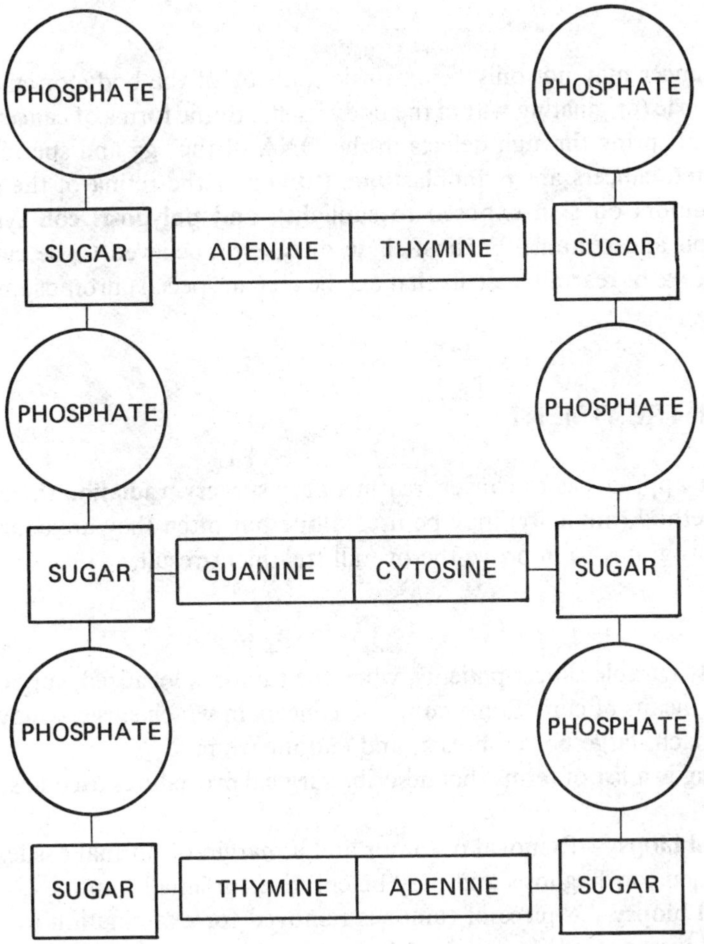

Figure 18-7 General pattern of nucleotide arrangement in a DNA molecule.

The effects of **radiation** (energy given off from radioactive or other substances) on cells can also lead to changes in DNA and malignant transformations. **Ionizing radiation** is energy given off by radioactive substances and x-rays. The radiation causes small particles called ions to be released in the cell. These particles may damage DNA. Thus, leukemia is an occupational hazard of radiologists, who are routinely exposed to x-rays. There is also a high incidence of leukemia among survivors of atomic bomb attacks, as in Hiroshima and Nagasaki. **Ultraviolet radiation** given off by the sun can cause skin cancer, especially in persons with lightly pigmented, or fair, skin.

There is now conclusive evidence that viruses cause both experimental and human cancer, as for example the human T-cell leukemia virus (HTLV), which causes a form of leukemia in adults. A related virus is thought to cause the acquired immunodeficiency syndrome (AIDS). *In vivo* studies (growing tumors in living animals) have shown that the SV-40 virus causes sarcomas in hamsters. *In vitro* studies (growing colonies of tumor cells on laboratory plates or in test tubes) have revealed the Epstein-Barr virus in cultured Burkitt's lymphoma cells. In addition to transmission of cancer by whole viruses, pieces of viral DNA (called **viral oncogenes**) or similar broken or dislocated pieces of human DNA (called **cellular oncogenes**) can cause normal cells to become malignant.

Heredity

Causes of cancer may not only be extrinsic (outside of the body, or environmental) but may also be intrinsic (originating within the body itself). Some forms of cancer are transmitted from parents to offspring through defects in the DNA of the egg and sperm cells. Examples of known inherited cancers are **retinoblastoma** (tumor of the retina of the eye); **xeroderma pigmentosum** (tumors on skin exposed to sunlight); and **polyposis coli syndrome** (polyps grow in the colon and rectum). Each of these diseases is believed to be caused by specific chromosomal breaks or rearrangements that can be seen in special chromosome pictures called karyotypes.

VII. CANCER TREATMENT

Three major approaches to cancer treatment are **surgery, radiation therapy**, and **chemotherapy**. Each method (**modality**) may be used alone but often they are coordinated in combined modality programs to improve the overall treatment result.

Surgery

In potentially curable cancer patients, when the tumor is localized, surgical excision may offer an effective means of cure. Some common cancers in which surgery may be curative are those of the stomach, large bowel, breast, and endometrium.

The following is a list of terms that describe surgical procedures used in staging and treating cancer:

1. **Excisional biopsy**—Removal of tumor and a margin of normal tissue. This procedure provides a specimen for diagnosis and may be curative for small tumors.
2. **Incisional biopsy**—A piece of tumor is removed for examination to establish a diagnosis. This procedure is used if excisional biopsy would create an unnecessary major defect (cosmetic or emotional), or if x-ray therapy is to be used to treat the bulk of the tumor.
3. **Needle biopsy**—A needle is inserted into the tissue in question and a core of tissue is removed. **Aspiration**, or suction, may be used to withdraw free cells from a fluid-filled cavity such as in cystic areas of the breast, or from a solid lump of tumor.
4. **Exfoliative cytology**—Cells are scraped (exfoliated) from the region of suspected disease and are examined under the microscope. The **Pap test**, to determine carcinoma of the cervix and vagina, is an example of exfoliative cytology.
5. **En block resection**—Tumor is removed along with a large area of surrounding tissues containing affected lymph nodes. This procedure is used with tumors which commonly metastasize to regional lymph nodes. Radical mastectomy, colectomy, and gastrectomy are examples.
6. **Exenteration**—A wide resection involving removal of tumor, its organ of origin, and all surrounding tissue in the body space, such as the pelvis.
7. **Cryosurgery**—Malignant tissue is frozen and thus destroyed. This procedure is often used to treat brain and bladder tumors.
8. **Electrocauterization**—Malignant tumors are destroyed (burned) by the passage of an electric current. Electrocauterization is often used in treating tumors of the rectum.

Radiation

The goal of radiation therapy is to deliver a maximal dose of ionizing radiation to the tumor tissue and a minimal dose to surrounding normal tissue. In reality, this goal is difficult to obtain, and usually one accepts a degree of residual normal cell damage (**morbidity**) as a sequel to destruction of the tumor. The effect of high-dose radiation to cells is to produce damage to DNA and thus inhibit cell replication and growth.

Some terms used in the field of radiation therapy for cancer are listed below:

1. **Radiosensitive tumor**—Tumor in which irradiation can cause death of cells without serious damage to surrounding normal tissue. Tumors of hematopoietic and lymphopoietic origin are radiosensitive.
2. **Radioresistant tumor**—Tumor that requires large doses of radiation to produce death of cells. The high doses of radiation may have a damaging effect on surrounding normal tissues. Connective tissue tumors are the most radioresistant tumors.
3. **Radiocurable tumor**—Tumor that can be completely eradicated by radiation therapy. These are usually localized tumors with no evidence of metastasis. Lymphomas and Hodgkin's disease are examples.
4. **Fractionation**—A method of giving radiation in small, repeated doses rather than a few large doses. This procedure allows larger total doses to be given without damaging normal tissue.
5. **Linear accelerator**—A large electronic device that produces high-energy x-ray beams for treatment of deep-seated tumors.
6. **Electron beams**—Low-energy beams for treatment of skin or surface tumors.
7. **Radiosensitizers**—Drugs that increase the sensitivity of tumors to x-rays.

Cancer Chemotherapy

Cancer chemotherapy is the treatment of cancer using drugs. It is probably the most important factor responsible for long-term survival in several types of cancer (choriocarcinoma, acute lymphocytic leukemia, Hodgkin's disease). Chemotherapy may be used alone or in combination with surgery and radiation.

Studies of **cell population kinetics** (the rate of tumor cell multiplication) are important in understanding how to use drugs to treat cancer. These studies provide information on the rate of cell division in normal and cancerous cells.

The term **growth fraction** refers to the percentage of cells in a tissue that are actively growing and dividing. A high tumor growth fraction means that a large percentage of tumor cells are actively dividing. Because most antitumor drugs have their major killing effect against cells that are undergoing DNA synthesis in preparation for cell division, a tumor with a large growth fraction will be more seriously damaged by those drugs than will a low growth fraction tumor. A highly **responsive tumor** is one that will be killed by drugs, while a **nonresponsive** or **resistant tumor** is not significantly affected by drug treatment.

The field of **pharmacokinetics** is concerned with the study of the distribution and disappearance of drugs in the whole animal. Obviously, the ideal is to develop drugs that kill large numbers of tumor cells without harming normal cells. Because some normal tissue cells, such as bone marrow and gastrointestinal lining cells, have large growth fractions, they suffer considerable damage from antitumor drugs. Scientists working in the field of pharmacokinetics of cancer chemotherapy are interested in the proper design of drug dosages, concentrations, and schedules of administration, so that they can achieve the greatest tumor kill with the least toxicity to normal cells.

Combination chemotherapy refers to the use of two or more antitumor drugs together to kill a specific type of malignant growth. In chemotherapy, drugs are given according to a written **protocol**, or plan, which details exactly how the drugs will be given. Usually drug therapy is continued until the patient achieves a complete **remission**, which is the absence of all signs of disease. At times, chemotherapy is given as an **adjuvant** (an aid) to surgery. This means that the drugs are used to kill possible hidden disease in patients who, after surgery, are otherwise free of any evidence of malignancy.

The following are categories of cancer chemotherapeutic agents:

1. **Alkylating agents**—These are synthetic compounds containing two or more chemical groups called alkyl groups. The drugs interfere with the process of DNA synthesis by attaching to DNA molecules. Toxic (poisonous) side effects include nausea and vomiting, diarrhea, bone marrow depression (myelosuppression), and alopecia (hair loss). These are common side effects because the cells in the gastrointestinal tract, bone marrow, and scalp are rapidly dividing cells (high growth fraction) which, along with tumor cells, are susceptible to the lethal effects of chemotherapeutic drugs. The side effects disappear after treatment is suspended.
2. **Antimetabolites**—These drugs inhibit the synthesis of substances (such as purines and pyrimidines) that are necessary for the replication of DNA. Antimetabolites that are effective in stopping cell division in this manner are called **antipurines**, **antipyrimidines**, and **antifolates** (antagonists of folic acid, which is involved in the synthesis of DNA). Side effects are myelosuppression, with leukopenia, thrombocytopenia, and bleeding; and oral and digestive tract toxicity, including stomatitis (sore mouth), nausea, and vomiting.
3. **Steroids**—It is known that the growth of some tumors (breast and prostate) is either accelerated or depressed by specific steroid hormones. Some tumor cells have **estrogen receptors (ER)**, which increase the likelihood that the tumor will respond to estrogen administration (in postmenopausal women) or to the removal of estrogen by oophorectomy (in premenopausal women). Fluid retention, masculinization, feminization, nausea, and vomiting are some possible side effects of various steroids. Tumor growth may also be inhibited by antiestrogen drugs such as **tamoxifen**, which block estrogen action.
4. **Antibiotics**—These drugs are produced by bacteria. Many of these drugs act by binding to DNA and RNA in the cell, thus preventing normal replication. Toxic effects from their use include alopecia, stomatitis, myelosuppression, and gastrointestinal disturbances.
5. **Plant alkaloids**—These drugs are chemicals derived from plants. They are used frequently in combination with other chemotherapeutic agents. Side effects include myelosuppression, alopecia, and nerve damage.
6. **Miscellaneous drugs**—The following drugs are also helpful in treating tumors: **L-asparaginase, dacarbazine, procarbazine,** and **lomustine**.
7. **Drug combinations**—Some drug combinations (combination chemotherapy) are effective in treating cancers such as Hodgkin's disease, acute leukemia, lymphoma, and breast cancer. Examples are **MOPP** (nitrogen **m**ustard, **O**ncovin, **p**rednisone, **p**rocarbazine), **POMP** (**p**rednisone, **O**ncovin, **m**ethotrexate, 6-mercapto**p**urine), **COP** (**C**ytoxan, **O**ncovin, **p**rednisone), **CMF** (**C**ytoxan, **m**ethotrexate, 5-**f**luorouracil); and **VPB** (**v**elban, cis-**p**latin, **b**leomycin).

Figure 18-8 reviews the major methods of cancer treatment, and Table 18-2 summarizes the categories of chemotherapeutic agents.

VIII. VOCABULARY

adenine	One of four bases in the DNA molecule.
adjuvant	Assisting or aiding.
alkylating agents	Synthetic chemicals containing alkyl groups that combine easily with other substances; used in cancer treatment and are carcinogenic as well.

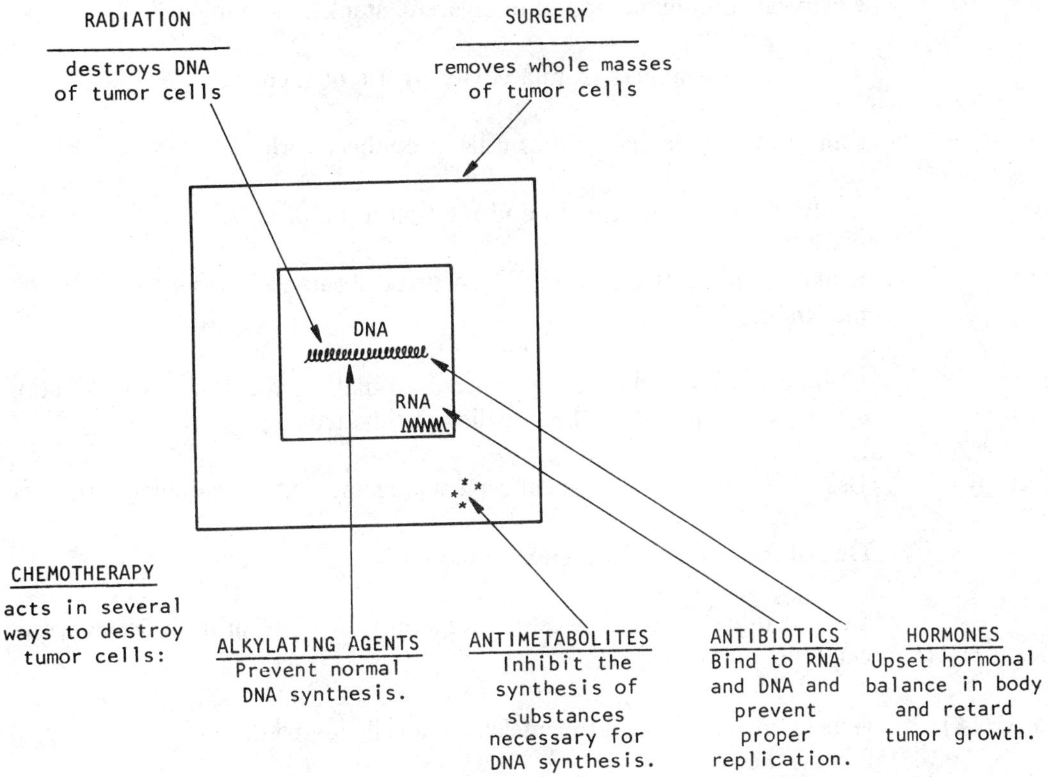

Figure 18-8 Methods of cancer treatment.

anaplasia — Loss of differentiation of cells; reversion to a more primitive cell type.

antibiotics — Chemical substances, produced by bacteria, that inhibit the growth of cells.

antimetabolites — Chemicals that prevent cell division by inhibiting the formation of substances necessary to make DNA.

TABLE 18-2 CATEGORIES OF CANCER CHEMOTHERAPEUTIC AGENTS

Alkylating agents	**Antimetabolites**
cyclophosphamide (Cytoxan)	cytosine arabinoside (ara-C)
melphalan (Alkeran)	5-fluorouracil (5-FU)
nitrogen mustard	methotrexate (MTX)
cis-platin	6-thioguanine (6-TG)
carmustine (BCNU)	**Antibiotics**
Steroids (hormones) and hormone antagonists	bleomycin sulfate
dexamethasone (Decadron)	daunorubicin HCl
diethylstilbestrol (DES)	doxorubicin HCl (Adriamycin)
prednisone	mithramycin
testosterone	actinomycin D
tamoxifen	**Miscellaneous drugs**
Plant alkaloids	dacarbazine
vinblastine sulfate (Velban)	L-asparaginase
vincristine sulfate (Oncovin)	lomustine
VF-16 (Etoposide)	procarbazine

aromatic hydrocarbons Chemical compounds found in cigarette smoke; carcinogenic.

aspiration To remove substances from a cavity by use of suction.

carcinoma Cancerous tumor made up of cells of epithelial origin.

cell population kinetics Study of the rate of growth and multiplication of cells.

cellular oncogenes Broken or dislocated pieces of DNA that can cause a normal cell to become malignant.

chemical carcinogens Chemical agents that cause cancer: aromatic hydrocarbons, alkylating agents, vinyl chloride, asbestos, diethylstilbestrol.

combination chemotherapy Use of several chemotherapeutic agents together in the treatment of tumors.

cytosine One of four bases in the DNA molecule.

dedifferentiation Loss of differentiation of cells; reversion to a more primitive, embryonic cell type; anaplasia.

deoxyribonucleic acid (DNA) Genetic material within the nucleus of a cell; controls cell division and protein synthesis.

deoxyribose Sugar found in DNA molecule.

differentiation Specialization of cells.

electron beams Low-energy beams of radiation for treatment of skin or surface tumors.

fractionation Giving radiation in small, repeated doses.

genetic code Arrangement of bases on the DNA strands.

grading Evaluating the microscopic appearance of tumor cells to determine the degree of dedifferentiation (anaplasia).

gross description of tumors Visual appearance of tumors: cystic, fungating, inflammatory, medullary, necrotic, polypoid, ulcerating, and verrucous.

growth fraction Percentage of cells in a tissue that are engaged in or will enter cell division.

guanine One of four bases in the DNA molecule.

helix Coiled structure; DNA consists of two coiled strands or helixes.

infiltrative Extending beyond normal tissue boundaries; invasive.

in vitro	In glass; an experiment performed in a laboratory with chemicals or isolated biological materials.
in vivo	In life; an experiment performed in a living animal.
ionizing radiation	Energy given off by radioactive atoms and x-rays.
lethal	Producing death.
linear accelerator	Device that produces high-energy x-ray beams for treatment of deep-seated tumors.
microscopic description (of tumors)	The appearance of tumors as seen under the microscope: alveolar, carcinoma *in situ,* diffuse, dysplastic, epidermoid, follicular, nodular, papillary, pleomorphic, scirrhous.
mitosis	A stage in the cell life cycle involving the production of two identical cells from a parent cell (replication).
mixed-tissue tumors	Tumors composed of different types of tissue (epithelial as well as connective tissue).
modality	Method of treatment, such as surgery, chemotherapy, or radiation.
morbidity	Damage to normal tissue (incapacitation).
mucinous	Containing mucus.
mutation	Change in the genetic material (DNA) of a cell; may be caused by chemicals, radiation, or viruses or may occur spontaneously.
nonresponsive tumor	Tumor that is not severely damaged by drug treatment.
nucleotide	Chemical compound composed of a base plus a sugar and phosphate part; building block of DNA.
pedunculated	Possessing a stem or stalk (peduncle); characteristic of some polypoid tumors.
pharmacokinetics	Study of the distribution and removal of drugs in the body over a period of time.
plant alkaloids	Chemicals derived from plants; used in cancer chemotherapy.
protocol	Plan for treatment of a type of illness.
purine	Substance (a base) found in DNA; examples are adenine and guanine.
pyrimidine	Substance (a base) found in DNA; examples are thymine and cytosine.

radiocurable tumor	A tumor that can be completely eradicated by radiation therapy.
radioresistant tumor	A tumor that requires large doses of radiation to destroy its cells.
radiosensitive tumors	A tumor in which radiation can cause death of cells.
radiosensitizers	Drugs that increase the sensitivity of tumors to x-rays.
replication	Cell division in which two identical cells are produced from a parent cell (mitosis).
responsive tumor	Tumor that can be eradicated by drug therapy.
ribonucleic acid (RNA)	Substance that, along with DNA, plays an important role in the synthesis of proteins in a cell.
sarcoma	Cancerous tumor derived from connective tissue.
serous	Pertaining to a thin, watery fluid (serum).
sessile	Having no stem; characteristic of some polypoid tumors.
solid tumor	Tumor composed of mass of cells.
staging	System of evaluating the extent of spread of tumors.
steroids	Complex, naturally occurring chemicals, such as hormones, that are used as chemotherapeutic agents.
surgical procedures to treat cancer	Methods of removing cancerous tissue: excisional biopsy, incisional biopsy, needle biopsy, exfoliative cytology, en block resection, cryosurgery, electrocauterization, exenteration.
thymine	One of four bases in the DNA molecule.
ultraviolet radiation	Rays given off by the sun.
viral oncogenes	Pieces of DNA from viruses that infect a normal cell and cause it to become malignant.

IX. COMBINING FORMS, SUFFIXES, AND PREFIXES

Combining Form	*Definition*	*Terminology*	*Meaning*
onc/o	tumor	oncology	________________
carcin/o	cancerous	adenocarcinoma	________________

sarc/o	flesh, connective tissue	osteosarcoma ______
leiomy/o	smooth muscle	leiomyosarcoma ______
rhabdomy/o	striated muscle	rhabdomyosarcoma ______
scirrh/o	hard	scirrhous ______
medull/o	soft, middle, marrow	medullary ______
papill/o	nipple-like	papillary ______
polyp/o	polyps; small growths	polypoid ______
cyst/o	sac of fluid	cystic ______
alveol/o	small sac	alveolar ______
follicul/o	small sac	follicular ______
ple/o	many, more	pleomorphic ______
terat/o	monster, malformed fetus	teratoma ______
mut/a	genetic change	mutation ______
mutagen/o	causing genetic change	mutagenic ______
radi/o	rays, x-rays	radiotherapy ______
		radioresistant ______
		radiosensitive ______
chem/o	chemical, drug	chemotherapy ______
pharmac/o	chemical, drug	pharmacology ______
tox/o	poison	toxic ______
cry/o	cold	cryosurgery ______
cauter/o	heat, burn	electrocauterization ______

therm/o	heat	hyperthermia ______ *An experimental form of cancer therapy.*
-plasia	formation, growth	hyperplasia ______
		dysplasia ______
-plasm	formation	neoplasm ______
ana-	backward, up	anaplasia ______
epi-	upon	epithelial ______
		epidermoid ______
meta-	beyond, change	metastasis ______
		metaplasia ______ *Change in form of tissue from normal to abnormal type.*

X. LABORATORY TESTS, CLINICAL PROCEDURES, AND ABBREVIATIONS

Laboratory Tests

CEA test

Carcinoembryonic antigen can be found in the bloodstream of patients with a variety of tumors of gastrointestinal origin. Measurement in the blood can lead to early identification, resection, and possible cure of some cases.

alpha-fetoprotein test

This test detects the presence of the protein antigen (alpha-fetoprotein) in the serum of patients with liver and testicular cancer.

beta-HCG test

This blood test detects the presence of a portion of human chorionic gonadotropin (HCG) in the serum of patients with testicular cancer and is used as a marker for the presence of tumor cells in the body.

estrogen (estradiol) receptor assay

This test measures the concentration of estrogen receptor sites in tumor cells of breast cancer patients. If a tumor is found to be estrogen receptor positive, a patient will likely respond to hormone therapy.

Clinical Procedures

scans

Radioactive substances are injected intravenously and pictures (scans) are taken of the organs in question. In liver and spleen scans, irregular distribution of radioactivity or absence of radioactivity indicates possible liver disease, while on bone scans, abnormal areas of concentration of radioactivity may indicate bone destruction and repair, processes which are associated with metastasis. Abnormalities in brain scans appear as increased accumulation of radioactivity (normal neural tissue does not take up radioactivity). Some of the radioactive substances used in obtaining scans are: **gallium-67**—whole-body scan (can detect head and neck tumors, Hodgkin's disease, lymphoma, lung tumors, bone tumors); **rose bengal**—liver scan; **technetium-99m**—liver and spleen scans; and **technetium-99m polyphosphate**—bone scan.

peritoneoscopy This procedure (also called laparoscopy) is used to inspect the abdominal (peritoneal) cavity for tumors. A peritoneoscope (laparoscope) is inserted into the peritoneal cavity through a small incision in the abdominal wall.

staging laparotomy This is a wide surgical incision of the abdomen which allows the physician to explore the abdominal cavity to determine the extent of disease.

lymphangiogram This is an x-ray record (after injection of contrast dye) of the lymph vessel system to detect enlarged lymph nodes, blockage of the lymphatic system, and presence of tumors.

bone marrow biopsy A small amount of bone marrow tissue is aspirated and examined under the microscope for evidence of cancerous cells.

Papanicolaou smear Tissue from the cervix and vagina is removed, stained, and examined under a microscope for early detection of cancer. Cells from the respiratory and gastrointestinal tracts may also be evaluated by this procedure.

Abbreviations

ara-C	Cytosine arabinoside
bx	Biopsy
Ca	Cancer
CEA	Carcinoembryonic antigen
chem	Chemotherapy
CMF	Cytoxan, methotrexate, 5-fluorouracil
DES	Diethylstilbestrol
DHL	Diffuse histiocytic lymphoma
DNA	Deoxyribonucleic acid
ER	Estrogen receptor
exc	Excision
5-FU	5-Fluorouracil
Ga	Gallium
Hd	Hodgkin's disease
mets	Metastases
MOPP	Nitrogen mustard, Oncovin, prednisone, procarbazine
MTX	Methotrexate
NED	No evidence of disease
NER	No evidence of recurrence
NERD	No evidence of recurrent disease
NPDL	Nodular, poorly differentiated lymphocytes
Pap smear	Papanicolaou smear
POMP	Prednisone, Oncovin, methotrexate, 6-mercaptopurine
prot.	Protocol
RAtx	Radiation therapy
RNA	Ribonucleic acid
st	Stage (of disease)
Tc	Technetium
TNM	Tumor, nodes, metastases

XI. PRACTICAL APPLICATIONS

Case Report

A 37-year-old white male underwent abdominal wall resection for a malignant melanoma arising in a nevus. One year later, he underwent bilateral axillary node dissection, which indicated 2 of 23 left axillary nodes positive for tumor. Two months later, his bone scan was positive at the right proximal humerus, and a biopsy revealed metastatic melanoma. The patient began having symptoms of involvement of the fourth lumbar nerve roots and received radiotherapy to the L-4 spine and the humerus with good response. However, several weeks later, he noted progressive right leg weakness and left leg sensory loss. Myelogram demonstrated two metastatic lesions at T-12/L-1 and L-4 that were not thought to be accessible surgically. The patient received further radiotherapy to the affected vertebral areas. The patient received one course of BCNU [a chemotherapeutic drug] from another physician who noted some optic disk edema. The patient was placed on dexamethasone (Decadron) therapy for 2 weeks, after which his course deteriorated progressively with numbness in his upper extremities bilaterally, left leg hypesthesia, and tremors. Decadron was continued and a neurosurgeon felt that little could be done surgically to reverse the deficits.

CAT scan was normal and a second myelogram demonstrated metastatic lesions at the L-4 and T-10 level. Radiation therapy was given to the cord and to the brain without measurable response. On August 7, 1981, the patient began having breathing difficulties and expired.

At autopsy metastatic melanoma was found in the pons, in the cerebellum, throughout the spinal cord with peripheral nerve extension, and in the lumbar vertebrae. There was extensive compression necrosis of the spinal cord in areas of tumor involvement. In the lungs, bilateral pulmonary emboli with lower lobe infarcts were found.

The Philadelphia Chromosome

The Philadelphia chromosome is found in the malignant cells of patient with chronic myelogenous leukemia. In these cells, chromosome 22 is unusually short, as though the end had broken off. The missing genetic material is usually found attached to chromosome 9. The shortened chromosome is referred to as the Philadelphia chromosome because it was first documented by researchers in that city.

XII. EXERCISES

A. Give four characteristics of cancerous tumors:

1. ______________________________

2. ______________________________

3. ______________________________

4. ______________________________

B. *Build medical terms:*

1. New growth ______
2. Excessive growth (numbers of cells) ______
3. Study of tumors ______
4. Tumor (benign) of a gland ______
5. Tumor (malignant) of striated muscle ______
6. Tumor (malignant) of bone ______
7. Tumor (malignant) of glandular tissue ______
8. Tumor (benign) of fat ______
9. Tumor (malignant) of melanocytes ______
10. Tumor (malignant) of smooth muscle ______

C. *Give the meaning of the following terms:*

1. carcinoma *in situ* ______
2. teratoma ______
3. anaplasia ______
4. infiltrative ______
5. TNM system ______
6. metaplasia ______
7. grading of malignant tumors ______
8. dedifferentiation ______
9. sessile ______
10. pedunculated ______
11. verrucous ______
12. epidermoid ______
13. mucinous ______

14. serous ______________________________

15. dysplastic ______________________________

D. *Match the following gross and microscopic descriptions of tumors with their meanings. Place a (G) or (M) next to the term to indicate whether it is a gross or microscopic description.*

1. scirrhous ( )	______	A.	Microscopic nipple-like projections.
2. medullary ( )	______	B.	Forming microscopic clusters of cells.
3. nodular ( )	______	C.	Forming small glandular sacs.
4. diffuse ( )	______	D.	Microscopic sacs within sarcomas.
5. alveolar ( )	______	E.	Hard, overgrown with fibrous tissue.
6. cystic ( )	______	F.	Projecting outward from a membrane base.
7. follicular ( )	______	G.	Cells spreading evenly throughout the tumor mass.
8. polypoid ( )	______	H.	Forming large open spaces filled with fluid.
9. papillary ( )	______	I.	Forming large, soft, fleshy tumors.
10. necrotic ( )	______	J.	Mushrooming pattern of tumor growth.
11. fungating ( )	______	K.	Producing open exposed surfaces.
12. inflammatory ( )	______	L.	Composed of many types of tumor cells.
13. ulcerating ( )	______	M.	Characterized by redness, swelling, and heat.
14. pleomorphic ( )	______	N.	Containing dead tissue.

E. *Select or supply the appropriate medical term:*

1. A (carcinoma/sarcoma) is a cancerous tumor composed of cells of epithelial tissue.

   An example of such a cancerous tumor is a ______________________________

   ____.

2. A (carcinoma/sarcoma) is a cancerous tumor composed of connective tissue. An example of such a cancerous tumor is a ______________________.

3. Genetic material inside the nucleus of a cell is called ______________________.

4. This material is composed of several parts. The sugar is called ______________ ______________, and the four base parts are called ______________ ______________, ______________ and ______________.

   There is also a ______________________ part within the structure of the genetic material.

5. Two important functions of a cell that are controlled by its genetic material are ______________________ and ______________________.
   These functions assure that the cell divides properly and that important substances are made for the growth of the cell.

6. A change in the genetic material of a cell that leads to an improper cell division or malignant growth is called a ______________________.

7. Some agents that can lead to changes in genetic material and cancerous tumors are ______________________, ______________________, and ______________________.

8. Some forms of cancer are transmitted from parents to offspring through defects in genetic material. Examples of such cancers are ______________________, ______________________, and ______________________.

F. *Give the meaning of the following medical terms:*

1. lethal ______________________
2. purine ______________________
3. mitosis ______________________
4. ionizing radiation ______________________

5. alkylating agents ______________________________

6. carcinogenesis ______________________________

7. *in vitro* ______________________________

8. *in vivo* ______________________________

9. diethylstilbestrol ______________________________

10. cellular oncogenes ______________________________

11. aromatic hydrocarbons ______________________________

12. morbidity ______________________________

13. viral oncogenes ______________________________

14. nucleotide ______________________________

15. ultraviolet radiation ______________________________

16. chemical carcinogens ______________________________

G. *Match the surgical procedure in Column I with a closely associated term in Column II:*

Column I		*Column II*
1. needle biopsy	______	Removal of tumor and a margin of normal tissue for diagnosis.
2. block resection	______	Burning lesion to kill cells.
3. incisional biopsy	______	Wide resection involving removal of tumor, its organ of origin, and surrounding tissue in the body space.
4. excisional biopsy		
5. exfoliative cytology	______	Scraping cells to examine microscopically.
6. cryosurgery	______	Removal of entire tumor and regional lymph nodes.
7. electrocauterization	______	Freezing lesion to kill cells.
8. exenteration	______	Withdrawal of a core of tissue from a tumor.
	______	Cutting into tumor to remove section for diagnosis.

H. *Supply answers for the following:*

1. The method of treating cancer by use of high-energy radiation waves is called ______________________________.

2. If tumor tissue requires large doses of radiation to kill cells, it is called a ______________________________ tumor.

3. If radiation can cause loss of tumor cells without much damage to surrounding regions, the tumor is called ______________________________.

4. A tumor that can be completely eradicated by irradiation is known as a ______________ tumor.

5. The method of giving radiation in short doses is called ______________________.

6. Treatment of cancerous tumors with drugs is called ______________________.

7. A tumor that will be killed by drugs is termed ______________________.

8. A tumor that is not significantly affected by drug treatment is termed ______________________________.

9. The study of drugs and their effect on the cell division of both normal and malignant tissues is called ______________________________.

10. The use of two or more drugs to kill tumor cells is called ______________________________.

11. Drugs that increase the sensitivity of tumors to high-energy x-ray beams are called ______________________.

12. Low-energy beams for treatment of skin or surface tumors are known as ______________________________.

13. A large electronic device that produces high-energy x-ray beams for treatment of deep-seated tumors is called a ______________________.

14. Some toxic side effects of cancer chemotherapy are ______________________, ______________________, ______________________, and ______________________.

15. Three types of antimetabolites are ______________________, ______________________, and ______________________.

I. Give meanings for the following medical terms:

1. modality ______________________
2. adjuvant ______________________
3. protocol ______________________
4. aspiration ______________________
5. remission ______________________
6. cell population kinetics ______________________
7. growth fraction ______________________
8. antimetabolite ______________________
9. myelosuppression ______________________
10. alopecia ______________________
11. plant alkaloids ______________________
12. antibiotics ______________________

J. Name five categories of cancer chemotherapeutic drugs and give an example of one drug in each category.

1. ______________________
2. ______________________
3. ______________________
4. ______________________
5. ______________________

K. Give the meanings for the following medical abbreviations:

1. CEA ____________________
2. DNA ____________________
3. TNM ____________________
4. MOPP ____________________
5. 5-FU ____________________
6. DES ____________________
7. MTX ____________________
8. mets ____________________
9. RAtx ____________________

L. Give the meaning of the following tests or procedures:

1. brain scan ____________________
2. laparotomy ____________________
3. alpha-fetoprotein ____________________
4. lymphangiogram ____________________
5. beta-HCG test ____________________
6. peritoneoscopy ____________________
7. estrogen receptor assay ____________________
8. bone marrow biopsy ____________________

ANSWERS

A.

1. Cells multiply rapidly.
2. Invasive and infiltrative growth.
3. Anaplasia (dedifferentiation) of cells.
4. Metastasis (spreading of tumor to secondary site).

B.

1. neoplasm
2. hyperplasia
3. oncology
4. adenoma
5. rhabdomyosarcoma
6. osteosarcoma (osteogenic sarcoma)
7. adenocarcinoma
8. lipoma
9. malignant melanoma
10. leiomyosarcoma

C.

1. Malignant growths that are localized.
2. Malignant neoplasm composed of cells derived from several types of tissue (monster-like appearance of the tumor).
3. Reversion of cells from a more complex form to a simpler, more primitive state; dedifferentiation.
4. Tending to extend beyond its boundaries.
5. Tumor staging system; T means tumor, N means lymph nodes, and M indicates metastases. The system allows physicians to evaluate the extent of spread of disease.
6. Change in the type of adult cells in a tissue to a form that is not normal for that tissue.
7. System of identifying the degree of anaplasia in tumor cells.
8. Anaplasia; reversion to a more primitive cell type.
9. Having no stem; characterizes some polypoid tumors.
10. Possessing a stem or stalk; as in some polypoid tumors.
11. Pertaining to wartlike growth of some tumors.
12. Resembling skin (epidermis) cells; characteristic of some tumors.
13. Full of mucus (contained in some cystic tumors).
14. Full of serum (contained in some cystic tumors).
15. Displaying a highly abnormal, but not clearly cancerous appearance.

D.

1. (M) E
2. (G) I
3. (M) B
4. (M) G
5. (M) D
6. (G) H
7. (M) C
8. (G) F
9. (M) A
10. (G) N
11. (G) J
12. (G) M
13. (G) K
14. (M) L

E.

1. carcinoma; thyroid adenocarcinoma, squamous cell carcinoma
2. sarcoma; liposarcoma, chondrosarcoma, osteogenic sarcoma
3. deoxyribonucleic acid; DNA
4. deoxyribose; adenine, guanine, cytosine, and thymine; phosphate
5. self-replication and protein synthesis
6. mutation
7. radiation, chemicals, and viruses
8. retinoblastoma, xeroderma pigmentosum, and polyposis coli syndrome.

F.

1. Pertaining to death or killing.
2. Type of base found in DNA; adenine and guanine are examples.
3. Cell division in which two identical cells are produced from a parent cell.
4. Energy given off by radioactive atoms and x-rays.
5. Chemicals that are known to be carcinogenic and that are also used in cancer treatment.
6. Production of cancerous tumors.
7. Experiment performed in a laboratory with chemicals.
8. Experiment performed in a living animal.
9. Synthetic estrogen compound; used in cancer treatment and a known carcinogen.
10. Broken or dislocated pieces of DNA that can cause a normal cell to become malignant.
11. Compounds known to be carcinogenic; benzpyrene (cigarette smoke).
12. Condition of being diseased.
13. Pieces of DNA from viruses that infect a normal cell and cause it to become malignant.
14. Building block of DNA; composed of a base, a sugar, and phosphate.
15. Rays given off by the sun; can be carcinogenic.
16. Chemical substances that can cause changes in DNA and produce cancer; examples are aromatic hydrocarbons, alkylating agents, vinyl chloride and asbestos, and hormones.

G.

4
7
8
5

2
6
1
3

H.

1. radiation therapy
2. radioresistant
3. radiosensitive
4. radiocurable
5. fractionation
6. chemotherapy
7. responsive
8. nonresponsive
9. pharmacokinetics
10. combination chemotherapy
11. radiosensitive
12. electron beams
13. linear accelerator
14. nausea and vomiting, myelosuppression, alopecia, and diarrhea
15. antipurines, antipyrimidines, and antifolates.

I.

1. Method of treatment.
2. That which aids or assists.
3. Report or plan of steps taken in an experiment or disease case.
4. Sucking out fluid from a cavity.
5. Absence of all signs of disease.
6. Study of what happens to a cell during cell division and how fast a group of cells is dividing in a total tissue mass.
7. Percentage of cells in a tissue that are going through cell division.
8. Type of chemotherapeutic agent; works by preventing cell division by inhibiting the formation of substances necessary to make DNA.
9. Inhibition of the formation of bone marrow tissue.
10. Baldness.
11. Chemicals derived from plants; used as cancer chemotherapeutic agents.
12. Substances produced by bacteria; inhibit the growth of cells.

J.

1. Alkylating agents; nitrogen mustard, cyclophosphamide, melphalan, cis-platin.
2. Antimetabolites; 5-fluorouracil, methotrexate, cytosine arabinoside, 6-thioguanine
3. Steroids; dexamethasone, diethylstilbestrol, prednisone, testosterone, tamoxifen
4. Antibiotics; bleomycin sulfate, mithramycin, daunorubicin HCl, doxorubicin HCl, actinomycin D
5. Plant alkaloids; vinblastine sulfate, vincristine sulfate, VF-16

K.

1. carcinoembryonic antigen
2. deoxyribonucleic acid.
3. tumor, node, and metastasis; staging system
4. nitrogen mustard, Oncovin, predisone, procarbazine
5. 5-fluorouracil
6. diethylstilbestrol
7. methotrexate
8. metastases
9. radiation therapy

L.

1. Pictures (scans) are taken of the brain after radioactive substance is injected intravenously.
2. Incision into the abdomen to determine the extent of disease.
3. Test for the presence of an antigen found in patients with liver and testicular cancer.
4. Record (x-ray) of lymph vessels.
5. Test for the presence of a portion of human chorionic gonadotropin hormone (a marker for testicular cancer).
6. Process of visually examining the peritoneum for evidence of tumor.
7. Test for the presence of estrogen receptor sites on tumor cells.
8. Removal and microscopic examination of a small amount of bone marrow tissue.

XIII. PRONUNCIATION OF TERMS

adenine	ĂD-ĕ-nēn
adenocarcinoma	ăd-ĕ-nō-kăr-sĭ-NŌ-mă
adjuvant	ĂD-jū-vănt
alkaloid	ĂL-kă-loyd
alkylating	ĂL-kĭ-lā-tĭng
alveolar	ăl-vē-Ō-lăr or ăl-VĒ-ō-lăr
anaplasia	ăn-ă-PLĀ-zē-ă
aspiration	ăs-pĭ-RĀ-shŭn
carcinogen	kăr-SĬN-ō-jĕn
cellular oncogenes	SĔL-ū-lăr ŎNGK-ō-jēnz
chemotherapy	kē-mō-THĔR-ă-pē
cryosurgery	krī-ō-SŬR-jĕr-ē
cystic	SĬS-tĭk

cytosine	SĪ-tō-sēn
differentiation	dĭf-ĕr-ĕn-shē-Ā-shŭn
dysplastic	dĭs-PLĂS-tĭk
electrocauterization	ē-lĕk-trō-kăw-tĕr-ĭ-ZĀ-shŭn
encapsulated	ĕn-KĂP-sū-lāt-ĕd
epidermoid	ĕp-ĭ-DĔR-moyd
exenteration	ĕks-ĕn-tĕ-RĀ-shŭn
exfoliative	ĕks-FŌ-lē-ā-tĭv
follicular	fō-LĬK-ū-lăr
fungating	fŭng-GĀ-tĭng or FŬNG-gā-tĭng
guanine	GWĂN-ēn
helix	HĒ-lĭks
hyperplasia	hī-pĕr-PLĀ-zē-ă
infiltrative	ĬN-fĭl-trā-tĭv or ĭn-FĬL-tră-tĭv
in vitro	ĭn VĒ-trō
in vivo	ĭn VĒ-vō
laparotomy	lăp-ă-RŎT-ō-mē
leiomyosarcoma	lī-ō-mī-ō-săr-KŌ-mă
lethal	LĒ-thăl
lymphangiogram	lĭm-FĂN-jē-ō-grăm
medullary	MĔD-ū-lăr-ē
metastasis	mĕ-TĂS-tă-sĭs
mitosis	mī-TŌ-sĭs
modality	mō-DĂL-ĭ-tē
morbidity	mŏr-BĬD-ĭ-tē
mucinous	MŪ-sĭ-nŭs
mutagenic	mū-tă-JĔN-ĭk
mutation	mū-TĀ-shŭn
necrotic	nĕ-KRŎT-ĭk
neoplasm	NĒ-ō-plăzm
nodular	NŎD-ū-lăr
nucleotide	NŪ-klē-ō-tīd

oncology	ŏn-KŎL-ō-jē
osteosarcoma	ŏs-tē-ō-săr-KŌ-mă
papillary	PĂP-ĭ-lăr-ē
pedunculated	pĕ-DŬNG-kū-lāt-ĕd
peritoneoscopy	pĕr-ĭ-tō-nē-ŎS-kō-pē
pharmacokinetics	făr-mă-kō-kĭ-NĔT-ĭks
pleomorphic	plē-ō-MŎR-fĭk
polypoid	PŎL-ĭ-poyd
protocol	PRŌ-tō-kŏl
purine	PŪ-rēn
pyrimidine	pĭ-RĬM-ĭ-dēn
rhabdomyosarcoma	răb-dō-mī-ō-săr-KŌ-mă
scirrhous	SKĬR-ŭs
serous	SĒ-rŭs
sessile	SĔS-ĭl
thymine	THĪ-mēn
toxic	TŎK-sĭk
ulcerating	ŬL-sĕ-rā-tĭng
verrucous	vĕ-RŌŌ-kŭs or VĔR-ōō-kŭs
viral oncogenes	VĪ-răl ŎNGK-ō-jēnz

REVIEW SHEET

Combining Forms

aden/o	______	onc/o	______
alveol/o	______	papill/o	______
carcin/o	______	pharmac/o	______
cauter/o	______	ple/o	______
chem/o	______	polyp/o	______
cry/o	______	radi/o	______
cyst/o	______	rhabdomy/o	______
follicul/o	______	sarc/o	______
leiomy/o	______	scirrh/o	______
medull/o	______	terat/o	______
mut/a	______	therm/o	______
mutagen/o	______	tox/o	______

Suffixes and Prefixes

ana-	______	-plasia	______
epi-	______	-plasm	______
hyper-	______		
meta-	______		

Additional Terms

adenine (550)

adjuvant (550)

alkylating agents (550)

alpha-fetoprotein test (556)

antibiotics (551)

antimetabolites (551)

aromatic hydrocarbons (552)

aspiration (552)

beta-HCG test (556)

bone marrow biopsy (557)

brain scan (557)

carcinoma (552)

carcinoma *in situ* (543)

CEA test (556)

cell population kinetics (552)

cellular oncogenes (552)

chemical carcinogens (552)

combination chemotherapy (552)

cytosine (552)

dedifferentiation (552)

deoxyribonucleic acid (552)

deoxyribose (552)

differentiation (552)

diffuse (543)

dysplastic (543)

electron beams (552)

estrogen receptor test (556)

excisional biopsy (548)

exfoliative cytology (548)

follicular (543)

fractionation (552)

fungating (542)

genetic code (552)

grading system (552)

growth fraction (552)

guanine (552)

helix (552)

incisional biopsy (548)

infiltrative (552)

inflammatory (542)

in vitro (553)

in vivo (553)

ionizing radiation (553)

lethal (553)

linear accelerator (553)

lymphangiogram (557)

medullary (542)

metastasis (539)

mitosis (553)

modality (553)

morbidity (553)

mutation (553)

necrotic (542)

needle biopsy (548)

nodular (543)

nonresponsive tumor (553)

nucleotide (553)

Papanicolaou smear (557)

papillary (543)

pedunculated (553)

peritoneoscopy (557)

pharmacokinetics (553)

plant alkaloids (553)

pleomorphic (543)

polypoid (542)

protocol (553)

purine (553)

pyrimidine (553)

radiocurable tumor (554)

radiosensitive tumor (554)

radiosensitizer (554)

remission (549)

replication (554)

responsive tumor (554)

ribonucleic acid (554)

sarcoma (554)

scirrhous (543)

serous (554)

sessile (554)

solid tumor (554)

staging laparotomy (557)

staging system (554)

steroids (554)

thymine (554)

ulcerating (542)

ultraviolet rays (554)

verrucous (543)

viral oncogenes (554)

CHAPTER 19

RADIOLOGY, NUCLEAR MEDICINE, AND RADIATION THERAPY

In this chapter you will:

- Learn the physical properties of x-rays;
- Become familiar with diagnostic and therapeutic techniques used by radiologists and radiotherapists;
- Identify the x-ray views and patient positions used in x-ray examinations;
- Learn about the role of radioactivity in the diagnosis and treatment of disease; and
- Become familiar with medical terms used in the specialties of radiology, nuclear medicine, and radiation therapy.

This chapter is divided into the following sections:

I. Introduction
II. Radiology
  A. Characteristics of X-Rays
  B. Diagnostic Techniques
  C. X-Ray Positioning
III. Nuclear Medicine
  A. Radioactivity and Radionuclides
  B. Diagnostic Imaging
IV. Radiation Therapy
V. Vocabulary
VI. Combining Forms and Terminology
VII. Abbreviations
VIII. Practical Applications
IX. Exercises
X. Pronunciation of Terms

I. INTRODUCTION

Radiology (also called **roentgenology** after its discoverer, Wilhelm Conrad Röntgen) is the medical specialty concerned with the study of x-rays. **X-rays** are invisible waves of energy that are produced by an energy source (x-ray machine or cathode tube) and are useful in diagnosis and treatment of disease.

Nuclear medicine is the medical specialty that studies the characteristics and uses of **radioactive substances** in the diagnosis and treatment of disease. Radioactive substances are materials that emit high-speed particles and energy-containing rays from the interior of their matter. The emitted particles and rays are called **radioactivity**, and can be of three types: **alpha particles, beta particles,** and **gamma rays. Gamma rays** are similar to x-rays and are used effectively as a diagnostic label to trace the path and uptake of chemical substances in the body.

Radiation therapy (radiotherapy) is the treatment of disease using an external source of high-energy x-rays and gamma rays or internally implanted radioactive substances. These rays and substances are effective in destroying tissue and stopping the growth of malignant cells.

The personnel involved in these medical fields are varied. A **radiologist** is a physician who specializes in the practice of diagnostic radiology. A **nuclear physician** is a radiologist who specializes in the practice of administering diagnostic nuclear medicine procedures. A **radiotherapist**, also a physician, specializes in the practice of radiotherapy (treatment of disease using radiation).

Allied health care professionals who work with physicians in the fields of radiology, nuclear medicine, and radiotherapy are called **radiologic technologists.** Radiologic technologists can be divided into three categories: **radiographers** (aid physicians in administering diagnostic x-ray procedures), **nuclear medicine technologists** (attend to patients undergoing nuclear medicine procedures and operate devices under the direction of a nuclear physician), and **radiation therapy technologists** (deliver courses of radiation therapy prescribed by a radiotherapist).

II. RADIOLOGY

A. Characteristics of X-Rays

Several characteristics of x-rays are useful to physicians in the diagnosis and treatment of disease. Some of these characteristics are:

1. **Ability to cause exposure of a photographic plate**. If a photographic plate is placed in front of a beam of x-rays, the x-rays, traveling unimpeded through the air, will expose the silver coating of the plate and cause it to blacken.

2. **Ability to penetrate different substances to varying degrees**. X-rays pass through the different types of substances in the human body (air in the lungs, water in blood vessels and lymph, fat around muscles, and metal such as calcium in bones) with varying ease. If the x-rays are absorbed (stopped) by the body substance (e.g., calcium in bones), they do not reach the photographic plate held behind the patient, and white areas are left in the x-ray film (plate). Figure 19-1 is an example of an x-ray photograph.

A substance is said to be **radiolucent** if it permits passage of most of the x-rays. Lung tissue (containing air) is an example of a radiolucent substance. **Radiopaque** substances (bones) are

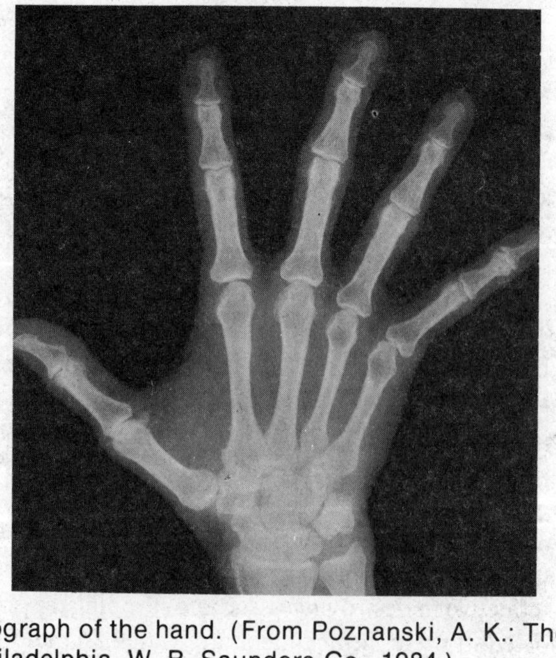

Figure 19-1 X-ray photograph of the hand. (From Poznanski, A. K.: The Hand in Radiologic Diagnosis. 2nd ed. Philadelphia, W. B. Saunders Co., 1984.)

those which absorb most of the x-rays they are exposed to, and thus only a small fraction of the x-rays penetrate.

3. **Invisibility**. X-rays cannot be detected by sight, sound, or touch. Workers exposed to x-rays must wear a **film badge** to detect and record the amount of radiation to which they have been exposed. The film badge contains a special film that is exposed by x-rays. The amount of blackness on the film is an indication of the amount of x-rays or gamma rays received by the wearer.

4. **Travel in straight lines**. This property allows the formation of precise shadow images on the x-ray plate and also permits x-ray beams to be directed accurately at a tissue site during radiotherapy.

5. **Scattering of radiation**. Scattering occurs when x-rays come in contact with any material. Greater scatter occurs with dense objects and less with those substances that are radiolucent. Scatter can be a serious occupational hazard to those in the vicinity of a source of x-rays, such as an x-ray machine. Also, because scatter can blur images and expose areas of film that otherwise would be in shadow, a grid (containing thin lead strips arranged parallel to the x-ray beams) is placed in front of the film to absorb scattered radiation before it strikes the x-ray film. The most frequently used grid is called a **Bucky grid**, and it tends to clarify x-ray images.

6. **Ionization**. X-rays have the ability to ionize substances through which they pass. Ionization is a chemical process in which the energy of an x-ray beam causes rearrangement and disruption within a substance so that previously neutral particles are changed to charged particles called **ions**. This strongly ionizing ability of x-rays is a double-edged sword. In x-ray therapy, the ionizing effect of x-rays can help kill cancerous cells and stop tumor growth; however, ionizing x-rays in small doses can affect normal body cells, leading to tissue damage and malignant changes. Thus, persons exposed to high doses of x-ray run an increased risk of developing leukemia, thyroid tumors, breast cancer, or other malignancies in their later years.

B. Diagnostic Techniques

X-rays are used in a variety of ways to detect pathological conditions. The most common use of the diagnostic x-ray is dental, to locate cavities (caries) in teeth. Other areas examined include the digestive, nervous, reproductive, and endocrine systems, and the chest and bones. Some special diagnostic x-ray techniques are:

Fluoroscopy. This x-ray procedure uses a fluorescent screen instead of a photographic plate to derive a visual image from the x-rays that pass through the patient. The fact that ionizing radiation such as x-rays can produce **fluorescence** (rays of light energy emitted as a result of exposure to and absorption of radiation from another source) is the basis for fluoroscopy. The fluorescent screen glows when it is struck by the x-rays. Opaque tissue, such as bone, appears as a dark shadow image on the fluorescent screen.

A major advantage of fluoroscopy over normal radiography is that internal organs, such as the heart and digestive tract organs, can be observed in motion. Also, the patient's position can be changed constantly to provide the right view at the right time so that the most useful diagnostic information can be obtained.

Image-intensifier systems for fluoroscopy can brighten fluoroscopic images and can be combined with still and movie cameras to obtain a permanent record of either a fluoroscopic or x-ray examination. This procedure is called **cineradiography** (cine- means motion).

Contrast Techniques. In a normal x-ray film and in fluoroscopy, the natural differences in the density of body tissues (e.g., air in lung, calcium in bone) produce contrasting shadow images on the x-ray film and fluorescent screen. However, when x-rays pass through two adjacent body parts composed of substances of the same density as, for example, the digestive organs in the abdomen, their images cannot be distinguished on the film or on the screen. It is necessary, then, to inject a **contrast medium** into the structure or fluid to be visualized so that the specific part, organ, tube, or liquid can be visualized as a negative imprint on the dense contrast agent.

Some artificial contrast material used in diagnostic radiological and fluoroscopic studies are:

Barium Sulfate. Barium sulfate is a metallic powder that is mixed in water and used for examination of the upper and lower GI (gastrointestinal) tract. A **barium swallow (upper GI series)** involves oral ingestion of barium sulfate so that the esophagus, stomach, and duodenum can be visualized. A **small bowel series (small bowel follow-through)** traces the passage of barium in a sequential manner as it passes through the small intestine. Figure 19-2 shows how barium outlines the small intestine on x-ray. A **barium enema** opacifies the lumen (passageway) of the large intestine using an enema containing barium sulfate.

Iodine Compounds. Radiopaque fluids containing up to 50 per cent iodine are used in the following tests:

1. **Angiocardiogram**—An x-ray image of blood vessels and heart chambers is obtained after injecting dye through a catheter (tube) into the appropriate blood vessel or heart chamber.

2. **Arteriogram**—A roentgenogram of an artery is obtained after injecting a radiopaque substance directly into the artery. Cerebral arteries are often examined in this manner in a search for aneurysm, blood clot, or tumor.

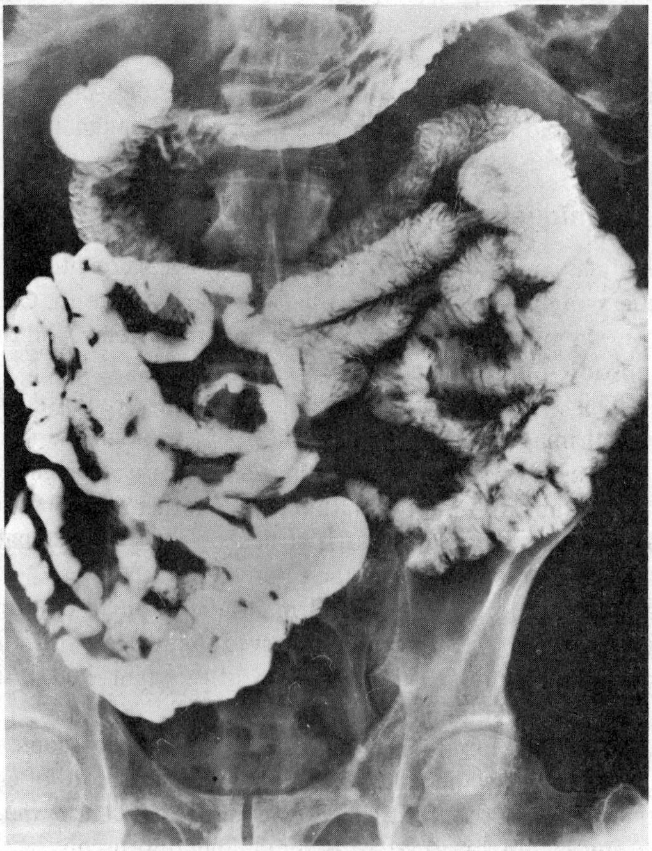

Figure 19-2 A radiograph of the normal small intestine 30 minutes after ingestion of barium. (From Marshak, R. H., and Lindner, A.E.: Radiology of the Small Intestine. 2nd ed. Philadelphia, W. B. Saunders Co., 1976.)

3. **Venogram**—An x-ray image of veins is taken after introducing contrast medium intravenously.

4. **Bronchogram**—A roentgenogram of the bronchial tubes is made after injecting dye into the bronchi through the trachea (windpipe).

5. **Cholecystogram**—A radiopaque substance is given orally; the substance collects in the gallbladder and x-rays are taken of the gallbladder and bile ducts. A fatty meal may then be given and follow-up x-rays taken to look for stones in the gallbladder and common bile duct.

6. **Intravenous cholangiogram (IVC)**—Dye is injected intravenously and directed by the liver into the bile ducts. X-rays are taken of the gallbladder and bile ducts. This test is frequently done after cholecystectomy to examine the patency of bile ducts.

7. **Hysterosalpingogram**—An x-ray record of the uterine tubes is obtained after injecting dye into the uterus via the vagina. This procedure can determine the **patency** (openness) of the uterine tubes.

8. **Intravenous pyelogram (IVP)**—An x-ray image of the renal pelvis and urinary tract is made after injecting dye into a vein. The dye is selectively concentrated by the kidneys and is excreted into the urine.

9. **Retrograde pyelogram (RP)**—This is an x-ray record of the renal pelvis and urinary tract made by injecting dye directly into the urethra, bladder, and ureters. The dye flows back up to the kidney through the ureters.

10. **Lymphangiogram**—An x-ray record of lymphatic vessels made after injecting dye into the lymphatic system.

11. **Myelogram**—An x-ray outline of the spinal canal is made after injecting radiopaque dye into the subarachnoid space surrounding the spinal cord. This test identifies protrusion of an intervertebral disk or bone pressing on the spinal cord or nerve roots. It can also identify tumors of the spinal cord.

12. **Sialogram**—This x-ray record of the salivary ducts is obtained after injection of radiopaque dye directly into the salivary ducts.

13. **Digital subtraction angiography (DSA)**—An x-ray image of contrast-injected blood vessels is produced by taking two x-rays (the first is without contrast) and using a computer to subtract obscuring shadows from the image. Figure 19-3 illustrates the final x-ray image produced by digital subtraction angiography.

Air and Other Gases. Air, carbon dioxide, and nitrous oxide may be used as radiolucent

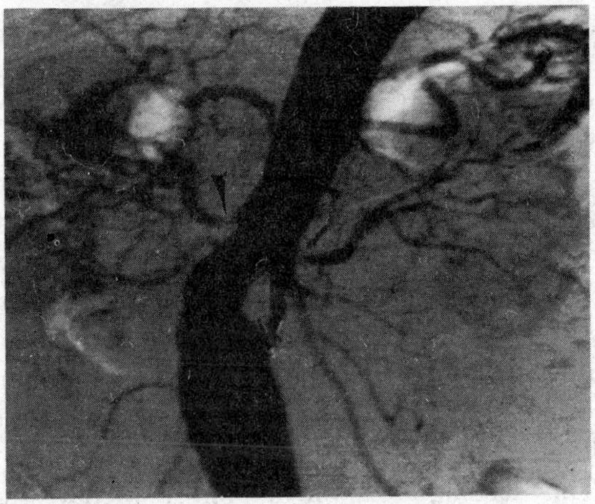

Figure 19-3 Digital subtraction angiography showing bilateral renal artery stenosis in a man with hypertension. (From Hillman, B. J.: Imaging and Hypertension. Philadelphia, W. B. Saunders Co., 1983.)

contrast media after fluid is removed from organs such as the brain ventricles and spinal cord. Examples are:

1. **Encephalogram (pneumoencephalogram)**—Air is injected into the lumbar portion of the spinal cord, and the brain and spinal cord are examined by x-ray.

2. **Arthrogram**—Dye or air or both are injected into a joint and x-rays are taken of the joint.

3. **Ventriculogram**—A neurosurgeon injects air or radiopaque dye into the lateral ventricles of the brain and x-ray films of the ventricles are taken.

Stereoscopy. Stereoscopy is a special radiographic technique in which an illusion of depth of an object is obtained. Two successive radiographs of the part of the body to be viewed are taken from different angles while the patient is immobilized. The resulting films are then examined simultaneously using a stereoscopic viewing device which merges the images, giving the appearance of depth to the picture. This technique is used in studies of the skull, as well as of other anatomical areas.

Tomography. Tomography (also called **laminagraphy**) is a technique for taking a series of x-ray pictures so that x-rays of a desired layer of the body are obtained, while at the same time structures in front of and behind that layer are blurred out. Multiple pictures, called **tomograms, laminagrams,** or **body sections,** are taken by changing the depth of focus of the x-ray machine while the patient remains still. Tomograms are thus x-ray "slices" taken at different depths of focus through the patient. Each tomogram obliterates all extraneous material and focuses on the one small slice which is to be viewed. Calcifications and other solid lesions that are missed on conventional x-rays can be picked up with tomography.

Computed Tomography (CT, CAT). This is a revolutionary technique in radiologic diagnosis. Machines called **CAT scanners** (also called **CT scanners**) beam ionizing x-rays through a patient at multiple angles around a specific section of the body. The absorption of the x-rays at these angles as they pass through the body is detected and relayed to a computer that is programmed with a knowledge of the absorption capacities of the different body tissues. The computer then synthesizes all the information it receives from the many different x-ray views and projects a single composite picture of a specific "slice" of the abdomen, chest, or head on a screen. The ability of CAT scanners to detect abnormalities is enhanced by the use of iodine-containing contrast agents, which outline blood vessels.

The CAT scanners are highly sensitive in detecting disease in soft body tissues and can actually provide images of internal organs which are impossible to visualize with ordinary x-ray technique. This special procedure, which may also involve the use of contrast dyes, can detect brain tumors, hematomas, spinal cord lesions, and masses in the chest, liver, kidneys, and pancreas. Figure 19-4 shows a CAT scan of the chest region and Figure 19-5 shows a CAT scan of the brain.

Xeroradiography. This radiographic technique uses the technology of the Xerox office copier to process x-ray images on Xerox paper instead of on an x-ray film. Ionizing radiation passes through the body and is detected on an electrically charged metal plate which is subsequently copied on paper. Within 90 seconds, an image of the soft tissues of the body can be obtained on specially treated Xerox paper and then observed under ordinary light. Because of the ability to visualize more detail in soft tissues, such as breast, **xeromammography** is thought to enhance the diagnosis of nonpalpable (unable to be felt) lesions and minute calcifications of the breast. Figure 19-6 shows examples of xeroradiograms.

Ultrasonography. This technique employs high-frequency, inaudible sound waves, which bounce off body tissues and are then recorded to give information about the anatomy of an internal organ. An instrument is placed near or on the skin, which is covered with a thin coating of mineral oil to assure good transmission of sound waves. This instrument emits sound waves in short, repetitive pulses. The ultrasound waves move with different speeds through body

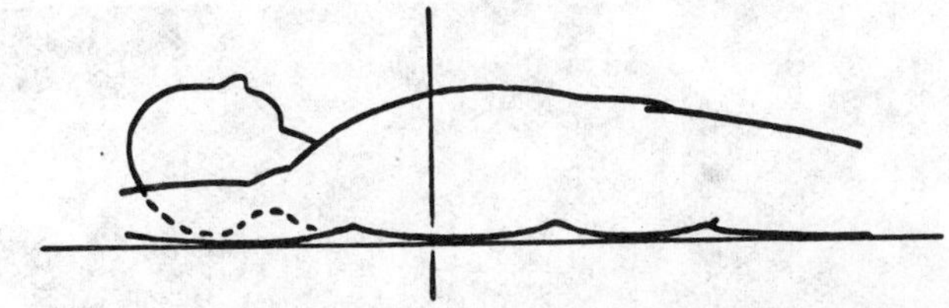

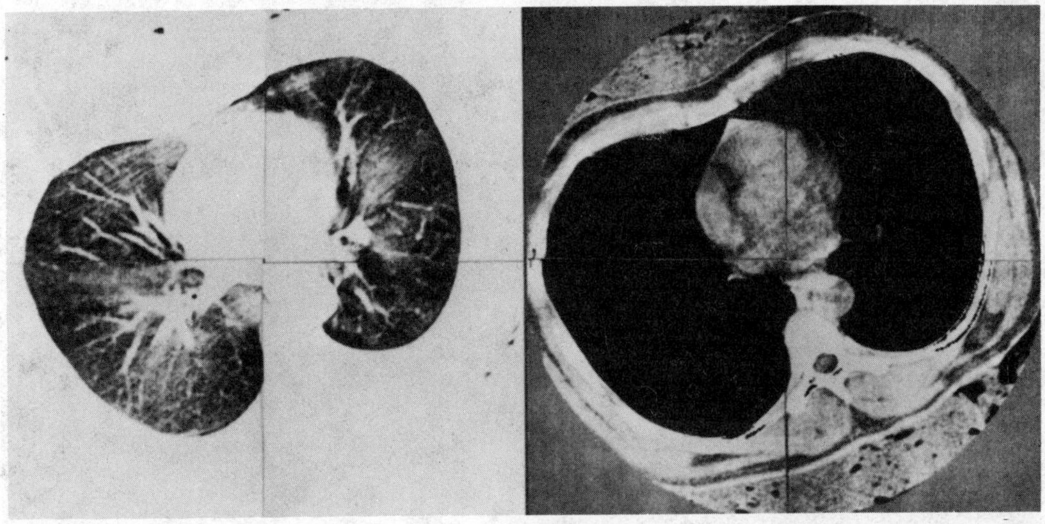

Figure 19-4 CT scan of the chest. On the left are the lungs, showing their blood vessels. On the right are the heart, spinal column, and rib cage. The diagram above shows the point on the human body where the images were taken. (Courtesy of EMI Medical Inc. X-Ray Systems, Northbrook, Illinois.)

tissues and detect interfaces between tissues of different density. An echo reflection of the sound waves is formed as the waves hit the various body tissues and pass back to the ultrasound monitor.

These ultrasonic echoes are then recorded as a composite picture of the area of the body over which the instrument has passed. The record produced by ultrasonography is called a **sonogram** or **echogram**.

Ultrasonography is used as a diagnostic tool not only by radiologists but also by neurosurgeons and ophthalmologists to detect intracranial and ophthalmic lesions, by cardiologists to

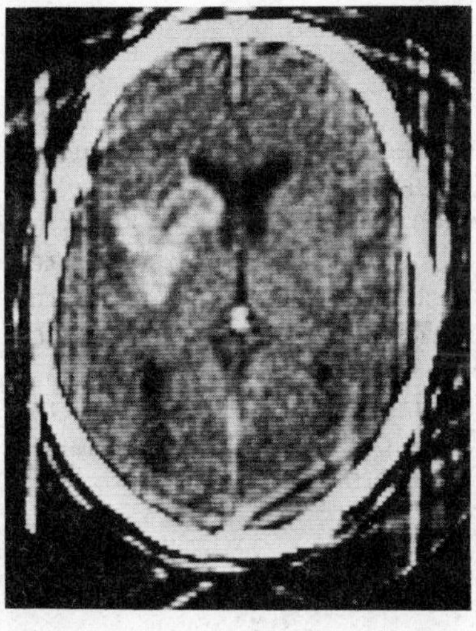

Figure 19-5 The white region on the left side of the brain is an area of cerebral infarction which resulted in the right hemiparesis and motor aphasia in the patient. The contrast material enters the infarcted tissue, giving it a dense appearance. (From Weisberg, L.A., Nice, C., and Katz, M.: Cerebral Computed Tomography: A Text-Atlas. 2nd ed. Philadelphia, W. B. Saunders Co., 1984.)

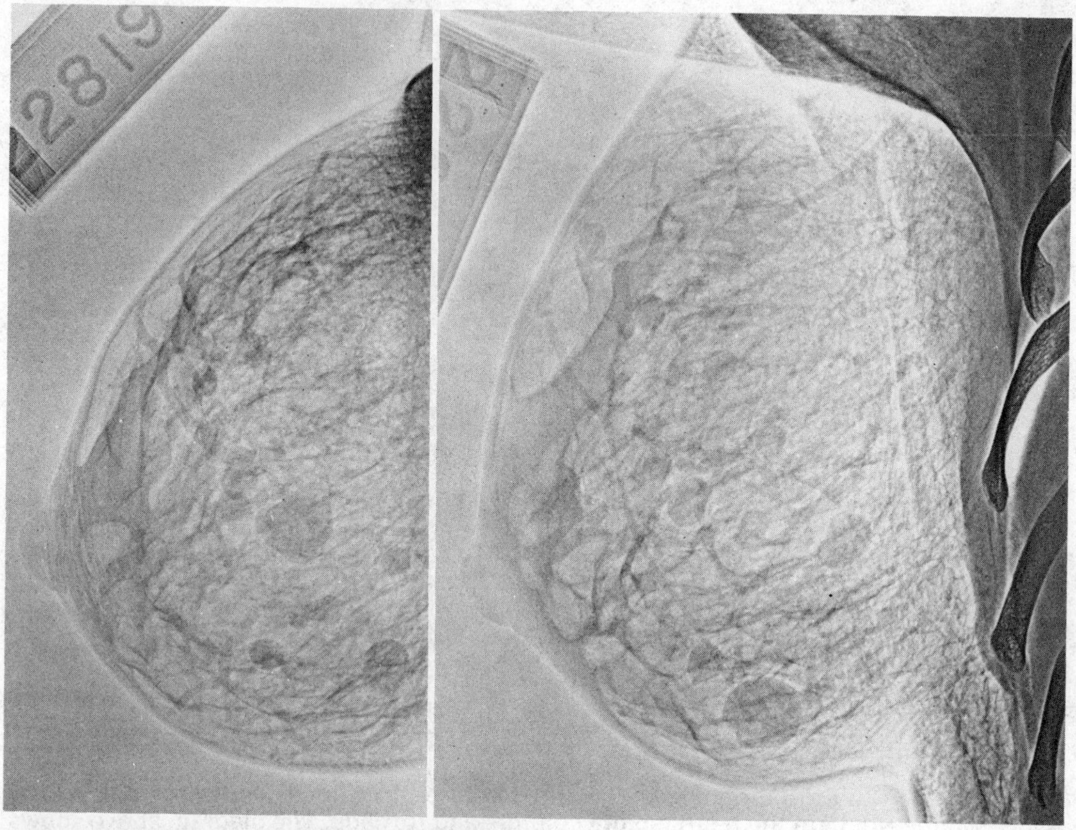

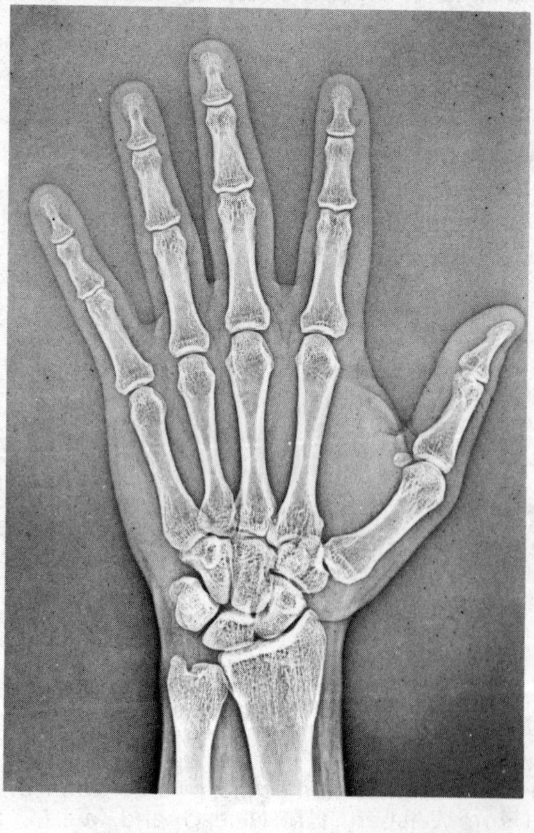

Figure 19-6 Xeroradiographs. Photographs above reveal multiple fibroadenomas with palpable masses in both breasts. Xeroradiograph of the hand shows bony structure detail and soft tissue as well. (Top, from Wolfe, J. N.: Mammography. Radiologic Clinics of North America, *12*:189, 1974; left, from Poznanski, A. K.: The Hand in Radiologic Diagnosis. 2nd ed. Philadelphia, W. B. Saunders Co., 1984.)

detect heart valve and blood vessel disorders, by gastroenterologists to locate abdominal masses outside the digestive organs, and by obstetricians and gynecologists to differentiate single and multiple pregnancies as well as to help in performing amniocentesis and in locating tumors or cysts.

The technique has several advantages in that the sound waves are nonionizing and noninjurious to tissues at the energy ranges utilized for diagnostic purposes. Since water is an excellent conductor of the ultrasonic beams, patients are requested to drink large quantities of water prior to examination, so that the urinary bladder will be distended and enable better viewing of pelvic and abdominal organs. Figure 19-7 is an example of an ultrasonogram.

Nuclear Magnetic Resonance (NMR) or Magnetic Resonance Imaging (MRI). This technique produces vertical and cross-sectional images, the latter being similar to CT scanning. NMR, however, uses no x-rays and does not require a contrast medium. The technique is based on the fact that the nuclei of some atoms behave like little magnets when a larger magnetic field is applied. The nuclei spin and emit radio waves which create an image as the nuclei move back to an equilibrium position. Hydrogen nuclei, present in water, and abundant in living tissue, are the nuclei used to create the image. NMR is useful in detecting edema in the brain, projecting a direct image of the spinal cord, detecting tumors in the chest and abdomen, and visualizing the cardiovascular system. Figure 19-8 shows three different NMR images (sagittal, coronal, and transverse).

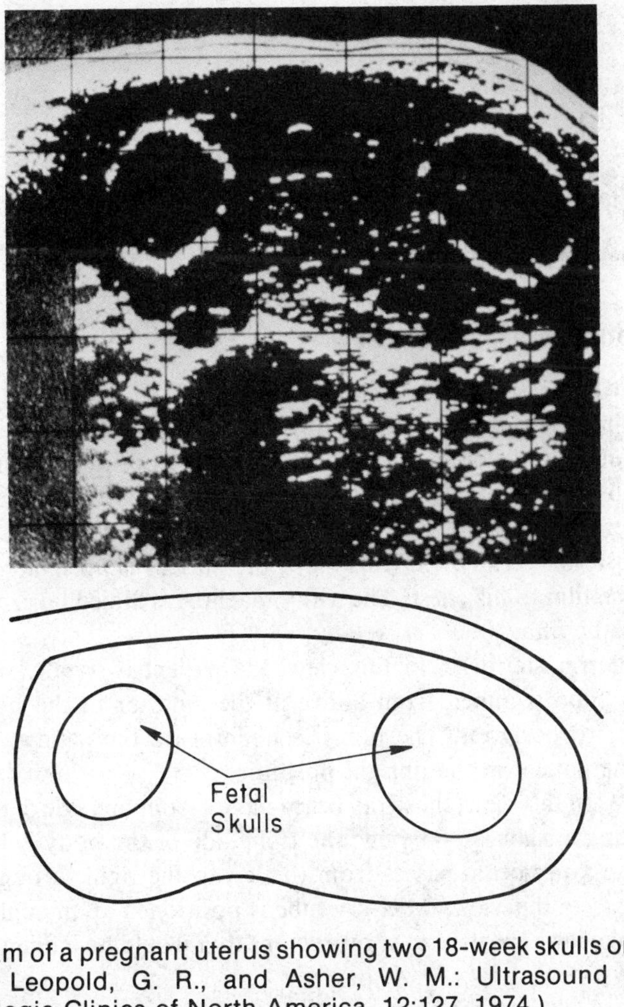

Figure 19-7 Sonogram of a pregnant uterus showing two 18-week skulls on opposite sides of the uterus. (From Leopold, G. R., and Asher, W. M.: Ultrasound in obstetrics and gynecology. Radiologic Clinics of North America, 12:127, 1974.)

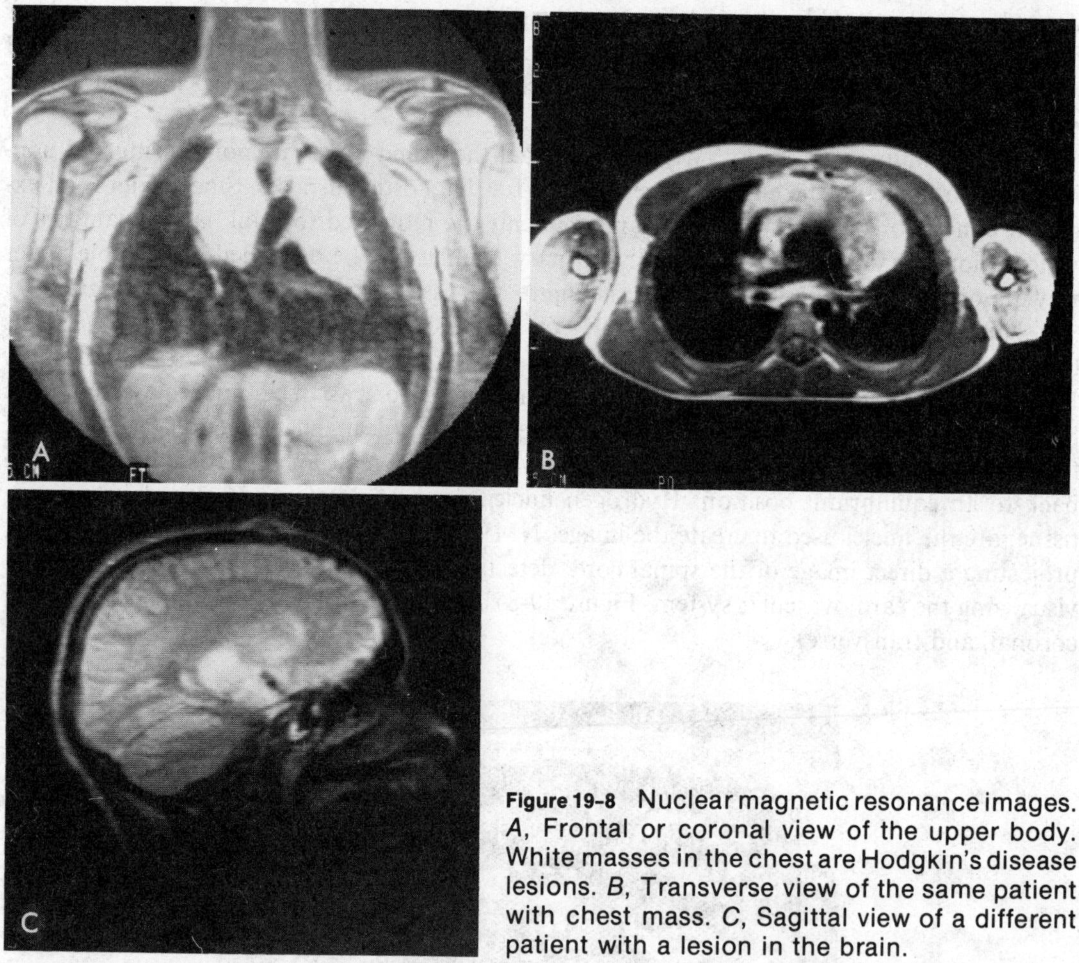

Figure 19-8 Nuclear magnetic resonance images. *A*, Frontal or coronal view of the upper body. White masses in the chest are Hodgkin's disease lesions. *B*, Transverse view of the same patient with chest mass. *C*, Sagittal view of a different patient with a lesion in the brain.

C. X-Ray Positioning

In order to take the best possible view of the part of the body being radiographed, the patient, film, and x-ray tube must be positioned in the most favorable alignment possible. There are special terms used by radiologists to designate the position or direction of the x-ray beam, the patient's position, and the motion and position of the part of the body to be examined. Some of the x-ray terms describing the position of the x-ray beam are:

1. **PA view** (**p**ostero**a**nterior). In this view, the patient is upright with his back to the x-ray machine and the film to his chest. The x-ray machine is aimed horizontally at a distance of about 6 feet from the film.

2. **AP view** (**a**ntero**p**osterior). In this view, the patient is usually supine (lying on the back) and the x-ray tube is aimed from above at the anterior of the body with the beam passing from anterior to posterior. The film lies underneath the patient. The AP view may also be taken with the patient in the upright position.

3. **Lateral view.** In this view, the x-ray beam passes from one side of the body toward the opposite side. In taking a right lateral view, the right side of the body is held closely against the x-ray film and the x-ray beam passes from the left to the right through the body.

4. **Oblique view.** In this view, the x-ray tube is positioned at an angle from the perpendicular plane. Oblique views are used to show regions that would be hidden and superimposed in routine AP and PA views.

The following terms are used to describe the position of the patient or part of the body in the x-ray examination:

1. **Abduction.** Moving the part of the body away from the midline or away from the body.
2. **Adduction.** Moving the part of the body toward the midline of the body or toward the body.
3. **Eversion.** Turning outward.
4. **Inversion.** Turning inward.
5. **Extension.** Lengthening or straightening a flexed limb.
6. **Flexion.** Bending a part of the body.
7. **Lateral decubitus.** Lying down on the side with the x-ray beam horizontally positioned; sometimes called **cross-table lateral**.
8. **Prone.** Lying on the belly (face down).
9. **Supine.** Lying on the back (face up).
10. **Recumbent.** Lying down (may be prone or supine).

III. NUCLEAR MEDICINE

A. Radioactivity and Radionuclides

The emission of energy in the form of particles or rays coming from the interior of a substance is called **radioactivity**. A **radionuclide** (or **radioisotope**) is a substance that gives off high-energy particles or rays as it disintegrates. **Half-life** is the time required for a radioactive substance (radionuclide) to lose half of its radioactivity by disintegration. Knowledge of a radionuclide's half-life is important in determining how long the radioactive substance will emit radioactivity when in the body.

Radionuclides emit three types of radioactivity: **alpha particles, beta particles,** and **gamma rays**. Gamma rays, which have greater penetrating ability than alpha and beta particles, and more ionizing power, are especially useful to physicians in both the diagnosis and treatment of disease.

B. Diagnostic Imaging

Diagnostic imaging is the use of radioactivity (gamma rays, for example) in the diagnosis of disease. Since substances that emit gamma rays can be detected and recorded when in the body, they can provide the physician with information and images of organs. For example, in **tracer studies**, a specific radionuclide is incorporated into a chemical substance and administered to the patient. The radionuclide plus pharmaceutical (together called a **labeled compound** or **radiopharmaceutical**) is traced with the use of an external detector to determine its distribution and localization in various organs, vessels, and fluids. The amount of radiopharmaceutical at a given location is proportional to the rate at which the gamma rays are emitted. The rays are measured and detected by a sensitive detection instrument called a **gamma camera** or **scintillation camera**.

The procedure of making an image to follow the distribution of radioactive substance in the body is called **scanning**, and the image produced by the gamma camera is called a **scan**. **Uptake** refers to the rate of absorption of the radiopharmaceutical into an organ or tissue.

Radiopharmaceuticals may be administered by many different routes to obtain a scan of a specific organ in the body. For example, in the case of a **lung scan**, the radiopharmaceutical can be given intravenously (**perfusion studies** which rely on passage of the radioactive compound through the capillaries of the lungs) or by inhalation (**ventilation studies**) of radioactive gas which fills the air sacs (alveoli). Figure 19-9 shows an example of a ventilation lung scan and a perfusion lung scan.

Other examples of diagnostic procedures that utilize radionuclides are:

1. **Bone scan.** **Technetium-99m**(^{99m}Tc) is used to label phosphate substances and is intravenously injected. The phosphate compound is taken up preferentially by bone, and the skeleton can be imaged in 2 or 3 hours by use of a gamma camera. Waiting 2 to 3 hours allows much of the radiopharmaceutical to be excreted in urine and allows for better visualization of the skeleton. Figure 19-10 is an example of a bone scan. The scan is useful in demonstrating malignant metastases to the skeleton, which appear as areas of high uptake ("hot spots") on the scan.

2. **Brain scan.** A radiopharmaceutical (technetium-99m pertechnetate) is injected intravenously, and about 2 hours later images of the brain are obtained via scanning. Normal scans would show no uptake of radiopharmaceutical in the brain because of the normal functioning of the blood-brain barrier (BBB) which prevents radiopharmaceuticals from entering the brain from the blood. However, if the BBB is broken down by tumor or disease, radiopharmaceutical enters the brain and shows up on the brain scan. Brain scans are useful in detecting infarctions, abscesses, tumors, and hematomas. Figure 19-11 shows a normal and abnormal brain scan.

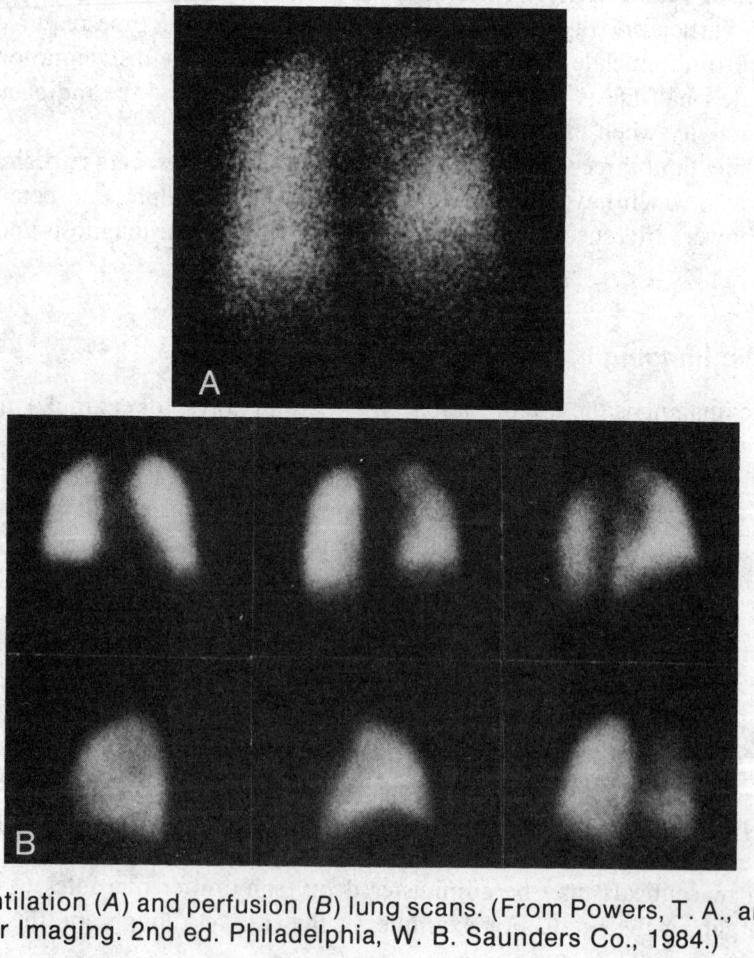

Figure 19-9 Ventilation (*A*) and perfusion (*B*) lung scans. (From Powers, T. A., and James, A. E., Jr.: Nuclear Imaging. 2nd ed. Philadelphia, W. B. Saunders Co., 1984.)

Figure 19-10 Total-body bone scan shows darkened areas of increased radiopharmaceutical uptake in the thoracic and lumbar spine. (From James, A. E., Jr., and Squire, L. F.: Nuclear Radiology. Philadelphia, W. B. Saunders Co., 1973.)

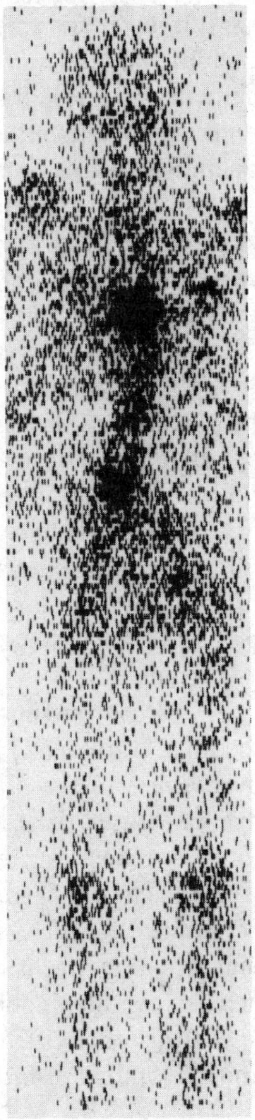

A

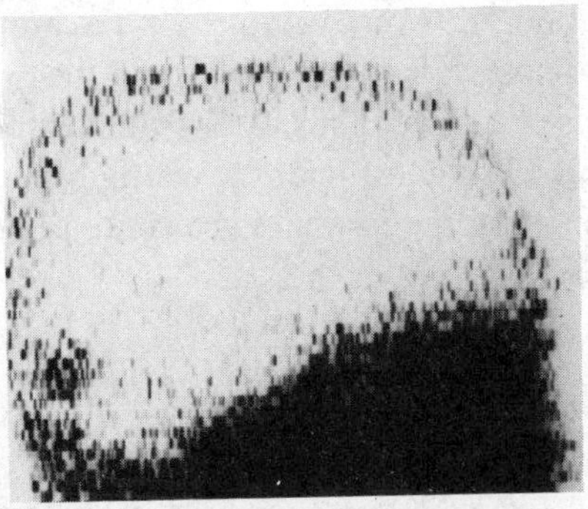

B

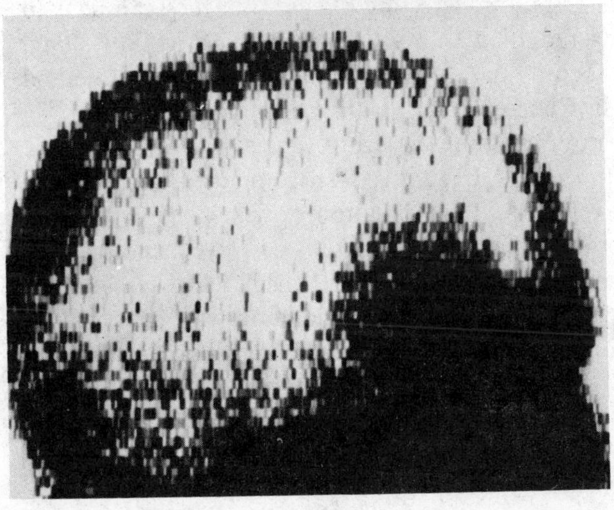

Figure 19-11 *A*, Normal lateral brain scan; *B*, mass (meningioma) in the inferior frontal area of the brain. (From James, A. E., Jr., and Squire, L. F.: Nuclear Radiology. Philadelphia, W. B. Saunders Co., 1973.)

3. **Liver and spleen scans.** To visualize the liver and spleen, a radiopharmaceutical (technetium-99m and sulfur colloid) is injected intravenously and images are taken with a gamma camera. Abnormalities such as cirrhosis, abscesses, tumor, hepatomegaly, and hepatitis can be detected by liver scanning, while splenomegaly due to tumor, cyst, abscess, or rupture can be diagnosed with spleen scanning.

4. **Radioactive iodine uptake by the thyroid gland.** Radioactive iodine compound (^{131}I) is given orally by capsule (the amount of radioactive substance in the capsule is measured earlier). The amount of radioactivity taken up by the thyroid gland during the process of making thyroid hormone can be measured at 6 and 24 hours and compared to normal values. This measurement reflects the rate of hormone synthesis by the thyroid gland.

5. **Thyroid scan.** Radionuclide is administered intravenously. The scan produced can help determine the size and shape of the thyroid gland. Hyperfunctioning thyroid nodules accumulate higher amounts of ^{131}I radioactivity and are termed "hot." Thyroid carcinoma does not concentrate radioiodine well and, therefore, is seen as a "cold" spot on the scan.

6. **Blood and heart scan.** Radiopharmaceutical (technetium-99m human serum albumin) is injected intravenously and the blood flow is imaged as the tracer passes through the chambers of the heart and large vessels. Sequential images can be recorded on film to give a motion picture of the passage of blood through the heart. Diagnosis of various forms of heart disease is possible.

7. **Positron-emission tomography (PET).** This radionuclide technique produces a cross-sectional (transverse) image of the distribution of radioactivity (through emission of positrons) in a region of the body. It is similar to the CAT scan but radioisotopes are used instead of dye and x-rays. The radionuclides are incorporated (by intravenous injection) into the tissues to be scanned, and an image is made showing where the radionuclide (such as carbon-11 glucose, oxygen-15 oxygen) is or is not being metabolized. For example, PET scanning has determined that schizophrenics do not metabolize glucose equally in all parts of the brain and that drug treatment can bring improvement to these regions. Thus, areas of metabolic deficiency can be pinpointed by PET, making it helpful in diagnosing and treating other neurological disorders such as stroke, epilepsy, and brain tumors, as well as cardiac, pulmonary, and abdominal disorders.

IV. RADIATION THERAPY

Not only are x-rays and radionuclides helpful in detecting disease, but they can be used as therapy as well. Large doses of ionizing radiation to body tissues can be **lethal** (killing) to the cells that are **irradiated**. Radiation therapy has been particularly helpful as a method for the treatment of cancers, as discussed in Chapter 18.

The machines used for radiation therapy are different from those used for diagnosis. Therapy machines deliver rays of many times higher intensity. These machines are of two general types. **Orthovoltage** machines deliver low-energy radiation, which in modern treatment centers is used in treatment of superficial skin cancers and in palliative treatment (relieving symptoms but not curing) of cancer patients. **Megavoltage** machines generate high-energy radiation and are used to treat deeper tissues in curative radiotherapy for cancer. Two examples of such machines are the **betatron** and the **linear accelerator;** they deliver a sharply defined radiation beam to a specific area of the body while sparing overlying superficial tissue.

Radiation may be applied to a tumor from some distance (**teletherapy**) or into or near the tumor itself (**brachytherapy**). Teletherapy machines (such as the linear accelerator) direct a beam of photons toward the tumor. The higher the energy of the photons, the greater the penetration of the beam. Photons can also be produced from a radioactive source (cobalt-60); both sources of high-energy photons (linear accelerator and cobalt) are well suited for the treatment of deep-seated tumors. Another form of external beam irradiation utilizes high-energy electrons that can be generated from a linear accelerator. Unlike high-energy photons, electrons do not penetrate as deeply into tissue and, therefore, are very useful for superficial cancers, such as skin tumors.

Brachytherapy includes **interstitial therapy** and **intracavitary therapy**. In order to deliver interstitial therapy, a radioactive element (such as radium, gold-198, iodine-125, or iridium-192) is surgically inserted into the tumor. This results in a very localized form of treatment, sparing normal tissues in the vicinity. The radionuclide is implanted in strands, in small sealed containers called seeds, or in removable needles. Intracavitary therapy is delivered by placing radioactive sources (radium, cesium-137, or phosphate-32) within a body cavity and adjacent to a tumor. This form of therapy is particularly suited for gynecological malignancies (uterus, cervix, or vagina).

Another form of radiotherapy is the administration of radioactive materials into the bloodstream. Iodine-131 is used to treat hyperthyroidism and thyroid carcinoma. In hyperthyroidism, the iodine-131, given orally, passes into the blood and accumulates in the thyroid gland, irradiating the tissue there and reducing the activity of the gland. ^{131}I is also taken up by thyroid tumors. In treating thyroid carcinoma, ^{131}I is used after partial or total thyroidectomy to inactivate any residual thyroid tissue and to treat metastases.

The dose unit of radiation absorbed by body tissue is called a **rad** (**r**adiation **a**bsorbed **d**ose). Tumors and body tissues are classified as **radiosensitive** and **radioresistant**, according to the number of rads necessary to kill or injure cells. Examples of radiosensitive organs are the ovaries and testes. Radioresistant organs (such as the pituitary and adrenal glands) are less susceptible to the effects of radiation. Lymphomas are generally radiosensitive, while sarcomas are generally very radioresistant.

Radiotherapy, although it is a palliative and curative agent, can produce undesirable side effects on normal body tissues. Some of these complications are reversible with time, and recovery takes place soon after the period of radiotherapy is completed. These acute reversible effects include:

1. Ulceration of mucous membranes (mucositis); for example, in the mouth, pharynx, vagina, bladder, or large and small intestine.
2. Nausea and vomiting as a reaction to radiotherapy to the brain or gastrointestinal organs.
3. Bone marrow suppression (myelosuppression), with leukopenia and thrombocytopenia.
4. Alopecia (baldness).

With higher doses of radiotherapy, these complications can be associated with permanent organ damage. In addition, radiotherapy delivered in therapeutic doses may produce chronic (long-lasting) injury to any body organ that happens to be in or near the path of the radiation beam. Examples of such chronic side effects are: nephritis, myelitis, pericarditis, pneumonitis, hepatitis, vasculitis (inflammation of blood vessels), and fibrosis of the skin and lungs.

V. VOCABULARY

betatron	Machine used in radiotherapy to deliver a dose of radiation to a patient.
brachytherapy	Radiation therapy using an implanted radioisotope radiation source (brachy = short).

Bucky grid	Lead strips placed near the x-ray film to absorb scattered radiation.
cineradiography	Use of motion picture techniques to record a series of x-ray images.
cobalt-60	A radioactive substance used in radiotherapy.
computed tomography	Diagnostic x-ray procedure whereby a cross-section image of a specific body segment is produced.
contrast techniques	Materials (contrast media) are injected to obtain contrast with surrounding tissue when shown on the x-ray film.
diagnostic imaging	Use of radioactivity to diagnose disease.
fluorescence	The emission of glowing light that results from exposure to absorption of radiation from x-rays.
fluoroscopy	The process of using x-rays to produce a fluorescent image on a screen.
gamma camera	Machine used to detect the presence of radiopharmaceuticals in the body in diagnostic imaging.
gamma rays	High-energy rays emitted by radioactive substances; similar to x-rays.
half-life	Time required for a radioactive substance to lose half its radioactivity by disintegration.
interstitial therapy	Radioisotopes are surgically inserted into a tumor.
intracavitary therapy	Radioisotopes are placed within a body cavity adjacent to a tumor.
ionization	The separation of stable substances into charged particles called ions.
irradiation	Administering radiation treatment to a patient.
laminagraphy	Diagnostic x-ray procedure in which a series of x-rays are taken, focusing on an organ at different depths; tomography.
lethal	Killing.
linear accelerator	Machine that delivers radiation therapy.
megavoltage	High-energy radiation generated by a machine and used in curative x-ray therapy for cancer.
nuclear magnetic resonance	A magnetic field and radio waves are used to form images of the body.
nuclear medicine	Medical specialty that studies the uses of radioactive substances in diagnosis and treatment of disease.

orthovoltage	Low-energy radiation used in palliative radiation therapy and superficial skin cancers.
perfusion studies	Radiopharmaceutical is injected intravenously and traced within the capillaries of an organ such as the lung.
positron emission tomography	Radioactive substances emit positrons, which create a cross-sectional image of the metabolism of the body.
rad	Radiation absorbed dose; a unit of absorbed radiation in the body.
radiation therapy	Treatment of disease using high energy radiation. Also called radiotherapy or radiation oncology.
radioisotope	A radioactive form of a substance; radionuclide.
radiology	Medical specialty concerned with the study of x-rays.
radiolucent	Permitting the passage of most x-rays. Radiolucent structures appear black on x-ray film.
radionuclide	Radioisotope.
radiopaque	Obstructing the passage of x-rays. Radiopaque structures appear white on the x-ray film.
radiopharmaceutical	A radioactive drug (radionuclide plus chemical) that is administered safely for diagnostic and therapeutic purposes.
radium	A radioactive substance used in radiation therapy.
scan	A general term for images of organs, parts, or transverse sections of the body produced in various ways. Most frequently used to describe images obtained from ultrasound, diagnostic imaging, or computed tomography.
scintillation camera	Gamma camera (scinti- means spark).
stereoscopy	Visualizing an organ in depth (three dimensions) by taking two successive x-rays and viewing both simultaneously through a viewer.
tagging	Attaching a radionuclide to a chemical and following its course in the body.
teletherapy	Radiation therapy using an external radiation source (tele- means far).
tomography	Diagnostic radiographic technique in which a series of pictures are taken at different depths of an organ.
tracer studies	Radionuclides are used as tags, or labels, attached to chemicals and followed as they migrate through the body.

ultrasonography Diagnostic technique that projects and retrieves high-frequency sound waves as they echo off of parts of the body.

uptake The rate of absorption of a radionuclide into an organ or tissue.

ventilation studies Radiopharmaceutical is inhaled and its passage through the respiratory tract is imaged.

xeroradiography A technique in which an x-ray image is made on a charged plate and then photographed subsequently on Xerox paper.

VI. COMBINING FORMS AND TERMINOLOGY

Combining Form	*Definition*	*Terminology*	*Meaning*
radi/o	rays, radio-activity	radiologist	______________
		radionuclides	______________
			______________
roentgen/o	x-rays	roentgenology	______________
tele/o	distant	teletherapy	______________
is/o	same, equal	radioisotope	______________
			______________
		top/o means place; isotopes of an element have similar structures but different weights and electric charges.	
ion/o	to wander	ionization	______________
xer/o	dry	xeroradiography	______________
			______________
ech/o	sound	echocardiography	______________
			______________
fluor/o	luminous	fluoroscopy	______________
			______________

cine/o	movement	cineradiography ________________
		________________
tom/o	to cut	tomography ________________

VII. ABBREVIATIONS

AP	Anteroposterior
^{198}Au	Radioactive gold (used in interstitial radiotherapy)
Ba	Barium
CAT	Computerized axial tomography
CT	Computed tomography
CXR	Chest x-ray
DI	Diagnostic imaging
DSA	Digital subtraction angiography
^{167}Ga	Radioactive gallium (used in whole-body and brain scans)
^{131}I	Radioactive iodine (used in thyroid uptake, liver, and kidney scans, and treatment of malignant and nonmalignant conditions of the thyroid)
IVC	Intravenous cholangiogram
IVP	Intravenous pyelogram
mCi	Millicurie (measure of radiation)
MRI	Magnetic resonance imaging
NMR	Nuclear magnetic resonance
PA	Posteroanterior
PET	Positron emission tomography
^{226}Ra	Radium (used in radiotherapy)
rad	Radiation absorbed dose
RP	Retrograde pyelogram
SBFT	Small bowel follow-through
^{99m}Tc	Radioactive technetium (used in brain, skull, thyroid, liver, spleen, bone, and lung scans)
μCi	Microcurie (measure of radiation)

VIII. PRACTICAL APPLICATIONS

CT Upper Abdomen Using IV Contrast

Comparison was also made with prior examination. The extensive retroperitoneal and mesenteric lymphadenopathy has shown marked reduction in size. The celiac lymph nodes are also reduced and the outlines of the lymph nodes are in the top limits of normal at this point. In images 8 and 9 the celiac lymph nodes are no longer visible. Previously described right pleural effusion is also not present. The obstructed right kidney shows atrophy and now measures approximately 7–8 cm in size. The left kidney remains much the same as before. The adrenal glands are symmetrical with normal aorta and inferior vena cava as well as abdominal wall.

General Hospital—Diagnostic Radiology Dept.—Schedule of Exams

CXR (A.P., P.A., lateral)	Hand	Cholecystogram
Chest fluoroscopy	Wrist	Intravenous cholangiogram
Skull	Elbow	IVP
Sinuses	Shoulder	Upper G.I. with SBFT
Sella turcica	Humerus	Barium enema
Cervical spine	Forearm	CAT (abd., brain)
Thoracic spine	Foot	Chest tomos
Lumbar spine	Ankle	Abd u/s of liver
Abdomen	Knee	Mammogram
Pelvis	Hip	Myelogram
Femur	Lower leg	Lymphangiogram

General Hospital—Nuclear Medicine Dept.—Radionuclides Available

Radionuclide	*Radiopharmaceutical*	*Admission Route*	*Target Organ*
Xe-133 (xenon)	xenon gas	inhaled	lungs
Tc-99m (technetium)	albumin microspheres	intravenous	lungs
Sr-87m (strontium)	solution	intravenous	bone
Tc-99m	diphosphonate	intravenous	bone
Tc-99m	pertechnetate	intravenous	brain
Tc-99m	sulfur colloid	intravenous	liver/spleen
Au-198 (gold)	colloid	intravenous	liver
Au-199	colloid	intravenous	spleen
I-131 (iodine)	rose bengal	intravenous	colon
Tc-99m	DTPA* or HIDA**	intravenous	kidney
Hg-197 (mercury)	chlormerodrin	intravenous	kidney
I-131	iodide	oral	thyroid
K-42 (potassium)	solution	intravenous	heart
Tl-201 (thallium)	thallium chloride	intravenous	heart
Tc-99m	pyrophosphate	intravenous	heart
Ga-67 (gallium)	citrate	intravenous	tumors and abscesses

*DTPA = diethylenetriaminepentaacetic acid
**HIDA = *N*-(2,6-dimethyl)iminodiacetic acid

IX. EXERCISES

A. *List six characteristics of x-rays:*

1. ______________________________

2. ______________________________

3. ______________________________

4. ______________________

5. ______________________

6. ______________________

B. Give the meaning of the following terms:

1. radiopaque ______________________
2. radiolucent ______________________
3. roentgenology ______________________
4. gamma rays ______________________
5. irradiation ______________________
6. ionization ______________________
7. nuclear medicine ______________________
8. Bucky grid ______________________
9. film badge ______________________
10. lethal ______________________
11. radiotherapy ______________________
12. radiologist ______________________
13. radiologic technologist ______________________
14. radiotherapist ______________________
15. nuclear physician ______________________

C. Give the name of the special diagnostic technique which fits each of the following definitions:

1. Radiopaque substances are given and x-rays taken ______________________
2. Use of motion picture techniques to record x-ray images ______________________
3. X-ray technique of blurring out all planes except the one to be seen in detail

   ____

4. Use of echoes of high-frequency sound waves to diagnose disease ____________

____

5. X-ray beams are focused from the body onto a screen which glows as a result of the ionizing effect of x-rays ____________

6. Three-dimensional x-ray views are produced by taking two successive x-rays and viewing both simultaneously with a three-dimensional viewer ____________

____

7. A magnetic field and radio waves are used to form images of the body ____________

____

8. X-ray images are recorded on a metal plate and photographed on Xerox paper

____

9. Hundreds of successive x-ray pictures are taken circularly around an area of the body and a computer synthesizes the information into a composite cross-section picture

____

D. *Give meanings for the following terms:*

1. pneumoencephalogram ____________
2. myelogram ____________
3. intravenous pyelogram ____________
4. arteriogram ____________
5. cholecystogram ____________
6. retrograde pyelogram ____________
7. lymphangiogram ____________
8. ventriculogram ____________
9. barium swallow ____________

10. intravenous cholangiogram ____________________

11. bronchogram ____________________

12. sialogram ____________________

13. barium enema ____________________

14. hysterosalpingogram ____________________

15. pneumoarthrogram ____________________

16. digital subtraction angiography ____________________

E. *Match the following x-ray views or positions in Column I with their meanings in Column II (insert correct letter in blank space):*

Column I		*Column II*
1. PA	________	A. On the side.
2. supine	________	B. Turned inward.
3. prone	________	C. Movement away from the midline.
4. AP	________	D. Lying on the belly.
5. lateral	________	E. X-ray tube positioned on an angle.
6. oblique	________	F. Bending a part.
7. decubitus	________	G. Straightening a limb.
8. adduction	________	H. Lying on the back.
9. inversion	________	I. Lying down on the side; cross-table lateral position.
10. abduction	________	J. Lying down; prone or supine.
11. recumbent	________	K. Anterior to posterior view.
12. eversion	________	L. Turning outward.
13. flexion	________	M. Posterior to anterior view.
14. extension	________	N. Movement toward the midline.

F. *Supply the medical term to fit the definition below:*

1. High-energy radiation used in curative x-ray therapy ____________________
2. Low-energy radiation used in treating superficial skin cancers and in palliative therapy ____________________
3. A radioactive form of an element ____________________
4. Compound that contains a radionuclide ____________________
5. A unit of absorbed radiation in the body ____________________
6. Radiation therapy from a shielded distant unit ____________________
7. Relieving, but not curing ____________________
8. Studies in which radiopharmaceuticals are followed through the body and in organs ____________________
9. Technetium-99m is used as a label for phosphate substances in this study ____________________
10. A radionuclide inserted into the body in rods, pellets, or beads as treatment for cancer of the bladder ____________________
11. Radiopharmaceutical is injected intravenously and traced within the lung ____________________
12. Radiopharmaceutical is inhaled and traced within the lung ____________________
13. Radionuclides are surgically inserted into the tumor ____________________
14. Tumors that are susceptible to the lethal effects of radiation are called ____________________
15. A form of radiotherapy in which radionuclides are placed within a cavity or adjacent to a tumor ____________________
16. Tumors that are not susceptible to the effects of radiotherapy are called ____________________

G. Give meanings for the following terms that describe side effects produced by radiotherapy:

1. alopecia ______________________
2. dysphagia ______________________
3. hyperemesis ______________________
4. leukopenia ______________________
5. mucositis ______________________
6. pericarditis ______________________
7. nephritis ______________________
8. myelosuppression ______________________
9. hepatitis ______________________
10. pneumonitis ______________________

H. Give the meanings of the following combining forms:

1. xer/o ______________ 3. cine/o ______________
2. ion/o ______________ 4. tom/o ______________

I. Give the meanings for the following terms and abbreviations:

1. half-life ______________________
2. gamma camera ______________________
3. diagnostic imaging ______________________
4. linear accelerator ______________________
5. perfusion study ______________________
6. CT ______________________
7. ^{99m}Tc ______________________
8. IVP ______________________
9. ^{131}I ______________________

10. DI ______________________________

11. PET ______________________________

12. brachytherapy ______________________________

ANSWERS

A.

1. Invisible.
2. Travel in straight lines.
3. Expose a photographic plate.
4. Ionize atoms.
5. Scattered by the material through which they pass.
6. Penetrate different substances in varying degrees.

B.

1. Obstructing the passage of x-rays.
2. Permitting the passage of x-rays.
3. Study of x-rays.
4. Rays that are similar to x-rays and are emitted by radioactive substances in tracer studies.
5. Administering radiation to a patient.
6. Separation of stable substances into charged particles called ions.
7. Study of the characteristics and uses of radioactive substances in the diagnosis and treatment of disease.
8. Series of lead strips used near x-ray film to absorb scattered radiation.
9. Radiation detection device.
10. Pertaining to killing.
11. The treatment of disease (usually malignant disease) by means of radiation—high-energy x-rays and gamma rays or internally implanted radioactive substances.
12. A physician who specializes in diagnostic radiology.
13. An allied health professional who works with physicians in the fields of radiology, nuclear medicine, and radiation therapy.
14. A physician who specializes in radiation therapy.
15. A radiologist who administers diagnostic nuclear medicine procedures.

C.

1. contrast techniques
2. cineradiography
3. tomography (laminagraphy)
4. ultrasonography
5. fluoroscopy
6. stereoscopy
7. nuclear magnetic resonance
8. xeroradiography
9. computed tomography

D.

1. Air is injected into a portion of the spinal cord and the brain and spinal cord are viewed by x-ray.
2. Radiopaque dye is injected into the membranes around the spinal cord and x-rays are taken.
3. Dye is injected into a vein and x-rays are taken of the renal pelvis.
4. Dye is injected into an artery and x-rays are taken.
5. A radiopaque substance is given orally and x-rays are taken of the gallbladder and bile ducts.
6. Dye is injected, via catheter, into the urethra, bladder, and ureters and x-rays are taken of the urinary tract.
7. Dye is injected into the lymphatic system and x-rays are taken to show the lymph vessels and nodes.
8. Air is injected into the ventricles of the brain and x-ray films of the ventricles are taken.
9. Barium sulfate is swallowed and x-rays are taken of the upper gastrointestinal region.
10. Dye is injected into a vein and concentrates in the gallbladder and bile ducts and x-rays are taken.
11. Dye is injected into the bronchial tubes and x-rays are taken of the lungs.
12. Dye is injected into the salivary ducts and x-rays are taken.
13. Barium sulfate is administered by enema and the lower gastrointestinal tract is viewed by x-ray study.
14. Dye is injected into the uterus, via the vagina, and x-rays are taken of the uterine tubes and uterus.
15. Air is injected into a joint and x-rays are taken of the joint.
16. An x-ray image of blood vessels (injected with contrast material) is produced by using a computer to subtract obscuring shadows from the image.

E.

1. M
2. H
3. D
4. K
5. A
6. E
7. I
8. N
9. B
10. C
11. J
12. L
13. F
14. G

F.

1. megavoltage
2. orthovoltage
3. radioisotope or radionuclide
4. radiopharmaceutical
5. rad
6. teletherapy
7. palliative
8. tracer studies
9. bone scan
10. cobalt-60
11. perfusion studies (lung scan)
12. ventilation studies (lung scan)
13. interstitial therapy (brachytherapy)
14. radiosensitive
15. intracavitary therapy (brachytherapy)
16. radioresistant

G.

1. Baldness
2. Difficult swallowing
3. Excessive vomiting
4. Deficiency of white blood cells
5. Inflammation of mucous membranes
6. Inflammation of the membrane surrounding the heart
7. Inflammation of the kidney
8. Stopping the formation of blood cells in the bone marrow
9. Inflammation of the liver
10. Inflammation of the lungs

H.

1. heat
2. dryness
3. to wander
4. motion
5. to cut

I.

1. Time that it takes a radioactive substance to lose half its radioactivity by disintegration.
2. Machine used to detect the presence of radiopharmaceuticals in the body.
3. Use of radioactivity to diagnose disease.
4. Machine that delivers high-energy radiation for radiotherapy.
5. Radioactive material is injected into a vein and scans are taken of the lungs.
6. Computed tomography.
7. Technetium-99m (radioactive substance used in diagnostic imaging).
8. Intravenous pyelogram.
9. Radioactive iodine used in diagnostic imaging.
10. Diagnostic imaging.
11. Positron emission tomography (areas of metabolic activity are imaged).
12. Radiotherapy using implanted radioisotopes.

X. PRONUNCIATION OF TERMS

abduction	ăb-DŬK-shŭn
adduction	ă-DŬK-shŭn
angiocardiogram	ăn-jē-ō-KĂR-dē-ō-grăm
angiogram	ĂN-jē-ō-grăm
anteroposterior	ăn-tĕr-ō-pōs-TĔ-rē-ŏr
arteriogram	ăr-TĒ-rē-ō-grăm
arthrogram	ĂR-thrō-grăm
betatron	BĀ-tă-trŏn
brachytherapy	brā-kē-THĔR-ă-pē or brăk-ē-THĔR-ă-pē
cholangiogram	kō-LĂN-jē-ō-grăm
cholecystogram	kō-lē-SĬS-tō-grăm
cineradiography	sĭn-ē-rā-dē-ŎG-ră-fē
decubitus	dē-KŪ-bĭ-tŭs

echogram	ĔK-ō-grăm
encephalogram	ĕn-SĔF-ă-lō-grăm
eversion	ē-VĔR-zhŭn
extension	ĕk-STĔN-shŭn
flexion	FLĔK-shŭn
fluorescence	flū-RĔS-ĕns
fluoroscopy	flū-RŎS-kō-pē
hysterosalpingogram	hĭs-tĕr-ō-săl-PĬNG-gō-grăm
inversion	ĭn-VĔR-zhŭn
ionization	ī-ŏn-ĭ-ZĀ-shŭn
irradiation	ĭ-rā-dē-Ā-shŭn
laminagraphy	lăm-ĭ-NĂG-ră-fē
lumen	LŌŌ-mĕn
lymphangiogram	lĭm-FĂN-jē-ō-grăm
megavoltage	MĔG-ă-vōl-tăj
myelogram	MĪ-ĕ-lō-grăm
oblique	ŏ-BLĒK
orthovoltage	ŎR-thō-vōl-tăj
pneumoencephalogram	nū-mō-ĕn-SĔF-ă-lō-grăm
posteroanterior	pōs-tĕr-ō-ăn-TĒ-rē-ŏr
prone	prōn
pyelogram	PĪ-ĕ-lō-grăm
radioisotope	rā-dē-ō-Ī-sō-tōp
radiolucent	rā-dē-ō-LŪ-sĕnt
radionuclide	rā-dē-ō-NŪ-klīd
radiopaque	rā-dē-ō-PĀK
radiopharmaceutical	rā-dē-ō-făr-mă-SŪ-tĭ-kăl
recumbent	rē-KŬM-bĕnt
roentgenology	rĕnt-gĕ-NŎL-ō-jē
scintillation	sĭn-tĭ-LĀ-shŭn
sialogram	sī-ĂL-ō-grăm
sonogram	SŎN-ō-grăm

stereoscopy	stě-rē-ŎS-kō-pē
supine	SŪ-pīn
technetium-99m	tĕk-NĒ-shē-ŭm
teletherapy	tĕl-ĕ-THĔR-ă-pē
tomography	tō-MŎG-ră-fē
ultrasonography	ŭl-tră-sō-NŎG-ră-fē
venogram	VĒ-nō-grăm
ventriculogram	vĕn-TRĬK-ū-lō-grăm
xeromammography	zē-rō-mă-MŎG-ră-fē
xeroradiography	zē-rō-rā-dē-ŎG-ră-fē

REVIEW SHEET 19

Combining Forms

cine/o	____________	radi/o	____________
ech/o	____________	roentgen/o	____________
fluor/o	____________	tele/o	____________
ion/o	____________	tom/o	____________
is/o	____________	xer/o	____________
myel/o	____________		

Additional Terms

abduction (583)

adduction (583)

alpha particles (583)

angiocardiogram (576)

AP view (582)

arteriogram (576)

arthrogram (578)

barium enema (576)

beta particles (583)

betatron (587)

bone scan (584)

brachytherapy (587)

brain scan (584)

bronchogram (577)

Bucky grid (588)

cholecystogram (577)

cineradiography (588)

cobalt-60 (588)

computed tomography (588)

contrast techniques (588)

decubitus (583)

diagnostic imaging (588)

digital subtraction angiography (577)

echogram (579)

encephalogram (578)

eversion (583)

extension (583)

film badge (575)

flexion (583)

fluorescence (588)

fluoroscopy (588)

gamma camera (588)

gamma rays (588)

half-life (588)

hysterosalpingogram (577)

interstitial therapy (588)

intracavitary therapy (588)

intravenous cholangiogram (577)

intravenous pyelogram (577)

inversion (583)

ionization (588)

irradiation (588)

laminagraphy (588)

linear accelerator (588)

liver scan (586)

lymphangiogram (577)

megavoltage (588)

myelogram (577)

nuclear magnetic resonance (588)

nuclear medicine (588)

nuclear physician (573)

oblique view (582)

orthovoltage (589)

PA view (582)

perfusion studies (589)

positron emission tomography (589)

prone (583)

rad (589)

radioactivity (583)

radioisotope (589)

radiologic technologist (574)

radiology (589)

radiolucent (589)

radiopaque (589)

radiopharmaceutical (589)

radioresistant (587)

radiosensitive (587)

radiotherapist (574)

radiotherapy (573)

recumbent (583)

retrograde pyelogram (577)

roentgenology (573)

scan (589)

scintillation camera (589)

sialogram (577)

small bowel follow-through (576)

sonogram (579)

spleen scan (586)

stereoscopy (589)

supine (583)

teletherapy (589)

thyroid scan (586)

tomography (589)

tracer studies (589)

ultrasonography (590)

upper GI series (576)

uptake (590)

venogram (577)

ventilation studies (590)

ventriculogram (578)

xeromammogram (578)

xeroradiography (590)

x-rays (573)

CHAPTER 20

PHARMACOLOGY

In this chapter you will:

- Learn of the various subspecialty areas of pharmacology;
- Identify the various routes of drug administration;
- Differentiate between the different classes of drugs and their actions and toxicities; and
- Define medical terms using combining forms, prefixes, and suffixes that relate to pharmacology.

This chapter is divided into the following sections:

I. INTRODUCTION

Drugs are chemical or biological substances used in the prevention or treatment of disease, or to alter bodily functions in a beneficial way. Drugs can come from many different sources. Some drugs are obtained from various parts of **plants**, such as the roots, leaves, and fruit. Examples of such drugs are digitalis (from the foxglove plant) and antibiotics such as penicillin and streptomycin (from lower plants called molds). Drugs can also be obtained from **animals**; for example, hormones are secretions from the glands of animals. Drugs can be made from chemical substances that are **synthesized** in the laboratory. Anticancer drugs, such as methotrexate and prednisone, are examples of laboratory-synthesized drugs. Some drugs are contained in food substances; these drugs are called **vitamins**. Drugs are dispensed by a **pharmacist**, and stored in an area known as a **pharmacy**.

The field of medicine that studies drugs—their nature, origin, and effect on the body—is called **pharmacology**. Pharmacology is a broad medical specialty and contains many subdivisions of study, including **medicinal chemistry**, **pharmacodynamics**, **pharmacokinetics**, **molecular pharmacology**, **chemotherapy**, and **toxicology**.

Medicinal chemistry is the study of new drug synthesis and the relationship between chemical structure and biological effects. **Pharmacodynamics** involves the study of drug effects in the body. Scientists may also study the processes of drug **absorption** (how drugs pass into the bloodstream), **metabolism** (changes drugs undergo within the body), and **excretion** (removal of the drug from the body). The mathematical description of drug disposition (appearance and disappearance) in the body is called **pharmacokinetics**. It is a measurement of the way a drug enters and leaves the blood and tissues over time.

Molecular pharmacology concerns the study of the interaction of drugs and subcellular entities, such as DNA, RNA, and enzymes. These studies provide important information about the mechanism of action of the drug.

PHARMACOLOGY

MEDICINAL CHEMISTRY	PHARMACODYNAMICS	PHARMACOKINETICS	MOLECULAR PHARMACOLOGY
New drug synthesis	Drug effects on the body	Drug concentration in tissues and blood is measured over a period of time	Interaction of drugs and subcellular components

CHEMOTHERAPY	TOXICOLOGY
Use of drugs in treatment of disease	Study of harmful chemicals and their effects on the body

Figure 20-1 Subspecialty areas of pharmacology.

Chemotherapy is the study of drugs that destroy microorganisms, parasites, or malignant cells within the body. Chemotherapy includes treatment of infectious diseases and cancer.

Toxicology is the study of harmful chemicals and their effects on the body. Toxicological studies in animals are required by law before new drugs can be tested in humans. A toxicologist is also interested in finding proper **antidotes** to any harmful effects of drugs. Antidotes are substances given to neutralize unwanted effects of drugs.

Figure 20-1 reviews the subspecialty areas of pharmacology.

II. DRUG NAMES, STANDARDS, AND REFERENCES

Names

A drug can have three different names. The **chemical name** is the chemical formula for the drug. This name is often long and complicated.

The **generic** or **official name** is a shorter, less complicated name that is recognized as identifying the drug for legal and scientific purposes. The generic name becomes public property after 17 years of use by the original manufacturer and any drug manufacturer may use it thereafter. There is only one generic name for each drug.

The **brand name** or **trade name** is the private property of the individual drug manufacturer and no competitor may use it. Brand names often have the superscript ® after or before the name. Most drugs have several brand names because each manufacturer producing the drug gives it a different name. When a specific brand name is ordered on a prescription by a physician, it must be dispensed by the pharmacist; no other brand name may be substituted. It is usual practice to capitalize the first letter of a brand name.

The following lists give the chemical, generic, and brand names of the antibiotic drug ampicillin; note that the drug can have several brand names but only generic, or official, name:

Chemical Name	*Generic Name*	*Brand Name*
alpha-aminobenzyl P	ampicillin	Amcill capsules
		Omnipen
		Penbritin
		Polycillin
		Principen/N

Standards

While the **Food and Drug Administration (FDA)** has the legal responsibility for deciding whether a drug may be distributed and sold, there are definite standards for drugs set by an independent committee of physicians, pharmacologists, pharmacists, and manufacturers. This committee is called the **United States Pharmacopeia (U.S.P.)**. Two important standards of the U.S.P. are that the drug must be clinically useful (useful for patients) and available in pure form (made by good manufacturing methods). If a drug has U.S.P. after its name, it has met with the standards of the Pharmacopeia. The **National Formulary (N.F.)** was another legally recognized book of standards and specifications for drugs. The U.S.P. acquired the N.F. in 1974 and since 1980 the two books have been published as a single volume that is revised every 5 years.

References

Libraries and hospitals have two large reference listings of drugs. The most complete and up-to-date is the **Hospital Formulary**, which gives information about the characteristics of drugs and their clinical usage (application to patient care).

The **Physician's Desk Reference (PDR)** is published by a private firm, and drug manufacturers pay to have their products listed. The PDR is a useful reference with several different indices to identify drugs; full descriptions, precautions, and warnings; and information about recommended dosage and administration for each drug.

III. ADMINISTRATION OF DRUGS

The route of administration of a drug (how it is introduced into the body) is very important in determining the rate and completeness of its absorption into the bloodstream and the speed and duration of the drug's action in the body.

The various methods of administering drugs are described below:

Oral Administration. Drugs may be given by mouth and are absorbed into the bloodstream through the stomach or intestinal wall. This method, although convenient for the patient, has several disadvantages. If the drug is destroyed in the digestive tract by digestive juices, or if the drug is unable to pass through the intestinal mucosa, it will be ineffective. Oral administration is also disadvantageous if time is a factor in therapy.

Sublingual Administration. Drugs are not swallowed but are placed under the tongue and allowed to dissolve in the saliva. For some agents absorption may be rapid. Nitroglycerin tablets are taken in this way to treat attacks of angina pectoris.

Rectal Administration. Suppositories (cone-shaped objects containing drugs) and aqueous solutions are inserted into the rectum. At times, drugs are given by rectum when oral administration presents difficulties, such as when the patient is nauseated and vomiting.

Parenteral Administration. This type of administration is accomplished by injection through a **syringe** (syring/o = tube) under the skin, into muscle, into a vein, or into a body cavity. There are several types of parenteral injections:

1. Subcutaneous injection. This is also called a **hypodermic injection**, and is given just under the skin. The outer surface of the arm is a usual location for this injection.

2. Intradermal injection. This shallow injection is made into the upper layers of the skin and is used chiefly in skin testing for allergic reactions.

3. Intramuscular injection (IM). The buttock or upper arm is usually the site for this injection into muscle. When drugs are irritating to the skin or when a large volume of a long-acting drug is needed, IM injections are advisable.

4. Intravenous injection (IV). This injection is given directly into the veins. It is given when an immediate effect from the drug is desired or when the drug cannot be safely given into other tissues. Good technical skill is needed in administering this injection, since leakage of drugs into surrounding tissues may result in damage to tissues.

5. Intrathecal injection. This injection is made into the space underlying the membranes (meninges) that surround the spinal cord and brain. Methotrexate (a cancer chemotherapeutic drug) is injected intrathecally for treatment of leukemia.

6. Intracavitary injection. This injection is made into a body cavity, such as the peritoneal or pleural cavity. For example, nitrogen mustard is injected into the pleural cavity in people who have pleural effusions due to malignant disease. The drug causes the pleural surfaces to adhere, thus obliterating the pleural space and preventing the accumulation of fluid.

Inhalation. Vapors, or gases, are taken into the nose or mouth and are absorbed into the bloodstream through the thin walls of the air sacs in the lungs. **Aerosols** (particles of drug suspended in air) are administered by inhalation, as are many anesthetics.

Topical Application. Drugs are locally applied on the skin or mucous membranes of the body. **Antiseptics** (against infection) and **antipruritics** (against itching) are commonly used as ointments, creams, and lotions.

Figure 20-2 is a chart summarizing the various routes of drug administration.

IV. TERMINOLOGY OF DRUG ACTION

The following terms describe the action and interaction of drugs in the body after they have been absorbed into the bloodstream:

Potentiation (Synergism). A combination of two drugs can sometimes cause an effect that is **greater** than the sum of the individual effects of each drug alone. For example, penicillin and streptomycin, two antibiotic drugs, are given together in treatment for bacterial endocarditis because of their synergistic action.

Additive Action. The combination of two similar drugs is equal to the **sum** of the effects of each. For example, if drug A gives 10 per cent tumor kill as a chemotherapeutic agent and drug B gives 20 per cent tumor kill, using A and B together would give 30 per cent tumor kill. If these drugs were synergistic in their action, a combination of both would give greater than 30 per cent tumor kill.

Cumulation. After administration of certain drugs, concentrations of the drug or its toxic effect on tissue may increase with each dose. The drug dosage may have to be reduced to prevent accumulation to toxic concentrations.

Oral	Sublingual	Rectal	Parenteral	Inhalation	Topical
Tablets	Tablets	Suppositories	Injections:	Aerosols	Lotions
			Subcutaneous		Creams
			Intradermal		Ointments
			Intramuscular		
			Intravenous		
			Intrathecal		
			Intracavitary		

Figure 20-2 Routes of drug administration.

Tolerance. The effects of a given dose diminish as treatment goes on, and larger doses must be given to maintain the desired effect. Tolerance is a feature of addiction to drugs such as morphine and meperidine (Demerol).

Idiosyncrasy. This is any unexpected effect that may appear in the patient following administration of a drug. Idiosyncratic reactions are produced in very few patients but may be life-threatening in those few instances. For example, in some individuals penicillin is known to cause an idiosyncratic reaction such as **anaphylaxis** (acute type of hypersensitivity, including asthma and shock).

V. DRUG TOXICITY

Drug toxicity is the poisonous and potentially dangerous effects of some drugs. Idiosyncrasy is an example of an unpredictable type of drug toxicity.

Other types of drug toxicity are more predictable and based on the dosage of the drug given. Physicians are trained to be aware of the potential toxic effects of all drugs that they prescribe. **Iatrogenic** (produced by treatment) disorders can occur, however, as a result of mistakes in diagnosis and treatment and the effects of drug toxicity.

Side effects are toxic effects that routinely result from the use of a drug. They often occur with the usual therapeutic dosage of a drug and are usually tolerable. For example, nausea, vomiting, and alopecia are common side effects of the chemotherapeutic drugs used to treat cancer.

Contraindications are factors in a patient's condition that make the use of a drug dangerous and ill advised. For example, in the presence of renal failure, it is unwise to administer a drug that is normally eliminated by the kidneys.

VI. CLASSES OF DRUGS

A. Neuropharmacologic Drugs

These drugs act on the nervous system. There are two main types: autonomic drugs and central nervous system drugs.

1. Autonomic Drugs. Autonomic drugs influence the body in a manner similar to the normal action of autonomic nerves. Some examples of autonomic drugs are:

a) Sympathomimetics. These **adrenergic** (working like Adrenalin) drugs increase heart rate and increase blood pressure (vasoconstriction of peripheral arterioles), relax gastrointestinal tract muscles, open air passages, and dilate arterioles that supply skeletal muscles. An example is **epinephrine (Adrenalin)**, which is used in bronchial asthma, allergic conditions, shock, and cardiac and respiratory failure, and to prolong the action of local anesthetics.

b) Sympatholytics. These drugs are antagonistic to epinephrine and other sympathomimetics. They cause vasodilation (lowering of blood pressure) and increase the tone (peristalsis) of gastrointestinal tract muscles, and other smooth muscles. An example is **reserpine**, which is used to lower blood pressure and as a general tranquilizer since it depresses the central nervous system as well as the sympathetic branch of the autonomic system. Also, **propranolol (Inderal)**, a beta-adrenergic blocker is used to decrease heart rate, dilate vessels, and treat angina and hypertension. **Beta-blocker drugs** block the action of epinephrine at receptor sites in heart muscle and in muscles in the walls of blood vessels.

c) Parasympathomimetics. These **cholinergic** drugs act like the neurotransmitter substance **acetylcholine** to stimulate the parasympathetic branch of the autonomic system. They decrease the heart rate, cause contraction of smooth muscles and the pupils of the eye, and increase the secretions of most exocrine glands. Examples are: **bethanechol**—used to stimulate release of fluid from the urinary bladder when there is postoperative retention; and **pilocarpine**—used as miotic (to contract the pupils in patients with glaucoma).

d) Parasympatholytics (Anticholinergics). These drugs have effects opposite to those of the parasympathomimetics. They dilate pupils (mydriasis), relax smooth muscle tissue (in cases of muscle cramps or spasms), and increase the rate of the heart. Drugs containing **atropine**, such as Donnatal and Lomotil, are examples of anticholinergic and antispasmodic parasympatholytics.

Figure 20-3 summarizes the various types of autonomic drugs, and gives examples of each type.

2. Central Nervous System Drugs. These drugs influence the body in two general ways: as **stimulants** and **depressants**.

a) Stimulants. These drugs are used to speed up vital processes (heart and respiration) in cases of shock and collapse. They also increase alertness, and they inhibit hyperactive behavior in children. High doses can produce restlessness, insomnia, and hypertension. Examples are: **amphetamines**—used to prevent narcolepsy (seizures of sleep), as an appetite depressant, and in hyperkinetic children; and **caffeine**—used as a general cerebral stimulant. It is a diuretic and will help relieve certain types of headache by constricting cerebral blood vessels.

b) Depressants. These drugs depress the CNS and can range in effect from mild sedation and somnolence (producing sleep) to general anesthesia and death. Some categories of depressants and examples of specific drugs are:

Alcohol. At first, alcohol increases heart and respiratory rate and produces talkativeness and lack of inhibition, but its later effect is depression of the CNS with a sedative-like effect.

Analgesics. These agents are used to relieve pain, induce sleep, suppress cough, and relieve dyspnea. Examples of **narcotic** (habit-forming) **analgesics** are those containing morphine and codeine. **Morphine** and **codeine** are **opiates** (derived from opium). Some narcotic analgesics containing codeine are Tylenol/Codeine and Fiorinal/Codeine. Semisynthetic and synthetic drugs with narcotic analgesic effects similar to those of morphine are methadone (used as a substitute for dependency on heroin), Demerol, and Percodan. **Endorphins** are opiate-like substances released at nerve endings within the body. Like morphine, endorphins produce euphoria and sedation, and lessen the transmission of pain perceptions. The term, endorphin, was created by combining the words "endogenous" and "morphine."

Non-narcotic analgesics are not habit-forming and are used for mild to moderate pain. An example of a non-narcotic analgesic is propoxyphene (Darvon).

Some analgesics are also anti-inflammatory agents, and are used to relieve joint pain.

AUTONOMIC DRUGS

SYMPATHOMIMETIC (adrenergic)	PARASYMPATHOMIMETIC (cholinergic)	SYMPATHOLYTIC	PARASYMPATHOLYTIC (anticholinergic)
Epinephrine	Bethanechol	Reserpine	Belladonna alkaloids
Norepinephrine	Pilocarpine	Propranolol	Atropine
		Methyldopa	

Figure 20-3

Examples of these **antiarthritic** drugs are **acetylsalicylic acid** (aspirin), **acetaminophen** (Tylenol), ibuprofen (Motrin), sulindac (Clinoril), and phenylbutazone (Butazolidin).

Sedatives and *Hypnotics.* Sedatives relax without necessarily producing sleep, while hypnotics actually produce sleep. **Chloral hydrate** is a weak hypnotic particularly useful for elderly patients; **barbiturates** such as **phenobarbital**, **pentabarbital**, and **secobarbital** are effective as "sleeping pills." These latter drugs can produce tolerance and become habit-forming.

Anticonvulsants. These drugs are used to treat epilepsy. Ideally, these drugs depress spontaneous activity of the brain emanating from areas of scar or tumor, without affecting normal brain function. An example is **phenytoin (Dilantin).**

Tranquilizers. These agents are useful in controlling anxiety. Minor tranquilizers are **chlordiazepoxide (Librium)**, **diazepam (Valium)**, and **meprobamate (Miltown, Equanil).** Major tranquilizers, such as **phenothiazines (Thorazine**, **Mellaril**, and **Stelazine**) and **lithium**, are used for control of more severe disturbances of behavior, such as psychoses.

Anesthetics. General anesthetics, such as **ether** and **nitrous oxide** produce loss of sensation throughout the entire body. Local anesthetics, such as **procaine (Novocain)** and **lidocaine (Xylocaine)**, are used to relieve or prevent pain in specific areas of the body.

Figure 20-4 summarizes the different categories of CNS drugs and gives examples of each.

B. Antihistamines

These drugs block the action of histamine, which is normally released in the body when foreign antigens enter. Histamine causes allergic symptoms such as hives, bronchial asthma, hay fever, and in severe cases, **anaphylactic shock** (dyspnea, hypotension, and loss of consciousness). Antihistamines cannot cure the allergic reaction, but they can relieve its symptoms. Examples of antihistamines are **diphenhydramine (Benadryl)** and **chlorpheniramine (ChlorTrimeton).**

CENTRAL NERVOUS SYSTEM DRUGS

STIMULANTS	DEPRESSANTS
Caffeine	Alcohol
Amphetamines	Analgesics narcotic—morphine and codeine non-narcotic—Darvon antiarthritics—acetylsalicylic acid (aspirin), acetaminophen (Tylenol)
	Sedatives and hypnotics chloral hydrate, barbiturates
	Anticonvulsants phenytoin (Dilantin)
	Tranquilizers minor—chlordiazepoxide (Librium) major—phenothiazines
	Anesthetics general—ether, nitrous oxide local—procaine (Novocain)

Figure 20-4

CARDIOVASCULAR DRUGS

HEART			BLOOD PRESSURE		
Cardiotonics	Antiarrhythmics	Antianginal Preparations	Vasodilators	Vasoconstrictors	Diuretics
Digoxin (Lanoxin)	Beta-blockers	Nitroglycerin	Beta-blockers	Epinephrine	Chlorothiazide (Diuril)
	Quinidine (Quinaglute)	Beta-blockers	Methyldopa (Aldomet)		
	Procainamide	Calcium channel blockers			

Figure 20-5

Other histamine antagonists block a specific action of histamine on the stomach, and thereby prevent acid secretion in patients with ulcers of the stomach and duodenum. An example of such a drug is **cimetidine (Tagamet)**.

C. Cardiovascular Drugs

Cardiovascular drugs can **act on the heart** or **affect blood pressure.**

1. Drugs Acting on the Heart. **Cardiotonic** drugs such as digoxin (Lanoxin) increase the force and the efficiency of the heart beat. These drugs are useful in congestive heart failure and in correcting abnormal heart rhythms. Other **antiarrhythmic drugs** include the beta-blocker propranolol (Inderal), and quinidine (Quinaglute). **Antianginal preparations** prevent angina by dilating coronary vessels. Nitroglycerin, beta-blockers, and calcium channel blockers are all antianginal drugs.

2. Drugs Affecting Blood Pressure. These drugs can relax **(vasodilators)** or contract **(vasoconstrictors)** the muscles in blood vessel walls and thereby lower or raise blood pressure. Examples of vasodilators (antihypertensives) are beta-blockers such as propranolol and nadolol (Corgard) and drugs such as methyldopa (Aldomet). Epinephrine is an example of a vasoconstrictor. **Diuretics**, drugs that promote the excretion of fluid from the kidney, also lower blood pressure. An example of a diuretic is chlorothiazide (Diuril).

Figure 20-5 reviews the different categories of cardiovascular drugs and gives examples of each type of drug.

D. Anticoagulants

These drugs, which affect blood clotting, are used to prevent the formation of clots (thrombi and emboli) in veins and arteries, and to prevent coagulation in preserved blood used for transfusions. Examples of anticoagulants are **heparin** and **warfarin (Coumadin)**. Heparin is used to prolong the clotting time of blood and to treat thrombophlebitis and pulmonary embolism. It prevents the extension of old clots and the formation of new ones. Coumadin acts by depressing the synthesis in the liver of several clotting factors that are known to be active in coagulation and the formation of thrombi.

E. Gastrointestinal Drugs

These drugs are used mainly to relieve uncomfortable and potentially dangerous symptoms, rather than as cures for specific diseases. Some examples of gastrointestinal drugs are:

1. **Antacids.** These agents neutralize the hydrochloric acid in the stomach to relieve symptoms of peptic ulcer, esophagitis, and any epigastric discomfort.

2. **Emetics.** These agents produce vomiting.

3. **Cathartics.** These agents relieve constipation and promote defecation for prediagnostic and preoperative procedures, and are used in the treatment of disorders of the gastrointestinal tract. They work in several ways: Some increase the intestinal salt content to cause fluid to fill the intestines; others increase the bulk of the intestinal contents to promote peristalsis; and those of a third type lubricate the intestinal tract to produce soft stools. Examples are **laxatives** (mild cathartics) and **purgatives** (strong cathartics), which should not be used chronically.

4. **Antinauseants (Antiemetics).** These drugs relieve nausea and vomiting and overcome vertigo, dizziness, motion sickness, and labyrinthitis.

5. **Antidiarrheals.** These agents relieve diarrhea and decrease the rapid movement of the bowels.

Figure 20-6 reviews the types of gastrointestinal drugs.

F. Antibiotics

An antibiotic is a chemical substance produced by a microorganism (bacterium, yeast, or mold). Antibiotics are able to stop the growth (**biostatic** function) or kill (**biocidal** function) bacteria, fungi, or parasites. The use of antibiotics (penicillin was first in general use in 1945) has largely controlled many diseases such as pneumonia, rheumatic fever, and mastoiditis. Caution about the use of antibiotics is warranted because they are powerful agents. With indiscriminate use, pathogenic organisms can develop resistance to the antibiotic and thus destroy the antibiotic's disease-fighting capability. Examples of antibiotics are:

Penicillin (Ampicillin, Penicillin G, Penicillin V). This drug is effective, for example, in treating pneumococci, gonococci, meningococci, and some aerobic and anaerobic staphylococci and in the treatment of syphilis. Semisynthetic penicillins **(oxacillin, nafcillin)** are resistant to bacterial enzymes that destroy penicillin and ampicillin.

Streptomycin. This drug is used chiefly against **gram-positive** (stained by the Gram stain) and **acid-fast** (not readily discolored by acids after staining) bacteria. It is often given in conjunction with other antibiotics. **Kanamycin (Kantrex)** and **gentamicin (Garamycin)** are other antibiotics that are closely related to streptomycin, but used against gram-negative bacteria.

Tetracyclines. These are broad-spectrum antibiotics; that is, they are effective against both gram-positive and gram-negative organisms.

Sulfonamides. These are bacteriostatic agents that are general anti-infectives.

GASTROINTESTINAL DRUGS

ANTACIDS	EMETICS	CATHARTICS	ANTINAUSEANTS	ANTIDIARRHEALS
Maalox	Syrup of ipecac	Laxatives	Dramamine	Lomotil
Gelusil	Table salt	Purgatives	Antivert	Kaopectate
Milk of magnesia			Compazine	

Figure 20-6

Sulfisoxazole (Gantrisin) and **sulfamethoxazole (Gantanol)** are used to combat urinary tract infection caused by a variety of bacteria.

Cephalosporins. These are potent new antibiotics that also are effective against penicillin-resistant organisms. Examples are **cephalexin (Keflex)** and **cephalothin (Keflin)**.

G. Anticancer Drugs

These drugs are discussed in Chapter 18.

H. Endocrine Drugs

These drugs act in much the same manner as the naturally occurring (endogenous) hormones discussed in Chapter 17. The following list gives the type of hormone, a specific example of a drug, and indications for its use in the body:

Type	*Drug*	*Indications*
Androgen	testosterone	Impotence; eunuchism (failure of development of male sex characteristics)
Estrogen	diethylstilbestrol	Menopausal vasomotor symptoms; atrophic vaginitis; ovarian failure; palliative therapy in breast and prostate carcinoma
	conjugated estrogens (Premarin)	See indications for diethylstilbestrol
Progestin	medroxyprogestrone (Provera)	Abnormal uterine bleeding due to hormonal imbalance; amenorrhea in a woman who has previously menstruated
Thyroid hormone	levothyroxine (Synthroid)	Reduced or absent thyroid function; myxedema coma
Glucocorticoid	dexamethasone (Decadron)	Adrenal gland insufficiency; rheumatic disorders and other inflammatory diseases; neoplastic and hematologic disorders
	prednisone (Deltasone)	See indications for dexamethasone

I. Vitamins

Vitamins are **micronutrient** substances which, along with micronutrients such as minerals (calcium, phosphorus, and potassium), are essential for proper health and growth. A balanced daily diet should include foods containing vitamins as well as **macronutrients**, such as carbohydrates, fat, and proteins.

The names of the vitamins are listed below with a principal food source containing the vitamin and the disease or symptoms resulting from deficiency of the vitamin.

Name	*Food Source*	*Deficiency Symptom*
Vitamin A	green leafy vegetables, egg yolks, cod liver oil	night blindness, xerophthalmia
Vitamin B_1 (thiamine)	yeast, liver, whole grains	beriberi (neurological disorder)
Vitamin B_2 (riboflavin)	milk, cheese, eggs, poultry, liver	cheilosis, stomatitis, dermatosis
Niacin (nicotinic acid)	yeast, liver, peanuts, wheat germ	pellagra (skin, digestive, and mental disturbances)
Vitamin B_6 (pyridoxine)	liver, yeast, fish	anemias, neuropathy, convulsions in infancy
Vitamin B_{12} (cobalamin)	liver, dairy products	pernicious anemia
Vitamin C (ascorbic acid)	citrus fruits, vegetables	scurvy (gingivitis, hemorrhages)
Vitamin D	cod liver oil, milk, egg yolks	rickets; osteomalacia
Vitamin E	green leafy vegetables, wheat germ	hemolysis
Folic acid	meat, green leafy vegetables	pancytopenia
Vitamin K	liver, vegetable oils, leafy vegetables	hemorrhages

VII. VOCABULARY

additive — Drug action in which the combination of two similar drugs is equal to the sum of the effects of each.

alcohol — A central nervous system depressant.

amphetamine — A central nervous system stimulant.

anaphylaxis — Hypersensitive reaction of the body to a drug or foreign organism. Symptoms may include hives, asthma, and rhinitis.

androgen	Hormone that promotes male characteristics.
antacid	Gastrointestinal drug that neutralizes the acid in the stomach.
antiarrhythmic	Cardiovascular drug that helps restore heart rhythm to a regular cycle.
antibiotic	Chemical substance, produced by a microorganism, that has the ability to inhibit or kill foreign organisms in the body.
anticoagulant	A drug that prevents the clotting of blood.
anticonvulsant	A drug used to prevent convulsions.
antidiarrheal	A drug used to prevent diarrhea.
antidote	An agent given to counteract an unwanted effect of a drug.
antihistamine	A drug that blocks the action of histamine and helps prevent allergic symptoms.
antinauseant	An agent that relieves nausea and vomiting.
barbiturate	A sedative and hypnotic drug.
beta-blockers	Drugs that block the action of epinephrine at sites on receptors of heart muscle cells, the muscle lining of blood vessels, and bronchial tubes.
brand name	Commercial name for a drug; trade name.
caffeine	A central nervous system stimulant; from coffee or tea.
cardiotonic	A drug that promotes the force and efficiency of the heart.
cathartic	A drug that relieves constipation.
cephalosporins	Antibiotics that are effective against penicillin-resistant organisms.
chemical name	Chemical formula for a drug.
cholinergic	A drug that has the same effect as acetylcholine; parasympathomimetic.
contraindications	Factors in the patient's condition that prevent the use of a particular drug or treatment.
cumulation	The concentration or toxic effect of a drug may increase with each dose.
depressant	An agent that reduces functional activity.

diuretic	An antihypertensive drug that increases production of urine and reduces the volume of fluid in the body.
emetic	An agent that promotes vomiting.
estrogens	Female sex hormones.
Food and Drug Administration (FDA)	Governmental agency having the legal responsibility for enforcing proper drug manufacture and clinical use.
generic name	The legal, noncommercial name for a drug.
glucocorticoids	Hormones from the adrenal cortex that raise blood sugar and reduce inflammation.
Hospital Formulary	Reference listing of drugs and their appropriate clinical usage.
hypnotic	An agent that produces sleep.
idiosyncrasy	A rare type of toxic effect produced in a particularly sensitive individual but not seen in most patients.
laxative	A weak cathartic.
molecular pharmacology	Study of the interaction of drugs and subcellular entities such as DNA, RNA, and enzymes.
narcotic	A habit-forming drug that relieves pain and produces stupor or insensibility.
parasympatholytic	Anticholinergic; producing effects resembling interruption of the parasympathetic nervous system.
parasympathomimetic	Cholinergic; producing effects resembling stimulation of the parasympathetic nervous system.
parenteral administration	Administration of drugs by injection into the skin, muscles, or veins.
penicillins	Antibacterial antibiotics derived from strains of fungi (genus penicillium) and effective in treating many bacterial infections.
pharmacodynamics	Study of drug effects in the body.
pharmacokinetics	The calculation of drug concentration in tissues and blood over a period of time.
phenothiazines	Major tranquilizers used for control of psychoses.
Physicians' Desk Reference (PDR)	Reference book that lists drug products.

potentiation	Drug action in which the effect of using two drugs together is greater than the sum of the effects of using each one alone; synergism.
progestins	Progesterone compounds.
purgative	A strong cathartic.
sedative	A mild hypnotic drug; relaxing without necessarily producing sleep.
side effect	A toxic effect that routinely results from the use of a drug.
stimulant	An agent that excites and promotes functional activity.
streptomycin	An antibiotic derived from streptomyces griseus.
sulfonamides	Bacteriostatic agents.
suppository	A cone-shaped object containing medication which is inserted into the rectum, vagina, or urethra.
sympathomimetic	A drug that acts like the sympathetic nervous system (increases heart rate and blood pressure and opens air passages); adrenergic.
synergism	Potentiation.
tetracyclines	Broad-spectrum antibiotics.
tolerance	Condition of becoming resistant to the action of a drug as treatment progresses so that larger and larger doses must be given to achieve the desired effect.
toxicity	Harmful effects of a drug.
toxicology	Study of harmful chemicals and their effects on the body.
tranquilizers	Drugs used to control anxiety.
United States Pharmacopeia (U.S.P.)	An authoritative list of drugs, formulas, and preparations that sets a standard for drug manufacturing and dispensing.

VIII. COMBINING FORMS

Combining Form	*Definition*	*Terminology*	*Meaning*
pharmac/o	drug	pharmacology	________________
chem/o	drug	chemotherapy	________________

tox/o	poison	toxic ________________
toxic/o	poison	cytotoxicity ________________
		toxicology ________________
lingu/o	tongue	sublingual ________________
derm/o	skin	intradermal ________________
enter/o	intestines	parenteral ________________ *par(a) means beside*
ven/o	vein	intravenous ________________
thec/o	sheath (of brain and spinal cord)	intrathecal ________________
aer/o	air	aerosol ________________ *sol- means solution*
erg/o	work	synergism ________________
		adrenergic ________________
		cholinergic ________________
idi/o	individual, distinct, own	idiopathic ________________ ________________
iatr/o	physician, treatment	iatrogenic ________________
cras/o	mixture, temperament	idiosyncrasy ________________ ________________
narc/o	numbness, stupor	narcotic ________________
		narcolepsy ________________ *-lepsy means seizure*
hypn/o	sleep	hypnogenic ________________
pyr/o	fever	antipyretic ________________

esthesi/o	feeling, nervous sensation	anesthesia ____________
algesi/o	sensitivity to pain	analgesia ____________
hist/o	tissue	antihistamine ____________ *-amine means an organic (containing carbon) nitrogen compound*
vas/o	vessel	vasoconstrictor ____________
myc/o	mold	erythromycin ____________
vit/o	life	vitamin ____________ *The first vitamins discovered were nitrogen-containing substances called amines.*
-cidal	pertaining to killing	bacteriocidal ____________ *Also spelled bactericidal.*
-static	pertaining to stopping, controlling	bacteriostatic ____________
-phylaxis	protection	anaphylaxis ____________ *Ana- means excessive in this word.* prophylaxis ____________
-mimetic	mimic, copy	sympathomimetic ____________
-lytic	reduce, destroy	sympatholytic ____________
anti-	against	antibiotic ____________
contra-	against	contraindication ____________ *Indication means to point out.*

IX. ABBREVIATIONS

The following are abbreviations you may encounter with reference to drugs and their administration:

Abbreviation	*Derivation*	*Meaning*
ac	*ante cibum*	before meals

ad lib	*ad libitum*	freely as desired
aq	*aqua*	water
bid	*bis in die*	two times a day
bin	*bis in noctis*	two times a night
c	*cum*	with
caps	*capsula*	capsule
cc		cubic centimeter
comp	*compositus*	compound
dil	*dilutus*	dilute
FDA		Food and Drug Administration
Gm	*gramme*	gram
gr.	*granum*	grain
gt, gtt.	*gutta*	drops
h	*hora*	hour
hs	*hora somni*	bedtime
IM		intramuscular
IV		intravenous
mg		milligram
N.F.		National Formulary
NPO	*nulla per os*	nothing by mouth
od	*omni die*	every day
oh	*omni hora*	every hour
ol	*oleum*	oil
om	*omni mane*	every morning
on	*omni nocte*	every night

os	*os*	mouth
oz.		ounce
pc	*post cibum*	after meals
PDR		Physicians' Desk Reference
po	*per os*	by mouth
prn	*pro re nata*	when requested
Q (q)	*quaque*	every
qd	*quaque die*	every day
qh	*quaque hora*	every hour
qid	*quater in die*	four times a day
qsuff	*quantum sufficit*	as much as suffices
s	*sine*	without
sos	*si opus sit*	if necessary
subq		subcutaneous injection
syr	*syrupus*	syrup
tab		tablet
tid	*ter in die*	three times a day
ung	*ungentum*	ointment
U.S.P.		United States Pharmacopeia

X. PRACTICAL APPLICATIONS

The drugs listed here are used as examples in the text. Their trade names, categories, and indications for use are reviewed.

Generic Name	*Trade Name*	*Category*	*Indications*
acetaminophen	Tylenol	analgesic	pain

acetylsalicyclic acid (aspirin)	various	analgesic	pain
atropine/ diphenoxylate	Lomotil	antidiarrheal	diarrhea
atropine/ phenobarbital/ scopolamine	Donnatal	parasympatholytic	duodenal ulcer/ irritable bowel syndrome
bethanechol	various	parasympathomimetic	urinary retention
butalbital/aspirin/ caffeine/codeine	Fiorinal/ Codeine	narcotic analgesic	pain
chlordiazepoxide	Librium	minor tranquilizer	anxiety
chlorpheniramine	ChlorTrimeton	antihistamine	allergic symptoms
chlorpromazine	Thorazine	major tranquilizer	psychosis
cimetidine	Tagamet	histamine antagonist	ulcer
dexamethasone	Decadron	glucocorticoid	endocrine/other disorders
diazepam	Valium	minor tranquilizer	anxiety
digoxin	Lanoxin	cardiotonic	congestive heart failure
dimenhydrinate	Dramamine	antinauseant	motion sickness
diphenhydramine	Benadryl	antihistamine	allergic rhinitis
epinephrine	Adrenalin	sympathomimetic	asthma/cardiac conditions
estrogens, conjugated	Premarin	hormone/estrogen	menopausal vasomotor symptoms
flurazepam	Dalmane	sedative/hypnotic	insomnia
ibuprofen	Motrin	analgesic	arthritis
meperidine	Demerol	narcotic analgesic	pain

meprobamate	Miltown	minor tranquilizer	anxiety
methyldopa	Aldomet	antihypertensive	hypertension
nadolol	Corgard	antihypertensive	hypertension
nitroglycerin	various	antianginal	angina
oxycodone	Percodan	narcotic analgesic	pain
phenobarbital	various	sedative/hypnotic	sedation/epilepsy
phenylbutazone	Butazolidin	analgesic/anti-inflammatory	arthritis
phenytoin	Dilantin	anticonvulsant	epilepsy
pilocarpine	various	parasympathomimetic	glaucoma
prednisone	various	glucocorticoid	endocrine/other disorders
procaine	Novocain	local anesthetic	prevention of pain
propoxyphene	Darvon	non-narcotic analgesic	mild/moderate pain
propranolol	Inderal	sympatholytic/beta-blocker	hypertension/angina/arrhythmias
reserpine	various	sympatholytic	hypertension
sulfisoxazolde	Gantrisin	sulfonamide	urinary tract infection
sulindac	Clinoril	anti-inflammatory	arthritis
thioridazine	Mellaril	major tranquilizer	psychosis
thyroxine	various	thyroid hormone	decreased thyroid function
trifluoperazine	Stelazine	major tranquilizer	psychosis
warfarin	Coumadin	anticoagulant	thrombosis

XI. EXERCISES

A. Name the pharmacological specialty from its description below:

1. Use of drugs in the treatment of disease ____________________
2. Study of new drug synthesis ____________________
3. Study of how drugs interact with subcellular parts ____________________
4. Study of the harmful effects of drugs ____________________
5. Study of drug effects on the body ____________________
6. Measurement of drug concentrations in tissues and in blood over a period of time

   ____

B. Build medical words:

1. Pertaining to against fever ____________________
2. Poisonous to cells ____________________
3. Pertaining to disease without a recognizable cause ____________________
4. Pertaining to within a vein ____________________
5. Study of drugs ____________________
6. Pertaining to under the tongue ____________________
7. Pertaining to under the skin ____________________
8. Seizure of sleep ____________________
9. Produced by a physician or by treatment ____________________
10. Pertaining to within the sheath around the spinal cord ____________________

C. Give four routes of drug administration:

1. ____________________ 3. ____________________

2. ____________________ 4. ____________________

D. Give the meaning of the following terms:

1. parenteral ______
2. pharmacopeia ______
3. idiosyncrasy ______
4. synergism ______
5. contraindications ______
6. anaphylaxis ______
7. antidote ______
8. drug toxicity ______
9. aerosol ______
10. side effect ______

E. Match the terms in Column I with associated terms in Column II:

Column I		*Column II*
1. pharmacy	______	A. Combination of two drugs together is equal to the sum of the effects of each.
2. molecular pharmacology	______	B. Drug name that gives the chemical formula.
3. brand name	______	C. Combination of two drugs together gives an effect that is greater than the sum of the effects of each.
4. generic name	______	
5. chemical name	______	D. Drugs passing into the bloodstream.
6. cumulation	______	E. Concentrations or toxic effects of a drug build up with each dose.
7. additive action	______	
8. potentiation	______	F. Effects of a drug diminish as larger and larger doses are needed to produce desired effect.
9. tolerance	______	G. Area to prepare, store, and dispense drugs.
10. absorption	______	H. Official name; legal and noncommercial name.

I. Trade name of drug privately owned by manufacturer.

J. Study of drug interaction with subcellular entities.

F. *Give the meanings of the following abbreviations:*

1. PDR ________________
2. FDA ________________
3. IV ________________
4. U.S.P. ________________
5. IM ________________
6. N.F. ________________

G. *Match the routes of administration of drugs in Column I with the medications and procedures in Column II:*

Column I		*Column II*
1. intravenous	______	A. Lotions, creams, ointments.
2. rectal	______	B. Tablets and capsules.
3. oral	______	C. Used for allergy skin tests.
4. topical	______	D. Lumbar puncture.
5. inhalation	______	E. Deep injection, usually in buttock.
6. intrathecal	______	F. Suppositories.
7. intramuscular	______	G. Used for blood transfusions.
8. intradermal	______	H. Aerosols.

H. *Give the meanings of the following terms that relate to autonomic neuropharmacologic drugs:*

1. sympathomimetic ________________

2. adrenergic agents ______

3. parasympathomimetic ______

4. cholinergic agents ______

5. acetylcholine ______

6. epinephrine ______

7. parasympatholytic ______

8. sympatholytic ______

I. *Match the autonomic acting drug in Column I with a term in Column II that describes its function:*

Column I		*Column II*
1. atropine	______	A. cholinergic
2. epinephrine	______	B. sympatholytic
3. reserpine	______	C. parasympatholytic (anticholinergic)
4. bethanecol	______	D. adrenergic
5. acetylcholine	______	
6. pilocarpine	______	
7. propranolol	______	
8. methyldopa	______	
9. norepinephrine	______	

J. *Give the meaning of the following terms that describe drugs affecting the central nervous system:*

1. depressants ______

2. stimulants ______

3. analgesic ______

4. anesthetic ______

5. anticonvulsant ______________________________

6. hypnotic ______________________________

7. endorphin ______________________________

8. narcotic ______________________________

9. sedative ______________________________

10. barbiturate ______________________________

11. tranquilizer ______________________________

12. phenothiazines ______________________________

K. *Match the name of the drug in Column I with an appropriate drug category in Column II:*

Column I		*Column II*
1. chloral hydrate	______	A. anesthetic
2. morphine	______	B. tranquilizer
3. acetylsalicyclic acid	______	C. sedative
		D. anticonvulsant
4. caffeine	______	E. narcotic analgesic
5. Dilantin	______	F. stimulant
6. amphetamine	______	G. analgesic
7. nitrous oxide	______	
8. codeine	______	
9. Thorazine	______	
10. Novocain	______	

L. *Give the meaning of the following terms:*

1. antihistamine ______________________________

2. anaphylactic shock ______________________________

3. antiarrhythmic ____________________

4. vasodilator ____________________

5. vasoconstrictor ____________________

6. diuretic ____________________

7. anticoagulant ____________________

M. *Name the type of action of the following drugs:*

1. Benadryl ____________________

2. ChlorTrimeton ____________________

3. heparin ____________________

4. lidocaine ____________________

5. digoxin ____________________

6. propranolol ____________________

7. nitroglycerin ____________________

8. Coumadin ____________________

9. Diuril ____________________

10. quinidine ____________________

N. *Give the meanings for the following types of gastrointestinal drugs:*

1. antidiarrheal ____________________

2. emetic ____________________

3. cathartic ____________________

4. antinauseant ____________________

5. antacid ____________________

6. purgative ____________________

7. laxative ____________________

O. Give the meanings of the following terms:

1. antibiotic ______
2. bacteriocidal ______
3. bacteriostatic ______
4. penicillin ______
5. streptomycin ______
6. macronutrients ______
7. vitamins ______
8. cephalosporins ______
9. tetracycline ______
10. glucocorticoids ______
11. progestins ______
12. androgens ______
13. estrogens ______

P. Give the other name of each of the vitamins listed:

1. cobalamin ______
2. thiamine ______
3. ascorbic acid ______
4. riboflavin ______
5. pyridoxine ______
6. nicotinic acid ______

Q. The following diseases are associated with what vitamin deficiency?

1. beriberi ______
2. pernicious anemia ______
3. night blindness ______
4. scurvy ______
5. pellagra ______
6. rickets ______

R. Give the meanings for the following abbreviations:

1. tid ____________
2. pc ____________
3. bid ____________
4. NPO ____________
5. hs ____________
6. qid ____________
7. ung ____________
8. qd ____________
9. gt. ____________
10. aq ____________

ANSWERS

A.

1. Chemotherapy
2. Medicinal chemistry
3. Molecular pharmacology
4. Toxicology
5. Pharmacodynamics
6. Pharmacokinetics

B.

1. Antipyretic
2. Cytotoxicity
3. Idiopathic
4. Intravenous
5. Pharmacology
6. Sublingual
7. Hypodermic or subcutaneous
8. Narcolepsy
9. Iatrogenic
10. Intrathecal

C.

1. Oral
2. Sublingual
3. Rectal
4. Parenteral

D.

1. Drugs are administered by injection through any route other than via the alimentary tract.
2. An authorized list of drugs and their preparation.
3. A rare type of toxic effect of a drug that is seen in a particularly sensitive individual.
4. Drug action in which the effect of using two drugs together is greater than the sum of the effects of using each one alone.
5. Factors in a patient's condition that prevent the use of a particular drug or treatment.
6. Hypersensitive reaction of the body to a drug or foreign organism.
7. An agent given to counteract an unwanted effect of a drug.
8. Harmful effects of a drug.
9. Particles of drug suspended in air.
10. A toxic effect that routinely occurs from the use of a drug.

E.

1. G
2. J
3. I
4. H
5. B
6. E
7. A
8. C
9. F
10. D

F.

1. Physician's Desk Reference
2. Food and Drug Administration
3. Intravenous
4. United States Pharmacopeia
5. Intramuscular
6. National Formulary

G.

1. G
2. F
3. B
4. A
5. H
6. D
7. E
8. C

H.

1. A drug that acts like the sympathetic nervous system (adrenergic).
2. Sympathomimetics; acting like Adrenalin.
3. Drugs that act like the parasympathetic nervous system; cholinergic.
4. Parasympathomimetics; acting like acetylcholine.
5. A neurotransmitter substance.
6. A sympathomimetic drug; hormone produced by the adrenal glands.
7. Drugs having an opposite effect to parasympathomimetics.
8. Drugs having an opposite effect to sympathomimetics.

I.

1. C
2. D
3. B
4. A
5. A
6. A
7. B
8. B
9. D

J.

1. Drugs that reduce functional activity.
2. Drugs that excite and promote functional activity.
3. An agent that reduces sensitivity to pain.
4. An agent that reduces feeling and sensation.
5. A drug that is used to prevent convulsions.
6. A drug that produces sleep or trance.
7. Produces euphoria and sedation.
8. A habit-forming drug that relieves pain and can produce stupor.
9. A drug that relaxes without producing sleep.
10. A drug that can have sedative and hypnotic effects.
11. A drug used to control anxiety.
12. Major tranquilizers used for control of the symptoms of severe mental illness (psychosis).

K.

1. C
2. E, G
3. G
4. F
5. D
6. F
7. A
8. E, G
9. B
10. A

L.

1. A drug that blocks the action of histamine and helps prevent allergic symptoms.
2. Severe hypersensitivity reaction resulting in a state of collapse and loss of consciousness.
3. A drug used to prevent abnormalities in heart rhythm.
4. An agent that causes dilation of blood vessels.
5. An agent that causes constriction (narrowing) of blood vessels.
6. A substance that stimulates production of urine and lowers blood pressure.
7. An agent used to prevent the formation of blood clots.

M.

1. Antihistamine.
2. Antihistamine.
3. Anticoagulant.
4. Local anesthetic.
5. Cardiotonic (promotes the strength and proper rate of the heart).
6. Antiarrhythmic, vasodilator, antianginal beta-blocker.
7. Antianginal preparation.
8. Anticoagulant.
9. Diuretic.
10. Antiarrhythmic.

N.

1. Drug used to prevent diarrhea.
2. Drug that stimulates vomiting.
3. Drug that relieves constipation.
4. Drug that relieves nausea and vomiting.
5. Drug that neutralizes acid in the stomach.
6. Drug that is a strong cathartic.
7. Drug that relieves mild constipation.

O.

1. Chemical that has the ability to inhibit or kill foreign organisms in the body.
2. Pertaining to the killing of bacteria.
3. Pertaining to inhibiting or retarding bacterial growth.
4. An antibiotic effective in treating many bacterial infections and derived from strains of fungi (genus Penicillium).
5. An antibiotic chiefly used against gram-positive and acid-fast bacteria.
6. Major food substances such as carbohydrates, proteins, and fats.
7. Micronutrient substances necessary for proper health and growth.
8. Antibiotics that are effective against penicillin-resistant organisms.
9. Antibiotic effective in treating a broad-spectrum (many kinds) of bacteria.
10. Hormones from the adrenal cortex; they raise blood sugar and reduce inflammation.
11. Progesterone compounds.
12. Male hormones.
13. Female hormones.

P.

1. Vitamin B_{12}.
2. Vitamin B_1.
3. Vitamin C.
4. Vitamin B_2.
5. Vitamin B_6.
6. Niacin.

Q.

1. Thiamine (vitamin B_1).
2. Cobalamin (vitamin B_{12}).
3. Vitamin A.
4. Vitamin C.
5. Niacin (nicotinic acid).
6. Vitamin D.

R.

1. Three times a day.
2. After meals.
3. Two times a day.
4. Nothing by mouth.
5. Bedtime.
6. Four times a day.
7. Ointment.
8. Every day.
9. Drops.
10. Water.

XII. PRONUNCIATION OF TERMS

adrenergic	ăd-rĕn-ĔR-jĭk
amphetamine	ăm-FĔT-ă-mēn
analgesic	ăn-ăl-JĒ-zĭk
anaphylaxis	ăn-ă-fĭ-LĂK-sĭs
anesthesia	ăn-ĕs-THĒ-zē-ă
antacid	ănt-ĂS-ĭd
antiarrhythmic	ăn-tĭ-ă-RĬTH-mĭk
anticoagulant	ăn-tĭ-kō-ĂG-ū-lănt
anticonvulsant	ăn-tĭ-kŏn-VŬL-sănt
antidiarrheal	ăn-tĭ-dī-ă-RĒ-ăl
antidote	ĂN-tĭ-dōt
antihistamine	ăn-tĭ-HĬS-tă-mēn
antinauseant	ăn-tĭ-NAW-zē-ănt
antipyretic	ăn-tĭ-pī-RĔT-ĭk
ascorbic acid	ăs-KŌR-bĭk ĂS-ĭd
bacteriocidal	băk-tē-rē-ō-SĪ-dăl

bacteriostatic	băk-tē-rē-ō-STĂT-ĭk
barbiturate	băr-BĬT-ū-rāt
cathartic	kă-THĂR-tĭk
cephalosporin	sĕf-ă-lō-SPŌR-ĭn
cholinergic	kō-lĭn-ĔR-jĭk
cobalamin	kō-BĂL-ă-mĭn
cumulation	kū-mū-LĀ-shŭn
cytotoxicity	sī-tō-tŏk-SĬS-ĭ-tē
diuretic	dī-ū-RĔT-ĭk
emetic	ĕ-MĔT-ĭk
erythromycin	ĕ-rĭth-rō-MĪ-sĭn
generic	jĕ-NĔR-ĭk
glucocorticoid	glōō-kō-KŌR-tĭ-koyd
histamine	HĬS-tă-mēn
hypnogenic	hĭp-nō-JĔN-ĭk
hypnotic	hĭp-NŎT-ĭk
iatrogenic	ī-ăt-rō-JĔN-ĭk
idiopathic	ĭd-ē-ō-PĂTH-ĭk
idiosyncrasy	ĭd-ē-ō-SĬN-kră-sē
intrathecal	ĭn-tră-THĒ-kăl
laxative	LĂK-să-tĭv
narcolepsy	NĂR-kō-lĕp-sē
narcotic	năr-KŎT-ĭk
niacin	NĪ-ă-sĭn
parasympatholytic	pă-ră-sĭm-pă-thō-LĬT-ĭk
parasympathomimetic	pă-ră-sĭm-pă-thō-mĭ-MĔT-ĭk
parenteral	pă-RĔN-tĕr-ăl
pharmacodynamics	făr-mă-kō-dī-NĂM-ĭks
pharmacology	făr-mă-KŎL-ō-jē
pharmacopeia	făr-mă-kō-PĒ-ă
phenothiazines	fē-nō-THĪ-ă-zēns
potentiation	pō-tĕn-shē-Ā-shŭn

progestin	prō-GĔS-tĭn
prophylaxis	prō-fĭ-LĂK-sĭs
purgative	PŬR-gă-tĭv
pyridoxine	pĭr-ĭ-DŎK-sēn
riboflavin	rī-bō-FLĀ-vĭn
streptomycin	strĕp-tō-MĪ-sĭn
sulfonamide	sŭl-FŎN-ă-mīd
sympatholytic	sĭm-păth-ō-LĬ-tĭk
sympathomimetic	sĭm-păth-ō-mĭ-MĔT-ĭk
synergism	SĬN-ĕr-jĭzm
syringe	sĭ-RĬNJ
tetracycline	tĕt-ră-SĪ-klēn
thiamine	THĪ-ă-mĭn
toxicity	tŏk-SĬS-ĭ-tē
toxicology	tŏk-sĭ-KŎL-ō-jē
vasoconstriction	văz-ō-kŏn-STRĬK-shŭn
vasodilation	văz-ō-dī-LĀ-shŭn

REVIEW SHEET 20

Combining Forms

aer/o	______	lingu/o	______
algesi/o	______	myc/o	______
chem/o	______	narc/o	______
cras/o	______	pharmac/o	______
derm/o	______	pyr/o	______
enter/o	______	thec/o	______
erg/o	______	tox/o	______
esthesi/o	______	toxic/o	______
hist/o	______	vas/o	______
hypn/o	______	ven/o	______
iatr/o	______	vit/o	______
idi/o	______		

Suffixes

-cidal	______	-mimetic	______
-lepsy	______	-phylaxis	______
-lytic	______	-static	______

Prefixes

ana-	______	para-	______
anti-	______	pro-	______
contra-	______	syn-	______

Additional Terms

additive (615)

alcohol (615)

amphetamine (615)

anaphylaxis (615)

antacid (616)

antidote (616)

ascorbic acid (615)

barbiturate (616)

beta-blockers (616)

brand name (616)

caffeine (616)

cardiotonic (616)

cathartic (616)

cephalosporins (616)

chemical name (616)

cholinergic (616)

cobalamin (615)

contraindications (616)

cumulation (616)

depressant (616)

diuretic (617)

emetic (617)

FDA (617)

generic name (617)

glucocorticoids (617)

hypnotic (617)

idiosyncrasy (617)

laxative (617)

medicinal chemistry (605)

molecular pharmacology (617)

narcotic (617)

nicotinic acid (615)

parasympatholytic (617)

parasympathomimetic (617)

parenteral (617)

penicillin (617)

pharmacodynamics (617)

pharmacokinetics (617)

phenothiazines (617)

potentiation (618)

purgative (618)

pyridoxine (615)

riboflavin (615)

sedative (618)

side effect (618)

stimulant (618)

sulfonamides (618)

sympatholytic (609)

sympathomimetic (618)

synergism (618)

syringe (607)

thiamine (615)

tolerance (618)

toxicology (618)

tranquilizer (618)

U.S.P. (618)

CHAPTER 21

PSYCHIATRY

In this chapter you will:

- Differentiate between a psychiatrist, psychologist, and other psychiatric specialists;
- Learn of tests used by clinical psychologists to evaluate a patient's mental health and intelligence;
- Define terms that describe major psychiatric disorders;
- Identify terms that describe psychiatric symptoms;
- Compare different types of therapy for psychiatric disorders; and
- Define combining forms, suffixes, prefixes, and abbreviations related to psychiatry.

This chapter is divided into the following sections:

I. INTRODUCTION

You will find this chapter different from others in the book. Psychiatric disorders are not readily explainable in terms of abnormalities in the structure or chemistry of an organ or tissue, as are other illnesses. In addition, the etiology of mental disorders is complex. While a chemical basis for psychiatric disorders cannot be excluded, psychological and social factors play an important role in mental illness. Our purpose here will be to provide a simple outline and definition of major psychiatric terms. For more extensive and detailed information, you may wish to consult the **Diagnostic and Statistical Manual III** (American Psychiatric Association, Washington, D.C., 1980), as well as other textbooks of psychiatry.

Psychiatry (psych/o = mind, iatr/o = treatment) is the branch of medicine that deals with the diagnosis, treatment, and prevention of mental illness. It is a specialty of clinical medicine comparable to surgery, internal medicine, pediatrics, and obstetrics.

Psychiatrists complete the same medical training (4 years of medical school) as other physicians and receive an M.D. degree. Then they spend a varying number of years training in the methods and practice of **psychotherapy** (treatment of mental disorders). Psychiatrists can also take additional years of training to specialize in certain aspects of psychiatry. **Child psychiatrists** specialize in the treatment of children; **forensic psychiatrists** specialize in the legal aspects of psychiatry, such as determination of mental competence in criminal cases. **Psychoanalysts** complete 3 to 5 years of training in a special psychotherapeutic technique called **psychoanalysis** in which the patient freely relates his or her thoughts to the analyst, who does not interfere in the flow of thoughts.

A **psychologist** is a nonmedical person who is trained in methods of psychotherapy, analysis, and research and completes a master's or doctor of philosophy (Ph.D.) degree in a specific field of interest, such as **clinical** (patient-oriented) **psychology**, **educational psychology**,

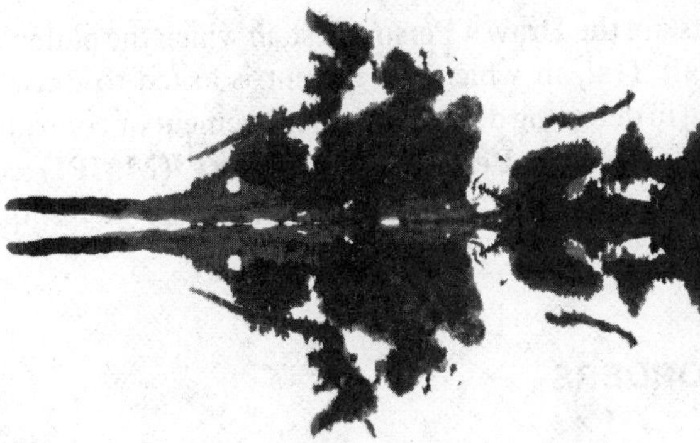

Figure 21-1 Inkblots like this one are presented on ten cards in the Rorschach test. The patient describes images seen in the blot.

experimental psychology, or **social psychology**. A clinical psychologist, like a psychiatrist, can use various methods of psychotherapy to treat patients but, unlike the psychiatrist, cannot use drugs or electroshock without the permission of a physician.

Clinical psychologists are trained in the use of tests to evaluate various aspects of a patient's mental health and intelligence. Examples are intelligence (I.Q.) tests such as the **Wechsler Adult Intelligence Scale (WAIS)** and the **Stanford-Binet Intelligence Scale**. Projective (personality) tests are the **Rorschach technique** (inkblots as in Figure 21-1 are used to bring out associations) and the **Thematic Apperception Test (TAT)**, in which pictures are used as stimuli for making up a story (see Figure 21-2). Both tests are especially revealing of personality structure.

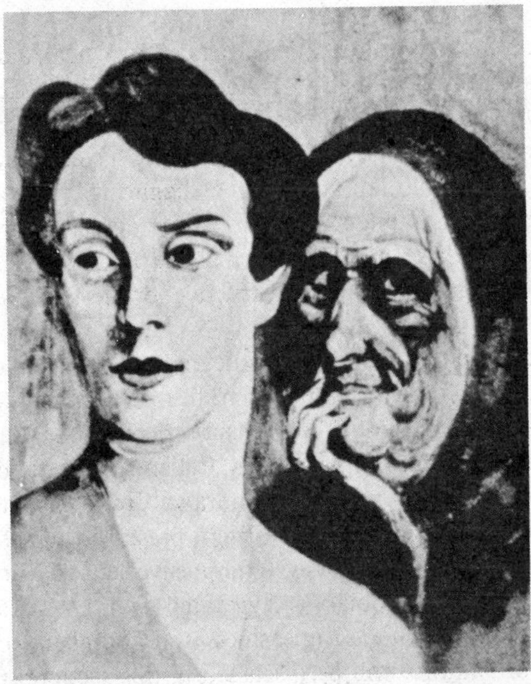

Figure 21-2 A sample picture from the Thematic Apperception Test. A patient is asked to tell the story that the picture illustrates. (Reprinted by permission from Murray, H.A.: Thematic Apperception Test. Cambridge, Mass., Harvard University Press. Copyright 1943 by the President and Fellows of Harvard College; copyright 1971 by Henry A. Murray.)

Graphomotor projection tests are the **Draw a Person Test**, in which the patient is asked to draw a body, and the **Bender-Gestalt Test**, in which the patient is asked to draw certain geometric designs. These tests are useful in detecting deficiencies in movement or coordination due to brain damage. The **Minnesota Multiphasic Personality Inventory (MMPI)** contains true-false questions that reveal aspects of personality, such as sense of duty or responsibility, ability to relate to others, and dominance.

II. PSYCHIATRIC DISORDERS

Sigmund Freud's ideas of personality structure play an important role in the understanding of many types of psychiatric disorders. Freud believed that personality is made up of three major parts: the **id**, the **ego**, and the **superego**. The **id** represents the unconscious instincts and psychic energy present at birth and thereafter. From the id arises basic drives which, operating according to the pleasure principle, seek immediate gratification regardless of the reality of the situation. The id is believed to predominate in the thinking of infants and to be manifest in the uncontrolled actions of certain mentally ill patients.

The **ego** is the central coordinating branch of the personality. It is the mediator between the id and the outside world. It is the part of the personality that evaluates and assesses the reality of a situation (**reality testing**) and, if necessary, postpones the gratification of a need or drive (id) until a satisfactory object or situation arises. The ego is perceived as being "self" by the individual.

The **superego** is the internalized conscience and moral part of the personality. It encompasses the sense of discipline derived from parental authority and society. Guilt feelings, for example, arise from behavior and thoughts that do not conform to the standards of the superego.

Freud believed that certain psychological disorders occur when conflicts arise between two or more of these aspects of the personality. **Defense mechanisms**, such as denial, are the techniques people employ to ward off the anxiety produced by these conflicts. For example, a person afflicted with a serious illness may avoid confronting his present or future problems by denial. Thus, he or she may refuse to believe the diagnosis, miss appointments, neglect medication, or ignore symptoms. While all persons utilize defense mechanisms to cope with difficult problems, the use of these mechanisms may be regarded as abnormal or normal according to whether their use makes a constructive or destructive contribution to the individual's personality.

Two general terms used to describe differing degrees of mental illness are **psychosis** and **neurosis**. A psychosis involves significant impairment of reality testing with symptoms such as **delusions** (false beliefs), **hallucinations** (false sensory perceptions), and bizarre behavior. Schizophrenic disorders are examples of psychoses. Patients exhibit a disturbed sense of self, inappropriate affect (emotional reactions) and withdrawal from the external world. Neurosis indicates a milder mental illness in which reality testing is preserved and psychotic symptoms are absent. Some examples of neuroses are obsessive-compulsive neurosis (uncontrollable thoughts and actions dominate behavior), phobias (exaggerated fears), and anxiety neurosis (unconscious fears provoke periods of intense uneasiness and apprehension).

Some psychiatric disorders that will be discussed in this section are: **affective disorders**, **anxiety disorders**, **somatoform disorders**, **dissociative disorders**, **psychosexual disorders**, **personality disorders**, **organic brain syndromes**, **schizophrenic disorders**, **paranoid disorder**, **chronic alcoholism**, and **drug dependence**.

1. Affective Disorders

An affective disorder is a disorder of mood. Examples are **manic-depressive illness, major depression, cyclothymic disorder**, and **dysthymic disorder**.

Manic-depressive illness is characterized by alternating moods of **mania** (excessive excitement, activity, exalted feelings, and decrease in need for sleep) and **depression** (sadness, loss of appetite, decreased activity, inability to sleep). The manic mood is a prominent part of the illness. Mood swings vary in length, changing daily or at longer intervals. Currently, the term **bipolar disorder** is used to describe a condition in which major manic and depressive episodes are intermixed or rapidly alternating every few days. Depressive symptoms are prominent in bipolar disorders.

Major depression involves severe **dysphoric** mood (sadness, hopelessness, irritability, worry, discouragement). Other symptoms are: poor appetite or significant weight loss, a sleep disorder such as insomnia or hypersomnia, recurrent thoughts of death or suicide, slowness in thinking and decisiveness, and fatigue. Psychotic features, such as delusions or hallucinations, can also be present as well.

Involutional melancholia is a depressive condition which occurs in late or middle age (involutional period). The patient is often severely depressed, and is preoccupied with excessive or inappropriate guilt. Insomnia and weight loss are prominent symptoms.

Cyclothymic disorder (cycl/o = cycle, thymic = mind) is a condition marked by numerous periods of both manic and depressive episodes, but not as severe or of as long duration as in manic-depressive illness. Psychotic features, which may be present in manic-depressive illness, are absent in cyclothymic disorder.

Dysthymic disorder (previously called depressive neurosis) involves depressive periods and mood, but not of the same severity and duration as in a major depressive episode. There are also no psychotic features (delusions, hallucinations, incoherent thinking), as are sometimes found in major depression.

2. Anxiety Disorders

These disorders are characterized by the experience of unpleasant tension, distress, and troubled feelings. Examples are **phobias** and **anxiety states**.

Phobias are irrational fears associated with some specific type of stimulus or situation. The phobic person usually goes to extreme length to avoid the object of his or her fear. Some common phobias are:

agoraphobia—fear of open, public places (agora means marketplace).
social phobia—fear of situations in which the individual is open to public scrutiny.
acrophobia—fear of high places (acr means extremities, heights).
claustrophobia—fear of being closed in (claustr means barrier).
zoophobia—fear of animals (zoo means animal life).

Anxiety states are exemplified by **panic disorder, generalized anxiety disorder, obsessive-compulsive disorder**, and **post-traumatic stress disorder**. A **panic disorder** is marked by episodes of panic (apprehension and fear) that are not precipitated by a phobic object, life-threatening situation, or physical exertion. The patient may have physical symptoms such as palpitations, dyspnea, dizziness, faintness, or choking sensations. A **generalized anxiety disorder** is characterized by persistent anxiety over a period of at least 1 month. The patient may have many of the following symptoms: apprehension, fearfulness, motor tension (jitteriness, trembling, eyelid twitch), sweating, dry mouth, dizziness.

Obsessive-compulsive disorder (previously called obsessive-compulsive neurosis) involves recurrent thoughts (**obsessions**) and repetitive acts (**compulsions**) that dominate the patient's behavior. The patient experiences anxiety if he or she is prevented from performing special rituals, which are used as a shield against overwhelming anxiety or fear. Compulsive hand-washing and preoccupation with unlikely dangers are examples of obsessive-compulsive disorders.

Post-traumatic stress disorder is a condition in which the patient has anxiety related to the re-experiencing (by recollection, dreams, or association) of a serious trauma in his or her life. Specific symptoms are sleep disturbance, guilt about surviving when others have not, memory impairment, and avoidance of activities that suggest recollection of the traumatic event.

3. Somatoform Disorders

These are disorders in which the patient's mental conflicts are expressed as physical symptoms. The physical symptoms are not adequately explained by any physical disorder or injury, and are not side effects of medication, drugs, or alcohol. Examples of somatoform symptoms are: gastrointestinal (abdominal pain, nausea, vomiting, diarrhea), cardiopulmonary (chest pain, palpitations), loss of function in a part of the body (difficult swallowing, loss of voice, deafness, blindness, paralysis). In **conversion disorder** (previously known as hysterical neurosis, conversion type), the predominant disturbance is a loss of physical functioning. The patient usually has a feared but unconscious conflict which threatens to escape from **repression** (a defense mechanism in which a person removes unacceptable ideas or impulses from consciousness), but the energies associated with this conflict are experienced as a physical symptom. The conversion symptom, in fact, enables the individual to avoid the conflict and get support from the environment around him or her. For example, a person with repressed anger and desire to physically harm a close family member may suddenly develop paralysis of the arm (conversion symptom).

Hypochondriasis (previously called hypochondriacal neurosis) is a somatoform disorder in which the patient has preoccupation with bodily aches, pains, and discomforts (in the absence of real disease). The hypochondriac has irrational fear and anxiety about his or her health.

Certain illnesses are recognized to be precipitated by emotional factors. These illnesses are called **psychosomatic**; examples are migraine headaches, ulcers, insomnia, neurodermatitis, hypertension, irritable bowel syndrome, and Crohn's disease.

Anorexia nervosa and **bulimia** are examples of eating disorders with a psychosomatic basis. Anorexia nervosa is a lack of appetite (or refusal to eat, with change in eating patterns) due to psychological factors such as anxiety, anger, and fear. The condition predominantly affects adolescent females and its principal symptom is a conscious, relentless attempt to diet, with significant loss of body weight. There is usually significant distortion of body image, as the individual misperceives her body as obese, even when she is obviously emaciated. Excessive, compulsive overactivity, such as exercise, running, or gymnastics, often occurs as well. Bulimic (bulimia means an abnormal increase in hunger) patients usually maintain normal body configuration and do not display the severe body-image distortion seen with anorexia. Bulimics, also almost exclusively female, have a fear of obesity and at the same time engage in eating binges. Following the eating binge (usually of foods high in calories) patients become depressed and lethargic and may induce vomiting.

4. Dissociative Disorders

Dissociative disorders (previously known as hysterical neurosis, dissociation type) involve mental symptoms that, like the physical somatoform symptoms, serve to hide the pain and anxiety of unconscious conflicts. Examples are **psychogenic amnesia** (inability to remember important personal information), **psychogenic fugue** (sudden unexpected travel away from home or work, with amnesia), and **multiple personality**, which is the existence within the individual of two or more distinct personalities (illustrated in literature by Dr. Jekyll and Mr. Hyde).

5. Psychosexual Disorders

These disorders are sexual perversions (deviations from the norm) or conditions in which the patient's psychological sexual identity is different from his or her anatomical sex (gender identity). Examples are:

transsexualism—the desire to change one's sex. Some transsexuals have been treated by sex-changing surgical procedures, intensive hormonal therapy, and psychotherapy.

fetishism—achieving sexual gratification by substituting in inanimate object for a human love object.

transvestism—dressing in the clothes of the opposite sex.

exhibitionism—compulsive need to expose one's body, particularly the genitals.

voyeurism—an abnormal desire to look at sexual organs or acts.

sexual masochism—achievement of sexual pleasure from suffering physical or psychological pain.

sexual sadism—achievement of sexual pleasure by inflicting physical or psychological pain.

6. Personality Disorders

These are lifelong patterns of behavior that are acceptable to the individual but produce conflict with others who interact with the individual. Some examples of character disorders are:

schizoid—emotionally cold and aloof; indifferent to praise or criticism, or to the feelings of others; few friendships.

paranoid—continually suspicious and mistrustful of other people; jealous and overly concerned with hidden motives of others; quick to take offense.

histrionic—emotional, immature, and dependent; irrational outbursts and tantrums; flamboyant and theatrical; having general dissatisfaction with themselves and angry feelings about the world.

antisocial—no loyalty or concern for others, and without moral standards; acts only in response to desires and impulses; cannot tolerate frustration and blames others when he is at fault.

passive-aggressive—shows aggressive feelings in passive ways, such as pouting, helplessness, stubbornness, obstructionism, and procrastination.

narcissistic—grandiose sense of self-importance or uniqueness and preoccupation with fantasies of success and power.

7. Organic Brain Syndromes

These are mental disturbances caused by or associated with illness such as strokes or tumors that affect the brain. Organic brain syndromes may produce the following symptoms:

Delirium. This disturbance involves disorientation, mental cloudiness, garbled thinking (dreamlike or nightmarish), visual **hallucinations** (false sensory perceptions), and abnormal emotions and mood (swinging from apathy to rage or sudden panic). The most common causes of delirium are head injury, fever, and drug intoxication or withdrawal, but it can also occur with a wide variety of infections, gland dysfunctions, and poisoning. **Delirium tremens** is a condition brought on by withdrawal after prolonged bouts of heavy alcohol ingestion.

Dementia. This syndrome is characterized by loss of memory and intelligence. The patient may have difficulty with learning, understanding, calculation, reasoning, and problem-solving, and may have lost the ability to make judgments. The most common causes are loss of blood supply to the brain due to blood vessel narrowing (arteriosclerosis) or clots. **Senile** (old-age) **dementia** occurs when there is progressive loss or atrophy of cells of the outer layer (gray matter) of the brain.

8. Schizophrenic Disorders

Schizophrenia is an important type of psychiatric disorder characterized by withdrawal from reality into an inner world of disorganized thinking and conflict. Some symptoms frequently present in schizophrenic patients are bizarre delusions, with no possible basis in fact, and auditory hallucinations in which the patient hears imaginary voices. Other symptoms are illogical thinking and incoherent speech. There also may be marked deterioration of the patient from a previous level of functioning in areas of work and social relations.

Types of schizophrenia described by physicians are: **disorganized type** (marked by frequent incoherence, indifferent or silly affect), **catatonic type** (marked by catatonic stupor in which the patient is mute and does not move or react to his environment), and **paranoid type** (marked by delusions of grandeur or persecution and hallucinations).

9. Paranoid Disorder

Individuals with paranoid disorder have persistent and unsubstantiated feelings of persecution and jealousy. Their symptoms are not as bizarre as those of a paranoid schizophrenic and their thinking is not incoherent. The term **paranoia** refers to a chronic state of persecutory delusions, lasting for many months.

10. Chronic Alcoholism

Excessive, long-term consumption of alcohol can lead to severe **addiction** (physical dependence on a habit) and to psychological symptoms such as hallucinations, amnesia, and paranoia, as well as physical ailments such as cirrhosis of the liver and brain damage. **Korsakoff's psychosis** is a condition that can result from chronic alcoholism. In this disorder, alcoholism leads to brain damage so that the patient is unable to remember and resorts to **confabulation** (lying).

11. Drug Dependence (Substance-Induced Disorders)

Continued or periodic administration of certain drugs produces a state of dependence. Two types of dependence occur: **psychological dependence** is a compulsion to continue taking a drug despite adverse consequences; **physical dependence** is indicated by the onset of symptoms when the drug is withdrawn abruptly. **Tolerance** is the declining effect of the drug so that the dose must be increased to give the same effect.

Some drugs that can lead to dependence and tolerance are:

Opioids. These drugs are derived from opium and can produce both physical and psychological dependence. Examples of opioids are **heroin**, **morphine**, **meperidine (Demerol)**,

dihydromorphinone (Dilaudid), **codeine**, and **methadone**. Typical symptoms of opioid intoxication are pupillary constriction, euphoria, slowness in movement, drowsiness, and slurred speech. Symptoms of opioid withdrawal (recent stoppage or reduction of opioid use) are tearing, rhinorrhea, pupillary dilation, abdominal cramps and diarrhea, and muscle and joint pain.

Sedatives. These drugs have a soothing or tranquilizing effect. Dependence, which can be both physical and psychological, is produced by **barbiturates** such as **phenobarbital**, **secobarbital**, and **amobarbital**. Other drugs which produce a barbiturate-like effect are **diazepam (Valium)**, **chlordiazepoxide (Librium)**, and **meprobamate (Miltown, Equanil)**. Intoxication is characterized by feelings of relaxation and euphoria ("high"), ataxia, confusion, disorientation, and depressed reflexes. Psychotic behavior can accompany withdrawal of the drug in a physically dependent person.

Cannabis (Marijuana). This drug and its derivatives come from the flowering tops and leaves of the hemp plant. Its effects depend upon the quantity consumed and the strength of the substance used. Normally, marijuana produces no physical dependence, but psychological dependence may occur. The most common effects of taking the drug are a "dreamy" state, euphoria, disjointed speech, and impairment of memory and judgment. High (toxic) doses may cause hallucinations and delusions or drowsiness and coma.

Amphetamine-Type Drugs. These central nervous system stimulants taken orally or intravenously ("speed") are **amphetamine (Benzedrine), dextroamphetamine (Dexedrine), methamphetamine (Desoxyn)**, and **phenmetrazine (Preludin)**. **Methylphenidate (Ritalin)** is not an amphetamine, but its action is similar. Amphetamines produce euphoria, impression of increased mental and physical energy, and decreased appetite (in some people). As tolerance develops with higher doses, depression and fatigue occur between doses. Judgment becomes faulty, and persecutory delusional ideas may develop, as well as visual and auditory hallucinations. Abrupt cessation of drug intake can result in somnolence and depression and, in some cases, suicide.

Cocaine. Cocaine is a stimulant drug that induces euphoria and hallucinations. It comes from the leaves of the coca tree in South America and has been used by native Indians to increase physical endurance. The drug is taken by sniffing or intravenous injection and users often combine cocaine with other drugs. A strong psychological dependence develops, but physical dependence, tolerance, and withdrawal symptoms do not occur. Symptoms of chronic use are persecutory delusions, anxiety, hallucinations, diarrhea, nausea, anorexia, and insomnia.

Hallucinogen-Type Drugs. These drugs produce a state of central nervous system excitement, hyperactivity, hallucinations, delusions, hypertension, and mood changes. Examples are **lysergic acid diethylamide (LSD)**, **mescaline (peyote)**, and **phencyclidine (PCP)**. While there is no evidence of physical or psychological dependence, these drugs have a high degree of **cross-tolerance** (use of one drug induces tolerance to another drug). Psychotic reactions such as depression and paranoia often occur after the drug experience.

Figure 21-3 reviews the various types of drug dependences.

III. PSYCHIATRIC SYMPTOMS

The following terms are often found in psychiatric literature and are used to describe abnormalities in behavior:

amnesia Loss of memory.

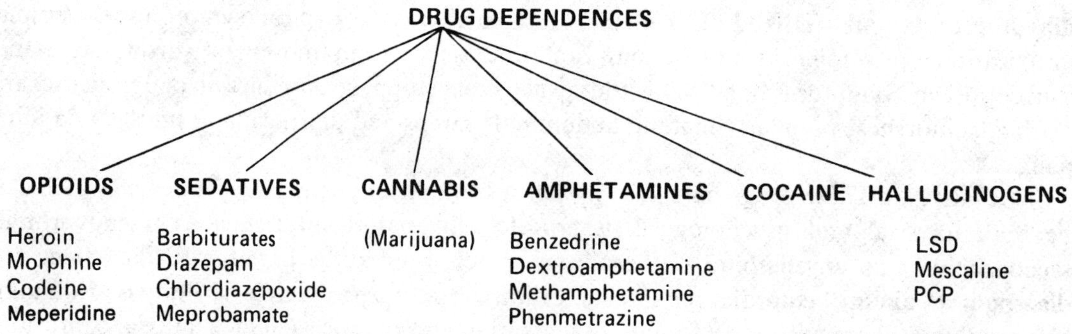

Figure 21-3

anxiety Troubled feelings, distress.

apathy Want of feeling; lack of interest or emotional involvement.

autism Pervasive lack of responsiveness to other people. If autism occurs in childhood accompanied by decreased language development, it is known as **infantile autism**.

compulsion Uncontrollable urge to perform an act repeatedly.

confabulation Lying; reciting imaginary experiences.

conversion An unconscious defense mechanism by which anxiety is converted into a bodily symptom.

cyclothymic State of exhibiting cycles of exhilaration and depression.

delusion A false belief or idea that cannot be changed by logical reasoning or evidence.

dissociation An unconscious defense mechanism by which uncomfortable feelings are separated from their real object and are redirected toward a second object or behavior pattern.

dysphoria Sadness, hopelessness, depressive mood.

euphoria Exaggerated feeling of well-being.

hallucination False or unreal sensory perception as, for example, hearing voices when none are present.

illusion False perception or misinterpretation of an actual sensory stimulus.

labile Unstable; undergoing rapid emotional change.

mania State of excessive excitability, hyperactivity, and agitation.

mutism Nonreactive state; stupor.

narcissism Self-love.

obsession Persistent idea, emotion, or urge.

paranoia Delusions of grandeur or persecution.

IV. THERAPEUTIC TERMINOLOGY

Some major therapeutic techniques for psychiatric disorders are **psychotherapy**, **electroshock therapy**, and **drug therapy**. A surgical procedure called **lobotomy** (also called leucotomy, prefrontal lobotomy, or transorbital lobotomy) is rarely used now. It involves severing some of the connections in the frontal lobes of the brain and was claimed to be effective in calming anxiety and aggressive behavior in schizophrenic patients.

Psychotherapy

This is the treatment of emotional problems by psychological techniques. The following are some of the many psychotherapeutic techniques used by both psychiatrists and psychologists.

Behavior Therapy. This type of therapy focuses on actual behavior patterns rather than on subconscious thoughts or feelings. It aims at improving symptoms and eliminating anxiety through **conditioning** (changing behavior and responses by training and repetition). Behavior therapy is used to treat phobias.

Group Therapy. A therapeutic method in which a group of patients discuss their problems and gain insight into their own personalities through these group discussions and interaction. **Psychodrama** is a form of group therapy in which patients express their feelings by acting roles along with other patient-actors on a stage. After a scene has been presented, the audience (composed of other patients) is asked to make comments and offer interpretations about what they have observed.

Play Therapy. Therapy in which a child, through play, uses toys to express conflicts and feelings which she or he is unable to communicate in a direct manner.

Hypnosis. In this therapy, a **trance** is created to increase the speed of psychotherapy or to help recovery of deeply repressed memories.

Psychoanalysis. Developed by Sigmund Freud, this long-term and intense form of psychotherapy seeks to influence behavior and resolve internal conflicts by allowing the patients to bring their unconscious emotions to the surface. Through techniques such as **free association** (speaking one's thoughts one after another without censorship), **transference** (relating to the therapist as one had done to a person who figured prominently in early childhood, such as a parent or sibling), and **dream interpretation**, the patient is able to bring to awareness his unconscious emotional conflicts and thus can overcome these problems.

Family Therapy. An entire family meets regularly with a therapist in order to resolve and understand their conflicts and problems.

Sex Therapy. This form of therapy helps individuals to overcome sexual dysfunctions such as **frigidity** (inhibited sexual response in women), **impotence** (inability of man to achieve erection), and **premature ejaculation** (release of semen before coitus can be achieved).

Electroshock Therapy

An electric current applied to the brain produces convulsions (involuntary muscular contractions) and sometimes unconsciousness. This treatment is used chiefly for serious depression. With the introduction of drug therapy, there are fewer indications for electroshock therapy.

Drug Therapy

Many agents are used to relieve the symptoms of psychiatric disorders. Some of these are:

Antianxiety Agents. These drugs (minor tranquilizers and sedatives) lessen anxiety. Examples are **diazepam (Valium)**, **chlordiazepoxide (Librium)**, and **barbiturates**.

Phenothiazines. These are **antipsychotic tranquilizers (neuroleptic drugs)** which can reduce excitement and control hostile and aggressive behavior in psychotic (schizophrenic) patients. Examples are **chlorpromazine (Thorazine)**, and **thioridazine (Mellaril)**.

Lithium. Lithium carbonate is used in the control of the manic phase of manic-depressive illness.

Antidepressants. These drugs are used to reverse depressive symptoms and produce feelings of well-being. Three examples of antidepressant drugs are:

Tricyclic antidepressants—synthetic drugs that resemble the antipsychotic tranquilizers and are commonly used in the treatment of severe depression. Examples are **amitriptyline (Elavil)**, **imipramine (Trofranil)**, and **protriptyline (Vivactil)**.

Monoamine oxidase (MAO) inhibitors—drugs that are used in depressed patients who do not respond to tricyclic antidepressants. They inhibit an enzyme (monoamine oxidase) that is important in breaking down neurotransmitters, such as norepinephrine and tyramine. An example of an MAO inhibitor is phenelzine (Nardil). The use of MAO inhibitors requires that numerous medications (those that increase blood pressure) and foods (those high in tyramine) be avoided so that a hypertensive crisis does not occur.

Amphetamines—these antidepressants produce mood elevation and are central nervous system stimulants. They are also used to reduce appetite in obese patients and for treatment of hyperkinetic children.

Figure 21-4 reviews the different types of drug therapies for psychiatric disorders.

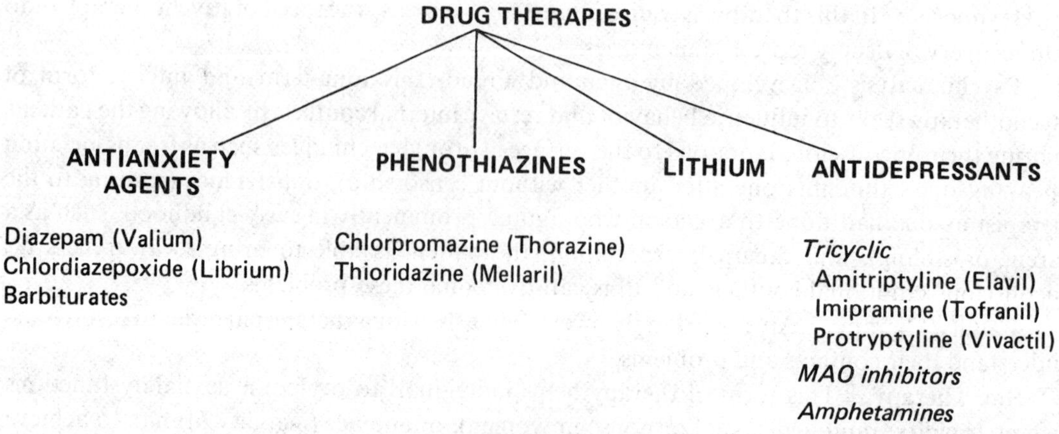

Figure 21-4

V. VOCABULARY

affect	The emotional reactions of a patient.
affective disorders	Disorders of mood.
alcoholism	Excessive dependence on alcohol.
amphetamines	Central nervous system stimulants; chronic, heavy use can lead to hallucinations, psychoses, and dependence.
anorexia nervosa	A psychosomatic eating disorder marked by excessive dieting and distortion of body image.
anxiety disorders	Mental disorders marked by troubled feelings, unpleasant tension, and distress.
behavior therapy	Psychotherapy focusing on actual behavior rather than on unconscious thoughts.
bipolar disorder	Frequent, intermixed periods of mania and depression.
bulimia	A psychosomatic eating disorder characterized by binge eating followed by vomiting and depression.
cocaine	A stimulant drug that causes euphoria and hallucinatory experiences.
conversion disorder	A condition in which physical symptoms appear as a defense against overwhelming anxiety and an unconscious conflict.
cyclothymic disorder	An affective disorder marked by alternating periods of elation and depression.
defense mechanism	An unconscious technique a person might use to resolve or conceal conflicts and anxiety.
delirium	Confusion in thinking; an organic brain syndrome marked by faulty perceptions and irrational behavior.
delirium tremens	An acute psychotic state that occurs during alcohol withdrawal.
depression	A major affective disorder marked by severe dysphoria, loss of energy, slowness in thinking, and possible psychotic features.
dementia	An organic brain syndrome marked by loss of higher mental functioning, judgment, and reasoning.
dissociative disorder	A condition marked by mental symptoms that hide the anxiety of unconscious conflicts.

dysthymic disorder An affective disorder with depressive periods and mood.

ego The conscious, coordinating element of the personality; it modifies and compromises between the id and the superego.

electroshock therapy A form of psychiatric treatment in which an electric current produces a convulsive seizure and unconsciousness; also called electroconvulsive treatment.

forensic psychiatry The legal aspects of psychiatry.

free association Psychoanalytic technique devised by Freud in which the patient verbalizes, without censorship, the passing contents of his mind.

group therapy A type of psychotherapy in which a group is used as the principal therapeutic agent.

hallucinogens Drugs that produce hallucinations.

hypnosis A therapist induces a trancelike state of altered consciousness to increase the pace of psychotherapy.

hypochondriasis Exaggerated concern with one's physical health.

id The major unconscious part of the personality; composed of energy that comes from instinctual drives and desires.

involutional melancholia Depression occurring in late or middle age, characterized by insomnia, anxiety, and sometimes paranoid ideas.

Korsakoff's psychosis A psychotic syndrome (confusion, amnesia, disorientation, confabulation) usually associated with alcoholism.

lithium A substance used to treat the manic stage of manic-depressive illness.

lobotomy A neurosurgical procedure in which cerebral nerve tracts are severed to treat hostility and aggression in schizophrenic patients. Not in current use.

manic-depressive illness A major affective disorder in which there are severe changes of mood (mania and depression).

marijuana Dried leaves and flowers from the hemp plant; produces physical and psychological changes when smoked in sufficient quantity.

monoamine oxidase (MAO) inhibitors Agents that inhibit the enzyme monoamine oxidase and are used as antidepressants.

neuroleptic drugs Drugs used to treat psychoses; phenothiazines.

neurosis	A mental disorder characterized by irrational anxiety. This term is used less frequently recently; it has been replaced by terms such as affective, somatoform, dissociative, and anxiety disorders.
opioids	Drugs (derived from opium) that can produce both physical and psychological dependence. Examples are heroin, morphine, and codeine.
organic brain syndromes	Mental symptoms caused by impaired brain function.
paranoid disorder	Condition in which patients have persistent delusions of persecution and jealousy.
personality disorder	A lifelong personality pattern which may be acceptable to the individual, but presents conflict with others.
phenothiazines	Antipsychotic tranquilizers.
phobia	An irrational fear of an object or situation.
physical dependence	A state in which severe symptoms occur when use of a drug is withdrawn abruptly.
play therapy	Use of toys and a playroom setting to enable a child to express feelings and conflicts.
psychoanalysis	A psychotherapy that allows the patient to explore inner (unconscious) emotions in an effort to understand and change current behavior.
psychodrama	A form of group therapy in which a patient expresses feelings by acting out roles with other patients.
psychological dependence	Compulsion to continue taking a drug despite adverse consequences.
psychosis	Severe mental disorder in which the patient withdraws from reality into an inner world of disorganized thinking and feeling.
psychosexual disorders	Disorders involving sexual deviation or gender identity.
psychosomatic	Pertaining to interrelationship of mind and body.
reality testing	The ability to perceive fact from fantasy; severely impaired in psychoses.
repression	A defense mechanism by which unacceptable thoughts, feelings, and impulses are pushed into the unconscious.
schizophrenia	A psychosis involving delusions, hallucinations, and bizarre and illogical thinking.
sedatives	Drugs that lessen anxiety.

senile dementia	Dementia occurring in old age.
sex therapy	Treatment in which physical and psychological methods are used to treat sexual disorders.
somatoform disorders	Disorders in which the patient has physical symptoms that cannot be explained by any actual physical disorder.
superego	Internalized conscience and moral part of the personality.
tolerance	The development of insensitivity to a drug. Increasing doses of a drug are needed to produce the desired effect.
transference	Psychoanalytic process in which the patient relates to the therapist as he or she had done to a prominent childhood figure.
tricyclic antidepressants	A class of drugs used to treat severe depression.

VI. COMBINING FORMS AND TERMINOLOGY

Combining Form	*Definition*	*Terminology*	*Meaning*
psych/o	mind	psychologist	______________
ment/o	mind	mental	______________
phren/o	mind	schizophrenia *schiz/o means split*	______________
somat/o	body	psychosomatic	______________
aut/o	self	autism	______________
iatr/o	treatment	psychiatrist	______________
-thymia	mind	cyclothymia *cycl/o means circle*	______________
		dysthymia	______________
-phobia	fear	xenophobia *xen- means stranger*	______________
		gamophobia *gam- means marriage*	______________

-phoria	feeling	dysphoria ______________
		euphoria ______________
-mania	obsessive preoccupation	pyromania ______________ *pyr/o means fire*
		kleptomania ______________ *klept/o means to steal*
-kinesia	movement	hyperkinesia ______________
-genic	produced by	psychogenic ______________
-pathy	emotion, diseased condition	apathy ______________
		sympathy ______________
-somnia	sleep	insomnia ______________
para-	abnormal	paranoia ______________ *no- comes from the Greek word "nous" meaning mind*
dys-	difficult	dyskinesia ______________
cata-	down	catatonic ______________ *ton- means tension*

VII. ABBREVIATIONS

C.A.	Chronological age
CNS	Central nervous system
DT	Delirium tremens
ECT	Electroconvulsive therapy
EST	Electroshock therapy
I.Q.	Intelligence quotient. The average person is considered to have an I.Q. of between 90 and 110. Those who score below 70 are considered mentally retarded
LSD	Lysergic acid diethylamide (hallucinogen)
MAO	Monoamine oxidase
M.A.	Mental age (as determined by psychological tests)
MMPI	Minnesota Multiphasic Personality Inventory
OBS	Organic brain syndrome
TAT	Thematic Apperception Test
WAIS	Wechsler Adult Intelligence Test
WISC	Wechsler Intelligence Scale for Children

VIII. PRACTICAL APPLICATIONS

Drug Description: Amitriptyline (Elavil)

Amitriptyline is an antidepressant with antianxiety action and has a sedative component. Its precise mechanism of action is unknown; it is not a monoamine oxidase inhibitor and does not act primarily by stimulating the central nervous system.

Indications: Used for relief of symptoms of depression.

Preparations: Tablets: 10, 25, 50, 75, 100, and 150 mg. Sterile solution for intramuscular injection.

Dosage: The initial daily dosage for adults is 75 mg in divided doses, which may be increased to 150 if necessary. An adequate response may take 30 days to develop. Maintenance dosage is 50 to 100 mg daily.

Contraindications and Precautions: This drug is contraindicated in patients with known hypersensitivity. Also, it should not be used concomitantly with MAO inhibitors. (Wait 14 days between the last dose of an MAO inhibitor if Elavil is being started.) Elavil is contraindicated during the acute recovery phase following myocardial infarction.

Adverse Reactions: Adverse reactions include side effects affecting the central nervous system (drowsiness, confusion, delusions, hallucinations, paresthesias of the extremities, ataxia, tinnitus, headache, insomnia), the cardiovascular system (arrhythmias, hypotension, myocardial infarction, palpitations), the gastrointestinal system (nausea, epigastric distress, vomiting, anorexia, stomatitis, diarrhea, parotid swelling, hepatitis), the hematologic system (myelosuppression, including leukopenia, eosinophilia, purpura, thrombocytopenia), the endocrinologic system (testicular swelling and gynecomastia in males, breast enlargement and galactorrhea in females), as well as anticholinergic effects (dry mouth, increased intraocular pressure, paralytic ileus, urinary retention) and allergic reactions (skin rash, urticaria, edema of face and tongue, photosensitization).

Drug Interactions: Elavil may block the antihypertensive action of guanethidine (Ismelin) and other similar drugs and enhance the response to alcohol and the effects of barbiturates and other CNS depressants.

Catatonic Schizophrenia: Case Report

A young, unmarried woman, aged 20, was admitted to a psychiatric hospital because she had become violent toward her parents, had been observed gazing into space with a rapt expression, and had been talking to invisible persons. She had been seen to strike odd poses. Her speech had become incoherent. The patient received voice messages telling her to do certain things. Then, pictures began to appear on the wall, most of them ugly and sneering. These pictures had names—one was named shyness, another distress, another envy.

The patient was agitated and noisy and uncooperative in the hospital for several weeks after she arrived, and she required sedation. She was given several courses of electroconvulsive treatment, which failed to influence the schizophrenic process to any significant degree. Ten years later, when neuroleptic drugs became available, she received pharmacotherapy.

Despite therapeutic efforts, her condition throughout her many years of stay in a mental hospital has remained one of chronic catatonic stupor. She is mute and practically devoid of any spontaneity, but she responds to simple requests. She stays in the same position for many hours or sits in a chair in a curled up position. Her facial expression is fixed and stony.

IX. EXERCISES

A. Give meanings for the following terms:

1. psychiatrist ________________
2. psychologist ________________
3. psychoanalyst ________________
4. forensic psychiatry ________________
5. id ________________
6. ego ________________
7. superego ________________
8. reality testing ________________
9. defense mechanism ________________
10. clinical psychology ________________

B. Name seven tests used by clinical psychologists to evaluate various aspects of a person's mental health:

1. ________________
2. ________________
3. ________________
4. ________________
5. ________________
6. ________________
7. ________________

C. *Give the meanings for the following terms:*

1. psychosis ______
2. neurosis ______
3. affective disorders ______
4. manic-depressive illness ______
5. major depression ______
6. cyclothymic disorder ______
7. dysthymic disorder ______
8. involutional melancholia ______
9. bipolar disorder ______
10. dysphoric mood ______

D. *Identify the anxiety disorder:*

1. Irrational fear associated with a specific situation or stimulus ______

   ______

2. Recurrent thoughts and repetitive acts dominate the patient's behavior

   ______

3. Episodes of apprehension and fear that are not associated with fear of a specific object or situation ______
4. Recollecting the experience of a serious traumatic event ______

E. *Give meanings for the following terms:*

1. somatoform disorders ______
2. conversion disorder ______
3. repression ______
4. amnesia ______

5. hypochondriasis ______

6. dissociative disorders ______

7. multiple personality ______

8. fugue ______

9. agoraphobia ______

10. acrophobia ______

11. anorexia nervosa ______

12. bulimia ______

F. *Describe the following psychosexual disorders:*

1. voyeurism ______

2. transvestism ______

3. transsexualism ______

4. sexual sadism ______

5. fetishism ______

6. exhibitionism ______

7. sexual masochism ______

G. *Name the personality disorder from its description below:*

1. No loyalty or concern for others; does not tolerate frustration and blames others when he or she is at fault ______

2. Fantasies of success and power, and grandiose sense of self-importance ______

3. Flamboyant, theatrical, emotionally immature ______

4. Pervasive, unwarranted suspiciousness and mistrust of people ______

5. Stubbornness, obstructionism, and procrastination are used to show aggressive feelings ______

6. Emotionally cold, aloof, indifferent to praise or criticism or to the feelings of others ______

H. *Give the meanings of the following terms:*

1. Organic brain syndromes ______
2. Delirium ______
3. Dementia ______
4. Delirium tremens ______
5. Senile dementia ______
6. Schizophrenic disorders ______
7. Disorganized schizophrenia ______
8. Catatonic schizophrenia ______
9. Paranoid schizophrenia ______
10. Paranoid disorder ______
11. Paranoia ______
12. Chronic alcoholism ______
13. Korsakoff's psychosis ______
14. Confabulation ______

I. *Give answers for the following:*

1. What is psychological drug dependence? ______
2. What is physical drug dependence? ______
3. Explain tolerance to a drug. ______
4. What are opioids? ______

5. Give three examples of opioids. ______

6. What are amphetamines? ______

7. Give three examples of amphetamines. ______

8. What are hallucinogens? ______

9. Give two examples of hallucinogens. ______

10. What are sedatives? ______

11. Give three examples of sedative-type drugs. ______

12. What is cocaine? ______

13. What is marijuana? ______

14. What is cross-tolerance? ______

J. Name the psychiatric symptom from its description below:

1. Uncontrollable urge to perform an act repeatedly ______

2. Feelings of sadness and hopelessness ______

3. Delusions of grandeur or persecution ______

4. Self-love ______

5. Pervasive lack of responsiveness to other people ______

6. A false belief or idea ______

7. A false or unreal perception, as hearing voices when none are present ______

______

8. A persistent idea, emotion, or urge ______

9. Anxiety is converted into a bodily symptom ______

10. Exaggerated feeling of well-being ______

11. A false perception or misinterpretation of actual sensory stimuli ______

______

12. Nonreactive state; stupor ______________________

13. Unstable; undergoing rapid emotional change ______________________

14. Lack of interest in or emotional involvement with others ______________________

K. *Identify the psychotherapeutic technique:*

1. Patients express their feelings by acting out roles on stage ______________________

2. A state of semiconsciousness helps the recovery of deeply repressed feelings ______________________

3. Long-term individual exploration of unconscious feelings ______________________

4. Therapy involves toys that a child uses to express conflicts and feelings ______________________

5. Therapy aims at changing actual behavior patterns rather than focusing on subconscious thoughts and feelings ______________________

6. Therapists use techniques to help people overcome sexual dysfunctions ______________________

7. Speaking one's thoughts without censorship ______________________

8. Relating to the therapist as one had done to a person in one's childhood ______________________

9. Convulsions are produced to reverse serious depressive states ______________________

L. *Give the meanings for the following terms:*

1. MAO inhibitors ______________________

2. phenothiazines ______________________

3. lithium ______________________

4. tricyclic antidepressants ______________________

5. antianxiety drugs ______________________

M. Give the meanings for the following combining forms or suffixes:

1. iatr/o ____________________
2. phren/o ____________________
3. somat/o ____________________
4. ment/o ____________________
5. cycl/o ____________________
6. -mania ____________________
7. -phoria ____________________
8. -phobia ____________________
9. -thymia ____________________
10. -kinesia ____________________
11. -somnia ____________________

N. Give meanings for the following terms:

1. dyskinesia ____________________
2. euphoria ____________________
3. claustrophobia ____________________
4. kleptomania ____________________
5. apathy ____________________
6. pyromania ____________________
7. psychosomatic ____________________
8. xenophobia ____________________
9. insomnia ____________________
10. hallucinogenic ____________________

O. Give meanings for the following abbreviations:

1. WAIS ____________________
2. ECT ____________________
3. MMPI ____________________
4. TAT ____________________
5. OBS ____________________

6. DT ______________________________

7. C.A. ______________________________

8. M.A. ______________________________

ANSWERS

A.

1. A physician who specializes in the treatment, diagnosis, and prevention of mental illness.
2. One who is trained in methods of psychological therapy, analysis, and research.
3. One who practices psychoanalysis; a psychiatrist or a psychologist.
4. A branch of psychiatry dealing with legal matters.
5. Major unconscious part of the personality; composed of instinctual drives and desires.
6. The conscious, coordinating branch of the personality; mediates between the id (instinct and drives) and the superego (internal moral and social prohibitions).
7. Internalized conscience or moral part of the personality.
8. The ability to perceive fact from fantasy.
9. Unconscious technique a person employs to ward off anxiety or conceal conflicts.
10. A branch of psychology dealing with patient care.

B.

1. Wechsler Adult Intelligence Scale
2. Stanford-Binet Intelligence Scale
3. Rorschach technique
4. Thematic Apperception Test
5. Draw a Person Test
6. Bender-Gestalt Test
7. Minnesota Multiphasic Personality Inventory

C.

1. A severe mental disorder in which the patient withdraws from reality into a world of disorganized thinking and feeling. Delusions and hallucinations are common.
2. A mental disorder characterized by irrational anxiety; reality testing is not impaired and psychotic symptoms (delusions and hallucinations) are absent.
3. Disorders of mood.
4. An affective disorder in which there are severe changes in mood from mania to depression.
5. A condition marked by severe dysphoria, loss of energy, slowness in thinking; psychotic features are sometimes present.
6. An affective disorder marked by alternating periods of elation (mania) and depression; psychotic features are absent.
7. An affective disorder involving depressive mood but not as severe or of as long duration as a major depressive episode. Psychotic features such as delusions, hallucinations, and incoherence are absent.
8. Depression occurring in late or middle age; characterized by anxiety, insomnia, and often paranoid ideas.
9. Frequent, intermixed periods of mania and depression; depressive mood is prominent.
10. Characterized by overwhelming sadness and hopelessness.

D.

1. Phobia.
2. Obsessive-compulsive disorder.
3. Panic disorder.
4. Post-traumatic stress disorder.

E.

1. Disorders in which the patient's mental conflicts are expressed as physical symptoms.
2. A somatoform disorder in which the predominant disturbance is a loss of physical functioning.
3. A defense mechanism in which a person removes unacceptable ideas and impulses from consciousness.
4. Loss of memory.
5. A somatoform disorder in which the patient is preoccupied with bodily aches, pains, and discomforts.
6. These disorders involve mental symptoms that mask the anxiety of an unconscious conflict.
7. A dissociative disorder in which there exist two or more distinct personalities in one individual.
8. A dissociative disorder in which the patient suddenly leaves home or work and is unable to recall recent past events.
9. Fear of public places from which escape might not be possible.
10. Fear of heights.
11. Eating disorder marked by excessive dieting and distortion of body image.
12. Binge eating followed by vomiting and depression.

F.

1. An abnormal desire to look at sexual organs or acts.
2. Dressing in clothes of the opposite sex.
3. Desire to change one's sex.
4. Achievement of sexual pleasure by inflicting physical or psychological pain.
5. Achievement of sexual pleasure by substituting an inanimate object for a human love object.
6. Compulsive need to expose one's body, particularly the genital organs.
7. Achievement of sexual pleasure from suffering physical or psychological pain.

G.

1. Antisocial.
2. Narcissistic.
3. Histrionic.
4. Paranoid.
5. Passive-aggressive.
6. Schizoid.

H.

1. Mental disturbances caused by or associated with illness such as stroke or tumors that affect the brain.
2. Disorientation, mental cloudiness, garbled thinking, visual hallucinations, and abnormal emotions (violent mood swings).
3. Loss of memory and intelligence due to lack of adequate blood supply to the brain.
4. A condition of delirium brought on by withdrawal after prolonged ingestion of alcohol.
5. Dementia that occurs with old age.
6. Disorders that are characterized by withdrawal from reality, delusions, hallucinations, and illogical and incoherent thinking.
7. This type of schizophrenia is marked by an indifferent or silly affect and frequent incoherence.
8. This type of schizophrenia is marked by stupor and mutism.
9. Paranoid schizophrenics have persistent delusions of grandeur or persecution and hallucinations.
10. A condition in which the patient has persecutory delusions or jealousy with none of the major psychotic symptoms (bizarre, delusions, incoherence of thinking and speech, hallucinations) of paranoid schizophrenics.
11. A chronic state of persecutory delusions, lasting at least 6 months.
12. Excessive, long-term consumption of alcohol.
13. A psychotic condition that results from chronic alcoholism.
14. Lying; reciting falsehoods.

I.

1. A compulsion to continue taking a drug despite adverse consequences.
2. The onset of physical symptoms when a drug is withdrawn abruptly.
3. The declining effect of the drug so that the dose must be increased to give the same effect.
4. Drugs derived from opium.
5. Heroin, morphine, and codeine.
6. Central nervous system stimulants that produce euphoria and an impression of increased mental and physical energy.
7. Benzedrine, dextroamphetamine, and methamphetamine.
8. Drugs that produce hallucinations, hyperactivity, delusions, and mood changes.
9. Lysergic acid diethylamide (LSD) and phencyclidine (PCP).
10. Sedatives are drugs that produce an overall soothing and tranquilizing effect.
11. Barbiturates, diazepam (Valium), and chlordiazepoxide (Librium).
12. A stimulant drug that induces euphoria and hallucinations.
13. A drug that produces a euphoric "dreamy" state, disjointed speech, and some impairment of memory; comes from the tops and leaves of the hemp plant, Cannabis.
14. A condition in which the use of one drug induces tolerance to another drug.

J.

1. Compulsion
2. Dysphoria
3. Paranoia
4. Narcissism
5. Autism
6. Delusion
7. Hallucination
8. Obsession
9. Conversion
10. Euphoria
11. Illusion
12. Mutism
13. Labile
14. Apathy

K.

1. Psychodrama
2. Hypnosis
3. Psychoanalysis
4. Play therapy
5. Behavioral therapy
6. Sex therapy
7. Free association
8. Transference
9. Electroshock or electroconvulsive treatment

L.

1. Drugs used to alleviate depressive symptoms; they inhibit the enzyme monoamine oxidase.
2. Antipsychotic tranquilizers that control hostile and aggressive behavior in psychotic patients.
3. A drug used to control symptoms of patients in the manic phase of manic-depressive illness.
4. Synthetic drugs used in the treatment of severe depression.
5. Minor tranquilizers and sedatives that lessen anxiety.

M.

1. Treatment
2. Mind
3. Body
4. Mind
5. Cycle
6. Obsessive preoccupation
7. Feeling
8. Fear
9. Mind
10. Movement
11. Sleep

N.

1. Difficult movement.
2. Good feeling; "high."
3. Fear of being closed in.
4. Obsessive preoccupation with stealing.
5. Lack of feeling; little emotional involvement.
6. Obsessive preoccupation with fire.
7. Pertaining to the mind and body; illness in which some part of the etiology is due to emotional factors.
8. Fear of strangers.
9. Inability to sleep.
10. Pertaining to producing hallucinations.

O.

1. Wechsler Adult Intelligence Test.
2. Electroconvulsive therapy.
3. Minnesota Multiphasic Personality Inventory.
4. Thematic Apperception Test.
5. Organic Brain Syndrome.
6. Delirium tremens.
7. Chronological age.
8. Mental age.

X. PRONUNCIATION OF TERMS

acrophobia	ăk-rō-FŌ-bē-ă
affect	ĂF-fĕkt
agoraphobia	ăg-ŏ-ră-FŌ-bē-ă
amnesia	ăm-NĒ-zē-ă
amphetamine	ăm-FĔT-ă-mēn
anorexia nervosa	ăn-ō-RĔK-sē-ă nĕr-VŌ-să
apathy	ĂP-ă-thē
autism	ĂW-tĭzm
bulimia	bū-LĒ-mē-ă
catatonic	kăt-ă-TŎN-ĭk
claustrophobia	klaws-trō-FŌ-bē-ă
compulsion	kŏm-PŬL-shŭn
confabulation	kŏn-făb-ū-LĀ-shŭn
conversion	kŏn-VĔR-zhŭn
cyclothymic	sī-klō-THĪ-mĭk
delirium	dĕ-LĬR-ē-ŭm
delirium tremens	dĕ-LĬR-ē-ŭm TRĔ-mĕnz
delusion	dĕ-LŪ-zhŭn

dementia	dē-MĔN-shē-ă
dipsomania	dĭp-sō-MĀ-nē-ă
dissociation	dĭs-sō-sē-Ā-shŭn
dyskinesia	dĭs-kĭ-NĒ-zē-ă
dysthymic	dĭs-THĪ-mĭk
ego	Ē-gō
euphoria	ū-FŎR-ē-ă
fetishism	FĔT-ĭsh-ĭzm
forensic	fŏ-RĔN-sĭk
fugue	fūg
gamophobia	găm-ō-FŌ-bē-ă
hallucination	hă-lū-sĭ-NĀ-shŭn
hallucinogen	hă-LŪ-sĭ-nō-jĕn
hypnosis	hĭp-NŌ-sĭs
hypochondriasis	hī-pō-kŏn-DRĪ-ă-sĭs
id	ĭd
illusion	ĭ-LŪ-zhŭn
involutional melancholia	ĭn-vō-LŪ-shŭn-ăl mĕl-ăn-KŌ-lē-ă
Korsakoff's psychosis	KŎR-să-kŏfs sī-KŌ-sĭs
labile	LĀ-bīl
lobotomy	lō-BŎT-ō-mē
mania	MĀ-nē-ă
marijuana	măr-ĭ-HWĂ-nă
masochism	MĂS-ō-kĭzm
mutism	MŪ-tĭzm
narcissism	NĂR-sĭ-sĭzm
opioid	Ō-pē-ŏyd
paranoia	păr-ă-NOY-ă
paranoid	PĂR-ă-noyd
phenothiazines	fē-nō-THĪ-ă-zēnz
psychiatry	sī-KĪ-ă-trē
psychoanalysis	sī-kō-ă-NĂL-ĭ-sĭs

psychosomatic	sī-kō-sō-MĂT-ĭk
pyromania	pī-rō-MĀ-nē-ă
sadism	SĀ-dĭzm
schizoid	SKĬZ-ŏyd or SKĬT-sŏyd
schizophrenia	skĭz-ō-FRĒ-nē-ă or skĭt-sō-FRĒ-nē-ă
senile dementia	SĒ-nīl dē-MĔN-shē-ă
transvestism	trăns-VĔS-tĭzm
voyeurism	VOY-yĕr-ĭzm
xenophobia	zĕn-ō-FŌ-bē-ă

REVIEW SHEET 21

Combining Forms

aut/o ____________________

gam/o ____________________

iatr/o ____________________

ment/o ____________________

phren/o ____________________

psych/o ____________________

pyr/o ____________________

schiz/o ____________________

somat/o ____________________

xen/o ____________________

Suffixes

-genic ____________________

-kinesia ____________________

-mania ____________________

-pathy ____________________

-phobia ____________________

-phoria ____________________

-somnia ____________________

Prefixes

anti- ____________________

cata- ____________________

dys- ____________________

para- ____________________

Additional Terms

affect (651)

affective disorders (651)

amnesia (647)

amphetamines (651)

anorexia nervosa (651)

anxiety disorders (651)

apathy (648)

autism (648)

behavior therapy (651)

bulimia (651)

cocaine (651)

compulsion (648)

confabulation (648)

conversion disorder (651)

cyclothymic disorder (651)

defense mechanism (651)

delirium (651)

delirium tremens (651)

delusion (648)

dementia (651)

depression (651)

dissociation disorder (651)

dysphoria (648)

dysthymic disorder (652)

ego (652)

electroshock therapy (652)

euphoria (648)

exhibitionism (645)

fetishism (645)

forensic psychiatry (652)

free association (652)

fugue (645)

group therapy (652)

hallucination (648)

hallucinogens (652)

hypnotherapy (649)

hypochondriasis (652)

id (652)

illusion (648)

involutional melancholia (652)

Korsakoff's psychosis (652)

labile (648)

lithium (652)

mania (649)

manic-depressive illness (652)

marijuana (652)

monoamine oxidase inhibitors (652)

multiple personality (645)

mutism (649)

narcissism (649)

neurosis (653)

obsession (649)

opioids (653)

organic brain syndrome (653)

paranoid disorder (653)

personality disorder (653)

phenothiazines (653)

psychoanalysis (653)

psychosis (653)

reality testing (653)

repression (653)

schizophrenia (653)

sedatives (653)

senile dementia (654)

sexual sadism (645)

somatoform disorders (654)

superego (654)

tolerance (654)

transference (654)

transsexualism (645)

transvestism (645)

tricyclic antidepressants (654)

voyeurism (645)

CHAPTER 22

ANALYSIS OF A MEDICAL PAPER

In this chapter you will:

- Gain practice in reading and understanding the medical language in context;
- Acquire knowledge of the anatomy and physiology of the lymphatic system in the body; and
- Find the meanings for combining forms, prefixes, and suffixes, and use them in building and giving the meaning of medical terms.

This chapter is divided into the following sections:

I. Introduction: Background Information
II. Terminology: Combining Forms, Suffixes, and Prefixes
III. Clinical Paper: *Shaking Chills Related to Occult Lymphoma*
IV. Questions about the Paper
V. Exercises
VI. Pronunciation of Terms

I. INTRODUCTION: BACKGROUND INFORMATION

The clinical medical paper included in this chapter describes the course of an illness called **lymphosarcoma**. The term lymph/o/sarc/oma is analyzed in the following manner:

-oma = **tumor**. A tumor is a new growth, or **neoplasm**. (**Neo** is a prefix meaning new, and **-plasm** is a suffix meaning formation or growth.)

lymph/o = **lymph**. Lymph is a clear fluid which is formed in all body tissues. Lymph flows from tissue spaces into small channels called lymph vessels which then lead through filters called lymph nodes (glands) and into special veins in the neck and chest where the lymph enters the bloodstream (Figure 22-1). Major sites of lymph node concentration are the **axillary** (armpit), **cervical** (neck), and **inguinal** (groin) regions of the body.

sarc/o = **flesh**. The root **sarc** indicates that this is a special type of tumor, a "flesh tumor." This means that the tumor, or new growth, originated from connective tissue, such as lymph, fat, muscle, and blood.

A lymphosarcoma, then, is a flesh tumor of the lymph nodes. Sarcomas, as well as carcinomas, are **malignant** tumors. Reviewing material already presented in Chapter 18, Cancer Medicine (Oncology), malignant (mal = bad) means that the tumor grows rapidly and may eventually display **metastasis** (meta = beyond; stasis = stopping, control). Metastasis means that the tumor spreads from its primary location to secondary sites around the body. Hence, the tumor is literally "beyond control." A **benign** (bene = good) tumor is slow growing and does not metastasize. Benign tumors are limited in extent and often are surrounded by a capsule. An example of a benign tumor is a thyroid adenoma.

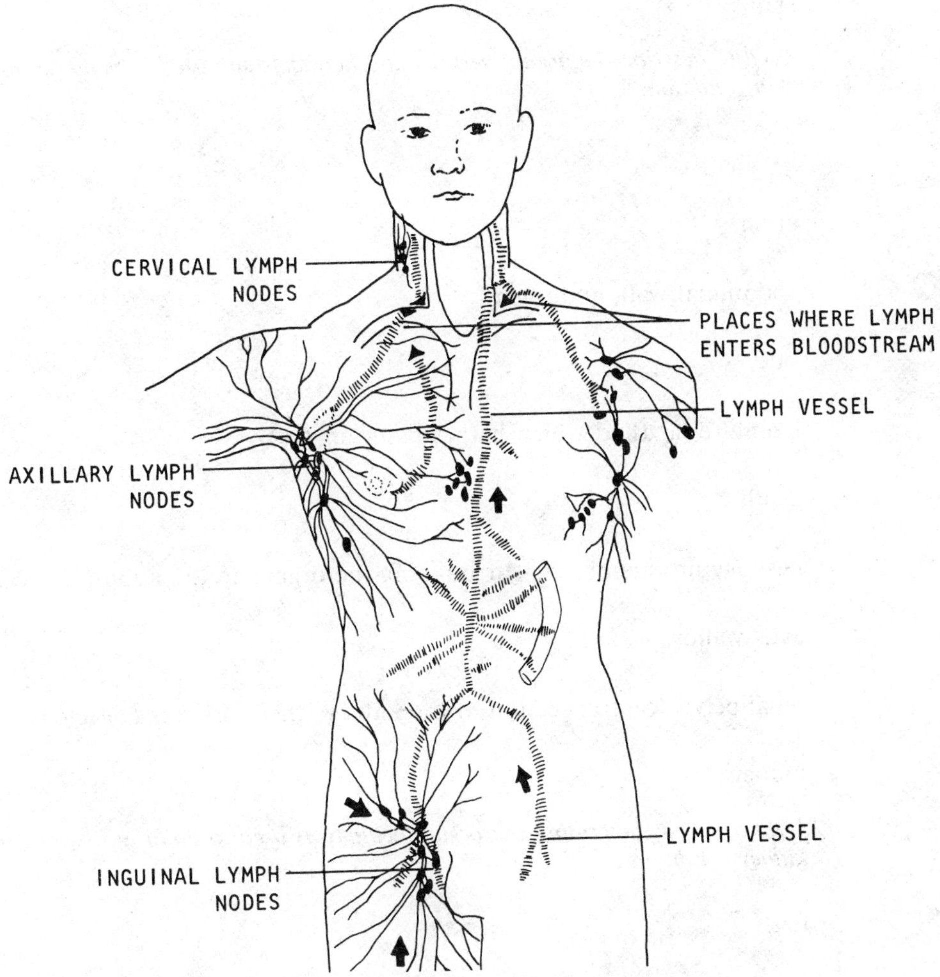

Figure 22-1 Lymph seeps out of tiny blood vessels, bathes the tissue spaces, and enters tiny branches of lymph vessels. It then flows through the lymph nodes into the bloodstream. Most of the lymph enters the bloodstream through veins in the left and right upper chest regions of the body.

II. TERMINOLOGY

Use this list as a guide as you explore the medical paper that follows.

Combining Forms

abdomin/o	abdomen
aden/o	gland
angi/o	vessel
axill/o	armpit
cervic/o	neck *Cervic/o can mean the neck of the body or the neck (cervix) of the uterus (womb).*

cutane/o — skin

Used to describe the organ; derm/o and dermat/o are used to build words about skin conditions.

hepat/o — liver

inguin/o — groin

lapar/o — abdominal wall, abdomen

later/o — side

lymph/o — lymph (clear fluid which bathes tissue spaces)

necr/o — death

peritone/o — peritoneum (membrane surrounding the organs in the abdominal cavity)

phag/o — eat, swallow

pyel/o — renal pelvis (central section of the kidney where urine is collected)

ren/o — kidney

Used in words describing the organ; nephr/o is used to build most words about kidney conditions.

sarc/o — flesh

thromb/o — clot

tom/o — to cut

ureter/o — ureters (tubes carrying urine from kidneys to bladder)

urin/o — urine

ven/o — vein

Suffixes

-crit — to separate

-gram — record

-lysis — to break down, destroy, separate out

-megaly — enlargement

-osis	abnormal condition (in blood cells, an increase in number)
-ous	pertaining to
-pathy	disease process
-plasia	condition expressing growth, formation
-plasm	growth, formation
-penia	decreased number (of blood cells)
-stasis	control, stop
-tomy	incision, to cut into
-um	a thing (noun ending)
-us	a thing (noun ending)

Prefixes

ana-	up, apart
bi-	two
endo-	within
eso-	inward
hyper-	above, excessive
hypo-	below, deficient
inter-	between
intra-	within
meta-	beyond, near, change
neo-	new
pan-	all
per-	through
peri-	surrounding
post-	after

re-	back
retro-	behind

Additional Terms

bilirubin SGOT alkaline phosphatase	indicators of liver function.
cephalothin kanamycin	antibiotic drugs used to treat infections.
chlorambucil prednisone	drugs used to treat malignant tumors.
culture	growing bacteria in a food medium.
diaphoresis	sweating.
fatigue	tiredness.
fulminant	severe and sudden with great rapidity.
hematocrit	percentage of red cells in a sample of blood.
hemoglobin	iron-containing substance in erythrocytes; enables the red cell to carry oxygen.
IVP	intravenous pyelogram, a record of the renal pelvis made by taking x-ray pictures of the kidney (renal pelvis) after dye is injected into a vein.
liver scan	radioactive material is injected into a vein and its concentration in the liver is recorded.
lyse	to break, disintegrate.

malaise	vague feeling of bodily discomfort.
neutrophils eosinophils monocytes bands	types of white blood cells (leukocytes).
occult	hidden; hard to find.
platelet	thrombocyte (clotting cell).
postmortem	after death; autopsy.
relapse	recurrence of disease after apparent recovery.
remission	lessening of symptoms of disease; return to better health.
rigors	chills.
sepsis	infection.
sputum	material coughed up from the lungs, windpipe, or throat.
tomogram	a method of taking x-ray pictures so that "cuts" or "slices" of regions of the body are obtained by special processing of the x-ray machine.
toxoplasma hemagglutination titer; fungal and PPD skin tests	indicate the presence of infection or past exposure to infection.

III. CLINICAL PAPER: *SHAKING CHILLS RELATED TO OCCULT LYMPHOMA*

Use the list of terms given above and your medical dictionary as you read the medical paper on the following pages. (Figure 22-2). Then answer the questions that follow it.

Reprinted from MEDICAL ANNALS OF THE DISTRICT OF COLUMBIA
Vol. 38, No. 1, January, 1969
Printed in U.S.A.

Shaking Chills Related to Occult Lymphoma

Report of a Case

BRUCE A. CHABNER, M.D.,* JOHN EASTON, M.D.,† AND VINCENT T. DeVITA, M.D.‡

SHAKING CHILLS have long been considered one of the most reliable signs of infection and can be a helpful clue in evaluating unexplained fever. In the case to be discussed the patient's course and autopsy findings indicate that lymphosarcoma may also be the cause of extreme rigors in association with spiking fevers, thus mimicking the clinical picture of occult infection.

Report of Case

A 63-year-old retired Negro engineer entered the Clinical Center on July 7, 1967 because of chills and fever (NIH No. 07-11-16). In 1963 a prostatic mass was resected and found to be a poorly differentiated lymphosarcoma. The patient was well thereafter until December 1966, when he was found to have massive retroperitoneal adenopathy, scalp nodules, and partial bilateral ureteral obstruction. Intravenous Cytoxan® led to apparent complete remission except for persistence of several small scalp nodules. Maintenance therapy consisting of prednisone and chlorambucil was continued for 6 months.

In late June of 1967 the patient began to have marked fatigue and malaise followed several days later by daily episodes of intense rigors, spiking fevers, and profuse diaphoresis. On admission his temperature was 40°C. Positive physical findings included only several 2 cm. scalp nodules which were unchanged since previous evaluations.

The hematocrit was 36.5 per cent, and the white blood cell count was 4,200 per cu. mm. with 63 per cent neutrophils, 14 per cent bands, 2 per cent lymphocytes, 1 per cent eosinophil, and 19 per cent monocytes. Urinalysis revealed 11 to 20 red blood cells and white blood cells per high-power field. All blood chemistries were normal, including liver and renal function tests and uric acid.

Twelve blood cultures, plus urine, sputum, and spinal-fluid cultures and smears were negative. A toxoplasma hemagglutination titer was negative, as were fungal and PPD skin tests. A chest X-ray film and IVP tomograms were normal. Abdominal and pelvic lymph nodes, as demonstrated by residual lymphangiogram dye, were of normal size.

During the first 4 weeks of hospitalization the patient experienced daily shaking chills, usually at 11:00 a.m., lasting 15 to 30 minutes, succeeded by a spiking fever to 39–40°C and several hours later profuse diaphoresis as the fever lysed. In the absence of demonstrable tumor and because of the presence of severe chills, occult infection was suspected, but routine diagnostic measures, including bone-marrow and percutaneous liver biopsies, yielded negative results. Two weeks of cephalothin (Keflin®) and kanamycin (Kantrex®) failed to affect the patient's course. Laparotomy for diagnostic purposes was strongly considered but was ultimately rejected when pancytopenia (white blood cells 1,500 per cu. mm., hemoglobin 8 Gm. per 100 c.c., platelet count 19,000 per cu. mm.) developed in the third hospital week. Bone-marrow biopsy showed hypoplasia of all cellular elements, and chlorambucil was discontinued. The fever and chills continued unabated.

During the fifth hospital week hepatomegaly and rapidly progressive hepatic failure became evident. SGOT rose to 310 units, alkaline phosphatase to 29 King-Armstrong units, and bilirubin to 23.1 mg. per 100 c.c. direct and 31.2 mg. per 100 c.c. total. A second liver scan now showed generally diminished uptake with several large filling defects. Hepatorenal failure supervened, and the patient expired on the forty-second hospital day.

Postmortem examination (A67-208) revealed massive lymphosarcomatous infiltration of the liver (figure 1), which weighed 1,760 Gm. A moderate degree of infiltration of the spleen (weight 350 Gm.) and bone marrow was present. Lymph nodes, though normal in size, also demonstrated a moderate degree of tumor invasion. Focal infiltrates were found in the skin, kidneys, lungs, esophagus, endocardium, and pericardium.

Other findings included a chronic penetrating ulcer in the first portion of the duodenum, cholemic nephrosis, and 4 gallstones, 1 mm. in size. There was no evidence of an acute or chronic septic process which might explain the patient's clinical symptoms. Cultures of the heart's blood taken several hours after death yielded 3 organisms (group D streptococcus, diphtheroids, and *Corynebacterium acnes*), all thought to represent contaminants or terminal sepsis.

*Clinical Associate, Laboratory of Chemical Pharmacology, National Cancer Institute, National Institutes of Health.

†Pathologist, Pathologic Anatomy, Clinical Center, National Institutes of Health.

‡Senior Investigator, Medicine Branch, National Cancer Institute, National Institutes of Health, Bethesda, Md. 20014. (Reprint requests to Dr. DeVita.)

Figure 22–2

Discussion

Several previous studies[1,2] have dealt with the difficult problem of differentiating between infection and tumor as the cause of fever in patients with cancer. Few observations, aside from positive bacteriologic evidence and a response to antibiotics, can identify the source of fever. However, according to Fenster and Klatskin,[3] shaking chills may be a "noteworthy" sign pointing toward infection. In reviewing the case histories of 81 patients with hepatic metastases due to a variety of tumors these authors found 19 cases in which fever appeared to be secondary to malignancy. In none of these cases were chills present.

In the case under discussion the uncommon association of shaking chills with malignancy is documented. Frank chills have been observed in at least 1 previous case of rapidly growing lymphoma. The patients described by Aledort et al[4] developed sudden renal failure along with spiking fever and chills, and at autopsy massive renal invasion by lymphosarcoma without evidence of infection was found. Rare and less well documented reports of the occurrence of chills in association with renal,[5] stomach,[6] and bowel[6] carcinomas are also to be found in the older literature.

We conclude that, although uncommon, malignant lymphoma and probably other forms of cancer should be considered in the differential diagnosis of a patient having rigors and fever Aggressive diagnostic measures, including early laparotomy, should be undertaken in the hope that a treatable infection or tumor will be found.

The mechanism by which the tumor led to chills in this patient is obscure. Although extensive hepatocellular necrosis was found at autopsy, tissue necrosis does not appear to have been a factor, since severe rigors were present at a time when liver chemistries, biopsy, and scan were all normal. The extreme rapidity of tumor growth is indicated by the progression to hepatic failure 3 weeks after these negative liver studies.

Death due to massive hepatic invasion and parenchymal necrosis as in this patient has been reported in 1 previous case of malignant lymphoma. In 1934 the Viennese physician, Carl Sternberg,[7] described a 32-year-old man who died of hepatic failure after a fulminant 7-week illness.

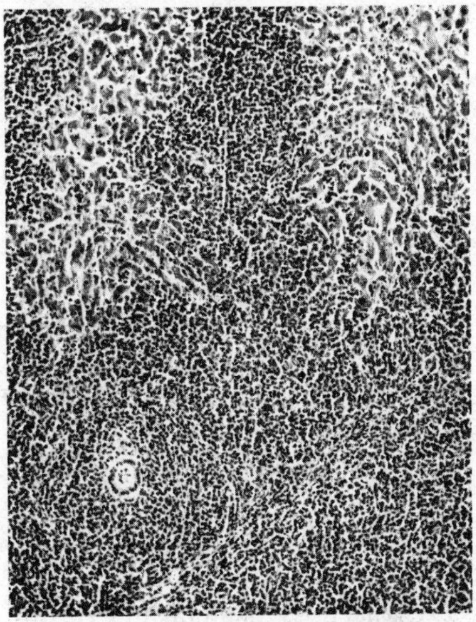

FIG. 1. Section of liver showing massive lymphosarcoma infiltrates in the portal-tract tissues and hepatic lobules. The hepatic cells adjacent to the tumor are degenerated and necrotic, and in other sections of the liver there were even larger areas of hepatocellular necrosis.

Summary

A case has been presented of a 63-year-old man in apparent remission from lymphosarcoma who had shaking chills and fever and who died of fulminant hepatic failure. At autopsy massive hepatic invasion by lymphosarcoma was found; no source of infection was uncovered that might explain the patient's presenting complaints. It is concluded that shaking chills may occur secondary to lymphoma and that an infectious etiology cannot be assumed in evaluating a patient with these complaints.

References

1. Boggs, D. R., and Frei, E., III: Clinical studies of fever and infection in cancer. Cancer, 1960, **13**, 1240.
2. Browder, A. A., Huff, J. W., and Petersdorf, R. G.: Significance of fever in neoplastic disease. Ann. Intern. Med., 1961, **55**, 932.
3. Fenster, L. F., and Klatskin, G.: Manifestations of metastatic tumors of the liver: a study of 81 patients subjected to needle biopsy. Amer. J. Med., 1961, **31**, 238.
4. Aledort, L. M., Hodges, M., and Brown, J. A.: Irreversible renal failure due to malignant lymphoma. Ann. Intern. Med., 1966, **65**, 117.
5. Israel, J.: Ueber Fieber bei malignen Nieren-und Nebennierengeschwülsten. Deutsche med. Wchnschr., Leipz. u. Berl., 1911, **37**, 57.
6. Finlayson, J.: On the occurrence of pyrexia, shiverings, and pyaemia in cases of malignant disease. Lancet, 1888, **2**, 710.
7. Sternberg, C.: Über Lymphosarkomatose der Leber. Wien. med. Wchnschr., 1934, **84**, 417.

Figure 22-2 (Continued)

IV. QUESTIONS ABOUT THE PAPER

1. (a) On admission the patient had "retroperitoneal adenopathy." The peritoneum is a membrane that surrounds the organs in the abdominal cavity (Figure 22-3). What are some of the organs in the abdominal cavity?

   ____

   ____

   (b) What does retroperitoneal mean? ______________________________

   ____

   (c) What does adenopathy mean? ______________________________

2. What does "bilateral ureteral obstruction" mean? ______________________________

   ____

3. By what route was Cytoxan given? ______________________________

4. What was the effect of giving the patient Cytoxan? ______________________________

5. In late June of 1967 the patient returns to the hospital. What term indicates his feeling of discomfort? ______________________________

   What term indicates his feeling of tiredness? ______________________________

6. What is the hematocrit? ______________________________

   ____

   ____

7. What is a lymphocyte? ______________________________

8. Where were 11 to 20 erythrocytes found? (See paragraph 3 under Report of Case.)

   ____

9. All chemical tests of blood were normal, including liver and kidney function tests.

   Which term means pertaining to the kidney? ______________________________

10. What is a blood culture? ______________________________

11. What is an IVP tomogram? ______________________________

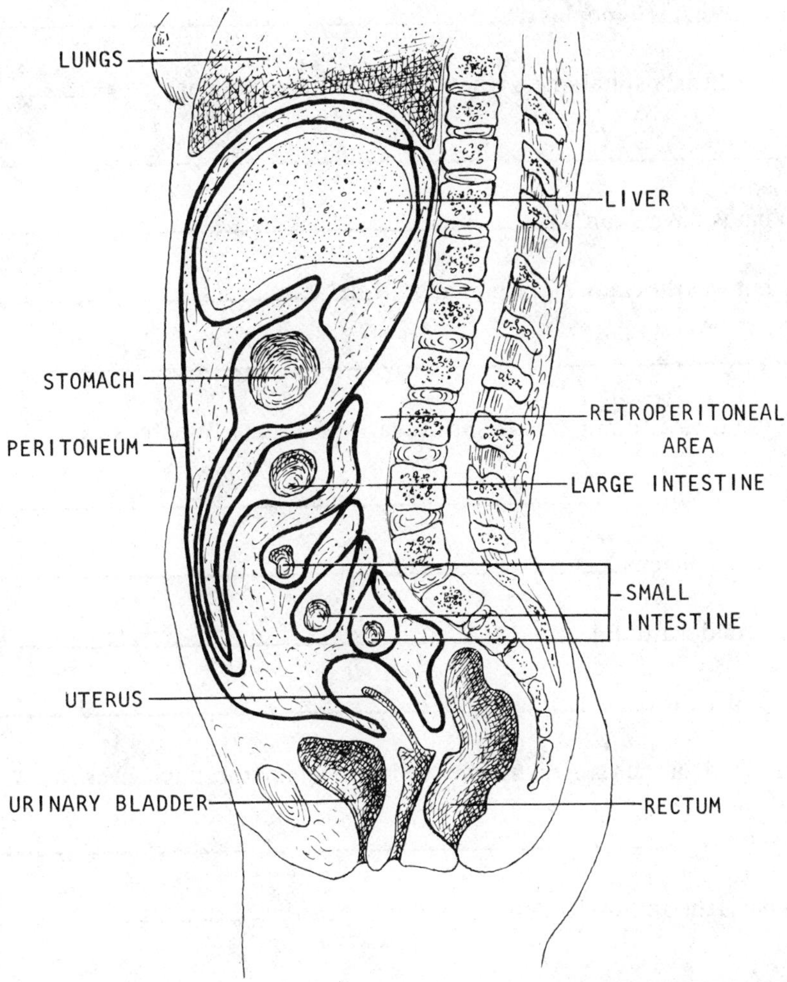

Figure 22-3 The peritoneum surrounds the organs in the abdominal cavity.

12. What recording (x-ray) showed the condition of the patient's abdominal and pelvic lymph nodes? ______

13. Why was a laparotomy not performed in the third hospital week?

______

14. What is hemoglobin? ______

15. Platelet counts tell the number of thrombocytes. What are thrombocytes?

______

16. (a) How was hypoplasia of all bone marrow cellular elements detected? ______

______

(b) What is hypoplasia? ______

17. In the fifth hospital week, what happened to the patient's liver? ______

______

18. What is a liver scan? ______

19. What was the cause of the patient's death? ______

______

20. On autopsy, tumor was found in various organs. Where is the:

(a) spleen ______

(b) esophagus ______

(c) endocardium ______

(d) pericardium ______

21. In Fig. 1 in the paper, the liver cells show hepatocellular necrosis. What does that mean? ______

22. What is the authors' conclusion about the case? ______

______

V. EXERCISES

A. Build medical words:

1. Blood vessel tumor ______
2. Inflammation of the liver ______
3. Incision of abdominal wall ______
4. Decreased number of red blood cells ______
5. Process of visually examining the peritoneum ______
6. Inflammation of the renal pelvis ______
7. Abnormal condition of white cells (too many) ______

8. Platelet ______________________________

9. Heart enlargement ______________________________

10. Excessive formation ______________________________

B. *Give the meaning of the following medical terms:*

1. percutaneous ______________________________
2. esophagotomy ______________________________
3. phagocyte ______________________________
4. lymphosarcoma ______________________________
5. resection ______________________________
6. ureterectomy ______________________________
7. hematocrit ______________________________
8. osteolysis ______________________________
9. intravenous ______________________________
10. bilateral ______________________________

C. *Give the answers called for:*

1. What are the medical terms for three regions of the body where there are large collections of lymph nodes? ______________________________
2. What is **metastasis**? ______________________________
3. What is the difference between a **benign** and a **malignant** tumor? ______________________________
____
4. What is a **neoplasm**? ______________________________
5. What is an **IVP tomogram**? ______________________________
6. What is a **necropsy**? ______________________________
7. What is the difference between a **relapse** and a **remission**? ______________________________

8. (a) **Malaise** means ______________________

   (b) **Fatigue** means ______________________

9. Where is **hemoglobin** found? ______________________

D. Match the term in Column I with a term of similar meaning in Column II:

Column I		*Column II*
1. lapar/o	______	A. intra-
2. cutane/o	______	B. section
3. ren/o	______	C. -penia
4. endo-	______	D. nephr/o
5. platelet	______	E. abdomin/o
6. hypo-	______	F. autopsy
7. -ectomy	______	G. biopsy
8. -tomy	______	H. thrombocyte
9. necropsy	______	I. -oma
10. neoplasm	______	J. malignant
		K. erythrocyte
		L. resection
		M. derm/o

ANSWERS

Answers to medical paper

1. (a) Stomach, intestines, liver, gallbladder, pancreas, spleen.
   (b) Pertaining to behind the peritoneum.
   (c) Disease of glands. The glands that are diseased are lymph glands.
2. Both ureters were obstructed by the tumor (bilateral means two or both sides).
3. Cytoxan was given intravenously (within a vein).
4. The effect of giving Cytoxan was to promote a remission (symptoms of disease disappear) except for the presence of several small scalp nodules (small nodes or growths).
5. Malaise means discomfort, uneasiness. Fatigue means tiredness.
6. Hematocrit literally means "to separate blood." It is actually the percentage of erythrocytes within a given blood volume. The hematocrit is measured by spinning blood very quickly in a machine (centrifuge) so that the red cells become separated from the rest of the blood and fall to the bottom of the test tube or container.
7. A lymph cell (type of white blood cell).
8. In urinalysis (word was shortened from urinanalysis). Urinalysis is separating apart urine to investigate its contents.
9. Renal (ren/o means kidney).
10. Blood is placed on growth media (food) and later examined for evidence of bacteria.
11. Intravenous pyelogram. A tomogram is a "slice" view of the organ taken by focusing the x-ray machine at several different levels. Dye is first injected into veins and tomograms are taken of the renal pelvis of the kidney.
12. Lymphangiogram (x-rays of lymph vessels after dye is injected into the lymphatic system of vessels). Note that the combining vowel "o" is dropped when lymph is followed by a "a" or "e."
13. Pancytopenia developed (decrease in number of all blood cells).
14. Hemoglobin (hem/o = blood; globin = protein) is the iron-containing protein substance in erythrocytes.
15. Clotting cells (a platelet is a thrombocyte).
16. (a) Bone marrow biopsy (microscopic examination of bone interior where blood cells are formed).
    (b) Decrease in growth, formation (hypo = deficient; -plasia = formation).
17. It became enlarged (hepatomegaly) and began to fail to function (hepatic failure).
18. Radioactive material is injected intravenously and measurements of its concentration in the liver are recorded. Diminished uptake indicates poor liver functioning.
19. Hepatorenal failure (lack of functioning of the liver and kidneys).
20. (a) Oval body lying below and behind the stomach on the upper left side of the abdomen. Blood cells are made and stored there.
    (b) Tube leading from the throat to the stomach (eso = inward; phag/o = swallowing).
    (c) Inner membrane within the heart.
    (d) Outer membrane surrounding the heart.
21. Abnormal condition of dead liver cells.
22. Shaking chills may not always be associated with infection but may be secondary to (occur with) a lymphosarcoma.

Answers to exercises

A.

1. hemangioma
2. hepatitis
3. laparotomy (abdominal section)
4. erythrocytopenia
5. peritoneoscopy
6. pyelitis
7. leukocytosis
8. thrombocyte (clotting cell)
9. cardiomegaly
10. hyperplasia

B.

1. Through the skin.
2. Incision into the esophagus.
3. Cell that eats other cells. Some leukocytes fight disease by phagocytosis.
4. Tumor (flesh) of lymph (a malignant tumor).
5. To cut out, remove.
6. Excision of a ureter.
7. Separation of blood (percentage of red blood cells).
8. Destruction of bone.
9. Pertaining to within a vein.
10. Pertaining to two (both) sides.

C.

1. Axillary (armpit); cervical (neck); inguinal (groin).
2. Metastasis (plural: metastases) is the spreading of malignant tumors away from their primary (first) location to distant (secondary) sites all over the body.
3. Benign tumors are limited in growth, are encapsulated, and do not metastasize. Malignant tumors are rapid and unlimited in their growth, are not encapsulated, and metastasize.
4. New growth; tumor.
5. IVP means intravenous pyelogram. This is an x-ray record (-gram) of the renal pelvis (pyel/o). It is taken by first injecting contrast dye into a vein (intravenous) and then taking x-ray pictures of the kidney region. Tomograms are a series of special x-ray pictures showing different depths or levels of a structure by blurring detail in the images of structures not in the specific plane to be viewed.
6. View of a dead body (autopsy) to determine the cause of death. Also called a postmortem examination.
7. A relapse is the reappearance of symptoms of disease. A remission is the lessening or disappearance of disease symptoms.
8. (a) Discomfort
   (b) Tiredness
9. Hemoglobin is an iron-containing substance in red blood cells. It helps the erythrocyte carry oxygen all over the body to all cells. Oxygen is necessary for the release of energy in cells. Can you understand why people are tired if they suffer from iron-deficiency anemia?

D.

1. E
2. M
3. D
4. A
5. H
6. C
7. L
8. B
9. F
10. I

VI. PRONUNCIATION OF TERMS

abdominal	ăb-DŎM-ĭ-năl
adenopathy	ăd-ĕ-NŎP-ă-thē
axillary	ĂK-sĭ-lăr-ē
benign	bē-NĪN
bilateral	bī-LĂT-ĕr-ăl
cardiomegaly	kăr-dē-ō-MĔG-ă-lē
cervical	SĔR-vĭ-kăl
endocardium	ĕn-dō-KĂR-dē-ŭm
erythrocytopenia	ĕ-rĭth-rō-sī-tō-PĒ-nē-ă
esophagotomy	ĕ-sŏf-ă-GŎT-ō-mē
esophagus	ĕ-SŎF-ă-gŭs
fatigue	fă-TĒG
hemangioma	hĕ-măn-jē-Ō-mă
hematocrit	hē-MĂT-ō-krĭt
hemoglobin	HĒ-mō-glō-bĭn
hepatic	hĕ-PĂT-ĭk
hepatitis	hĕp-ă-TĪ-tĭs
hepatomegaly	hĕp-ă-tō-MĔG-ă-lē
hepatorenal	hĕp-a-tō-RĒ-nal
hyperplasia	hī-pĕr-PLĀ-zē-ă
hypoplasia	hī-pō-PLĀ-zē-ă
inguinal	ĬNG-gwĭ-năl
intravenous	ĭn-tră-VĒ-nŭs
laparotomy	lăp-ă-RŎT-ō-mē
leukocytosis	lo͞o-kō-sī-TŌ-sĭs
lymphangiogram	lĭm-FĂN-jē-ō-grăm

lymphocyte	LĬM-fō-sīt
lymphosarcoma	lĭm-fō-săr-KŌ-mă
malaise	mă-LĀZ
malignant	mă-LĬG-nănt
metastasis	mĕ-TĂS-tă-sĭs
necrosis	nĕ-KRŌ-sĭs
neoplasm	NĒ-ō-plăzm
osteolysis	ŏs-tē-ŎL-ĭ-sĭs
pancytopenia	păn-sī-tō-PĒ-nē-ă
percutaneous	pĕr-kū-TĀ-nē-ŭs
pericardium	pĕr-ĭ-KĂR-dē-ŭm
peritoneoscopy	pĕr-ĭ-tō-nē-ŎS-kō-pē
peritoneum	pĕr-ĭ-tō-NĒ-ŭm
phagocyte	FĂG-ō-sīt
platelet	PLĀT-lĕt
prostate	PRŎS-tāt
pyelitis	pī-ĕ-LĪ-tĭs
pyelogram	PĪ-ĕ-lō-grăm
relapse	RĒ-lăps or rē-LĂPS
remission	rē-MĬSH-ŭn
renal	RĒ-năl
resection	rē-SĔK-shŭn
retroperitoneal	rĕ-trō-pĕr-ĭ-tō-NĒ-ăl
tomogram	TŌ-mō-grăm
ureter	ū-RĒ-tĕr or Ū-rĕ-tĕr
ureteral	ū-RĒ-tĕr-ăl
ureterectomy	ū-rē-tĕr-ĔK-tō-mē
urinalysis	ū-rĭ-NĂL-ĭ-sĭs

REVIEW SHEET 22

Combining Forms

abdomin/o	______________	lymph/o	______________
aden/o	______________	necr/o	______________
angi/o	______________	peritone/o	______________
axill/o	______________	phag/o	______________
cervic/o	______________	pyel/o	______________
cutane/o	______________	ren/o	______________
hemat/o	______________	sarc/o	______________
hepat/o	______________	thromb/o	______________
inguin/o	______________	tom/o	______________
lapar/o	______________	ureter/o	______________
later/o	______________	urin/o	______________

ven/o ______________

Suffixes

-crit	______________	-osis	______________
-gram	______________	-ous	______________
-lysis	______________	-penia	______________
-pathy	______________	-stasis	______________
-plasia	______________	-tomy	______________
-plasm	______________	-um	______________
-megaly	______________	-us	______________

Prefixes

ana- ____________

bi- ____________

endo- ____________

eso- ____________

hyper- ____________

hypo- ____________

inter- ____________

intra- ____________

meta- ____________

neo- ____________

pan- ____________

per- ____________

peri- ____________

post- ____________

re- ____________

retro- ____________

GLOSSARY

PLURALS

The rules for commonly forming plurals of medical terms are as follows:

1. For words ending in **is**, drop the **is** and add **es**:

   Examples:

Singular	*Plural*
anastomosis	anastomoses
metastasis	metastases
epiphysis	epiphyses
prosthesis	prostheses

2. For words ending in **um**, drop the **um** and add **a**:

   Examples:

Singular	*Plural*
bacterium	bacteria
diverticulum	diverticula
ovum	ova

3. For words ending in **us**, drop the **us** and add **i**:

   Examples:

Singular	*Plural*
calculus	calculi
bronchus	bronchi
nucleus	nuclei

   Two exceptions to this rule are viruses and sinuses.

4. For words ending in **a**, retain the **a** and add **e**:

   Examples:

Singular	*Plural*
vertebra	vertebrae
bursa	bursae
bulla	bullae

5. For words ending in **ix** and **ex**, drop the **ix** or **ex** and add **ices**:

   Examples:

Singular	*Plural*
apex	apices
varix	varices

6. For words ending in **on**, drop the **on** and add **a**:

Examples:

Singular	*Plural*
ganglion	ganglia
spermatozoon	spermatozoa

ABBREVIATIONS

AAL	Anterior axillary line.
abd	Abdomen.
ABO	Three main blood types.
AC	Air conduction.
a.c.	Before meals (*ante cibum*).
Accom.	Accommodation.
ACh	Acetylcholine.
ACTA	Automated computerized transverse axial scanner (machine for computerized axial tomography).
ACTH	Adrenocorticotropic hormone.
AD	Right ear (*auris dextra*).
ad lib.	As desired.
ADH	Antidiuretic hormone; vasopressin.
AFB	Acid-fast bacillus.
AFP	Alpha-fetoprotein.
AHF	Antihemophilic factor.
AI	Aortic insufficiency.
AIDS	Acquired immunodeficiency syndrome.
AKA	Above-knee amputation.
ALL	Acute lymphocytic leukemia.
ALP	Alkaline phosphatase.
ALT	Alanine transaminase (liver and heart enzyme). Formerly SGPT.
AML	Acute myelocytic (myelogenous) leukemia.
amp	Amplue; ampere.
AP	Anteroposterior.
A&P	Auscultation and percussion.
aq.	Water (*aqua*).
ara-C	Cytosine arabinoside.
ARDS	Acute respiratory distress syndrome.
AS	Left ear (*auris sinistra*); aortic stenosis.
ASD	Atrial septal defect.
ASH	Asymmetrical septal hypertrophy.
ASHD	Arteriosclerotic heart disease.
AST	Aspartate amino transferase (liver and heart enzyme). Formerly SGOT.
Astigm.	Astigmatism.
Au	Gold.
ausc.	Auscultation.
A-V	Arteriovenous; atrioventricular.
AVR	Aortic valve replacement.
Ba	Barium.
BaE	Barium enema.
baso	Basophils.
BC	Bone conduction.
B-cells	Lymphocytes produced in the bone marrow.
BCNU	Bischloroethylnitrosourea.
BE	Barium enema.
b.i.d.	Twice a day (*bis in die*).
BMR	Basal metabolic rate.
BP	Blood pressure.
BPH	Benign prostatic hypertrophy.
Broncho	Bronchoscopy.
BSP	Bromsulphalein (dye used in liver function test; its retention is indicative of liver damage or disease).
BT	Bleeding time.
BUN	Blood urea nitrogen.
bx	Biopsy.
c̄	With (*cum*).
C-1, C-2	First, second cervical vertebra.
C_{cr}	Creatinine clearance.
C.A.	Chronological age.
Ca	Calcium; cancer.
CAD	Coronary artery disease.
CAPD	Continuous ambulatory peritoneal dialysis.
CAT scan	Computed (axial) tomography.
CBC, c.b.c.	Complete blood count.
cc	Cubic centimeter (unit of mass; 1/1000 liter).
CCU	Coronary care unit.
CEA	Carcinoembryonic antigen.
Chem	Chemotherapy.
CHF	Congestive heart failure.
chr	Chronic.
μCi	Microcurie.
c. gl.	Correction with glasses.
CK	Creatine kinase.
Cl	Chlorine.
CLL	Chronic lymphocytic leukemia.
cm	Centimeter (1/100 meter).

CMF Cytoxan, methotrexate, and 5-fluorouracil.
CMG Cystometrogram.
CML Chronic myelogenous leukemia.
CNS Central nervous system.
Co Cobalt.
CO_2 Carbon dioxide.
COP Cytoxan, Oncovin, and prednisone (antineoplastic drugs given in combination chemotherapy).
COPD Chronic obstructive pulmonary disease.
CPC Clinicopathological conference.
CPK Creatinine phosphokinase (enzyme released into blood following injury to heart or skeletal muscles).
CPR Cardiopulmonary resuscitation.
CRF Chronic renal failure.
CS Cesarean section.
C-section Cesarean section.
CSF Cerebrospinal fluid.
CT scan Computed tomography.
ct. Count.
CVA Cerebrovascular accident.
CVP Cytoxan, vincristine, and prednisone (antineoplastic drugs given in combination chemotherapy).
CVS Cardiovascular system.
C/W Compare with.
CXR Chest x-ray.
cyl. Cylindrical lens.
cysto Cystoscopy.
CZI Crystalline zinc insulin.

D&C Dilation and curettage.
DD Discharge diagnosis.
Derm. Dermatology.
DES Diethylstilbestrol.
DHL Diffuse histiocytic lymphoma.
DI Diabetes insipidus; diagnostic imaging.
diff. differential count (white blood cells).
DLE Discoid lupus erythematosus.
DM Diabetes mellitus.
DNA Deoxyribonucleic acid.
DOB Date of birth.
DSA Digital subtraction angiography.
DT Delirium tremens.
DTR Deep tendon reflexes.
DUB Dysfunctional uterine bleeding.
D_x Diagnosis.

e Without.
EBV Epstein-Barr virus.
ECC Extracorporeal circulation.
ECF Extended-care facility.
ECG (EKG) Electrocardiogram.
ECT Electroconvulsive therapy.
EEG Electroencephalogram.
EM Electron microscope.
Em Emmetropia.
EMG Electromyogram.
ENT Ear, nose, and throat.
eos., eosins Eosinophils.
ER Emergency room; estrogen receptor.
ESR Erythrocyte sedimentation rate.
EST Electroshock therapy.
ETF Eustachian tube function.
exc Excision.

F Fahrenheit.
FACP Fellow, American College of Physicians.
FACS Fellow, American College of Surgeons.
Fb Fingerbreadth.
FBS Fasting blood sugar.
FDA Food and Drug Administration.
Fe Iron.
FH Family history.
FHT Fetal heart tones.
FSH Follicle-stimulating hormone.
FTA-ABS Fluorescent treponemal antibody absorption test.
FTS Fetal heart tones.
F/u Follow-up.
5-FU 5-Fluorouracil.
FUO Fever of undetermined origin.

μg Microgram (one-millionth of a gram).
Ga Gallium.
GB Gallbladder.
GBS Gallbladder series (x-rays).
GC Gonorrhea.
GFR Glomerular filtration rate.
GH Growth hormone.
GI Gastrointestinal.
Gm, gm Gram.
gr. Grain(s).
Grav. 1, 2, 3 First, second, third pregnancy.
GTT Glucose tolerance test.
gtt. Drops (*guttae*).
GU Genitourinary.
Gyn Gynecology.

H Hydrogen.
Hb (Hgb) Hemoglobin.
HCG (hCH) Human chorionic gonadotropin.

HCl Hydrochloric acid.
HCO_3 Bicarbonate.
Hct (HCT) Hematocrit.
HD Hearing distance; hemodialysis.
Hd Hodgkin's disease.
h.d. At bedtime (*hora decubitus*).
HDL High density lipoproteins.
He Helium.
Hg Mercury.
Hgb Hemoglobin.
hGH Human growth hormone.
h/o History of.
H_2O Water.
h.p.f. High power field (microscope).
h.s. At bedtime (*hora somni*).
HSG Hysterosalpingography.
h-s megaly Hepatosplenomegaly.
HVD Hypertensive vascular disease.
hx History.

I Iodine.
^{131}I Radioactive isotope of iodine.
IADH Inappropriate antidiuretic hormone.
ICU Intensive care unit.
IDDM Insulin dependent diabetes mellitus.
IgA, IgD, IgG, IgM, IgE Immunoglobulins.
IHSS Idiopathic hypertrophic subaortic stenosis.
IM Intramuscular (injection).
inf. Infusion; inferior.
INH Isoniazid (drug used to treat tuberculosis).
inj. Injection.
IPPB Intermittent positive-pressure breathing.
I.Q. Intelligence quotient.
IUD Intrauterine device.
IV (i.v.) Intravenous (injection).
IVC Intravenous cholangiogram.
IVP Intravenous pyelogram.

K Potassium.
Kg; kg Kilogram (1000 grams).
KUB Kidney, ureter, and bladder (abdominal x-ray).

L Liter; left; lower.
L-1, L-2 First, second lumbar vertebra.
LA Left atrium.
lap. Laparotomy.
LAT; lat. Lateral.
LB Large bowel.
LCM Left costal margin.
LD; LDH Lactic dehydrogenase.
LDL Low density lipoproteins.
LE Lupus erythematosus.
LFT Liver function test.
LH Luteinizing hormone.
Lin. ac. Linear accelerator.
LLL Left lower lobe (lung).
LLQ Left lower quadrant (abdomen).
LMP Last menstrual period.
LN; l.n. Lymph node.
LP Lumbar puncture.
l.p.f. Low power field.
LPN Licensed practical nurse.
LSD Lysergic acid diethylamide.
LSK Liver, spleen, and kidneys.
LTH Prolactin.
LUL Left upper lobe (lung).
LUQ Left upper quadrant (abdomen).
LV Left ventricle.
L&W Living and well.
lymphs Lymphocyte.

M Monocytes; meter.
M.A. Mental age.
MAO Monoamine oxidase.
MCH Mean corpuscular hemoglobin (amount of hemoglobin in each red blood cell).
MCHC Mean corpuscular hemoglobin concentration (amount of hemoglobin per unit of blood).
mCi Millicurie.
μCi Microcurie.
MCL Midclavicular line.
MCV Mean corpuscular volume (measurement of size of individual red cell).
mEq/L Milliequivalent per liter (measurement of the concentration of a solution).
metamyl Metamyelocyte.
mets Metastases.
mg Milligram (1/1000 gram).
μg Microgram (one-millionth of a gram).
MH Marital history.
MI Myocardial infarction; mitral insufficiency.
ml Milliliter (1/1000 liter).
mm Millimeter (1/1000 meter; 0.039 inch).
mm Hg Millimeters of mercury.
MMPI Minnesota Multiphasic Personality Inventory.
mμ Millimicron (1/1000 micron; a micron is 10^{-3} mm.).
mon, mono Monocyte.

MOPP	Nitrogen mustard, Oncovin, prednisone, and procarbazine (combination chemotherapy).
6-MP	6-Mercaptopurine (antineoplastic drug).
MRI	Magnetic resonance imaging.
mRNA	Messenger RNA.
MS	Mitral stenosis; multiple sclerosis; morphine sulfate.
MSL	Midsternal line.
MTX	Methotrexate.
MVP	Mitral valve prolapse.
MVR	Mitral valve replacement.
myelocyt	Myelocyte.
Myop.	Myopia.

N	Nitrogen.
Na	Sodium.
NB	Newborn.
NBS	Normal bowel or breath sounds.
NED	No evidence of disease.
neg.	Negative.
NER	No evidence of recurrence.
NERD	No evidence of recurrent disease.
N.F.	National Formulary.
n/f	Negro female.
NG tube	Nasogastric tube.
NIDDM	Non-insulin dependent diabetes mellitus.
n/m	Negro male.
NMR	Nuclear magnetic resonance.
NOS	Not otherwise specified.
NPDL	Nodular, poorly differentiated lymphocytes.
NPH	Neutral protamine Hagedorn insulin.
NPO	Nothing by mouth (*nulla per os*).
NTP	Normal temperature and pressure.

O_2	Oxygen.
OB	Obstetrics.
OBS	Organic brain syndrome.
OCG	Oral cholecystogram.
OD	Right eye (*oculus dexter*).
17-OH	17-Hydroxycorticosteroids.
Ophth.	Ophthalmology.
OR	Operating room.
ORTH; Ortho.	Orthopedics.
OS	Left eye (*oculus sinister*).
os	Opening; mouth; bone.
OSB	Organic brain syndrome.
OT	Old tuberculin; occupational therapy.
Oto.	Otology.
OU	Each eye (*oculus uterque*).
OV	Office visit.
oz.	Ounce.

P	Phosphorus; pulse.
PA	Posteroanterior.
P&A	Percussion and auscultation.
PAC	Premature atrial contractions.
$PaCO_2$	Carbon dioxide pressure.
palp.	Palpable; palpation.
PaO_2	Oxygen pressure.
Pap smear	Papanicolaou smear.
Para 1, 2, 3	Unipara, bipara, tripara (number of viable births).
PAT	Paroxysmal atrial tachycardia.
Path	Pathology.
PA view	Posteroanterior view (x-ray position).
PBI	Protein-bound iodine.
p.c.	After meals (*post cibum*).
PCO_2	Carbon dioxide pressure.
PD	Peritoneal dialysis.
PDA	Patent ductus arteriosus.
PDR	Physicians' Desk Reference.
PE	Physical examination.
PET	Positron emission tomography.
PE tube	Ventilating tube for eardrum.
PEG	Pneumoencephalography.
pH	Hydrogen ion concentration (alkalinity and acidity measurement).
PID	Pelvic inflammatory disease.
PKU	Phenylketonuria.
plts.	Platelets.
PM	Post mortem; petit mal; afternoon (post meridian).
PMN	Polymorphonuclear leukocyte.
p/o	Postoperative.
p.o.	Orally (*per os*).
PO_2	Oxygen pressure.
poly	Polymorphonuclear leukocyte.
POMP	Prednisone, Oncovin, methotrexate, and 6-mercaptopurine (combination chemotherapy).
pos.	Positive.
PP	Postprandial (after meals).
PPD	Purified protein derivative (test for tuberculosis).
pre-op	Preoperative.
PRL	Prolactin.
p.r.n.	As required (*pro re nata*).
prot.	Protocol.
Pro. time	Prothrombin time (test of blood clotting).
PSP	Phenylsulfonphthalein (dye test for kidney impairment).
PT	Prothrombin; physical therapy.
pt.	Patient.

PTA Prior to admission.
PTCA Percutaneous transluminal coronary angioplasty.
PTH Parathyroid hormone.
PTT Partial thromboplastin time.
PU Pregnancy urine.
PVC Premature ventricular contractions.
PZI Protamine zinc insulin.

q.d. Every day (*quaque die*).
q.h. Every hour (*quaque hora*).
q.i.d. Four times daily (*quater in die*).
q.n. Every night (*quaque nox*).
q.n.s. Quantity not sufficient.

R, r., rt. Right.
RA Rheumatoid arthritis; right atrium.
Ra Radium.
rad Radiation absorbed dose.
RAI Radioactive iodine.
RAIU Radioactive iodine uptake.
RAtx Radiation therapy.
RBC Red blood cell (corpuscle); red blood count.
RCM Right costal margin.
RDS Respiratory distress syndrome.
RF Rheumatoid factor.
Rh Rhesus (monkey) factor in blood.
RIA Radioimmunoassay.
RLL Right lower lobe (lung).
RLM Right middle lobe (lung).
RLQ Right lower quadrant (abdomen).
RNA Ribonucleic acid.
R/O Rule out.
RP Retrograde pyelogram.
RT Radiation therapy.
RUL Right upper lobe (lung).
RUQ Right upper quadrant (abdomen).
RV Right ventricle.
R_x Treatment; therapy.

s Without (*sine*).
S-1, S-2 First, second sacral vertebra.
S-A Sinoatrial.
SBE Subacute bacterial endocarditis.
SBFT Small bowel follow-through (x-ray study).
SCD Sudden cardiac death.
Sed. rate Sedimentation rate (rate of blood sedimentation.)
segs Segmented cells.
s. gl. Without correction (without glasses).
SGOT Serum glutamic-oxaloacetic transaminase.
SGPT Serum glutamic-pyruvic transaminase.
SH Serum hepatitis.
SI Sacroiliac joint.
SLE Systemic lupus erythematosus.
SOB Shortness of breath.
sol. Solution.
S/P Status post (refers to previous disease condition).
sp. gr. Specific gravity.
SPC Serum protein electrophoresis.
SR Sedimentation rate.
Sr Strontium.
st Stage (of disease).
Staph. Staphylococcus.
stat. Immediately (*statim*).
STH Somatotropin (growth hormone).
Strep. Streptococcus.
S.T.S. Serological test for syphilis.
Subcu. Subcutaneous.
SV-40 Simian vacuolating virus.
SVC Superior vena cava.
Sx Symptoms.

T Temperature.
T-1, T-2 First, second thoracic vertebra.
T_3 Triiodothyronine.
T_4 Thyroxine.
T&A Tonsillectomy and adenoidectomy.
tab Tablet.
TAH Total abdominal hysterectomy.
TAT Thematic Apperception Test.
TB Tuberculosis.
TBI Total-body irradiation.
Tc Technetium.
T-cells Lymphocytes produced in the thymus gland.
TIA Transient ischemic attack.
t.i.d. Three times daily (*ter in die*).
TNI Total nodal irradiation.
TNM Tumor, nodes, and metastases.
tomos Tomograms.
TP Testosterone propionate (male hormone).
TPI *Treponema pallidum* immobilization (test for syphilis).
TPN Total parenteral nutrition.
TPR Temperature, pulse, and respiration.
TSH Thyroid-stimulating hormone.
TUR, TURP Transurethral resection (for prostatectomy).
Tx Treatment.

U	Unit.
U/A	Urinalysis.
UC	Uterine contractions.
UGI	Upper gastrointestinal.
umb.	Navel (*umbilicus*).
ung.	Ointment.
Ur.	Urine.
URI	Upper respiratory infection.
Urol.	Urology.
u/s	Ultrasound.
U.S.P.	United States Pharmacopeia.
UTI	Urinary tract infection.
VA	Visual acuity.
VCU	Voiding cystourethogram.
VD	Venereal disease.
VDRL	Venereal Disease Research Laboratory (an antibody test for syphilis).
VF	Visual field.
VLDL	Very low density lipoproteins.
VSD	Ventricular septal defect.
WAIS	Wechsler Adult Intelligence Test.
WBC	White blood cell; white blood count.
W-E	Wide excision.
w/f	White female.
WISC	Wechsler Intelligence Scale for Children.
w/m	White male.
y/o	Year old.

MEDICAL TERMS → ENGLISH

Combining Form, Suffix, or Prefix	*Meaning*
a-	no; not; without
ab-	away from
abdomin/o	abdomen
-ac	pertaining to
acanth/o	spiny; thorny
acetabul/o	acetabulum (hip socket)
acou/o	hearing
acous/o	hearing
acr/o	extremities; top; extreme point
acu/o	sharp; severe; sudden
ad-	toward
aden/o	gland
adenoid/o	adenoids
adip/o	fat
adren/o	adrenal glands
adrenal/o	adrenal glands
aer/o	air
agglutin/o	clumping; sticking together
agor/a	marketplace
-agra	excessive pain
-al	pertaining to
alb/o	white
albin/o	white
albumin/o	albumin
algesi/o	excessive sensitivity to pain
-algia	pain
alveol/o	alveolus; air sac; small sac
ambly/o	dim; dull
-amine	nitrogen compound
amni/o	amnion
amyl/o	starch
an-	no; not; without
an/o	anus
ana-	up; apart; backward; excessive
andr/o	male
aneurysm/o	aneurysm
angi/o	vessel
ankyl/o	crooked; bent; stiff
ante-	before; forward
anter/o	front
anthrac/o	coal dust
anti-	against
aort/o	aorta
-apheresis	removal
aponeur/o	aponeurosis (type of tendon)
append/o	appendix
appendic/o	appendix
aque/o	water
-ar	pertaining to
-arche	beginning
arteri/o	artery
arteriol/o	arteriole
arthr/o	joint
articul/o	joint
-ary	pertaining to

Combining Form, Suffix, or Prefix	*Meaning*
-ase	enzyme
-asthenia	lack of strength
atel/o	incomplete
ather/o	plaque (fatty substance)
atri/o	atrium
audi/o	hearing
aur/i	ear
aur/o	ear
aut/o	self
auto-	self
axill/o	armpit
azot/o	urea; nitrogen
bacteri/o	bacteria
balan/o	glans penis
bar/o	pressure; weight
bartholin/o	Bartholin's glands
bas/o	base; opposite of acid
bi-	two
bi/o	life
bil/i	bile; gall
bilirubin/o	bilirubin
-blast	embryonic; immature
blephar/o	eyelid
bol/o	cast; throw
brachi/o	arm
brachy-	short
brady-	slow
bronch/o	bronchial tube
bronchi/o	bronchial tube
bronchiol/o	bronchiole
bucc/o	cheek
burs/o	bursa (sac of fluid near joints)
calc/o	calcium
calcane/o	calcaneus (heel bone)
cali/o	calyx
-capnia	carbon dioxide
carcin/o	cancerous
cardi/o	heart
carp/o	carpus (wrist bone)
cata-	down
caud/o	tail; lower part of body
caus/o	burn
cauter/o	heat; burn
cec/o	cecum
-cele	hernia
celi/o	belly; abdomen
-centesis	surgical puncture to remove fluid
cephal/o	head
cerebell/o	cerebellum
cerebr/o	brain; cerebrum

Combining Form, Suffix, or Prefix	*Meaning*
cerumin/o	cerumen
cervic/o	neck; cervix (neck of uterus)
-chalasis	relaxation
cheil/o	lip
chem/o	drug; chemical
chir/o	hand
chol/e	bile; gall
cholecyst/o	gallbladder
choledoch/o	common bile duct
cholesterol/o	cholesterol
chondr/o	cartilage
chori/o	chorion
choroid/o	choroid layer of eye
chrom/o	color
chron/o	time
chym/o	to pour
cib/o	meal
-cidal	pertaining to killing
cine/o	movement
cis/o	to cut
-clasis	break
-clast	break
claustr/o	barrier
clavicul/o	clavicle (collar bone)
-clysis	irrigation; washing
-coccus (-cocci, pl.)	berry-shaped bacterium
coccyg/o	coccyx (tailbone)
col/o	colon; large intestine
colon/o	colon; large intestine
colp/o	vagina
con-	together, with
coni/o	dust
conjunctiv/o	conjunctiva
contra-	against; opposite
cor/o	pupil
core/o	pupil
corne/o	cornea
coron/o	heart
cortic/o	cortex, outer region
cost/o	rib
crani/o	skull
cras/o	mixture; temperament
crin/o	secrete
-crine	secrete; separate
-crit	separate
cry/o	cold
crypt/o	hidden
culd/o	cul-de-sac
-cusis	hearing
cutane/o	skin
cyan/o	blue
cycl/o	ciliary body of eye; cycle
-cyesis	pregnancy

Combining Form, Suffix, or Prefix	*Meaning*
cyst/o	urinary bladder; cyst; sac of fluid
cyt/o	cell
-cyte	cell
-cytosis	condition of cells
dacry/o	tear; lacrimal duct; tear duct
dacryocyst/o	tear sac; lacrimal sac
dactyl/o	fingers; toes
de-	lack of; down
dent/i	tooth
derm/o	skin
dermat/o	skin
-desis	to bind, tie together
dia-	complete; through
diaphor/o	sweat
dipl/o	double
dips/o	thirst
dist/o	far
dors/o	back (of body)
-drome	to run
duct/o	to lead, carry
duoden/o	duodenum
dur/o	dura mater
-dynia	pain
dys-	bad; painful; difficult
-eal	pertaining to
ec-	out; outside
ech/o	sound
-ectasia	stretching; dilation
-ectasis	stretching; dilation
ecto-	out; outside
-ectomy	removal; excision
electr/o	electricity
em-	in
-emesis	vomiting
-emia	blood condition
emmetr/o	in due measure
en-	in; within
encephal/o	brain
endo-	in; within
enter/o	intestines (usually small intestine)
eosin/o	red; rosy; dawn-colored
epi-	above; upon; on
epididym/o	epididymis
epiglott/o	epiglottis
episi/o	vulva
-er	one who
erg/o	work

Combining Form, Suffix, or Prefix	*Meaning*
erythem/o	flushed; redness
erythr/o	red
eso-	inward
esophag/o	esophagus
esthesi/o	feeling (nervous sensation)
estr/o	female
ethm/o	sieve
eti/o	cause
eu-	good
ex-	out; away from
exo-	out; away from
extra-	outside
fasci/o	fascia
femor/o	femur (thigh bone)
fibros/o	fibrous connective tissue
fibul/o	fibula
fluor/o	luminous
follicul/o	follicle; small sac
furc/o	forking; branching
-fusion	to pour
galact/o	milk
gangli/o	ganglion
ganglion/o	ganglion
gastr/o	stomach
gen/o	producing; produced by
-genesis	producing; forming
-genic	produced by or in
gingiv/o	gum
glauc/o	gray
gli/o	glue; neuroglial tissue (supportive tissue of nervous system)
-globin	protein
-globulin	protein
glomerul/o	glomerulus
gloss/o	tongue
gluc/o	glucose; sugar
glyc/o	glucose; sugar
glycogen/o	glycogen; animal starch
gnos/o	knowledge
gon/o	seed
gonad/o	sex glands
-grade	to go
-gram	record
granul/o	granule(s)
-graph	instrument for recording
-graphy	process of recording
gravid/o	pregnancy
gynec/o	woman; female

Combining Form, Suffix, or Prefix	Meaning
hem/o	blood
hemat/o	blood
hemi-	half
hepat/o	liver
herni/o	hernia
hidr/o	sweat
hist/o	tissue
histi/o	tissue
home/o	sameness; unchanging; constant
humer/o	humerus (upper arm bone)
hydr/o	water
hyper-	above; excessive; beyond
hypn/o	sleep
hypo-	deficient; below; under
hyster/o	uterus; womb
-ia	condition
-iac	pertaining to
-iasis	abnormal condition
iatr/o	physician; treatment
-ic	pertaining to
ichthy/o	dry; scaly
idi/o	individual; own; distinct
ile/o	ileum
ili/o	ilium
immun/o	immune; protection; safe
in-	in; into; hot
infra-	below; inferior to
inguin/o	groin
inter-	between
intra-	within
ion/o	ion; to wander
-ior	pertaining to
ir/o	iris (colored portion of eye)
irid/o	iris (colored portion of eye)
is/o	same; equal
isch/o	to hold back
ischi/o	ischium (part of hip bone)
-ism	process
-ist	specialist
-itis	inflammation
-ium	structure; tissue
jejun/o	jejunum
kal/i	potassium
kary/o	nucleus
kerat/o	horny, hard; cornea
ket/o	ketones; acetones
keton/o	ketones; acetones
kinesi/o	movement
klept/o	to steal
labi/o	lip
lacrim/o	tear; tear duct; lacrimal duct
lact/o	milk
lamin/o	lamina (part of vertebral arch)
lapar/o	abdominal wall; abdomen
laryng/o	larynx (voice box)
later/o	side
leiomy/o	smooth (visceral) muscle
lept/o	thin, slender
leuk/o	white
-lexia	speech; word; phrase
ligament/o	ligament
lingu/o	tongue
lip/o	fat; lipid
lith/o	stone; calculus
lob/o	lobe
-logy	study of
lumb/o	lower back; loin
lymph/o	lymph
lymphaden/o	lymph gland
lymphangi/o	lymph vessel
-lysis	break down; separation destruction
-lytic	to reduce, destroy
macro-	large
mal-	bad
-malacia	softening
malleol/o	malleolus
mamm/o	breast
mandibul/o	mandible (lower jaw bone)
-mania	obsessive preoccupation
mast/o	breast
mastoid/o	mastoid process
maxill/o	maxilla (upper jaw bone)
meat/o	meatus
medi/o	middle
medull/o	medulla (inner section); middle; soft; marrow
-megaly	enlargement
melan/o	black
men/o	menses; menstruation
mening/o	membranes; meninges
meningi/o	membranes; meninges
ment/o	mind
meso-	middle
meta-	change; beyond
metacarp/o	metacarpals (hand bones)

Combining Form, Suffix, or Prefix	*Meaning*
-meter	measure
metr/o	uterus; womb
metri/o	uterus; womb
mi/o	smaller; less
micro-	small
-mimetic	mimic; copy
mon/o	one; single
morph/o	shape; form
mort/o	death
muc/o	mucus
multi-	many
mut/a	genetic change
my/o	muscle
myc/o	fungus
mydri/o	wide
myel/o	spinal cord; bone marrow
myocardi/o	myocardium (heart muscle)
myom/o	muscle tumor
myos/o	muscle
myring/o	tympanic membrane (eardrum)
myx/o	mucus
narc/o	numbness; stupor
nas/o	nose
nat/i	birth
natr/o	sodium
necr/o	death
nect/o	to bind, tie, connect
neo-	new
nephr/o	kidney
neur/o	nerve
neutr/o	neither; neutral
nid/o	nest
noct/i	night
norm/o	rule; order
nucle/o	nucleus
nulli-	none
nyctal/o	night
ocul/o	eye
odont/o	tooth
-oid	resembling
-ole	little; small
olecran/o	olecranon; elbow
olig/o	scanty
-oma	tumor; mass
om/o	shoulder
onc/o	tumor
onych/o	nail
oo/o	egg
oophor/o	ovary
ophthalm/o	eye

Combining Form, Suffix, or Prefix	*Meaning*
-opia	vision
-opsy	view of
opt/o	eye; vision
-or	one who
or/o	mouth
orch/o	testis
orchi/o	testis
orchid/o	testis
orth/o	straight
-ose	pertaining to
-osis	abnormal condition
-osmia	smell
oste/o	bone
ot/o	ear
-ous	pertaining to
ov/o	egg
ovari/o	ovary
ox/o	oxygen
pachy-	heavy; thick
palat/o	palate
palpebr/o	eyelid
pan-	all
pancreat/o	pancreas
papill/o	nipple-like
para-	near; beside; abnormal
-para	to bear, bring forth (live births)
parathyroid/o	parathyroid glands
-paresis	slight paralysis
-partum	birth; labor
patell/a	patella
patell/o	patella
path/o	disease
-pathy	disease; emotion
pector/o	chest
ped/o	child; foot
pelv/i	pelvic bone; hip
pelv/o	pelvic cavity; hip
-penia	deficiency
-pepsia	digestion
per-	through
peri-	surrounding
perine/o	perineum
peritone/o	peritoneum
perone/o	fibula
-pexy	fixation; to put in place
phac/o	lens of eye
phag/o	eat; swallow
-phagia	eating; swallowing
phak/o	lens of eye
phalang/o	phalanges (finger and toe
pharmac/o	drug
pharyng/o	throat; pharynx
phas/o	speech

Combining Form, Suffix, or Prefix	*Meaning*
phe/o	dusky
-pheresis	removal
phil/o	like; love; attraction to
-philia	attraction for
phleb/o	vein
phob/o	fear
-phobia	fear
-phonia	voice; sound
-phoresis	carrying; transmission
-phoria	to bear, carry; feeling (mental state)
phot/o	light
phren/o	diaphragm; mind
-phylaxis	protection
physi/o	nature
-physis	to grow
-phyte	plant
pil/o	hair
pineal/o	pineal gland
plas/o	development; formation
-plasia	formation; development; growth
-plasm	formation
-plastic	pertaining to formation
-plasty	surgical repair
ple/o	more; many
-plegia	paralysis; palsy
pleur/o	pleura
plex/o	plexus; network (of nerves)
-pnea	breathing
pneum/o	lung; air
pneumon/o	lung; air
pod/o	foot
-poiesis	formation
poikil/o	varied; irregular
polio-	gray matter of brain and spinal cord
poly-	many
polyp/o	polyp; small growth
pont/o	pons (a part of the brain)
-porosis	passage
post-	after; behind
poster/o	back (of body); behind
-prandial	meal
-praxia	action
pre-	before; in front of
presby/o	old age
primi-	first
pro-	before
proct/o	anus and rectum
prostat/o	prostate gland
prot/o	first
proxim/o	near
pseud/o	false

Combining Form, Suffix, or Prefix	*Meaning*
psych/o	mind
-ptosis	drooping; sagging; prolapse
-ptysis	spitting
pub/o	pubis (part of hip bone)
pulmon/o	lung
pupill/o	pupil
py/o	pus
pyel/o	renal pelvis
pylor/o	pylorus; pyloric sphincter
pyr/o	fever; fire
quadri-	four
rachi/o	spinal column; vertebrae
radi/o	radius (lateral lower arm bone); rays; x-rays; radioactivity
radicul/o	nerve root
re-	back
rect/o	rectum
ren/o	kidney
reticul/o	network
retin/o	retina
retro-	behind; back
rhabdomy/o	striated (skeletal) muscle
rhin/o	nose
roentgen/o	x-rays
-rrhage	bursting forth of blood
-rrhagia	bursting forth of blood
-rrhaphy	suture
-rrhea	flow; discharge
-rrhexis	rupture
sacr/o	sacrum
salping/o	uterine (fallopian) tube; oviduct; auditory (eustachian tube
-salpinx	uterine (fallopian) tube; oviduct
sarc/o	flesh (connective tissue)
scapul/o	scapula; shoulder blade
scirrh/o	hard
scler/o	sclera (white of eye)
-sclerosis	hardening
-scope	instrument for visual examination
-scopy	visual examination
scot/o	darkness
seb/o	sebum
secti/o	to cut
semi-	half

Combining Form, Suffix, or Prefix	*Meaning*
seps/o	infection
sial/o	saliva
sialaden/o	salivary gland
sider/o	iron
sigmoid/o	sigmoid colon
sinus/o	sinus
-sis	state of; condition
somat/o	body
somn/o	sleep
-somnia	sleep
son/o	sound
-spasm	sudden contraction of muscles
sperm/o	spermatozoa; sperm cells
spermat/o	spermatozoa; sperm cells
sphen/o	wedge; sphenoid bone
spher/o	globe-shaped; round
sphygm/o	pulse
-sphyxia	pulse
spin/o	spine (backbone)
spir/o	to breathe
splen/o	spleen
spondyl/o	vertebrae (backbone)
squam/o	scale
-stalsis	contraction
staped/o	stapes (middle ear bone)
staphyl/o	clusters; grapes
-stasis	stopping; controlling
-static	pertaining to stopping; controlling
steat/o	fat, lipid, sebum
-stenosis	tightening; stricture
ster/o	solid structure
stere/o	solid; three-dimensional
stern/o	sternum (breastbone)
steth/o	chest
-sthenia	strength
stomat/o	mouth
-stomy	new opening
strept/o	twisted chains
sub-	under; below
submaxill/o	mandible (lower jaw bone)
supra-	above
sym-	together; with
syn-	together; with
syndesm/o	ligament
synovi/o	synovia; synovial membrane
syring/o	tube
tachy-	fast
tax/o	order; coordination
tele/o	distant
ten/o	tendon

Combining Form, Suffix, or Prefix	*Meaning*
tend/o	tendon
tendin/o	tendon
terat/o	monster; malformed fetus
test/o	testis; testicle
tetra-	four
thalam/o	thalamus
thalass/o	sea
the/o	put; place
thec/o	sheath
thel/o	nipple
-therapy	treatment
therm/o	heat
thorac/o	chest
-thorax	pleural cavity; chest
thromb/o	clot
thym/o	thymus gland
-thymic	pertaining to mind
thyr/o	shield; thyroid gland
thyroid/o	thyroid gland
tibi/o	tibia (shin bone)
-tic	pertaining to
-tocia	labor; birth
-tocin	labor; delivery
tom/o	to cut
-tome	instrument to cut
-tomy	process of cutting
tone/o	to stretch
tonsill/o	tonsil
top/o	place; position; location
tox/o	poison
toxic/o	poison
trache/o	trachea (windpipe)
trans-	across
-tresia	opening
tri-	three
trich/o	hair
trigon/o	trigone
-trophy	nourishment; development
-tropia	to turn
tympan/o	tympanic membrane (eardrum); middle ear
-ule	little; small
uln/o	ulna (medial lower arm bone)
ultra-	beyond; excess
-um	structure; tissue; thing
ungu/o	nail
uni-	one
ur/o	urine; urinary tract
ureter/o	ureter
urethr/o	urethra
-uria	urination; urine

Combining Form, Suffix, or Prefix	*Meaning*
-us	thing
uter/o	uterus; womb
uve/o	vascular layer of eye (iris, choroid, ciliary body)
uvul/o	uvula
vagin/o	vagina
valv/o	valve
valvul/o	valve
vas/o	vessel; duct; vas deferens
ven/o	vein
ventr/o	belly side of body
ventricul/o	ventricle (of brain or heart)
venul/o	venule; small vein
-version	to turn
vertebr/o	vertebrae (backbone)
vesic/o	urinary bladder
vesicul/o	seminal vesicle
viscer/o	internal organs
vit/o	life
vitre/o	glassy
vulv/o	vulva
xanth/o	yellow
xer/o	dry
xiph/o	sword
-y	condition; process
zo/o	animal life

ENGLISH → MEDICAL TERMS

Meaning	*Combining Form, Prefix, or Suffix*
abdomen	abdomin/o
	celi/o
	lapar/o
abdominal wall	lapar/o
abnormal	para-
abnormal condition	-iasis
	-osis
above	epi-
	hyper-
	supra-
acetabulum	acetabul/o
acetones	ket/o
	keton/o
across	trans-
action	-praxia
adrenal glands	adren/o
	adrenal/o
after	post-
against	anti-
	contra-
air	aer/o
	pneum/o
	pneumon/o
air sac	alveol/o
albumin	albumin/o
all	pan-
alveolus	alveol/o
amnion	amni/o
aneurysm	aneurysm/o
animal life	zo/o
animal starch	glycogen/o
anus	an/o
anus and rectum	proct/o
apart	ana-
appendix	append/o
	appendic/o
arm	brachi/o
arm bone, lower, lateral	radi/o
arm bone, lower, medial	uln/o
arm bone, upper	humer/o
armpit	axill/o
arteriole	arteriol/o
artery	arteri/o
atrium	atri/o
attraction for	-philia
attraction to	phil/o
auditory tube	salping/o
away from	ab-
	ex-
	exo-
back	re-
	retro-
back, lower	lumb/o
back portion of body	dors/o
	poster/o
backbone	spin/o
	spondyl/o
	vertebr/o

Meaning	Combining Form, Prefix, or Suffix	Meaning	Combining Form, Prefix, or Suffix
backward	ana-	bring forth	-para
bacteria	bacteri/o	bronchial tube	bronch/o
bacterium, berry-shaped	-coccus		bronchi/o
bad	dys-	bronchiole	bronchiol/o
	mal-	bronchus	bronch/o
barrier	claustr/o		bronchi/o
base (not acidic)	bas/o	burn	caus/o
bear	-para		cauter/o
	-phoria	bursa	burs/o
before	ante-	bursting forth of blood	-rrhage
	pre-		-rrhagia
	pro-		
beginning	-arche		
behind	post-	calcaneus	calcane/o
	poster/o	calcium	calc/o
	retro-	calculus	lith/o
belly	celi/o	calyx	cali/o
belly side of body	ventr/o	cancerous	carcin/o
below	hypo-	carbon dioxide	-capnia
	infra-	carry	duct/o
	sub-		-phoria
bent	ankyl/o	carrying	-phoresis
beside	para-	cartilage	chondr/o
between	inter-	cast throw	bol/o
beyond	hyper-	cause	eti/o
	meta-	cecum	cec/o
	ultra-	cell	cyt/o
bile	bil/i		-cyte
	chol/e	cells, condition of	-cytosis
bilirubin	bilirubin/o	cerebellum	cerebell/o
bind	-desis	cerebrum	cerebr/o
	nect/o	cerumen	cerumin/o
birth	nat/i	cervix	cervic/o
	-partum	change	meta-
	-tocia	cheek	bucc/o
births, live	-para	chemical	chem/o
black	melan/o	chest	pector/o
blood	hem/o		steth/o
	hemat/o		thorac/o
blood condition	-emia		-thorax
blue	cyan/o	child	ped/o
body	somat/o	cholesterol	cholesterol/o
bone	oste/o	chorion	chori/o
bone marrow	myel/o	choroid layer	choroid/o
brain	encephal/o	ciliary body	cycl/o
	cerebr/o	clavicle	clavicul/o
branching	furc/o	clot	thromb/o
break	-clasis	clumping	agglutin/o
	-clast	clusters	staphyl/o
break down	-lysis	coal dust	anthrac/o
breast	mamm/o	coccyx	coccyg/o
	mast/o	cold	cry/o
breastbone	stern/o	collar bone	clavicul/o
breathe	spir/o	colon	col/o
breathing	-pnea		colon/o

Meaning	Combining Form, Prefix, or Suffix	Meaning	Combining Form, Prefix, or Suffix
color	chrom/o	drooping	-ptosis
common bile duct	choledoch/o	drug	chem/o
complete	dia-		pharmac/o
condition	-ia	dry	ichthy/o
	-sis		xer/o
	-y	duct	vas/o
condition, abnormal	-iasis	dull	ambly/o
	-osis	duodenum	duoden/o
connect	nect/o	dura mater	dur/o
connective tissue	sarc/o	dusky	phe/o
constant	home/o	dust	coni/o
controlling	-stasis		
contraction	-stalsis		
contraction of muscles, sudden	-spasm		
		ear	aur/i
coordination	tax/o		aur/o
copy	-mimetic	eardrum	myring/o
cornea	corne/o		tympan/o
	kerat/o	eat	phag/o
cortex	cortic/o	eating	-phagia
crooked	ankyl/o	egg	oo/o
cut	cis/o	elbow	olecran/o
	secti/o	electricity	electr/o
	tom/o	embryonic	-blast
cutting, process of	-tomy	enlargement	-megaly
cycle	cycl/o	enzyme	-ase
		epididymis	epididym/o
		epiglottis	epiglott/o
darkness	scot/o	equal	is/o
dawn-colored	eosin/o	esophagus	esophag/o
death	mort/o	eustachian tube	salping/o
	necr/o	excess	ultra-
deficiency	-penia	excessive	ana-
deficient	hypo-		hyper-
delivery	-tocin	excision	-ectomy
destroy	-lytic	extreme point	acr/o
destruction	-lysis	extremities	acr/o
development	plas/o	eye	ocul/o
	-plasia		ophthalm/o
	-trophy		opt/o
diaphragm	phren/o	eyelid	blephar/o
difficult	dys-		palpebr/o
digestion	-pepsia		
dilation	-ectasia		
	-ectasis		
dim	ambly/o	fallopian tube	salping/o
discharge	-rrhea		-salpinx
disease	path/o	false	pseudo-
	-pathy	far	dist/o
distant	tele/o	fascia	fasci/o
distinct	idi/o	fast	tachy-
double	dipl/o	fat	adip/o
down	cata-		lip/o
	de-		steat/o

Meaning	*Combining Form, Prefix, or Suffix*
fear	phob/o
	-phobia
feeling	esthesi/o
	-phoria
female	estr/o
	gynec/o
femur	femor/o
fever	pyr/o
fibrous connective tissue	fibros/o
fibula	fibul/o
	perone/o
finger and toe bones	phalang/o
fingers	dactyl/o
fire	pyr/o
first	prot/o
fixation	-pexy
flesh	sarc/o
flow	-rrhea
flushed	erythem/o
foot	pod/o
forking	furc/o
form	morph/o
formation	plas/o
	-plasia
	-plasm
	-poiesis
forming	-genesis
forward	ante-
four	quadri-
front	anter/o
fungus	myc/o
gall	bil/i
	chol/e
gallbladder	cholecyst/o
ganglion	gangli/o
	ganglion/o
genetic change	mut/a
gland	aden/o
glans penis	balan/o
glassy	vitre/o
globe-shaped	spher/o
glomerulus	glomerul/o
glucose	gluc/o
	glyc/o
glue	gli/o
glycogen	glycogen/o
go	-grade
good	eu-
granule(s)	granul/o
grapes	staphyl/o
gray	glauc/o
gray matter	polio-
groin	inguin/o

Meaning	*Combining Form, Prefix, or Suffix*
grow	-physis
growth	-plasia
gum	gingiv/o
hair	pil/o
	trich/o
half	hemi-
	semi-
hand	chir/o
hand bones	metacarp/o
hard	kerat/o
	scirrh/o
hardening	-sclerosis
head	cephal/o
hearing	acou/o
	acous/o
	audi/o
	-cusis
heart	cardi/o
	coron/o
heart muscle	myocardi/o
heat	cauter/o
	therm/o
heavy	pachy-
heel bone	calcane/o
hernia	-cele
	herni/o
hip	pelv/i
	pelv/o
hold back	isch/o
horny	kerat/o
humerus	humer/o
ileum	ile/o
ilium	ili/o
immature	-blast
immune	immun/o
in	em-
	en-
	endo-
	in-
in due measure	emmetr/o
in front of	pre-
incomplete	atel/o
individual	idi/o
infection	seps/o
inferior to	infra-
inflammation	-itis
instrument for recording	-graph
instrument to cut	-tome
instrument for visual examination	-scope
internal organs	viscer/o

Meaning	Combining Form, Prefix, or Suffix	Meaning	Combining Form, Prefix, or Suffix
intestine, small	enter/o	loin	lumb/o
into	in-	love	phil/o
ion	ion/o	luminous	fluor/o
iris	ir/o	lung	pneum/o
	irid/o		pneumon/o
iron	sider/o		pulmon/o
irregular	poikil/o	lymph	lymph/o
irrigation	-clysis	lymph gland	lymphaden/o
ischium	ischi/o	lymph vessel	lymphangi/o
		male	andr/o
jaw, lower	mandibul/o	malformed fetus	terat/o
	submaxill/o	malleolus	malleol/o
jaw, upper	maxill/o	mandible	mandibul/o
joint	arthr/o		submaxill/o
	articul/o	many	multi-
			ple/o
			poly-
ketones	ket/o	marketplace	agor/a
	keton/o	marrow	medull/o
kidney	nephr/o	mass	-oma
	ren/o	mastoid process	mastoid/o
killing	-cidal	maxilla	maxill/o
knowledge	gnos/o	meal	cib/o
			-prandial
		measure	-meter
labor	-partum	meatus	meat/o
	-tocia	medulla	medull/o
	-tocin	membranes	mening/o
lack of	de-		meningi/o
lack of strength	-asthenia	meninges	mening/o
lacrimal duct	dacry/o		meningi/o
	lacrim/o	menses	men/o
lacrimal sac	dacryocyst/o	menstruation	men/o
lamina	lamin/o	metacarpals	metacarp/o
large	macro-	middle	medi/o
larynx	laryng/o		medull/o
lead	duct/o		meso-
lens of eye	phac/o	middle ear	tympan/o
	phak/o	milk	galact/o
less	mi/o		lact/o
life	bi/o	mimic	-mimetic
	vit/o	mind	ment/o
ligament	ligament/o		phren/o
	syndesm/o		psych/o
like	phil/o		-thymic
lip	cheil/o	mixture	cras/o
	labi/o	monster	terat/o
lipid	lip/o	more	ple/o
	steat/o	mouth	or/o
little	-ole		stomat/o
	-ule	movement	cine/o
liver	hepat/o		kinesi/o
lobe	lob/o	mucus	muc/o
location	top/o		myx/o

Meaning	Combining Form, Prefix, or Suffix	Meaning	Combining Form, Prefix, or Suffix
muscle	my/o	out	ec-
	myos/o		ex-
muscle, heart	myocardi/o		exo-
muscle, smooth (visceral)	leiomy/o	outer region	cortic/o
muscle, striated (skeletal)	rhabdomy/o	outside	ec-
muscle tumor	myom/o		extra-
myocardium	myocardi/o	ovary	oophor/o
		oviduct	salping/o
			-salpinx
nail	onych/o	own	idi/o
	ungu/o	oxygen	ox/o
nature	physi/o		
near	para-		
	proxim/o	pain	-algia
neck	cervic/o		-dynia
neither	neutr/o	pain, excessive	-agra
nerve	neur/o	pain, excessive sensitivity	algesi/o
nerve root	radicul/o	to	
nest	nid/o	painful	dys-
network	reticul/o	palate	palat/o
network of nerves	plex/o	palsy	-plegia
neutral	neutr/o	pancreas	pancreat/o
night	noct/i	paralysis	-plegia
	nyctal/o	paralysis, slight	-paresis
nipple-like	papill/o	patella	patell/a
nitrogen	azot/o		patell/o
nitrogen compound	-amine	pelvic bone	pelv/i
no	a-	pelvic cavity	pelv/o
	an-	pelvis, renal	pyel/o
none	nulli-	perineum	perine/o
nose	nas/o	peritoneum	peritone/o
	rhin/o	pertaining to	-ac
not	a-		-al
	an-		-ar
	in-		-ary
nourishment	-trophy		-eal
nucleus	kary/o		-iac
	nucle/o		-ic
numbness	narc/o		-ior
			-ous
			-tic
obsessive preoccupation	-mania	phrase	-lexia
old age	presby/o	physician	iatr/o
olecranon	olecran/o	pineal gland	pineal/o
on	epi-	place	the/o
one	mon/o		top/o
	uni-	plant	-phyte
one who	-er	plaque	ather/o
	-or	pleura	pleur/o
opening	-tresia	pleural cavity	-thorax
opening, new	-stomy	plexus	plex/o
opposite	contra-	poison	tox/o
order	norm/o		toxic/o
	tax/o	polyp	polyp/o
organs, internal	viscer/o	pons	pont/o

Meaning	*Combining Form, Prefix, or Suffix*
position	top/o
potassium	kal/i
pour	chym/o
	-fusion
pregnancy	-cyesis
	gravid/o
pressure	bar/o
process	-ism
	-y
producing	gen/o
	-genesis
prolapse	-ptosis
prostate gland	prostat/o
protection	immun/o
	-phylaxis
protein	-globin
	-globulin
pubis	pub/o
pulse	sphygm/o
	-sphyxia
puncture to remove fluid	-centesis
pupil	cor/o
	core/o
	pupill/o
pus	py/o
put	the/o
put in place	-pexy
pyloric sphincter	pylor/o
pylorus	pylor/o
radioactivity	radi/o
radius	radi/o
rays	radi/o
record	-gram
recording, process of	-graphy
rectum	rect/o
red	eosin/o
	erythr/o
redness	erythem/o
reduce	-lytic
relaxation	-chalasis
removal	-apheresis
	-ectomy
	-pheresis
renal pelvis	pyel/o
resembling	-oid
retina	retin/o
rib	cost/o
rosy	eosin/o
round	spher/o
rule	norm/o
run	-drome
rupture	-rrhexis

Meaning	*Combining Form, Prefix, or Suffix*
sac, small	alveol/o
	follicul/o
sac of fluid	cyst/o
sacrum	sacr/o
safe	immun/o
sagging	-ptosis
saliva	sial/o
salivary gland	sialaden/o
same	is/o
sameness	home/o
scaly	ichthy/o
scanty	olig/o
sclera	scler/o
sea	thalass/o
sebum	seb/o
	steat/o
secrete	crin/o
	-crine
seed	gon/o
self	aut/o
	auto-
seminal vesicle	vesicul/o
separate	-crine
separation	-lysis
severe	acu/o
sex glands	gonad/o
shape	morph/o
sharp	acu/o
sheath	thec/o
shield	thyr/o
shin bone	tibi/o
short	brachy-
shoulder	om/o
side	later/o
sieve	ethm/o
sigmoid colon	sigmoid/o
single	mon/o
sinus	sinus/o
skin	cutane/o
	derm/o
	dermat/o
skull	crani/o
sleep	hypn/o
	somn/o
	-somnia
slender	lept/o
slow	brady-
small	micro-
	-ole
	-ule
small intestine	enter/o
smaller	mi/o
smell	-osmia
sodium	natr/o

Meaning	*Combining Form, Prefix, or Suffix*
soft	medull/o
softening	-malacia
sound	ech/o
	-phonia
	son/o
specialist	-ist
speech	-lexia
sperm cells	sperm/o
	spermat/o
spermatozoa	sperm/o
	spermat/o
spinal column	rachi/o
spinal cord	myel/o
spine	spin/o
spiny	acanth/o
spitting	-ptysis
spleen	splen/o
stapes	staped/o
starch	amyl/o
state of	-sis
steal	klept/o
sternum	stern/o
sticking together	agglutin/o
stiff	ankyl/o
stomach	gastr/o
stone	lith/o
stopping	-stasis
	-static
straight	orth/o
stretch	tone/o
stretching	-ectasia
	-ectasis
stricture	-stenosis
structure	-ium
	-um
structure, solid	ster/o
study of	-logy
stupor	narc/o
sudden	acu/o
sugar	gluc/o
	glyc/o
surgical repair	-plasty
surrounding	peri-
suture	-rrhaphy
swallow	phag/o
swallowing	-phagia
sweat	diaphor/o
	hidr/o
sword	xiph/o
synovia	synovi/o
synovial membrane	synovi/o
tail	caud/o
tailbone	coccyg/o

Meaning	*Combining Form, Prefix, or Suffix*
tear	dacry/o
	lacrim/o
tear duct	dacry/o
	lacrim/o
tear sac	dacryocyst/o
temperament	cras/o
tendon	ten/o
	tend/o
	tendin/o
testis	orch/o
	orchi/o
	orchid/o
	test/o
thick	pachy-
thigh bone	femor/o
thin	lept/o
thing	-um
	-us
thirst	dips/o
thorny	acanth/o
three	tri-
throat	pharyng/o
through	dia-
throw	bol/o
thymus gland	thym/o
thyroid gland	thry/o
	thyroid/o
tibia	tibi/o
tie	nect/o
tie together	-desis
tightening	-stenosis
time	chron/o
tissue	hist/o
	histi/o
	-ium
	-um
toes	dactyl/o
together	con-
	sym-
	syn-
tongue	gloss/o
	lingu/o
tonsil	tonsill/o
tooth	dent/i
	odont/o
top	acr/o
toward	ad-
trachea	trache/o
transmission	-phoresis
treatment	iatr/o
	-therapy
trigone	trigon/o
tube	syring/o
tumor	-oma
	onc/o

Meaning	*Combining Form, Prefix, or Suffix*
turn	-tropia
	-version
twisted chains	strept/o
two	bi-
tympanic membrane	myring/o
	tympan/o
ulna	uln/o
unchanging	home/o
under	hypo-
up	ana-
upon	epi-
urea	azot/o
ureter	ureter/o
urethra	urethr/o
urinary bladder	cyst/o
	vesic/o
urinary tract	ur/o
urination	-uria
urine	ur/o
	-uria
uterine tube	salping/o
	-salpinx
uterus	hyster/o
	metr/o
	metri/o
	uter/o
uvula	uvul/o
vagina	colp/o
	vagin/o
valve	valv/o
	valvul/o
varied	poikil/o
vascular layer of eye	uve/o
vein	phleb/o
	ven/o
vein, small	venul/o
ventricle	ventricul/o
vertebrae	rachi/o
	spondyl/o
	vertebr/o
vessel	angi/o
	vas/o
view of	-opsy
vision	-opia
	opt/o
visual examination	-scopy
voice	-phonia
voice box	laryng/o
vomiting	-emesis
vulva	episi/o
	vulv/o
wander	ion/o
washing	-clysis
water	aque/o
	hydr/o
wedge	sphen/o
weight	bar/o
well	eu-
white	alb/o
	albin/o
	leuk/o
wide	mydri/o
windpipe	trache/o
with	con-
	sym-
	syn-
within	en-
	endo-
	intra-
woman	gynec/o
womb	hyster/o
	metr/o
	metri/o
	uter/o
word	-lexia
work	erg/o
wrist bone	carp/o
x-rays	radi/o
yellow	xanth/o

NORMAL LABORATORY VALUES FOR SELECTED TESTS

The normal values listed in this table are only guidelines and are not to be taken as absolute. Normal values vary with the particular procedure employed and may vary from laboratory to laboratory.

mg = milligram (one thousandth of a gram)
dl = deciliter (one tenth of a liter or 100 ml)
mEq = milliequivalent
thou = thousand
mill = million

ml = milliliter
U = unit
l = liter
g = gram
cu mm = cubic millimeter (mm^3)

	Units	Normal range
albumin	g/dl	3.8–4.9
ALT/GPT	U/l	8–20
AST/GOT	U/l	8–20
bilirubin (total)	mg/dl	0.2–1.5
calcium	mEq/l	4.5–5.3
carbon dioxide (CO_2)	mEq/l	23–33
chloride (Cl)	mEq/l	100–110
cholesterol	mg/dl	163–263
creatinine	mg/dl	0.7–1.6
glucose	mg/dl	70–120
magnesium (Mg)	mEq/l	1.30–2.10
potassium (K)	mEq/l	3.3–4.6
sodium (Na)	mEq/l	137–145
urea nitrogen	mg/dl	7–23
Hematocrit	percent	M. 42–50
		F. 35–45
Hemoglobin	g/dl	M. 14.0–16.3
		F. 12.0–15.4
Platelet	thou/cu mm	145–364
RBC	mill/cu mm	M. 4.5–6.0
		F. 4.0–5.5
WBC	thou/cu mm	5.0–10.0

INDEX

Page numbers in *italics* indicate illustrations.